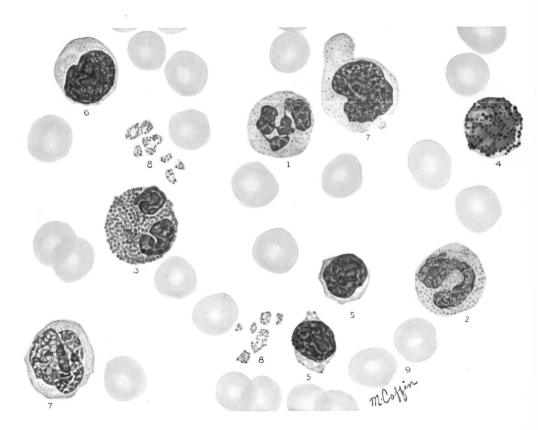

NORMAL CELLULAR CONSTITUENTS OF ADULT HUMAN BLOOD

1, Segmented (polymorphonuclear) neutrophil; 2, Band (stab) neutrophil; 3, Segmented eosinophil; 4, Basophil; 5, Small lymphocytes; 6, Large lymphocyte; 7, Monocytes; 8, Thrombocytes; and 9, Erythrocytes. (From Custer: An Atlas of the Blood and Bone Marrow.)

THIRD EDITION

Fundamentals of
CLINICAL
HEMATOLOGY

BYRD S. LEAVELL, M.D.

Professor of Internal Medicine,
School of Medicine, University of Virginia;
Hematologist and Attending Physician,
University of Virginia Hospital

OSCAR A. THORUP, Jr. M.D.

Professor and Head, Department of Internal Medicine,
College of Medicine, University of Arizona

W. B. SAUNDERS COMPANY
PHILADELPHIA · LONDON · TORONTO

W. B. Saunders Company: West Washington Square
                            Philadelphia, Pa.   19105

                            12 Dyott Street
                            London, WC1A   1DB

                            1835 Yonge Street
                            Toronto 7, Ontario

Listed here is the latest translated edition of this book together with the language of the translation and the publisher.

Spanish (*2nd Edition*) – Nueva Editorial Interamericana, S.A., deC.V.,
                        Mexico

Fundamentals of Clinical Hematology   ISBN 0-7216-5677-3

Print Number: 9   8   7   6   5   4   3   2

*To
our children
and other students of today,
our hope for the future.*

Preface

The aim of the third edition, like that of its predecessors, is to present a readable, concise, yet comprehensive volume on clinical hematology. Disease is viewed as an expression of derangement in normal metabolism. In order to provide a sound foundation for understanding the problems involved in hematological disorders, relevant physiological processes, such as iron metabolism and blood coagulation, are reviewed before the related clinical disorders are discussed. An attempt is made to relate each disease to a specific defect in metabolism or abnormality in some physiological process.

The general arrangement of the first two editions has been followed, but the continued increase in our knowledge of nearly every aspect of hematology has necessitated numerous changes. In order to provide space for much new material, the descriptions of laboratory procedures that formed a part of the first two editions have been omitted. A short section describing the relationship of the histologic details of the cells to the physiologic function has been incorporated into the first chapter. The discussions of iron metabolism, vitamin B_{12} and folic acid, as well as those of nearly all the other subjects, contain new information. The chapter on hemolytic anemia has been revised and expanded. The recent aggressive approach toward the diagnosis and treatment of patients with lymphoma and leukemia has prompted extensive revision of the chapters devoted to these subjects. New knowledge of leukocyte physiology and the recognition of qualitative abnormalities in leukocytes have brought the morphologic hematologists into closer contact with their colleagues in immunology and infectious diseases. The numerous developments in the field of hemostasis, particularly those concerning the platelets and blood coagulation, have brought better understanding of many disorders, but at times one wonders if there is not an infinite variety of coagulation problems. The mystery, or mysteries, of the disorders associated with plasma cell and serum globulins are being clarified gradually.

The many changes that have occurred over the past decade suggest that we are on the threshold of newer concepts and better understanding of the causes of malignant disorders and the interaction among infectious agents, the immunologic mechanism in the body, and malignancy. Such knowledge probably will lead to a unifying concept of many disorders that are now considered separately.

An extensive bibliography has again been included. It is hoped that the reading of the topics in the text will give an understanding of important fundamental aspects of the disorders and their management; the references in the bibliography should provide ready access to fuller and more detailed discussions of the different aspects of the disorders.

Throughout the text, references are made to the film strip "Hematology," a study of morphology prepared by Drs. Hyun, Blank, and Custer. For example, "F.S.:I, 4" means film strip No. I, picture number 4; "F.S.:III, 143" refers to picture 143 in film strip III.

Our colleagues have been of great assistance to us. We particularly appreciate the revision of the chapter on hemolytic anemias done by Dr. Daniel N. Mohler, Professor of Medicine at the University of Virginia School of Medicine.

We are grateful for the assistance given by other members of the faculties of the University of Virginia and the University of Arizona: Dr. Munsey S. Wheby, Dr. Johnson T. Carpenter, Jr., Dr. Charles Hess, Dr. William Porter, Dr. David Riddick, Dr. Rick Moore, Dr. Robert McGilvery, Dr. Gerald Goldstein, Dr. O. B. Bobbitt, Dr. Thomas Bithell, Dr. Diane Komp, and Dr. William Constable: Dr. William F. Denny and Dr. John Thomas Boyer.

Our special thanks go to Miss Barbara Marshall, Mrs. Marcia Novak, Mrs. Judith Huber, Miss Linda Durham, and Mrs. Susan Mikita; also to Miss Anne Russell of the Department of Medical Illustrations at the University of Virginia, Mr. Clyde Baker, the University of Arizona, Department of Medical Illustrations, and Mrs. Ruth Ogden, medical artist. The authors again appreciate the invaluable assistance that the staff of the W. B. Saunders Co. has given us.

Byrd S. Leavell, M.D.

Oscar A. Thorup, Jr., M.D.

A Filmstrip Presentation

HEMATOLOGY

A Morphologic Study

By

BONG HAK HYUN, M.D., D.Sc.
MINERVA BLANK, Ph.D.
R. PHILIP CUSTER, M.D.

As a teaching adjunct in Hematology, three 35mm filmstrips of fifty frames each (289 views in all) are obtainable separately from the publisher. Excellent photomicrographs in color correlate blood and bone-marrow findings in the anemias, leukemias and allied malignant diseases, hemorrhagic disorders, and a variety of other conditions. Both smears and sections of marrow are pictured in almost all instances. Accompanied by an explanatory booklet, the filmstrips provide a valuable visual aid for individual study or group teaching.

A sample set of six frames is available to teachers without charge from the Educational Department of the publisher.

Contents

I

THE ORIGIN AND MORPHOLOGY OF BLOOD CELLS 1

II

ERYTHROPOIESIS AND THE METABOLISM OF HEMOGLOBIN 26

Erythropoiesis 26
Abnormal Porphyrin Metabolism 41
Additional Factors Needed for Erythropoiesis 45

III

CLASSIFICATION, MECHANISMS, AND DIAGNOSIS OF ANEMIA 56

The Classification of Anemia 56
Mechanisms Responsible for Anemia 59
Diagnosis of the Patient with Anemia 68
　　Examination of the Bone Marrow 80

IV

DISORDERS OF VITAMIN B_{12} AND FOLIC ACID METABOLISM 86

Vitamin B_{12} 86
Folic Acid 89
Metabolic Functions of Vitamin B_{12} and Folic Acid 89
Classification of Megaloblastic Anemias 92
Vitamin B_{12} Deficiency 93
Folate Deficiency 107

V

DISORDERS OF IRON METABOLISM ... 116

Iron Metabolism ... 116
Anemia of Iron Deficiency ... 129
Anemias Associated with Abnormal Utilization of Iron ... 138
Iron Overload ... 147

VI

BONE MARROW FAILURE ... 156

Classification ... 156
Aplastic Anemia ... 157
Erythrocytic Hypoplasia (Pure Red Cell Anemia) ... 170
Aplastic Anemia in Children ... 172

VII

HEMOLYTIC ANEMIA ... 178

Erythrocyte Metabolism and Methemoglobinemia ... 179
Classification ... 184
Hereditary Hemolytic Disorders ... 186
    Erythrocyte Membrane Defects ... 186
    Pentose Phosphate Shunt-Glutathione System Enzyme
        Deficiencies ... 194
    Glycolytic Enzyme Deficiencies ... 197
    Hemoglobinopathies ... 198
Acquired Hemolytic Disorders ... 222
    Antibody Mediated ... 222
    Immune Drug-Induced Hemolytic Anemia ... 230
    Paroxysmal Nocturnal Hemoglobinuria ... 240
    Mechanical Hemolysis ... 242

VIII

ANEMIA RESULTING FROM OTHER DISORDERS ... 262

Anemia Associated with Chronic Disease ... 262
Anemia Associated with Myxedema ... 263
Anemia Associated with Acute Blood Loss ... 266
Anemia Associated with Pregnancy ... 267
Anemia Associated with Chronic Renal Disease ... 270
Anemia Associated with Chronic Liver Disease ... 272
Hypersplenism and Big Spleen Disease ... 274

IX

POLYCYTHEMIA ... 281

Polycythemia Vera ... 282

Secondary Polycythemia... 291
Benign Familial Polycythemia................................... 294

X

HEMOSTASIS: THEORY AND CLINICAL APPLICATIONS 302

Normal Hemostasis 302
Fibrinolysis.. 320
Anticoagulants... 327
Examination of the Patient with Hemorrhagic Diathesis............ 333

XI

DISORDERS OF HEMOSTASIS... 353

Thrombocytopenic Purpura... 354
Non-Thrombocytopenic Purpura.................................... 370
Hereditary Hemorrhagic Telangiectasia........................ 374
Abnormalities of Blood Coagulation............................. 376

XII

LEUKOCYTES 428

Granulocytes 428
Disorders Associated with Quantitative Defects in Granulocytes... 442
Neutropenia.. 448
Disorders Associated with Qualitative Defects in Granulocytes... 449
Infectious Mononucleosis 452

XIII

LEUKEMIA... 471

Acute Leukemia 478
Chronic Lymphocytic Leukemia................................... 487
Chronic Granulocytic Leukemia 496
Eosinophilic Leukemia.. 506
Monocytic Leukemia.. 507
DiGuglielmo Syndrome... 511
Myeloid Metaplasia... 512
Hemorrhagic Thrombocythemia 522

XIV

MALIGNANT LYMPHOMAS (LYMPHOMA, LYMPHOBLASTOMA) 529

The Diagnosis of the Patient with Enlarged Lymph Nodes 529
Classification... 533
Hodgkin's Disease 535

Lymphosarcoma and Reticulum Cell Sarcoma........................... 540
Giant Follicular Lymphoma.. 543
Other Disorders.. 544

XV

PROLIFERATIVE DISORDERS OF THE LYMPHORETICULAR SYSTEM
ASSOCIATED WITH PLASMA PROTEIN ABNORMALITIES...................... 569

Immunologic Mechanisms 580
Disorders of Plasma Cells and Lymphocytes Associated with
Immunoglobulin Abnormalities 584
Multiple Myeloma 584
Macroglobulinemia 601

XVI

THERAPEUTIC AGENTS USED IN THE TREATMENT OF HEMATOLOGIC
DISORDERS.. 611

Blood Transfusion.. 626

INDEX.. 647

I / The Origin and Morphology of Blood Cells

The important contributions made by Ehrlich can be considered the beginning of modern hematology.[20] The staining methods which he introduced became the cornerstone of morphologic hematology and cytochemistry. With the use of the new technique Ehrlich described many cellular details and developed a classification of blood cells.

In recent years there have been enormous gains in the knowledge of the structure and function of cells as the result of information derived from electron microscopy, biochemical analysis of cell fractions, differential staining techniques, and immunologic methods. These have provided a better understanding of the derangements that occur in many hematologic diseases and have greatly expanded the methods used in the diagnosis of hematological problems. Despite these advances, the study of the cells in the peripheral blood and bone marrow by means of light microscopy remains essential for the diagnosis of many hematologic disorders.

The Cell

Most cells contain a nucleus and cytoplasm. Both are complex structures which have numerous vital functions. In general the nucleus controls the development, function, and division of the cell and the cytoplasm carries out most of its synthetic activity.

The cell membrane. The cell membrane is one example of biological membranes that control many vital functions. When studied with electron microscopy, membranes from bacteria, plants, and animals appear to consist of two dark lines separated by a lighter zone. Danielli and Davson[15] and

1

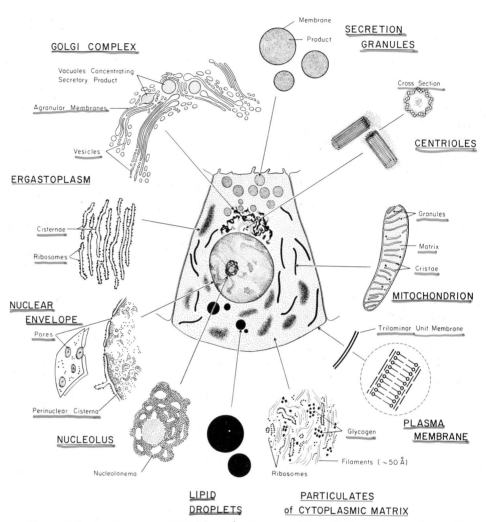

Figure 1–1. In the center of this figure is a diagram of the cell, illustrating the form of its organelles and inclusions as they appear by light microscopy. Around the periphery are representations of the finer structure of these same components as seen in electron micrographs. (From Bloom and Fawcett: A Textbook of Histology. Philadelphia, Saunders, 1968.)

Robertson[44] have proposed the unit membrane hypothesis that all biologic membranes have the same basic structure, consisting of a bimolecular lipid leaflet sandwiched between layers that are non-lipid and largely protein; the lipid molecules have their polar groups facing outward and the long chain hydrocarbons inward. Position of the layers is maintained by ionic binding of hydrophilic head groups of the phospholipids to the protein layer. Although the membranes have a uniform appearance in section, chemical data indicate that membranes in different cells, and in different parts of the same cell, vary greatly in chemical composition and function.[31, 59] Among the diversified tasks assigned to membranes are the following: protein biosynthesis; energy transduction (especially nerves); transport of amino acids, sugar, and other small molecules; flow of water; maintenance of specific ion balance; pinocytosis; phagocytosis; and a variety of reactions in intermediary metabolism and controlled growth and division.[59]

Nucleus. The nucleus, which is essential for growth and division of the cell, is found in nearly all cells; one important exception is the erythrocyte. The most important constituent of the nucleus is deoxyribonucleic acid (DNA), which in combination with structural proteins forms the chromatin material of the nucleus. The appearance of the chromatin, which stains deeply with basic dyes because of its DNA content, varies with different stages of development of the cell. During interphase the chromatin consists of clumps of deeply staining material, heterochromatin, and a lighter, staining portion, euchromatin. The DNA occurs in long thin threads in the form of a double helix that contains the genes and carries the biochemical, morphological, and metabolic characteristics of the cell when it divides. The matrix of the chromatin in the nucleus has been referred to as nuclear sap, nuclear matrix, or nuclear ground substance.

Most cells contain from one to four blue staining nucleoli surrounded by aggregates of chromatin. The nucleoli stain blue because of the presence of ribonucleic acid (RNA). The nucleolus often is unusually large in rapidly growing cells. Although evidence indicates that the nucleolus is important in nucleic acid metabolism and protein synthesis, its precise function remains to be established.

Electron microscopy has shown that the nuclear envelope consists of two parallel membranes which enclose a narrow perinuclear space. Numerous "nuclear pores" are formed where the two membranes touch each other, but the extent that material passes from the nucleus to the cytoplasm through these pores is uncertain. The outermost layer of the nuclear membrane, where ribosomes are usually attached, is often continuous with the endoplasmic reticulum.

Cytoplasm. Electron microscopy has revealed that a large portion of the cytoplasm consists of fluid-filled channels of granular and agranular endoplasmic reticulum that are often continuous with the outer layer of the nuclear membrane. Much of the endoplasmic reticulum is given a granular appearance by adhering ribosomes. Each ribosome consists of two ribonucleoprotein particles of unequal size. Usually several ribosomes are attached to a single strand of messenger RNA (mRNA) to form a polyribosome. Protein synthesis begins with enzymatic activation of amino acids by the attachment of the AMP moiety of ATP to the amino acid[53] and the subsequent transfer to a molecule of transfer RNA (tRNA or sRNA) specific for that particular amino acid. The molecules of tRNA are brought into line along the mRNA to form polypeptides in a sequence dictated by the code in the mRNA. The ribosome seems to read the message encoded into mRNA by moving along the mRNA from one end to the other. Ribosomes are situated near the endoplasmic reticulum in cells that produce protein destined to be secreted by the cell; the protein follows the reticular channels to the Golgi apparatus for further modification and temporary storage. The agranular reticulum, a tubular network without associated ribosomes, occupies varying amounts of cytoplasm in cells that differ greatly in function.

Mitochondria. Mitochondria, which can be seen with light microscopy when stained supravitally with Janus green, occur in all aerobic cells of higher animals.[53] These organelles have two membranes. The inner membrane, which has many infoldings termed "cristae mitochondriales," surrounds a protein and lipid containing matrix. The membranes consist of 35 to 40 per cent lipid, mainly enzymatic. Although mitochondria are usually slender rods, the number, size, shape, and distribution of mitochondria vary widely in different kinds of cells.

The main function of the mitochondria concerns oxidative processes, particularly those involved in lipid metabolism, the Krebs cycle, and phosphorylation. Mitochondria have been referred to as "power plants" because they supply energy for many chemical reactions and transport systems. Through the breakdown of carbohydrates, fats, and proteins, high energy phosphates (ATP) are formed which are important in many cellular functions including the transport of ions and molecules across subcellular and cellular membranes. Among the enzymes found in mitochondria are the cytochromes, coenzyme Q, flavoproteins, dehydrogenases, oxidative phosphorylation enzymes, Krebs cycle enzymes, glutamate dehydrogenase, and enzymes for protein and lipid synthesis.

Both DNA and RNA have been identified in mitochondria and constitute an extranuclear genetic system concerned with protein synthesis by a process that differs somewhat from cytoplasmic ribosomal synthesis: cyclophosphamide, for example, does not have the same inhibitory effect on protein synthesis in mitochondria that it has on cytoplasmic protein synthesis. Mitochondria are apparently formed by growth and division of existing mitochondria.[53]

Lysosomes. Lysosomes have been defined as a heterogeneous group of cytoplasmic organelles that mediate the digestive and lytic processes of the cell.[60] Lysosomes occur in most vertebrate cells; they contain a number of enzymes and other substances listed in Table 1–1. A number of histochemical and biochemical studies have resulted in the suggestion that any intracellular organelle contained in a single unit membrane and staining for acid phosphatase be considered a lysosome.

A variety of lysosomes that differ in function have been identified. One is the specific granule in leukocytes and macrophages that is so important in phagocytosis. The membrane of the lysosome fuses with the membrane of the "phagosome" formed by invagination of the cellular membrane when foreign bodies are engulfed; the subsequent discharge of enzymes from the lysosomes lyses the engulfed material. Because the enzymes remain confined within the fused membranes, the cell is not necessarily damaged by the reaction. The lysosomes may be important in the processing of antigens by macrophages, apparently a preliminary step for the stimulation of antibody production by antigens. Another form of lysosome is the "autophagic vacuole" that develops when a portion of the cytoplasm is destroyed in response to some injury. Cell death and destruction can be produced by the unrestricted release of the enzyme into the cytoplasm or by phagocytosis by other cells. In surviving cells, both phagosomes and autophagic vacuoles can form "residual bodies" that are filled with debris that is often lipid.

The membranes of lysosomes, which resemble those surrounding mitochondria and erythrocytes, are affected in living cells by a number of substances including streptolysins O and S, x-rays, vitamin A, and bacterial endotoxins.[60]

Table 1–1. *Enzymes and Other Substances Localized to Lysosomes*

ENZYMES	OTHER SUBSTANCES
Acid phosphatase	Phagocytin
Acid ribonuclease	Cationic "inflammatory" protein
Acid deoxyribonuclease	Mucopolysaccharides and glycoproteins
Acid protease (or proteases); cathepsins	Plasminogen activator
Phosphoprotein phosphatase	Permeability-inducing protease
Beta-glucuronidase	Hemolysin (or hemolysins)
Beta-N-acetylglucosaminidase	Unidentified basic proteins
Alpha-mannosidase	
Beta-galactosidase	
Alpha$_1 \rightarrow {}_4$glucosidase	
Hyaluronidase	
Lysozyme	
Phospholipase, acid lipase	
Phosphatidic acid phosphatase	
Collagenase	
Arylsulfatases A and B	
Nonspecific esterases	

(From Weissman: New England J. Med., 273:1085, 1965.)

It appears likely that the labilizing effect of substances on lysosomes is a result of their effect on the membranes, because many exert similar effects on membranes of erythrocytes and mitochondria. The anti-inflammatory steroids, cortisone, prednisone, and others, have a stabilizing effect on lysosomes, which may explain in part the pharmacologic action of these compounds.[60]

Golgi apparatus. The Golgi apparatus is located near the nucleus. It can be seen by light microscopy when stained with osmium or silver compounds. Research with radioactive tracers, special staining methods, and electron microscopy has shown that the Golgi apparatus is the primary site for the synthesis of large carbohydrates and for "packaging" the secretions, external and internal, formed in the cell. Protein is synthesized from amino acids on the ribosomes and moves to the Golgi apparatus where carbohydrates are added to the protein. The apparatus appears to contain a pile of saccules; as these saccules move upward in the apparatus they accumulate more carbohydrate and more of the cell's secretion product. The topmost saccules bud off, eventually make their way through the cell membrane, and release their enclosed glycoprotein. Although the Golgi apparatus is probably not the exclusive site of the formation of carbohydrate side chains in glycoproteins and mucopolysaccharides, it appears to be the main organelle involved.[35a]

The Blood Cells

Opinions about the origin of most of the blood cells have been a source of disagreements and polemical outbursts over the years; even now, after many years of study and discussion, there is no unanimity of opinion on many points. Ehrlich recognized that the granulocytic series of cells arose from a non-granular precursor in the bone marrow and thought that lymphocytes originated in the lymph glands.[20] This distinction formed the basis of his theory of the dual origin of white cells. Ehrlich considered this dualistic doctrine to be one of the most important results of his long continued studies in hematology, but it was not accepted by many hematologists. The dualistic theory was supported by Banti, Turk, Naegeli, and others,[20, 40] and was opposed by the monophyleticists, Maximow, Jordan, Bloom, and others, who believed that myeloid tissue could arise postembryonically from lymphocytes.[9, 27, 33] Still another theory, the polyphyletic, has been advanced by Cunningham, Sabin, and Doan, who concluded that each type of adult cell has its own particular blast precursor.[14] Detailed discussions of the different theories of the origin of the various cells are presented in Downey's Handbook of Hematology[19] and in review articles.[14, 33, 38, 45]

Much of the confusion regarding the identity of cells has been caused by lack of a uniform terminology. Different techniques and different types of material have been used by investigators who have given different names to the same cells and have employed the same term for different cells. Fortunately, unanimity of hematologic opinion as to the origin and relationship of the cells is not essential for the successful management of most clinical hematologic problems. There are enough points of agreement to allow the development of the workable concept of cellular relationships that is needed for an organized approach to clinical problems. A knowledge of morphology is necessary for the diagnosis of many hematologic diseases, and a terminology is essential for communication.

In selecting the terms to be used in this text the authors have chosen those that are used most commonly; in the classification of cells the terms recommended by the Committee for Clarification of the Nomenclature of Cells and Diseases of the Blood-Forming Organs have been included in every instance.[12]

The Stem Cell

Although the identity of the much discussed "stem cell" remains a mystery, the concept of such a cell is generally accepted. Considerable recent evidence supports the view that the cell in question is morphologically indistinguishable from the small or medium-sized lymphocyte found in the bone marrow.[13] It has been demonstrated that it is these cells, separated from other marrow cells by glass wool column filters, which can incorporate tritiated thymidine into the nucleus, repopulate the marrow, and form spleen colonies in guinea pigs with the development of lines of erythroblasts, granulocytes, and megakaryocytes. Small lymphocytes found in the peripheral blood or lymph nodes, reticulum cells, granulocytic cells, and erythroblastic cells do not possess this capacity. In addition, a study reported that in rats the injection of testosterone led to a diminution in marrow and thymic lymphocytes associated with increased hematopoiesis and retained immunologic capacity; the observations were interpreted as a reflection of the accelerated differentiation of lymphoid cells in the marrow into erythroid and granulocytic cell lines and those in the thymus into immunologically active cells.[20a]

The Granulocytic Series

The granulocytes, which are motile and phagocytic, constitute the main defense of the body against bacterial infection. The kinetics and functions of these cells are discussed in Chapter XII.

Origin

Under normal conditions the older granulocytic cells, the bands and segmented cells, develop from the myelocytes in the bone marrow. Various cells have been considered to be the non-granular ancestors of the granular myelocytes.[14, 27, 33, 40] Although these theories differ in details, all agree that in the adult under normal circumstances the older cells of the granulocytic series arise in the bone marrow and are derived from the myelocytes and their precursors, which are either myeloblasts or cells that have an identical appearance in fixed smears.

Morphology

Myeloblast. The myeloblast occurs in normal bone marrow but is not found in the circulating blood except in certain disease states. In fixed smears the diameter of myeloblasts ranges from 11 to 18 microns. With Wright's stain the nuclear material assumes a deep purplish blue color; the chromatin is finely divided, punctate, or strandlike, and appears condensed only around the rims of the nucleoli. The cytoplasm stains the same light blue color as the nucleolus, is variable in amount and often forms little more than a rim about the nucleus. Myeloblasts generally give a negative reaction when a peroxidase stain is used, but some cells that are classed as myeloblasts with Wright's stain give a positive reaction with peroxidase stain. The staining properties of the cells are related to the nucleoproteins. Ribonucleic acid (RNA) occurs both in the nucleoli and in the cytoplasm; deoxyribonucleic acid (DNA) is found mainly in the nucleus. Protein synthesis in the cell is thought to be under the control of the nucleoproteins and the presence of the nucleolus has been correlated with active cellular proliferation;[34, 61] cellular proliferation ceases when the nucleolus disappears and is replaced by the more deeply basophilic heterochromatin.[55]

Myeloblasts vary in size and other details. The nucleus is sometimes slightly indented and in acute leukemia it is occasionally deeply indented or lobulated. Rieder cells are myeloblasts that have trifoliate or quadrifoliate nuclei. The cytoplasm of myeloblasts and monoblasts sometimes contains Auer bodies. These structures, which appeared with Wright's stain and resemble a stained tubercle bacillus, give positive peroxidase and oxidase reactions. Histochemical study has revealed that these rods contain ribonucleic acid and a lipoid material, possibly a mucopolysaccharide.[1] When myeloblasts are stained supravitally with neutral red and Janus green, numerous small mitochondria can be seen in the cytoplasm.

Progranulocyte (promyelocyte). The progranulocyte is the next stage in development after the myeloblast and some may resemble myeloblasts with the addition of azurophilic cytoplasmic granules. Other cells at this stage have a coarser nuclear structure than the myeloblast, are larger, and contain numerous azurophilic granules in the cytoplasm and in the region overlying the nucleus. Nucleoli may or may not be visible at this stage. The appearance and development of the granules appear to be closely related to the differentiation of the cytoplasmic proteins. Thorell has shown that the myeloblast has a high concentration of cytoplasmic polynucleotides and a prominent nucleolus.[55]

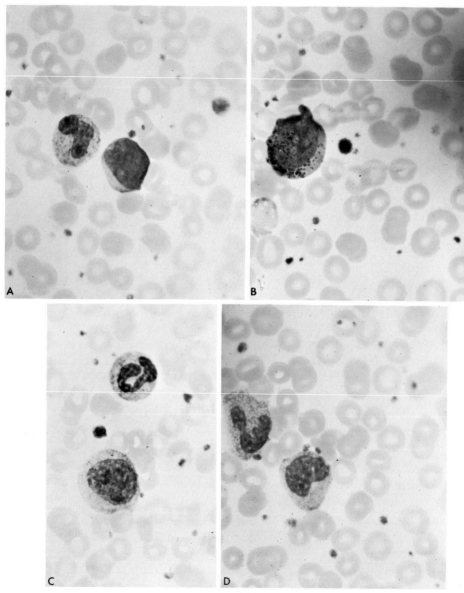

Figure 1–2. Early cells of the granulocytic series. *A*, Myeloblast. *B*, Progranulocyte. *C*, Myelocyte (early). *D*, Metamyelocyte.

When the cell matures to the progranulocytic stage the cytoplasmic polynucleotides decrease as the granules appear. Further development of the granules is associated with continued decrease in the polynucleotide content and none is demonstrable by the time the myelocyte stage is reached. The nucleolus, which has been thought to have considerable influence over the differentiation of the cytoplasmic proteins, contains ribonucleic acid; this material decreases gradually and is no longer detectable in the myelocytic stage. When the nucleolus disappears, further differentiation of the cytoplasmic protein cannot take place.

Myelocyte. Myelocytes are the first cells of the granulocytic series that contain specific granules, which are either neutrophilic, eosinophilic, or basophilic. Both neutrophilic and eosinophilic granules give a positive peroxidase reaction. As the myelocyte develops from the progranulocyte it becomes smaller and the nuclear chromatin becomes coarser. When supravital stains are used, numerous small mitochondria and a variable number of neutral red bodies can be demonstrated in the cytoplasm. The number, location, and arrangement of the neutral red bodies have been employed as a basis for classifying myelocytes according to different stages of development as myelocytes A, B, and C.[14]

Metamyelocyte (juvenile). As the myelocyte matures, the chromatin structure of the nucleus becomes coarser, specific granulation persists, and the nucleus becomes indented. At this stage the cell is termed a metamyelocyte.

Band cell (stab cell). According to the Committee on Nomenclature of Blood Cells, any cell of the granulocytic series is classed as a band cell "which has a nucleus which could be described as a curved or coiled band, no matter how marked the indentation, if it does not completely segment the nucleus into lobes connected by a filament."[12]

Segmented cell (polymorphonuclear). These are the fully developed cells of the granulocytic series whose nuclei contain two or more lobes that are joined by filamentous connections. The nuclear chromatin is coarse and has the appearance of blocks or knots connected by strands. The cytoplasm contains numerous granules that stain specifically with Wright's stain.

The neutrophil segmented cell (neutrophil) gives a positive peroxidase reaction. In supravital preparations numerous small refractile bodies fill the cytoplasm and active ameboid movement is prominent.

Various abnormal forms of granulocytes have been described. Macropolycytes, unusually large neutrophils with nuclei consisting of five to ten lobes, are seen in patients with a deficiency in vitamin B_{12} or folic acid. The Pelger-Huët anomaly, first described by Pelger in 1928,[41] is characterized by decreased segmentation of the nucleus and increased condensation of the nuclear chromatin. An abnormally large number of the cells (69 to 93 per cent) are two-lobed; they differ from band cells in that the individual lobes tend to be round and are joined by a narrow strand. The anomaly is inherited and involves the eosinophils and basophils as well as neutrophils.

A number of abnormalities have been described in the granules and cytoplasm of the granulocytes. Alder's constitutional granulation anomaly is characterized by the presence of large and numerous azurophil granulations in the neutrophils, eosinophils, and basophils; some of the monocytes and lymphocytes may be involved.[5] The heavy granulations may hide the nuclei of the cells. The blood of some but not all patients with gargoylism manifests

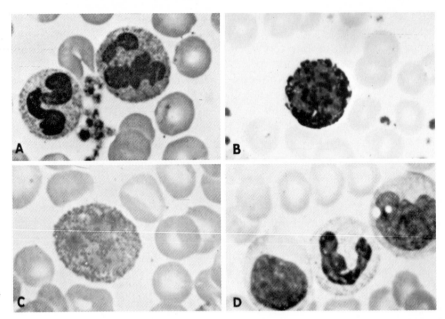

Figure 1–3. Later cells of the granulocytic series. *A*, Neutrophils. *B*, Basophil. *C*, Eosinophil. *D*, Comparison of lymphocyte, neutrophil, and monocyte.

this granulation anomaly.[23] "Toxic granulation" is the term given to changes in the granulocytes that occur in some patients with severe infections and other illnesses; the granules are dark, sometimes basophilic, and at times the cytoplasm is basophilic and vacuolated. Döhle inclusion bodies are round, blue-staining bodies sometimes seen in the cytoplasm of neutrophils; the bodies, which may measure 2 microns in diameter, are round or oval in shape; as many as three or four may be present in the periphery of the cell. They have been described in patients with various bacterial infections and also in burns.[38] The Chediak-Higashi syndrome, which is seen mainly in young children but also in young adults, is characterized by the presence of large eosinophilic, peroxidase positive inclusion bodies in myeloblasts and promyelocytes of the bone marrow; more mature cells of the granulocytic series contain abnormally large granules that stain normally.[9a, 23a] Patients with the syndrome have a predisposition for malignant lymphoma. The May-Heggelin anomaly is rare; it is characterized by Döhle bodies in the majority of the neutrophils, monocytes and eosinophils associated with giant platelets, and, at times, thrombocytopenia. (F.S.: III, 145.)

The eosinophil segmented cell (eosinophil) is a fully developed cell. The nucleus does not stain as heavily as that of the neutrophil. The eosinophil is characterized by the presence of large granules that fill the cytoplasm and stain a bright yellowish red color with Wright's stain. When stained supravitally with neutral red and Janus green the granules appear large, very refractile, and yellow. These cells give a positive peroxidase reaction. Histochemical studies indicate that the eosinophil granules are composed of protein and surrounded by phospholipid.[8] Verdoperoxidase is also present.[2, 3] Eosinophils contain about one-third of the histamine found in normal blood.[22]

The basophil segmented cell (basophil) is somewhat smaller than the neutrophil and eosinophil. The characteristic feature of this cell is the presence of large purplish black granules that almost completely fill the cell. The granules appear red when stained supravitally with neutral red. The cells are peroxidase negative. Basophils contain relatively large amounts of histamine,[10, 11] about one-half of the histamine content of normal blood.[22] The presence of heparin has been suspected but not proved. (F.S.: III, 142–144.)

The Lymphocytic Series

The lymphocytic series of cells, which probably includes cells with diverse potentials, is concerned with resistance to infection, antibody production, and tissue rejection; the cells have little motility. The kinetics and functions of these cells are discussed in Chapter XV.

Origin

Lymphocytes are produced in lymph nodes, in the periarterial pulp of the spleen, in nodules of the tonsils, in the mucous membranes of the gastro-intestinal, genitourinary, and respiratory tracts, and in the lymph nodules in the bone marrow.[19, 27, 33, 45] Various cellular origins of the lymphocytes have been suggested. Among these are pre-existing lymphocytes,[9, 27] reticulum cells,[9, 17, 45] hemocytoblasts,[9, 27] and "primitive white cells" intermediate between reticulum cells and lymphoblasts.[14] Much evidence suggests that some lymphocytes are not irreversible "end cells" as the granulocytes are, but instead cells that retain the potential for further differentiation, at least under special circumstances. The lymphocyte has been considered to be the source of plasma cells[33, 52] and also of wandering tissue phagocytes.[33, 43] The conclusion has also been reached that lymphocytes act as stem cells and produce myeloid cells,[17, 27, 28] erythrocyte precursors, and other marrow elements under the specific stimulus of special environmental factors.

Morphology

Lymphoblast. The lymphoblast occurs in the peripheral blood rarely, if at all, except in cases of leukemia. It is distinguished from the myeloblast with difficulty and the identity of a blast cell usually is assumed from the recognition of the older cells that accompany it. The nucleus of the lymphoblast is round and has a fine chromatin structure in which several nucleoli are often visible. The cytoplasm stains pale blue and contains no granules.

Prolymphocyte. Lymphocytic cells that are intermediate between lymphoblasts and lymphocytes are termed prolymphocytes. Although the nuclear chromatin appears coarser than that of the blast cells, it is finer than that of the lymphocytes. At times nucleoli or nucleolar remnants are visible. Usually the diameter of these cells is greater than 15 microns.

Lymphocyte. In dry smears the diameter of small lymphocytes varies from 7 to 10 microns, but the less common large lymphocytes may have a diameter of 20 microns. When Wright's stain is used the nucleus of the small lymphocytes, which is usually round but sometimes indented, appears almost to fill the entire cell. The nucleus has a prominent membrane, stains deeply, and contains large masses of chromatin. No nucleoli can be identified. In the large lymphocytes the nuclear chromatin stains less deeply and appears somewhat less compact. The cytoplasm, which is much more abundant in the larger lymphocytes, stains pale blue. A small number of reddish violet granules are scattered through the cytoplasm of many of the cells of this series. The lymphocytes do not give a positive reaction with the peroxidase stain. When stained supravitally with Janus green and neutral red, the lymphocytes are seen to contain a variable number of short, rodlike mitochondria that usually appear clumped in one part of the cytoplasm, often opposite the nuclear indentation. A few small neutral red vacuoles are also seen.

Lymphocytes at times show definite staining abnormalities in disease states, particularly in virus infections. The cytoplasm of the larger cells is sometimes deeply basophilic and opaque and at other times it is almost colorless. Nuclear fenestrations and cytoplasmic vacuoles are often present.

The Monocytic Series

The monocytes are phagocytic cells, probably related to the tissue macrophages. They function in the body defense against infection, particularly in the formation of granulomas and giant cells, and in the destruction of damaged tissue; they also play a role in immune reactions, probably by processing the antigen before it provokes a response from the lymphocytes.[39]

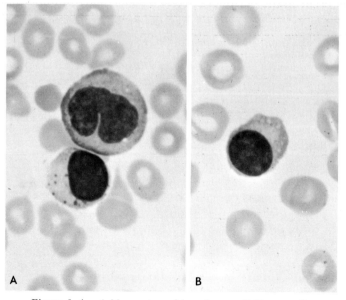

Figure 1-4. *A,* Monocyte and lymphocyte. *B,* Plasma cell.

Origin

In 1924 Maximow stated that "of all the cells in the circulating blood, the monocytes offer the greatest difficulty to elucidation of their relationship and origin."[33] Five decades later both their origin and their relationship to the histiocytes (macrophages) remain uncertain. At various times monocytes have been considered to arise from lymphocytes,[9, 27] endothelial cells,[32] histiocytes,[6, 33] myeloblasts,[40] and monoblasts.[46]

A relationship between monocytes, histiocytes, and lymphocytes is shown by the study of the reaction in inflammation. Maximow considered it proved that the tissue macrophages (polyblasts, mononuclear-phagocytic elements) arise partly through direct transformation of the free histiocytes of the tissue by mobilization and also through changes that occur in monocytes and lymphocytes that migrate from blood vessels into the field of inflammation. Rebuck and Crowley, who published an extensive review of the work on this subject, studied the cellular reactions occurring in sterile inflammation of the human skin and concluded that the main source of macrophages in the inflammation is the emigrated lymphocytes, and the monocytes and tissue cells play a subsidiary role because of their limited numbers.[43] Other evidence (Chaps. XII and XV) indicates that monocytes originate in the bone marrow and become macrophages on leaving the circulation.

Morphology

Monoblast. According to the Committee on the Nomenclature of Blood Cells (1949), the monoblast is any cell of the monocytic series that has a fine chromatin structure.[12] Nucleoli are usually visible, and such cells found in association with monocytes should be tentatively classed as monoblasts. These cells do not occur in the peripheral blood or bone marrow under normal conditions but may be seen in patients with monocytic leukemia. In such circumstances many of the "blast" cells appear identical with the myeloblast.

Promonocyte. Promonocytes are cells that have an indented nucleus and appear younger than the monocytes in that the nuclear chromatin appears more finely divided and contains nucleoli or nucleolar remnants. These cells are thought to be intermediate between the blast cells and adult monocytes. They are not seen in the peripheral blood normally but at times do occur in disseminated tuberculosis and other diseases involving the reticuloendothelial system, as well as in monocytic leukemia.

Monocyte. The monocyte is usually larger than the other cells of the peripheral blood. In dried smears the diameter measures from 16 to 22 microns. When stained with Wright's preparation, the monocyte possesses an abundant pale bluish gray cytoplasm which appears somewhat more opaque than the cytoplasm of the lymphocytes. The cytoplasm contains numerous fine reddish granules, and vacuoles are often present. The nucleus, which is often but not invariably indented, has a stringy chromatin structure that appears more condensed where the strands of chromatin meet. When these cells are stained supravitally with neutral red and Janus green, large numbers of short mitochondria can be seen in the cytoplasm. Neutral red regularly stains a group of cytoplasmic vacuoles near the indentation of the nucleus. This rosette of red vacuoles has been considered by some authors to be a characteristic peculiar to monocytes,[46] but others do not share this opinion. Although monocytes are usually easily distinguished from lymphocytes and myelocytes by their size and the appearance of the nucleus and cytoplasm, at times atypical cells are seen that cannot be identified with confidence by any of the staining methods; some such cells are considered to be "virocytes" and others are designated "lympho-reticular cells."

The Thromboyctic Series

The thrombocytes or blood platelets are an essential part of the hemostatic mechanism of the body; they are important in thrombosis and blood coagulation.[32a] The chemistry and function of these blood elements are discussed in Chapter XI.

Origin

Megakaryocytes are thought to arise from primitive mesenchymal cells by way of the hemocytoblast, the precursor of the megakaryoblast.[56]

Wright's hypothesis of the origin of the blood platelets as fragmented portions of the cytoplasm of the megakaryocytes of the bone marrow is generally accepted.[63] More recent studies that utilized antisera[7] and the electron microscope[4, 24] support the same conclusion.

Morphology

Megakaryoblast. Megakaryoblasts, which are found only in the bone marrow in special circumstances, are larger than the other blast cells. The cytoplasm is pale blue. The nucleus, which is round or oval, has a finely divided chromatin structure and a variable number of small nucleoli may be apparent.

Promegakaryocyte. Promegakaryocytes are considered to be intermediate between megakaryoblasts and megakaryocytes. The nucleus, which has a shape similar to that of the megakaryocyte, contains nucleoli surrounded by a rather coarse chromatin structure. The cytoplasm contains a number of fine purplish red granules.

Megakaryocyte. The megakaryocyte has now been demonstrated to circulate in small numbers in the venous blood of normal persons and in larger numbers in the venous blood of patients with cancer.[25, 30] It has been demonstrated in dogs and in humans that the lungs trap the great majority of these large cells. It has been estimated that from 9 to 26 per cent of the platelets are released in the pulmonary capillaries by these mature megakaryocytes.[29] Megakaryocytes are found in the bone marrow. They are very large cells that often have a diameter that varies from 50 to 100 microns. The nucleus, which is usually polyploid, stains dark blue with Wright's stain and contains no visible nucleoli. The abundant cytoplasm stains light blue and contains numerous purplish red granules. These granules often appear in aggregates.

Thrombocyte (platelet). Thrombocytes, or blood platelets, are the smallest stained elements in the peripheral blood. Ordinarily they have a diameter of from 2 to 4 microns, but in some disease states and on smears made from blood collected with an anticoagulant the platelets appear much larger. In such circumstances they may approach the small lymphocyte in size or may form a strand that stretches across an entire oil immersion field. These elements contain no nuclei, and when stained with Wright's stain appear to consist of a pale cytoplasm that contains numerous reddish purple granules.

The Plasmacytic Series

The plasma cells are an important part of the body's defense mechanism and are the main sources of the plasma globulins. These cells are discussed in more detail in Chapter XV.

Origin

Michels reviewed the rather extensive literature on the plasma cell that appeared prior to 1931 and noted that at least four different cellular origins had been suggested.[36] These were (1) histogenous origin from connective tissue cells, including tissue lymphocytes, fibroblasts, and resting wandering cells; (2) origin from emigrated lymphocytes; (3) origin from emigrated lymphocytes or pre-existing tissue lymphocytes; and (4) origin from immature blood cells such as myeloblasts or erythroblasts, through aberration. Sundberg reviewed the subject of the origin and function of the plasma cells[52] and pointed out that, although studies on the production of antibodies emphasize a close relationship between the plasma cells and the lymphocytes, the concept of multiple origin of plasma cells from lymphocytes, perivascular cells, mesothelial cells, macrophages, and fibroblasts, which was proposed by Downey in 1931, cannot be excluded with certainty.[18]

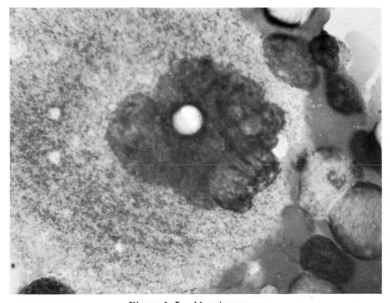

Figure 1–5. Megakaryocyte.

Morphology

Plasmablast (myeloma cell).   Plasmablasts do not occur normally in the peripheral blood or in the bone marrow and are seen only in plasmacytic leukemia or multiple myeloma. The nucleus, which is usually eccentric, has a fine chromatin structure and contains one or more large nucleoli. The cytoplasm stains blue and is more opaque than that of the myeloblast or lymphoblast.

Proplasmacyte.   These cells are intermediate between the plasmablasts and the plasmacytes. The chromatin of the nucleus appears more coarse than that of the plasmablast but is definitely more immature than that of the plasmacyte. Usually a single nucleolus is present, but at times more than one are seen.

Plasmacyte (plasma cell, Marschalko's plasma cell).   In fixed smears the plasma cells vary considerably in size, and diameters range from 10 to 20 microns. The characteristic feature of the cell is the eccentric location of the round or oval nucleus which has extremely coarse chromatin. The chromatin consists of blocks which stain deeply. The arrangement of the chromatin in the nucleus has been compared in appearance to the spokes of a wheel. The cytoplasm, which often has an irregular border, is abundant, stains dark blue, and is characterized by a perinuclear area of lighter staining. The cytoplasm is non-homogeneous and small vacuoles are often present. When supravital stains are used, numerous small mitochondria can be seen in the cytoplasm of the cell.

Plasmacytes are not usually seen in the peripheral blood but may appear in serum sickness, rubella, infectious mononucleosis, infectious hepatitis, multiple myeloma, plasma cell leukemia, and other conditions. Normally plasmacytes are present in the lymph nodes, the connective tissue, and the bone marrow.

The Erythrocytic Series

The erythrocytes contain hemoglobin, which is essential for transport of the oxygen from the lungs to the tissues in the body. The production and function of these cells are discussed in Chaps. II and VII.

Origin

Michels in 1931 published an extensive review of erythropoiesis.[37] He attributes the first observation of the red corpuscles to Jan Schwammerdam in 1658 and the first report of nucleated red corpuscles in the human species to Webber, who in 1838 observed them in a human fetus of 12 weeks. In 1857 Kölliker demonstrated erythropoiesis in the embryonic liver and recognized that the non-nucleated red corpuscles arose from the nucleated forms. He recognized that the spleen was also an organ of erythropoiesis but thought that nucleated red corpuscles did not occur in the blood or any of the organs of adults. Neumann in 1868 demonstrated that the mammalian red corpuscles arose throughout life from the nucleated elements in the bone marrow. He

Table 1–2. *Origin and Relationship of Blood Cells*

Stem Cell

Megakaryoblast —— Promegakaryocyte —— Megakaryocyte —————————————— Thrombocyte

Myeloblast —— Progranulocyte
— E. Myelocyte ——————————————— Eosinophil
— N. Myelocyte —— N. Metamyelocyte —— Band Cell —— Neutrophil segmented
— B. Myelocyte —————————————— Basophil

Monoblast —— Promonocyte ———————————————————————— Monocyte

Lymphoblast —— Prolymphocyte ——————————————————————— Lymphocyte

Plasmablast —— Proplasmacyte ——————————————————————— Plasmacyte

Pronormoblast (Rubriblast) —— Basophilic Normoblast (Prorubricyte) —— Polychromatic Normoblast (Rubricyte) —— Orthochromatic Normoblast (Metarubricyte) —— Reticulocyte —— Erythrocyte

Promegaloblast —— Basophilic Megaloblast —— Polychromatic Megaloblast —— Orthochromatic Megaloblast —— Reticulocyte —— Erythrocyte

Adapted from Diggs, Sturm and Bell: The Morphology of Human Blood Cells. Philadelphia, W. B. Saunders Co., 1956.

studied human cadaver material and observed erythropoiesis in many bones; he also noted that the red marrow increased at the expense of the yellow marrow to provide an additional source of erythrocyte production.

The identity of the precursors of the nucleated red cells has been a controversial subject. Maximow concluded that in the embryo the hemocytoblasts, which were derived from the mesenchyme, produce the nucleated precursors of the erythrocyte. He thought that hematopoiesis in the adult is homoplastic, that erythrocytes develop from nucleated precursors of fixed lineage, but he considered it possible that in abnormal conditions, when homoplastic production might be inadequate, heteroplastic formation might be called forth.[33] Jordan suggested that small lymphocytes that originate in the lymph nodes might leave the circulation in the bone marrow and serve as erythrocyte precursors.[27] Doan, Cunningham, and Sabin studied the bone marrows of pigeons recovering from starvation and the bone marrows of rabbits given repeated doses of dead typhoid bacilli[16] and concluded that the erythrocyte precursors arise from the endothelial cells of the capillaries and develop intravascularly, but that the granulocytes arise from reticular cells in the interspaces of the veins. Jordan and Johnson performed similar experiments on pigeons and concluded that, although erythropoiesis is mainly intravascular, the erythrocyte precursor is not an endothelial cell but instead is the hemocytoblast which sometimes develops extravascularly and migrates into the vessels.[28] Bloom and Bartelmez[9] and Gilmour[21] also have concluded that in human embryos erythropoiesis is extravascular.

In the embryo the main site of erythropoiesis during the first 2 months is the yolk sac, where the first blood cells arise from mesenchymal cells.[9] In the next phase of development erythropoiesis is chiefly in the liver and, to a lesser extent, in the spleen until about the sixth month. Hematopoiesis appears in the bone marrow at about the fifth month and increases in this tissue as it declines in the liver. After birth the bone marrow is essentially the only tissue concerned in the production of erythrocytes. In the first few years of postnatal life erythropoiesis is active in the marrow of practically all the bones, but in adults it is confined largely to the skull, thorax, vertebra, innominate bone, and the upper ends of the femur and humerus. In the normal bone marrow erythropoiesis is carried on mainly by division of the polychromatic and orthochromatic normoblast cells that comprise about 90 per cent of the erythrocyte precursors in the marrow. When erythropoiesis is accelerated, increased numbers of the earlier forms are evident. In disease states, when the hematopoietic tissue is displaced by metastatic cells or myelofibrosis, extramedullary erythropoiesis appears in the liver, spleen, and lymph nodes.

In postnatal life normally the blood cells are formed in the bone marrow and lymphoid tissues of the body. The bone marrow is the sole site of origin of the erythrocytic, granulocytic, and megakaryocytic cells. Transplant experiments indicate that formation of the microcirculation from reticular cells precedes hematopoietic repopulation.[54] Some of the lymphocytes also originate in the marrow; other morphologically similar cells that probably have different functions are produced in the thymus, lymph nodes, and other lymphoid tissue in the body. In certain hematologic disorders, extramedullary hematopoiesis appears in the spleen, liver, lymph nodes and other tissues.

Morphology

The terminology that has been used in discussion of the nucleated cells of the erythrocytic series has been the source of considerable confusion. Because different definitions have been given to the same term by different authors, the Committee for Clarification of the Nomenclature of Cells and Diseases of the Blood and Blood-Forming Organs has recommended an entirely new terminology for the nucleated cells of the erythrocytic series.[12] The terms recommended—rubriblast, prorubricyte, rubricyte, and metarubricyte—have not been used widely. The Committee felt that the recommended names indicated stages of differentiation in development of the adult erythrocyte. They recommended that the qualifying phrase "pernicious anemia type" be used to indicate the cells that showed the morphologic characteristics seen in patients with untreated pernicious anemia.

Usually the type of erythropoiesis is described as being either "normoblastic" or "megaloblastic." The term "megaloblast" has been used with different meanings in the literature. Ehrlich introduced the term to indicate the large nucleated precursor of the erythrocytes that is characterized by its much weaker affinity for nuclear stains.[20] He thought that the presence of this cell indicated an abnormal type of erythropoiesis that was seen in adults almost exclusively in pernicious anemia, and that it represented an embryonic type of cell. He considered it a line of cell maturation different from the "normoblastic" type which was seen in nearly all other types of anemia. The normoblastic type of maturation was characterized by erythrocyte precursors that contained a nucleus that gave an intense color with nuclear stains. Doan, Cunningham, and Sabin used the term "megaloblast" to indicate the first generation of cells in the red blood cell series that could be distinguished from endothelial cells in either the embryonic or adult types of erythropoiesis.[16] Thus, according to one usage of the term, "megaloblast" indicates an abnormal type of erythropoiesis that occurs only in special disease states when seen in postnatal human beings; according to the other usage the term indicates a very young erythrocyte precursor that may occur whenever erythropoiesis is markedly increased but otherwise normal. The term "erythroblast" has been used by some authors to refer to all forms of nucleated red corpuscles, but Doan, Cunningham, and Sabin have used this term to indicate an intermediate stage in the development of the erythrocyte.[16] The term "megaloblast" is used in this text as it has been used by Ehrlich, Downey, Jones, and Wintrobe.[19, 20, 26, 62]

Erythropoiesis is considered as being normal in type when the normoblastic series is present and abnormal when the megaloblastic series is present. Similar stages in the development of the nucleated red cells can be recognized in both series. In normoblastic maturation the cells of the different stages are termed pronormoblast, basophilic normoblast, polychromatic normoblast, and orthochromatic normoblast. In the megaloblastic type of maturation the corresponding cells are termed promegaloblast, basophilic megaloblast, polychromatic megaloblast, and orthochromatic megaloblast.

Pronormoblast (rubriblast). The pronormoblast is the youngest recognizable precursor of the erythrocyte. Its diameter varies from 12 to 19 microns. The nucleus, which is round and fills most of the cell, contains strands of

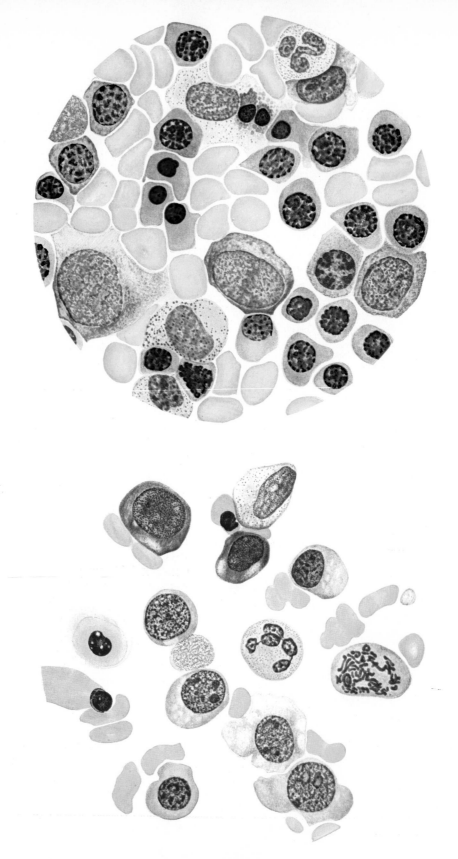

Figures 1–6 and 1–7. *See legends on opposite page.*

chromatin and several nucleoli. The nongranular cytoplasm stains blue. Usually these cells can be distinguished from myeloblasts by the coarser staining of the nuclear chromatin and the more opaque cytoplasm. Thorell[55] has demonstrated that during this and the next phase of development of the red blood cell a considerable portion of the proteins is being formed. The production of protein is accompanied by a marked decrease in the cytoplasmic nucleotides; by the time that the end of the basophilic normoblast stage is reached the cytoplasmic nucleotides have practically disappeared and protein production is greatly reduced.

Basophilic normoblast (prorubricyte). The basophilic normoblast differs from the pronormoblast in that the nuclear chromatin is more coarse, distinct nucleoli are not seen, and the cytoplasm is more densely basophilic.

Polychromatic normoblast (rubricyte). This stage covers a relatively wide range in the maturation of the erythrocyte, from the beginning of recognizable hemoglobin in the cytoplasm to the complete disappearance of basophilia. During this time the nucleus becomes smaller and the nuclear chromatin becomes more condensed. This stage of development is characterized by a remarkable production of hemoglobin. Thorell has reported that the concentration of hemoglobin increases from 1×10^{-6} micrograms during this phase, and has suggested that it is at this time that the formation of the iron porphyrin component and its coupling to globin takes place.[55]

Orthochromatic normoblast (metarubricyte). A normoblast is considered to reach the orthochromatic stage when the cytoplasm appears to contain its full complement of hemoglobin. The nuclear chromatin becomes more and more condensed; the nucleus diminishes in size and finally disappears. During this phase the quantity of hemoglobin of the cell reaches that contained at maturity, 28×10^{-6} micrograms. This is accompanied by a decrease in volume of the cell that amounts to 25 to 33 per cent.

Megaloblasts. The details, such as presence of nucleoli, basophilia, and degree of hemoglobinization, that distinguish a pronormoblast or a basophilic normoblast from a polychromatic normoblast are the same criteria that are used for differentiating a promegaloblast from a polychromatic megaloblast and the other cells in this series. In distinguishing megaloblastic erythropoiesis from normoblastic erythropoiesis in the smear stained with Wright's stain, it is well to remember the admonition of Ehrlich and Lazarus who wrote, "In order to gain a perfectly clear conception of the physiological and pathological import of the erythroblasts, it is absolutely necessary to consider, in the first place, only typical examples of both forms." There are, as would be expected, a large number of cells which cannot be classified either as normoblasts or as megaloblasts on account of the fact that some of the characteristics which Ehrlich described for these cells are wanting.[20]

The types of erythropoiesis are most easily distinguished at the third or "polychromatic" stage. Two details that aid in distinguishing megaloblasts from normoblasts at this stage are, first, an increase in the lighter staining parachromatin of the nucleus in the megaloblasts and, second, the appearance

---

Figure 1-6. (*opposite page—upper*). Normoblastic hyperplasia in hemolytic anemia.

Figure 1-7. (*opposite page—lower*). Megaloblastic hyperplasia in pernicious anemia. (From Heilmeyer and Bergemann: Atlas der klinischen Hämatologie und Cytologie. Berlin-Göttingen-Heidelberg, Springer, 1955.)

of hemoglobin in cells with nuclei that appear more immature than is ordinarily the case in the normoblastic type of erythropoiesis. The younger promegaloblasts and basophilic megaloblasts are also recognizably different from their normoblastic counterparts. The nucleus of the megaloblast stains lighter because the nuclear chromatin is usually more finely divided and appears more separated because of the increase in parachromatin. In the orthochromatic stage the megaloblast is often larger than the corresponding normoblast; the increase in parachromatin usually remains evident until the nuclear chromatin becomes almost completely condensed and pyknotic in appearance.

Different degrees of megaloblastosis occur and some hematologists employ a semi-quantitative graduation of from "one plus" to "four plus." "Megaloblastoid" is a term sometimes used to describe minor megaloblastic changes, usually an increase in the nuclear parachromatin, that occur in many patients with hematologic disorders, particularly leukemia, refractory anemia, and hemolytic anemia; the changes may be due to folate deficiency or some abnormality in folate—vitamin B_{12} metabolism, but often no satisfactory explanation is apparent.

Reticulocytes. Reticulocytes are young non-nucleated cells of the erythrocytic series that can be recognized only with supravital stains. When brilliant cresyl blue is used, the reticulocyte appears to contain granules or a fibrillar network that stains light blue in color; the structures stained in this way are mainly ribosomes. When the preparation is counterstained with Wright's stain these structures appear darker and are recognized more easily. Normally reticulocytes constitute less than 2 per cent of the circulating erythrocytes and the number is often less than 1 per cent. Determination of the percentage of reticulocytes in the peripheral blood affords one of the best measures of increased erythropoiesis because the number of reticulocytes reflects the effective increase in bone marrow activity better than the morphological appearance of the bone marrow does. The percentage of reticulocytes is nearly always increased after hemorrhage, during hemolysis, and after specific therapy is instituted for anemia. The reticulocytes released into the circulation mature to become erythrocytes within several days unless they are destroyed. (F.S.: I, 9.)

Erythrocytes. The erythrocytes are adult members of the erythrocytic series. They are nonnucleated biconcave discs that stain a pink or pinkish gray color with Wright's stain. The diameters of the erythrocytes on dried films were found by Price-Jones to have a mean of 7.2 microns and to range from 6.7 to 7.7 microns.[42] When erythrocytes that have been stained with Wright's stain appear grayish blue the condition is termed "diffuse basophilia," and when bluish granules are evident in the cells "punctate basophilia" is said to be present. Both of these staining reactions are signs of immaturity and reflect the persistence of ribose nucleoprotein in the cells. Punctate basophilia, or "stippling," is increased after exposure to lead and other metals.

In disease states the erythrocytes are often abnormal. The cells may show marked abnormalities in shape (poikilocytosis) or size (anisocytosis). The deformity may vary from a slight irregularity to a marked elongation; cells of the latter variety are sometimes referred to as "pencil forms." Erythrocytes that have a diameter of less than 6 microns are termed "microcytes." Microcytes that occur in iron deficiency often exhibit a distinct increase in central pallor and are termed "hypochromic microcytes." In other disorders, such as familial spherocytosis, the diameter of the erythrocytes is less than normal but the thickness of the cell is increased and the hemoglobin content is normal. Such cells, which are spoken of as "microspherocytes," appear small but stain deeply and do not have the central pallor that is seen in the hypochromic microcytes and normal cells. Macrocytes, defined by some authors as cells with a diameter greater than 9 microns, occur in deficiencies of folic acid or vitamin B_{12}, myxedema, and other disorders. The presence of large oval macrocytes in the peripheral blood smear strongly suggests a deficiency of vitamin B_{12} or folate. "Target cells" ("Mexican hat cells"), which are thinner than normal and have a relatively large diameter, resemble the concentric circles of a rifle target in appearance. They occur in various types of anemia, such as sickle cell anemia, hemoglobin C disease, and the thalassemias, and also during jaundice and after splenectomy. "Burr cells" are so called because the erythrocytes have numerous spinelike projections; they are seen in uremia. Acanthocytes (*acanthus*— thorn or sharp point) occur as part of a rare syndrome comprising atypical retinitis pigmentosa, steatorrhea, ataxia, and absent serum beta-lipopro- tein.[47, 49] Spinous erythrocytes, termed "burr cells" or "spur cells," have been described in a variety of disorders including uremia, microangiopathic hemolytic anemia, and thrombotic thrombocytopenic purpura; some of these abnormalities are the result of acquired damage to the red cell membrane, in some circum- stances from a factor present in the plasma.[48, 51] Other forms of poikilocytes are "helmet cells" and shistocytes (cell fragments), most often seen in patients with impact hemolysis. "Howell-Jolly bodies" are sometimes seen in erythrocytes of patients with anemia. These particles usually occur singly. They are larger than the usual granules and are thought to be nuclear particles because they take the nuclear stains. "Cabot rings," which may be single or double, occur in both nucleated and non-nucleated cells. Whether these structures, which some- times appear bright red in smears prepared with Wright's stain, are derivatives of nuclear material or products of cellular degeneration produced by toxic substances is uncertain. (F.S.: I, 7–12.)

"Siderocytes" are erythrocytes that contain particles of non-hemoglobin iron. Siderotic granules resemble those seen in punctate basophilia when smears are prepared with Wright's stain, but the difference between the par- ticles can be shown by the Prussian blue staining reaction. Siderocytes are seen most often in the peripheral blood in hemolytic anemia and after splenectomy. "Heinz bodies" are highly refractile particles of denatured hemoglobin 1 to 3 microns in diameter that can be visualized with supravital stains but not with Wright's stain. They occur in the peripheral blood of susceptible persons after exposure to certain drugs, particularly primaquine, acetanilid, and acetyl- phenylhydrazine. The observation that these bodies become more numerous after splenectomy suggests that the spleen may be able to remove these bodies from the intact cells.

Other abnormalities of the erythrocytes that can be seen on the stained smear are often of diagnostic significance. Erythrocytes that appear elongated with rounded ends are known as "ovalocytes" or "elliptocytes." Small numbers of such cells may occur on smears made from normal persons. This type of cell also develops as the result of a hereditary defect, in which case the vast majority of the cells have an oval or elliptical shape. The erythrocytes of pa- tients with sickle cell anemia or sickle cell trait assume a crescent form when the hemoglobin is in the reduced state. In patients with sickle cell anemia some of these forms may be apparent in a fixed smear prepared with Wright's stain, but usually this deformity can be demonstrated only in moist preparations.

References

1. Ackerman, G. A.: Microscopic and histochemical studies of the Auer bodies in leukemic cells. Blood, 5:847, 1950.
2. Agner, K.: Verdoperoxidase. Acta physiol. scandinav., Suppl. 8, 2, 1941.
3. Agner, K.: Detoxicating effect of verdoperoxidase on toxins. Nature, 159:271, 1947.
4. Albrecht, M.: Studies on the evolution of thrombocytes, experiences with megakaryocytes in vitro. Internat. Soc. Hem. Abstract 437, p. 346, 1956.
5. Alder, A.: Über Konstitutonell Bedingte Granulation-veränderungen der Leukozyten. Deutsches Arch. klin. Med., 183:372, 1939.
6. Aschoff, L., and Kiyono, K.: Zur Frage der grossen Mononuklearen. Folia haemat. (1. Teil), 15:383, 1913.
7. Bedson, S. P., and Johnston, M. E.: Further observations on platelet genesis. J. Path. & Bact., 28:101, 1925.
8. Bloom, L. M., and Wislocki, G. B.: The localization of lipids in human blood and bone marrow cells. Blood, 5:79, 1950.
9. Bloom, W., and Bartelmez, G. W.: Hematopoiesis in young human embryos. Am. J. Anat., 67:21, 1940.
9a. Chédiak, M.: Nouvelle anomalia leucocytaire de caractère constitutional et familial. Rev. Hemat., 7:362, 1952.
10. Code, C. F.: The histamine-like activity of white blood cells. J. Physiol., 90:485, 1937.
11. Code, C. F.: The source in blood of the histamine-like constituent. J. Physiol., 90:349, 1937.
12. Condensation of the First Two Reports of the Committee for Clarification of the Nomenclature of Cells and Diseases of the Blood and Blood-Forming Organs. Blood, 4:89, 1949.
13. Cudkowicz, G., Bennett, M., and Shearer, G. M.: Pluripotent stem cell function of the mouse marrow lymphocyte. Science, 144:866, 1964.
14. Cunningham, R. S., Sabin, F. R., and Doan, C. A.: The development of leukocytes, lymphocytes, and monocytes from a specific stem-cell in adult tissues. Contrib. Embryol., Carnegie Inst., 16:227, 1925.
15. Danielli, J. F., and Davson, H.: Contributions to theory of permeability of thin films. J. Cell & Comp. Physiol., 5:495, 1935.
16. Doan, C. A., Cunningham, R. S., and Sabin, F. R.: Experimental studies on the origin and maturation of avian and mammalian red blood-cells. Contrib. Embryol., Carnegie Inst., 16:163, 1928.
17. Downey, H.: The occurrence and significance of the "myeloblast" under normal and pathologic conditions. Arch. Int. Med., 33:301, 1924.
18. Downey, H.: Origin of monocytes in monocytic leukemia and leukemic reticuloendotheliosis. Anat. Rec., 48:16, 1931.
19. Downey, H.: Handbook of Hematology. Paul B. Hoeber, New York, 1938.
20. Ehrlich, P., and Lazarus, A.: Anemia, 2nd Ed. Rebman Ltd., London, 1910.
20a. Frey-Wettstein, M., and Craddock, C. G.: Testosterone-induced depletion of thymus and marrow lymphocytes as related to lymphopoiesis and hematopoiesis. Blood, 35:257, 1970.
21. Gilmour, J. R.: Normal haemopoiesis in the intra-uterine and neonatal life. J. Path. Bact., 52:25, 1941.
22. Graham, H. T., Lowry, O. H., Wheelwright, F., Lenz, M. A., and Parish, H. H., Jr.: Distribution of histamine among leukocytes and platelets. Blood, 10:467, 1955.
23. Griffiths, S. B., and Findlay, M.: Gargoylism: Clinical, radiological and haematological features in two siblings. Arch. Dis. Childhood, 33:229, 1958.
23a. Higashi, O.: Congenital gigantism of peroxidase granules. Tokoku Jour. Exper. Med., 59:315, 1954.
24. Hiraki, K.: The function of the megakaryocyte: Observations both in idiopathic thrombocytopenic purpura and normal adults. Internat. Soc. Hem. Abstract 436, p. 345, 1956.
25. Hume, R., West, J. T., Malmgren, R. A., and Chu, E. A.: Quantitative observations of circulating megakaryocytes in the blood of patients with cancer. New England J. Med., 270:111, 1964.
26. Jones, O. P.: Cytology of pathologic marrow cells with especial reference to marrow biopsies. In Downey, H., Ed.: Handbook of Hematology. Paul B. Hoeber, Inc., New York, 1938, p. 2045.

27. Jordan, H. E.: The significance of the lymphoid nodule. Am. J. Anat., *57*:1, 1935.
28. Jordan, H. E., and Johnson, E. P.: Erythrocyte production in the bone marrow of the pigeon. Am. J. Anat., *56*:71, 1935.
29. Kaufman, R. M., Airo, R., Pollack, S., and Crosby, W. H.: Pulmonary megakaryocytes: Their origin and significance. J. Clin. Invest., *44*:1063, 1965.
30. Kaufman, R. M., Airo, R., Pollack, S., Crosby, W. H., and Doberneck, R.: Origin of pulmonary megakaryocytes. Blood, *25*:767, 1965.
31. Korn, E. D.: Structure of biological membranes. Science, *153*:1491, 1966.
32. Mallory, F. B.: A histological study of typhoid fever. J. Exper. Med., *3*:611, 1898.
32a. Marcus, A. J.: Platelet function. N. England J. Med., *280*:1213, 1278, and 1330, 1969.
33. Maximow, A.: Relation of the blood cells to connective tissue and endothelium. Physiol. Rev., *4*:533, 1924.
34. Mazia, D., and Prescott, D. M.: Nuclear function and mitosis. Science, *120*:120, 1954.
35. McCulloch, E. A., Siminovitch, L., and Till, J. E.: Spleen-colony formation in anemic mice genotype WW^V. Science, *144*:845, 1964.
35a. Meuter, M., and Lebond, C. P.: The Golgi apparatus. Scientific American, *22*:100, 1969.
36. Michels, N. A.: The plasma cell. Arch. Path., *11*:775, 1931.
37. Michels, N. A.: Erythropoiesis: A critical review of the literature. Folio haemat., *45*:75, 1931.
38. Miner, R. W., Ed.: Leukocyte functions. Ann. N.Y. Acad. Sc., *59*:667–1069, 1955.
39. Mosier, D. E.: A requirement for two cell types for antibody formation in vitro. Science, *158*:1573, 1967.
40. Naegeli, O.: Blutkrankheiten und Blutdiagnostik. Verlag von Veit and Comp. Leipzig, 1908, p. 117.
41. Pelger, K.: Demonstratie van een paar zeldzaam voorkomende typen van bloedlichaampjes en bespreking der patienten. Nederl. tijdschr. geneesk., *72*:1178, 1928.
42. Price-Jones, C.: Red cell diameter in one hundred healthy persons and in pernicious anemia. The effect of liver treatment. J. Path. & Bact., *32*:479, 1929.
43. Rebuck, J. W., and Crowley, J. H.: A method of studying leukocyte functions in vivo. Ann. N.Y. Acad. Sc., *59*:757, 1955.
44. Robertson, J. D.: Ultrastructure of cell membranes and their derivatives. Biochem. Soc. Symp. (Cambridge, England), *16*:3. 1959.
45. Sabin, F. R.: On the origin of the cells of the blood. Physiol. Rev., *2*:38, 1922.
46. Sabin, F. R., Doan, C. A., and Cunningham, R. S.: Discrimination of two types of phagocytic cells in connective tissue by the supravital technique. Contrib. Embryol., Carnegie Inst., *16*:125, 1925.
47. Salt, H. B., Wolff, O. H., Lloyd, J. K., Fosbrooke, A. S., Cameron, A. H., and Hubble, D. V.: On having no beta-lipoprotein. A syndrome comprising a-beta-lipoproteinaemia, acanthocytosis and steatorrhoea. Lancet, *2*:325, 1960.
48. Silber, R.: Acanthocytes, spurs, burrs and membranes. Blood, *34*:111, 1969.
49. Simon, E. R., and Ways, P.: Incubation hemolysis and red cell metabolism in acanthocytosis. J. Clin. Invest., *43*:1311, 1964.
50. Skendzel, L. P., and Hoffman, G. C.: Pelger anomaly of leukocytes: 41 cases in seven families. Am. J. Clin. Path., *37*:294, 1962.
51. Smith, J. A., Lonergan, E. T., and Sterling, K.: Spur-cell anemia. N. England J. Med., *271*:396, 1964.
52. Sundberg, R. D.: Lymphocytes and plasma cells. Ann. N.Y. Acad. Sc., *59*:671, 1955.
53. Tapley, D. F.: Kimberg, D. V., and Buchanan, J. L.: The mitochondrion. New England J. Med., *276*:1124, 1182, 1967.
54. Tavassoli, M., and Crosby, W. H.: Transplantation of marrow to extramedullary sites. Science, *161*:55, 1968.
55. Thorell, B.: Studies on the formation of cellular substances during blood cell production. Acta med. scandinav., Suppl. 200, 1947.
56. Tocantins, L. M.: The mammalian blood platelets in health and disease. Medicine, *17*:155, 1938.
57. Valentine, W. N., Pearce, M. L., and Lawrence, J. S.: Studies on the histamine content of blood. Blood, *5*:623, 1950.
58. Weiner, W., and Topley, E.: Döhle bodies in the leukocytes of patients with burns. J. Clin. Path., *8*:324, 1955.
59. Weinstein, R. S.: The structure of cell membranes. New England J. Med., *281*:86, 1969.
60. Weissman, G.: Lysosomes. New England J. Med., *273*:1084, 1143, 1965.
61. White, J. C.: The cytoplasmic basophilia of bone marrow cells. J. Path. Bact., *59*:223, 1947.
62. Wintrobe, M. M.: Clinical Hematology, 4th Ed. Lea and Febiger, Philadelphia, 1956.
63. Wright, J. H.: The histogenesis of the blood platelets. J. Morphol., *21*:263, 1910.

II / Erythropoiesis and the Metabolism of Hemoglobin

Erythropoiesis

The primary function of the red blood cell is the transport of respiratory gases. In order to fulfill this function there must be sufficient circulating erythrocytes to meet the metabolic needs of the body. There is a compensatory increase in the number of peripheral red blood cells when there is a decrease in the amount of oxygen reaching the tissue cells of the body. If there is a surfeit of·oxygen available, a decrease in circulating erythrocytes occurs.

The Control of Erythropoiesis

The physiologic control of the number of circulating erythrocytes is maintained by regulation of erythropoiesis and not by regulation of their peripheral destruction.

The sequence of events that occurs in erythropoiesis and the factors that regulate the process are an aspect of the fundamental biological phenomena of cell reproduction and organ regeneration. The recognizable elements of the bone marrow are derived from pluripotential precursor cells which give rise to erythrocytic, granulocytic and megakaryocytic cells. These stem cells have not been identified, but studies of regeneration after irradiation strongly suggest that these cells can circulate in the peripheral blood and repopulate the marrow.[14] The existence of another compartment of "committed cells" between the pluripotential cells and the recognizable elements of the marrow has been proposed but not proved.[98, 132]

Lajtha has proposed a model of stem cell kinetics which fits many experimental observations and the theoretical mathematical considerations concerned with this problem.[108, 109] According to this concept, in response to an appropriate stimulus, stem cells can either reproduce themselves or differentiate into precursors of the specific cell lines — erythrocytic, granulocytic, or megakaryocytic. If stem cells are removed from the compartment by death or differentiation, a feedback mechanism is triggered off and stem cells divide to restore the stem cell population; the triggered cells cannot differentiate until they have completed the cell cycle. Such a mechanism would explain the maintenance of a stem cell pool in a relatively steady state in response to stimuli for differentiation or for replacement after damage to the cells. If the stimulus is for erythropoiesis, which may be an enzyme induction in the stem cell in response to erythropoietin,[109] the earliest recognizable specific red cell precursors, the pronormoblasts, are produced. These divide and mature, a process that is repeated by the intermediate basophilic and polychromatophilic normoblasts. The late orthochromatic normoblast does not divide but develops into a reticulocyte, the immediate precursor of the erythrocyte. The interval between mitosis of the cells is probably between 12 and 21 hours, and the average number of divisions during maturation in man is estimated at three or four.[4, 10, 106] Under normal conditions, about 4 days are required for the development of a pronormoblast into an erythrocyte. Iron is incorporated into all the erythrocyte precursors, but the intake is greatest in the pronormoblasts and least in the reticulocytes;[110] maximal hemoglobin production commences after the basophilic stage.

Erythropoietin

The theory that the well known effect of hypoxia, the stimulation of erythropoiesis, was mediated by a humoral factor which was produced outside the erythropoietic tissue in response to the hypoxia, was proposed by Carnot and DeFlandre in 1906.[20] In 1947 Grant and Root observed that the stimulation of erythropoiesis was not dependent on the oxygen saturation of the blood of the bone marrow.[58] Reissmann's demonstration in 1950 that hypoxia in only one of a parabiotic pair of rats caused increased erythropoiesis in both rats stimulated interest in a search for a plasma factor.[158] Erslev and others have amply demonstrated by numerous experiments and a variety of techniques that hemorrhage, hemolysis, hypoxia, and cobalt lead to the appearance of a plasma factor that stimulates erythropoiesis.[36] This factor, generally termed erythropoietin, has been the subject of comprehensive reviews.[54, 194]

The erythropoietic factor is heat-stable and non-dialyzable, contains sialic acid, and appears to be a glycoprotein that has an electrophoretic mobility characteristic of the $alpha_1$ or $alpha_2$ globulins. The mean half-life of erythropoietin in human plasma has been reported to be 24.9 hours.[164] Although this factor remains active in a pH range of 3 to 10, more erythropoietin is excreted into an alkaline urine. The mechanism responsible for this is unclear.[126] Erythropoietin is inactivated by proteolytic enzymes. The molecular weight has been estimated variously as 10,000, 29,000, and 62,000.[140]

Jacobson and his collaborators have shown that the main, though not the sole, site of production of erythropoietin is the kidney; they suggest that 10 per cent of the erythropoietin may be formed elsewhere.[83, 84] An erythrocyte stimulating factor, which is released in response to hypoxia and is believed to be identical to erythropoietin, has been demonstrated in the plasma of nephrectomized rats.[44] Studies of anephric patients have shown that man can support red cell production at a reduced level in the absence of renal tissue.[133]

Failure to find large amounts of erythropoietin in the kidney prompted a search for a precursor. An enzyme has been found in the mitochondrial fraction of kidney homogenates of the cortex and medulla which yields erythropoietin on incubation with normal serum.[100] The enzyme, termed renal erythropoietic factor or REF, is believed to act on a substrate which is produced in the liver and is carried as an alpha 2-globulin in normal serum.[195, 219, 223, 224] Little if any species specificity has been demonstrated.

The evidence indicates that the main action of erythropoietin is the stimulation of differentiation of stem cells into red cell precursors.[39] An increase in the synthesis of ribonucleic acid (RNA) in bone marrow cells in vitro is noted within 15 minutes of the addition of erythropoietin. This effect is abolished by actinomycin-D, which blocks DNA-dependent RNA synthesis.[95] The type of RNA produced is unknown.[74, 95]

The observation that stimulation of erythropoiesis causes the release of large reticulocytes with unusually dense reticulum probably indicates that such cells have been released earlier than normal. This has been interpreted as evidence that erythropoietin acts on differentiated red cell precursors to produce acceleration in the maturation of the erythrocytic series.[12] Stohlman has suggested that erythropoietin induces hemoglobin formation and can act either on the stem cell or on the early differentiated red cell precursors. When hemoglobin synthesis is accelerated, the critical hemoglobin concentration of the cell is reached more rapidly, a feedback mechanism shuts off further nucleic acid synthesis, and the terminal division is skipped. When this occurs, macrocytes, which are short-lived, are produced.[196]

Evidence for the suppression of erythropoiesis through the action of inhibitors of erythropoietin[213] and/or stem cell function[41] has been presented. There is also a reduction in the response to hypoxia once the hematocrit rises above 60 per cent. The mechanism by which this is mediated is not clear but appears to be related to the elevated hematocrit per se.[91]

Erythropoietin has been detected in the urine of normal persons;[42] increased levels have been demonstrated in the plasma and urine in a variety of clinical states accompanied by anemia. Whether erythropoietin is the normal regulator of erythropoiesis or an emergency mechanism has not been established. Various observations support the concept that erythropoietin is increased in circumstances in which there is diminished oxygen-carrying capacity of the blood in relation to the need of the tissues. However, the demonstration that plasma erythropoietin levels are increased in subjects with compensated hyperhemolysis, although there is no reduction in the oxygen-carrying capacity of the blood, indicates that there must be other regulators of erythropoietin production, possibly a feedback mechanism from the peripheral cells.[194, 196]

The mechanism by which androgenic steroids increase red cell mass and plasma volume is not clear. The effect has been shown to be independent of the virilizing capacity of the hormone and occurs despite already increased levels of erythropoietin.[3, 33, 46, 63, 129, 131]

Figures 2–1 to 2–4 indicate how a simple negative feedback system might operate to control erythropoiesis.

The physiological control of erythropoiesis in the normal person, assuming an adequate supply of necessary protein, vitamins, and minerals, is depicted in Figure 2–1. The daily destruction of approximately 2×10^{11} erythrocytes must be compensated by the release of an equal number of erythrocytes from the marrow. Present evidence indicates that the kidney is the main but not the sole site of the production of an enzyme, REF, which, through its action on a circulating plasma globulin, liberates erythropoietin.[55, 83, 84, 134, 143]

Hemorrhage or an increase in the rate of destruction of erythrocytes results in anemia if it is uncompensated. The total quantity of oxygen reaching the tissue cells is reduced because of the decreased number of circulating erythrocytes. An increase in erythropoietin activity of the plasma has been demonstrated under such conditions and is thought to be responsible for the increased erythropoiesis which compensates for the loss of red blood cells (Fig. 2–2).[36]

Decreased arterial oxygen saturation resulting from cardiopulmonary conditions has been found to increase erythropoietin activity and to be associated with increased erythropoiesis (Fig. 2–3). A secondary polycythemia results from the sustained stimulus.[25] A similar situation is thought to be obtained when cobaltous chloride is administered to a patient. Increased levels of erythropoietin have been demonstrated following administration of cobalt[52] but the mechanism through which this effect is produced is unknown.[105]

Anemia is associated with hypothyroidism in a high percentage of cases.

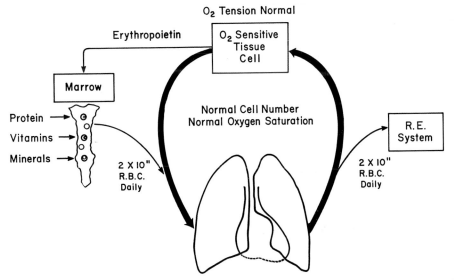

Figure 2–1. Schematic representation of the control of erythropoiesis under normal conditions.

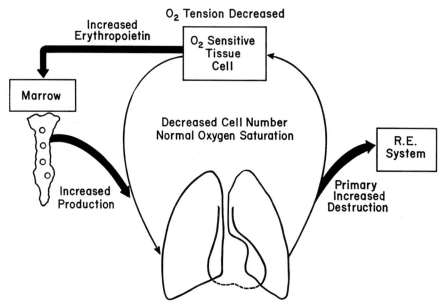

Figure 2-2. Schematic representation of the control of erythropoiesis with increased loss of red cells by bleeding or increased destruction.

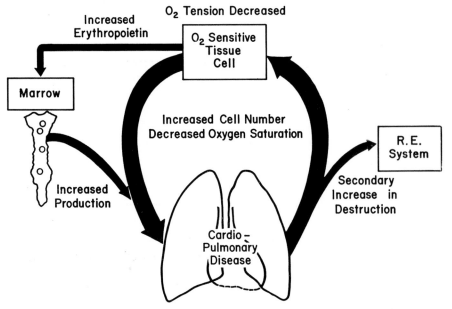

Figure 2-3. Schematic representation of the control of erythropoiesis in cardiopulmonary disease with decreased arterial oxygen saturation.

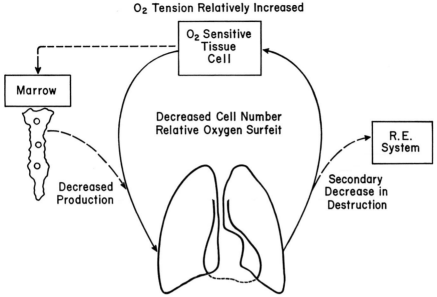

Figure 2–4. Schematic representation of the control of erythropoiesis under conditions of oxygen surfeit.

Decreased oxygen demand by the tissue cells might be expected to be reflected by diminished erythropoietin production and anemia (Fig. 2–4). The red blood cell count stabilizes at a level sufficient to meet the diminished metabolic demands of the body. It has been shown, however, that further reduction of the circulating red blood cells by bleeding results in a prompt reticulocytosis with a return of the red blood cell count to the prebleeding level in a normal period of time. These studies suggest that the anemia of myxedema occurs as the result of diminished metabolic demands rather than as an abnormality of the erythropoietic system.[115]

The Role of Hemoglobin

Hemoglobin is formed by the developing erythrocyte in the bone marrow. The most rapid hemoglobin formation is in the class III (polychromatophilic) normoblast when approximately 80 per cent of the hemoglobin carried by the mature cell is formed.[197] Though hemoglobin may be formed in the reticulocyte and, under exceptional circumstances, the immature non-reticulated erythrocyte, its formation under normal conditions is confined to the developing normoblasts in the marrow.[122, 201]

The level of hemoglobin in the blood represents the balance between production and destruction of the hemoglobin molecule. In the normal person the hemoglobin level is constant, as production and destruction are nicely balanced.

The total quantity of hemoglobin in the blood may be determined by multiplying the concentration of hemoglobin by the blood volume since hemoglobin production and destruction are in a state of equilibrium. If the concentration of hemoglobin is 15 gm. per cent (mean male equals 16.3 gm. per cent; mean female, 14.5 gm. per cent),[32] and the total volume roughly 5000 ml., the total quantity of hemoglobin is calculated as follows:

$$\text{Total hemoglobin} = \text{concentration of hemoglobin (gm./ml.)} \times \text{blood volume (ml.)}$$
$$\text{Total hemoglobin} = 0.15 \times 5000 = 750 \text{ gm. hemoglobin}$$

The life span of the hemoglobin molecule is approximately 120 days; its destruction occurs coincident with that of the erythrocyte. If the total amount of hemoglobin in the body at any one time is 750 gm., and the life span of the red blood cell is 120 days, the amount of hemoglobin formed each day can be calculated, since 1/120 of the total amount must be formed daily.

$$\frac{\text{Total hemoglobin}}{\text{life span in days}} = \text{rate of production/day}$$

$$\frac{750}{120} = 6.25 \text{ gm. hemoglobin/day}$$

Under normal conditions the body produces approximately 6.25 gm. of hemoglobin per day. The maximal effort of the body in the event of hemolytic disease has been calculated to be approximately 40 gm. per day.[26] This means that the survival time of the erythrocyte may be reduced to 18 or 19 days without the occurrence of anemia if the bone marrow functions at maximal capacity.

$$\frac{\text{Total hemoglobin}}{\text{life span in days}} = \text{rate of production/day}$$

$$\frac{750 \text{ gm.}}{X} = 40 \text{ gm./day} \qquad X = 18.8 \text{ days}$$

When hyperhemolysis is compensated, excessive destruction of red blood cells exists without the development of anemia. It is generally felt that the increase in the production of red blood cells and hemoglobin is brought about by increase in the mass of erythroid precursors rather than an increase in the rate of maturation in the individual red blood cell,[30] though the latter has not been ruled out as a contributing factor.

If the destruction of red blood cells exceeds the maximal effort of the bone marrow, anemia develops. The anemia becomes stabilized when erythrocyte production and erythrocyte destruction proceed at a constant rate. Although the values found for hemoglobin and red blood cells are not normal, they do not decrease progressively unless the life span of the cell is further shortened or unless there is interference with marrow production. The laboratory findings of patients with sickle cell anemia illustrate these points. The life span of the erythrocyte is shorter than can be compensated for by maximal marrow production, and in usual circumstances the subnormal hemoglobin value stabilizes at a level that depends on the life span of the erythrocyte and the maximal marrow output. This anemia is made more severe by a sudden increase in hemolytic activity or by a decrease in erythrocyte production. Either mechanism results in a further reduction of circulating erythrocytes.

The Chemistry of Hemoglobin

In recent years much has been learned of the synthesis of cellular protein.[27, 137] The genetic information needed to produce a specific protein is coded in the order of the base pairs in the deoxyribonucleic acid (DNA) of the cell nucleus. The DNA molecule is a double-stranded helix. The strands are composed of alternating units of the sugar deoxyribose and a phosphate compound and are bound together through each of the sugar units by the base pairs adenine and thymine or guanine and cytosine. The information is transferred by complementary base pairing of another macromolecule, ribonucleic acid (RNA), which is referred to as messenger RNA.[77] The process by which information is transferred from deoxyribonucleic acid (DNA) to ribonucleic acid (RNA) is referred to as transcription of the genetic message.

The RNA molecule is a single-stranded helix similar to DNA. Its structure differs from that of DNA in that the sugar in RNA is ribose, and where DNA contains the base thymine, RNA contains the base uracil. Messenger RNA leaves the nucleus and by virtue of its chemical template makes possible the synthesis of a specific protein by the ribosomes in the cytoplasm of the cell. Ribosomes are composed of protein and a high molecular weight ribonucleic acid termed ribosomal RNA. In order for protein synthesis to proceed amino acids of proper kind and amount must be delivered to the ribosomes. This is accomplished by another specialized form of low molecular weight RNA, which is termed soluble or transfer RNA. Each transfer RNA is specific for a certain amino acid though each amino acid may bind to more than one type of transfer RNA. In order for the binding of amino acid and transfer RNA to occur, a specific amino acid activating enzyme and energy in the form of ATP must be present. The transfer RNA carries the amino acid to a specific site on the ribosome determined by the relationship of the order of base pairs on the messenger RNA to those of the transfer RNA. As the ribosome moves along the messenger RNA template an ever lengthening polypeptide of precisely ordered amino acids emerges. The completed polypeptide is then released to enter into the formation of a complete protein molecule. These events are depicted in a highly schematic fashion in Figure 2–5.

Hemoglobin has a molecular weight of 66,700[1, 82] and is thought to be ellipsoid in shape.[29, 78] The results of x-ray crystallographic studies have indicated that the hemoglobin molecule is composed of two identical half molecules,[145] and this has been confirmed by the analysis of tryptic hydrolysates.[79] Each half molecule has now been shown to contain two different peptide chains which have been designated α and β.[159] The sequence of the amino acids which comprise the α and β peptide chains is under genetic control and their synthesis begins early in the development of the normoblast.[197] The importance of the proper organization of the amino acids during the synthesis of these proteins has been demonstrated by comparing the molecular structure of the hemoglobin from normal persons with that obtained from patients with one of the hemoglobinopathies.[79]

Of the approximately 30 peptide spots obtained from heat- and trypsin-digested hemoglobin by electrophoresis and chromatography, only one peptide from sickle cell hemoglobin differed from normal.[79] Analysis of the abnormal

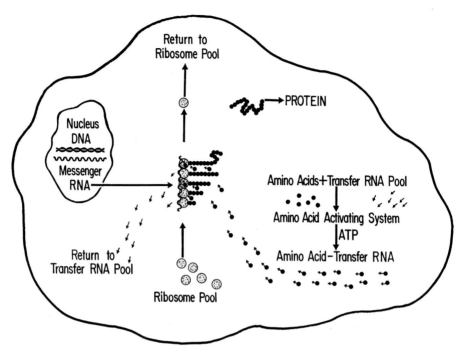

Figure 2-5.   Diagram of protein production in a cell.

peptide revealed that a glutamic acid residue had been replaced by valine.[80] A similar study of the C hemoglobin molecule indicated that the same peptide was again abnormal but in this instance the normal glutamic acid had been replaced by lysine.[76] In both instances the abnormal peptide was a component of the β peptide chain. Subsequent investigations of hemoglobins E, D, and I have revealed similar amino acid substitutions in other peptides of both the α and β chains.[81] These brilliant studies have revealed that a variation of but one amino acid out of more than 300 in the half molecule can mean the difference between normal health, a moderate disability, and a fatal illness.

It has been suggested[81] that the chemical structure of the two genes which appear to be involved in the production of hemoglobin determines the amino acid sequence of the peptide chains. Any alteration of the chemical structure of the genes would alter in turn the sequence of the amino acids of the hemoglobin molecule. Since the genes are self-replicating macromolecules, any structural abnormality would be transmitted from one generation to the next. Whether or not the effect of such an abnormality is clinically important depends on the portion of the peptide chain involved and the nature of the substitution.[81]

In addition to the protein moiety the hemoglobin molecule contains four heme groups. The enzymes necessary for the initial and terminal synthetic steps of heme reside in the mitochondria, whereas those enzymes needed for the intermediate steps are present in the cytoplasm. The synthesis of the final tetrameric form of hemoglobin is probably accomplished by the association of heme with alpha-beta dimers after ribosomal release of the individual globin chains.[206a] Heme is fitted into a highly hydrophobic pocket on the surface of each globin chain and is held in contact with histidine and other contiguous chemical groups in the pocket by van der Waal's forces.[208a] Oxygen is carried in these pockets in a ligand with the ferrous ion of heme and the distal histidine residue.[78, 90, 142, 144, 146, 162, 197, 208a]

Heme, a porphyrin ring structure containing a chelated iron atom, has been found to be part of the molecular structure of myoglobin, the cytochromes, peroxidase, and catalase as well as hemoglobin. Porphyrins are widely distributed in nature and are found in both plants and animals where they serve many vital metabolic processes. Chlorophyll, which is essential for photosynthesis and thus for the existence of life on earth, is a magnesium porphyrin compound. A porphyrin structure with a complexed cobalt atom forms part of the vitamin B_{12} molecule.[73, 99, 184]

The chemistry of porphyrins. Porphyrins differ from one another and are classified according to the nature and order of the side chains which may be substituted for the eight beta hydrogen atoms. One important group of porphyrins is that which has the same two side chains substituted for the replaceable hydrogen atoms in the 3 and 4 positions in each of the constituent pyrroles. Such an arrangement allows four possible isomers, the notations of which are I, II, III, IV. Uroporphyrin and coproporphyrin are examples of this group. Only types I and III are important to man.

The structural difference between uroporphyrin I and uroporphyrin III lies in the position of the acetic and propionic acid side chains in pyrrole ring IV (Fig. 2–6).

The structural difference between coproporphyrins I and II also lies in the position of the side chains located on pyrrole IV, and the difference between the uroporphyrins and coproporphyrins is in the presence of a methyl group in the coproporphyrins in the position occupied by the acetic acid side chain in the uroporphyrins (Fig. 2–7).

Uroporphyrin and coproporphyrin each occur in both urine and feces despite the impression to the contrary given by their names. The urine contains small amounts of uroporphyrin (5 to 10 micrograms per day) with both isomers present.[22] Larger quantities of coproporphyrin are found in the urine

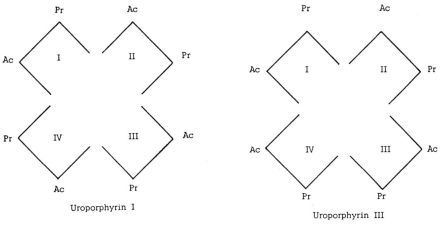

Figure 2–6. Schematic diagram of uroporphyrins I and III; acetic acid and propionic acid side chains.

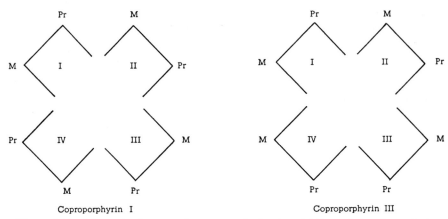

Figure 2–7.   Schematic diagram of coproporphyrins I and III; methyl and propionic acid side chains.

(100 to 300 micrograms per day) and the type III isomer predominates.[23, 155, 225] Inadequate data are available to determine a normal range of fecal uroporphyrin excretion. The quantity of fecal coproporphyrin excreted daily is from 150 to 400 micrograms.[115, 161]

When there are three different side chains substituted for the replaceable hydrogen atoms of the constituent pyrroles, a larger number of isomers are possible. Mesoporphyrin is a tetramethyl, diethyl, dipropionic acid porphyrin and 15 isomers have been enumerated. Protoporphyrin is similar but two vinyl are substituted for the two ethyl side chains. The isomer which is found in the hemoglobin molecule is classified as protoporphyrin IX, type III.

Porphyrin is composed of four monopyrroles. The elucidation of the synthesis of porphyrin has made it clear that glycine and succinyl-CoA are the basic building blocks.[153, 154, 185, 187, 190, 218] Succinyl-CoA, from the tricarboxylic acid cycle, with the addition of glycine forms α-amino, β-keto adipic acid which is then decarboxylated to form δ-aminolevulinic acid. The formation of δ-aminolevulinic acid from succinyl-CoA and glycine requires pyridoxyl phosphate,[176] CoA,[162] ferrous iron,[16] and the enzyme δ-aminolevulinic acid synthetase (ALA synthetase) in mitochondria.[4, 48] The iron requirement may reflect an effect of the metal on the synthesis of the enzyme system as intact cells are required to show the effect and none is noted when iron is added to mitochondrial suspensions.[18, 199] Outside the mitochondria, two molecules of δ-aminolevulinic acid condense to form porphobilinogen, a monopyrrole, which contains acetic and propionic acid side chains.[182, 188, 189] This reaction has been shown to be catalyzed by the soluble enzyme δ-aminolevulinic acid dehydrase which has been purified and found to contain—SH groups.[49, 175]

A cell-free extract of erythrocytes is capable of converting porphobilinogen to uroporphyrin.[9, 10, 26, 189] Two enzymes are required to catalyze this transformation. Porphobilinogen deaminase results in the formation of a linear tetrapyrrole which is then converted to type III isomer in the presence of an isomerase. In the absence of the isomerase only the type I isomer is formed.

The exact method by which the four pyrroles polymerize has not been settled though a variety of possibilities have been suggested.[118, 127, 128, 217] It is felt that the macrocyclic structures which are formed from porphobilinogen are porphyrinogens and that the porphyrins result from auto-oxidation of these compounds.[155, 162, 206] Although uroporphyrin is poorly utilized by hemolysates to form coproporphyrin, uroporphyrinogen III is easily transformed to coproporphyrinogen III by the soluble enzyme uroporphyrinogen decarboxylase.[139, 167] The decarboxylase is not specific and decarboxylates the side chains of type I and III isomers at random. In contrast, the enzyme coproporphyrinogen oxidative decarboxylase is highly specific for the type III coproporphyrinogen isomer and results only in the formation of protoporphyrinogen IX.[149] Protoporphyrinogen IX is converted to protoporphyrin IX by the enzyme protoporphyrinogen oxidase. The enzymes coproporphyrinogen oxidative decarboxylase and protoporphyrinogen oxidase are insoluble and located in the mitochondria.[40, 168] Ferrochetalase heme synthetase catalyzes the insertion of iron into protoporphyrin.[90]

Following its formation in the mitochondria, heme diffuses into the extramitochondrial space where it combines with the completed α and β chains to form hemoglobin.[50, 150, 177, 221]

The intermediates in the biosynthesis of heme are then uro- and coropor-

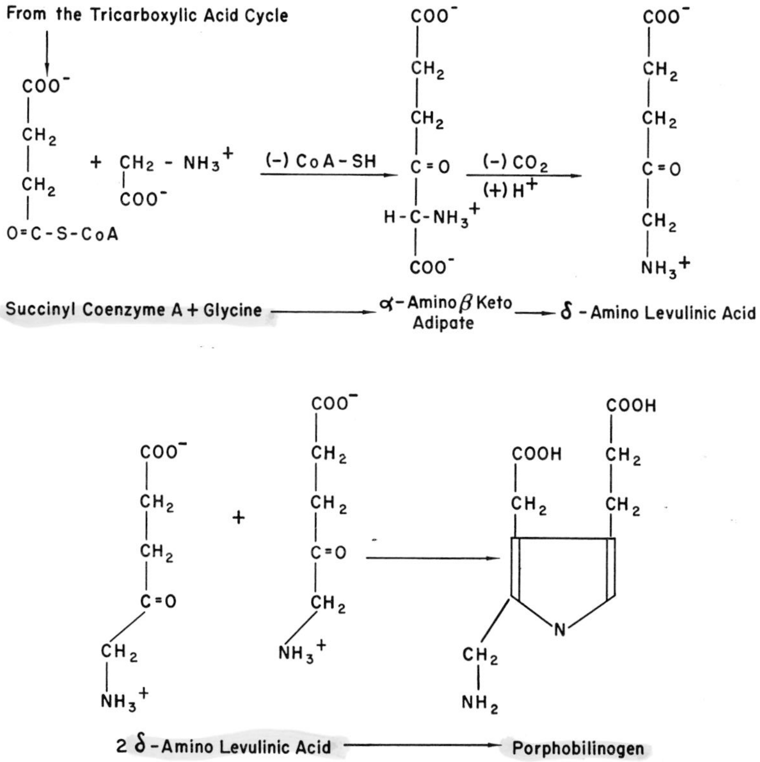

Figure 2–8. Formation of porphobilinogen from succinyl-coenzyme A and glycine.

phyrinogens and not uro- and coproporphyrins. It appears, however, that iron is incorporated into protoporphyrin and not protoporphyrinogen.[56]

Free protoporphyrin and coproporphyrin have been demonstrated in both the nucleated and non-nucleated erythrocytes. The concentration of both compounds increases just prior to reticulocytosis.[16, 179, 180] It has been suggested that they represent incomplete hemoglobin synthesis[225] or residuals left after hemoglobin synthesis.[136] The level of free erythrocyte protoporphyrin is from 13 to 139 micrograms per 100 ml. of erythrocytes.[202] Erythrocyte coproporphyrin concentration has been found to be from 0.5 to 1.5 micrograms per 100 ml. of erythrocytes.[16, 203]

Hemoglobin Catabolism

Senescent red cells are removed from the circulation by reticuloendothelial cells. The hemoglobin is liberated, but is not reutilized as such. Amino acids released from the degradation of globin return to the general amino acid pool.[67, 210, 211] The degradation of heme to bile pigment takes place in the microsomal fraction of the reticuloendothelial cells.[196a] Heme is first transformed to biliverdin by a microsomal enzyme, heme oxygenase, with the release of iron. This is the rate limiting step in the breakdown of hemoglobin

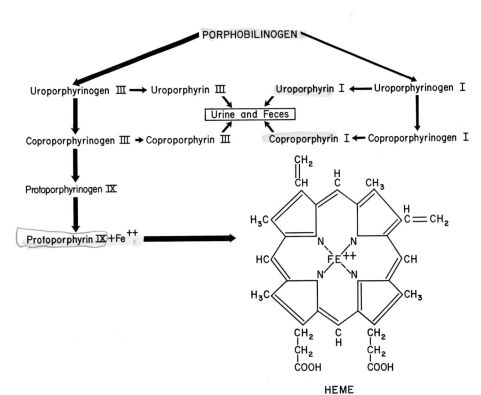

Figure 2–9.   Formation of heme from porphobilinogen.

and requires molecular oxygen and NADPH. The iron is returned to the iron pool and reutilized in the formation of hemoglobin. The biliveridin is next reduced to bilirubin by another microsomal NADPH-dependent enzyme, biliverdin reductase. The activity of both these enzymes is very high in the spleen and liver.[196a] Bilirubin is then released from the reticuloendothelial cells into the plasma where it is bound to albumin and transported to the parenchymal cells of the liver. There, in the liver microsomes, it is conjugated with glucuronic acid and excreted in the bile.[169, 170] Should the liver be unable to carry on this conjugation in the normal manner, a high "indirect acting" bilirubin level in the blood would result. Should there be obstruction to the excretion of the conjugated form via the biliary system, an increase in the "direct acting" bilirubin in the blood would result. Whether the bilirubin gives a "direct" or "indirect" van den Bergh reaction depends on the presence or absence of the glucuronic acid conjugation. The enzyme transferase found in the microsomes of the liver cells and uridine diphosphate glucuronic acid are both necessary for this reaction to occur. It has been suggested that the excess unconjugated bilirubin found in the newborn is due to inadequate development of the glucuronide conjugating system.[15]

In the bowel the action of the intestinal bacteria on bilirubin leads to several degradation products which are known collectively as fecal urobilinogen. Approximately 50 per cent of the urobilinogen is reabsorbed from the gut and recirculated in the blood to be reexcreted by the liver. This is the source of urobilinogen in liver bile and of the small amount lost through the kidney that is termed urinary urobilinogen. Normal daily excretion of urinary urobilinogen is from 0 to 3.5 mg.

The amount of fecal urobilinogen in the stool can be measured and has been found to vary from 40 to 280 mg. per day. Since the amount of fecal urobilinogen excreted depends on the amount of bilirubin secreted by the liver into the bile, it has been used as an index of hemoglobin breakdown. Hemoglobin from destroyed red blood cells is not the only source of urobilinogen, however, and the excretion of fecal urobilinogen does not always measure red cell destruction accurately. Studying the excretion of stercobilin, one of the components of fecal urobilinogen, investigators have found that as much as 11 per cent must come from sources other than the breakdown of mature red blood cells.[120] Whether this represents a breakdown of developing cells while still in the marrow or some non-hemoglobin porphyrin pathway is not known. In certain disease states, the amount of non-hemoglobin stercobilin rises to as high as 50 per cent.[119, 121]

Should intravascular hemolysis occur, hemoglobin is released into the plasma rather than into cytoplasm of the reticuloendothelial cell and is quickly bound by haptoglobin.[58, 138] Haptoglobin is an α-2-glycoprotein which combines stoichiometrically with hemoglobin, forming a stable complex.[85] As the plasma concentration of haptoglobin is 0.1 to 0.04 gm. per cent, approximately 100 mg. of hemoglobin is bound by 100 ml. of plasma.[113, 114] The haptoglobin-hemoglobin complex is too large to be filtered by the kidney and does not appear in the urine. It is taken up by the reticuloendothelial system and the hemoglobin is degraded in the usual fashion.

When intravascular hemolysis continues for long periods or the amount

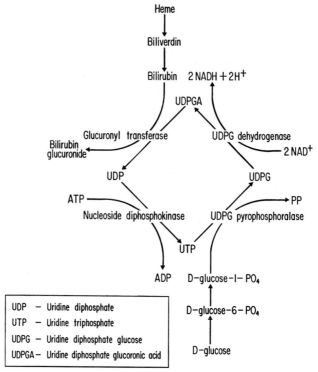

Figure 2–10.   Diagram indicating relationship of glucose metabolism and heme degradation.

of free hemoglobin is sufficiently large, the binding capacity of plasma hapto-globin is exceeded and free hemoglobin appears in the urine. Free hemoglobin is cleared from the plasma faster than the haptoglobin-hemoglobin complex. Although the permeability of the glomerulus to free hemoglobin is relatively low, it is considerably greater than for albumin and other proteins of similar molecular weights. This may be explained in part by the fact that hemoglobin tends to dissociate into alpha-beta dimers at the physiologic pH and ionic strength plasma.[16a] Earlier work indicated that a negligible amount of hemo-globin was reabsorbed by the renal tubules,[111, 113] but recent studies show that the bulk of the hemoglobin filtered by the glomerulus in most clinical disorders with hemoglobinemia is reabsorbed by the proximal tubules. There iron is released and reabsorbed into the plasma for reutilization. The globin and porphyrin moieties also are rapidly catabolized and reutilized. Thus the proxi-mal tubular cell resembles the reticuloendothelial cell in its ability to conserve hemoglobin iron.[16a]

Several types of haptoglobin have been identified by electrophoresis, and their transmission has been shown to be genetically determined.[138, 192] No selective advantage has been demonstrated and all have similar binding capa-cities. The half-life of haptoglobin appears to be in the order of 5.4 days.[86] The concentration of heptoglobin has been found to be decreased in all hemolytic states and in chronic hepatocellular disease. It is increased in the course of acute or chronic infection and in tissue destruction or proliferation.[138]

Abnormal Porphyrin Metabolism

Characterization of the precursors and intermediates involved in the biosynthesis of heme has laid the foundation for the understanding of the several disorders associated with abnormal porphyrin metabolism. Despite their rarity these disorders have evoked widespread interest and have afforded unique opportunities for the study of porphyrin metabolism. Current interest centers on the relationship of porphyrin synthesis to other metabolic pathways[103, 104, 136, 188] and mechanisms of detoxification of internal and external toxins. One of the difficult problems in the understanding of the pathophysiology of porphyria has been the failure to relate, in a constant fashion, the clinical symptoms of porphyria to the extent of pyrrole production. Granick[57] has suggested that heme synthesis is controlled by regulation of the production of ALA synthetase by a repressor-operator mechanism. The repressor is heme plus an aporepressor protein. The displacement of heme by a drug or steroid inactivates the repressor; the structural gene for ALA synthetase can then code more messenger RNA, and more enzyme is synthesized. Since the other enzymes in this system are not rate limiting, this would lead to an overproduction of heme precursors. Labbe[102] has suggested that a biochemical lesion in the energy forming system in the mitochondria may lead secondarily to derepression of the operator gene and overproduction of porphyrins. Thus, porphyrinogenesis would be secondary to some other metabolic defect.

There is no doubt that continued investigation of these disorders will widen our knowledge of mitochondrial and nuclear biochemistry and genetics.[163, 198]

The disease states which result from disordered porphyrin metabolism may be classified as follows:

I. Disorders of porphyrin synthesis in the erythrocyte
1. Porphyria (congenital) erythropoietica
2. Protoporphyria (congenital) erythropoietica
II. Disorders of porphyrin synthesis in the liver
1. Porphyria hepatica
a. Intermittent acute (Swedish porphyria)
b. Hereditary coproporphyria
c. Cutanea tarda
d. Mixed (South African porphyria, porphyria variegata)
III. Acquired (toxic) porphyria

Porphyria erythropoietica. Porphyria erythropoietica is a rare metabolic disorder of the erythrocyte which is probably transmitted as a recessive genetic abnormality.[200] Patients with this disorder appear to have both normal and abnormal erythroid cell lines in the marrow.[174] The nuclei and to a lesser extent the cytoplasm of cells of the affected line show a characteristic red fluorescence when studied with the fluorescence microscope. In addition they may have a dark nuclear inclusion body containing hemoglobin. As destruction of circulating erythrocytes cannot account for the quantity of porphyrin excreted by these patients it has been postulated that uroporphyrin may be released into the plasma at a rapid rate during the maturation of the nucleated red cells in the marrow.[173] The red fluorescence which has been demonstrated in the spleen is thought to result from the local destruction of red blood cells containing the abnormal porphyrin. The isomers found in the urine and blood of these patients are copro- and uroporphyrin I. These porphyrins are not complexed with a metal and the monopyrrole porphobilinogen is not found.

Recent studies have revealed that, when incubated with porphobilinogen, hemolysates prepared from the red cells of these patients had a greater porphyrin forming ability than hemolysates prepared from normal red cells.[207] The finding of protoporphyrin IX indicated that isomerase was not lacking.[162, 207]

The suggestion has been made that excessive production of porphyrin precursors may overwhelm the normal isomerase activity, resulting in the production of the usual amount of type III porphyrins but excessive quantities of the type I isomers. A variety of genetic defects which might produce such a result have been suggested.[94, 207] The alternate formation of excessive quantities of uroporphyrin I which cannot be used in heme synthesis is believed responsible for the clinical manifestations of the disorder.[61, 121, 135, 218]

The clinical picture is characterized by photosensitivity which leads to erythema, blisters, ulcer formation, and ultimate mutilation of exposed areas. Hemolytic anemia is usually present, and thrombocytopenia may occur.[62] Splenomegaly is expected. Because of the deposition of uroporphyrin I in the bones and teeth, these structures are often red-brown and will fluoresce under a Wood's light.[2, 20, 68]

Treatment is non-specific. Sunlight must be avoided. Splenectomy has relieved the hemolytic anemia in a number of patients.[174]

Congenital erythropoietic protoporphyria. Erythropoietic protoporphyria is an inborn error of metabolism characterized by a marked increase in the concentration of erythrocyte protoporphyrin IX and mild photosensitivity. Erythrocyte coproporphyrin III, fecal coproporphyrin, and fecal protoporphyrin concentration may be normal or increased and plasma protoporphyrin may be elevated. The most severe skin lesions accompany the greatest increases of plasma and erythrocyte protoporphyrin.[147] Urinary porphyrin excretion is normal. There are two populations of red cells. Less than half the circulating cells exhibit fluorescence and photohemolysis.[88] The disorder appears in childhood and is believed to be transmitted as a Mendelian dominant.[65, 151, 220]

Patients with erythropoietic protoporphyria have abnormal sensitivity to light and develop erythema, edema, and itching of the exposed skin.[125] Vesicle formation, hirsutism, and scarring have been reported[151] but are not characteristic.[65, 125] The one reported instance of hemolytic anemia was associated with hepatosplenomegaly, moderate leukopenia and thrombocytopenia and responded to splenectomy.[151]

The disorder appears to be the result of overproduction of normal protoporphyrin IX in the developing red cells in the marrow. A non-erythropoietic site for production of high plasma protoporphyrin levels has not been excluded.[157] The maximal skin sensitivity to monochromatic light has been shown to be 400 to 410 mμ which corresponds to the Soret band of maximal light absorption by the porphyrin.[125] It has been suggested that the higher energy state attained by the porphyrins on exposure to light is in some way responsible for the skin damage.[15] A large amount of hyaline material has been shown to be invariably associated with the blood vessels of the upper corium in areas of exposed skin.[147] After exposure to 400 mμ light, a thickening of the walls of subepidermal small blood vessels was found. Some of these small vessels were occluded.[6] Electron microscopy has revealed that the amorphous material noted in the small blood vessels in the upper part of the dermis appeared to be derived from constituents of the blood or from the vessel wall.[166]

A recent report indicates that the anionic exchange resin cholestyramine may block enterohepatic circulation of protoporphyrin, prevent potential liver damage, and reduce skin photosensitivity. Further studies of these effects should prove interesting.[87, 92, 93]

Porphyria hepatica. The site of deranged porphyrin metabolism in this disorder is not the bone marrow but the liver.[174] Porphyria hepatica may be the result of a metabolic defect in the synthesis of heme proteins other than hemoglobin. Catalase synthesis has, for example, been shown to be abnormal in experimental porphyria.[172] These disorders are more common than the erythropoietic type.

Intermittent acute type. The intermittent acute type of porphyria hepatica is a familial disorder inherited as an autosomal dominant. Evidence has been collected suggesting that it affected the royal houses of Stuart, Hanover, and Prussia and was responsible for the illness of King George III.[123, 124] It usually appears after puberty though in rare cases it may be evident in childhood.[200] In this disorder the erythrocyte porphyrins are normal, but excessive quantities of zinc complexed uroporphyrin I and III and coproporphyrin III are found in the urine. The porphyrin precursor, porphobilinogen, is found in the urine during the acute attacks and the finding of this monopyrrole is diagnostic. The liver contains large quantities of porphyrin precursors and increased amounts of porphyrin. Marrow porphyrins are normal. Hepatic δ-aminolevulinic acid synthetase levels have been found to be somewhat elevated.[222]

The clinical manifestations of the intermittent acute type of porphyria hepatica are varied, but abdominal colic—which can be of extreme severity— weakness and paresthesia of extremities, constipation, convulsions, coma, psychoses, and hypertension may occur. Fatalities are generally due to respiratory paralysis but may occur during coma or from cachexia.[160] Hypochloremia or hyponatremia noted during acute attacks has been demonstrated to be the result of inappropriate secretion of antidiuretic hormone.[72, 198]

Treatment includes avoidance of alcohol, barbiturates, or other liver toxins. Chlorpromazine has been reported effective in relief of symptoms[206] and this has been confirmed.[200] Splenectomy is not indicated.

Hereditary coproporphyria. There is persistent excretion of large amounts of coproporphyrin III in both urine and feces in this disorder, and porphyrin precursors occur in the urine during the acute episodes. The disorder is transmitted as a Mendelian autosomal dominant. Family studies have revealed that as many as 50 per cent of those with coproporphyria have no symptoms similar to those of acute intermittent porphyria. Photosensitivity is rare but has been noted.[24] Acute attacks may be precipitated or exacerbated by the same drugs noted to affect the course of acute intermittent porphyria.[24, 51, 66]

Cutanea tarda type. As its name suggests this disorder begins later in life, and its symptoms include photosensitivity. It is a familial disorder associated with parenchymal liver disease in a high percentage of cases. The photosensitivity is moderate in severity. The disease runs a mild course if the patients protect themselves from exposure to sunlight and hepatotoxins. A history of chronic alcoholism is not uncommon. The porphyrins excreted are the zinc complexed uroporphyrins I and III and coproporphyrin III. Porphyrins may be found in the blood and are elevated in the liver. Porphobilinogen is not found in the urine of these patients. The prognosis is generally good but depends on the degree of liver damage. Improvement has been reported following the administration of adenosine monophosphate and suggests that some aberration in purine synthesis may play a role in this disorder.[45, 156]

Several investigators have noted a tendency to high serum iron and transferrin values in a number of patients with porphyria cutanea tarda.[34] Though no consistent abnormality in iron metabolism has been demonstrated,[152] phlebotomy has resulted in markedly reduced porphyrin excretion and remission. Administration of iron results in a return of symptoms.[35] The precise role that iron may play in this disorder is unknown, but the effect of phlebotomy has been salutary.[7, 35]

Mixed type.   These patients have symptoms of both the cutanea tarda and the acute intermittent type of porphyria.[206] The high incidence of this disorder among the Boers of South Africa is responsible for the designation "South African porphyria." During the acute stage of the disorder, the urine contains δ-aminolevulinic acid, porphobilinogen, uroporphyrin, and coproporphyrin. The stool also contains large quantities of porphyrins. Between attacks the urine may be negative but the stools continue to be positive.

Acquired (toxic) porphyria.   Acquired porphyria with photosensitivity, marked porphyrinuria, and hepatomegaly has occurred as the result of the ingestion of the fungicide hexachlorobenzene.[19] The bullous lesions of the skin often progressed to ulceration and healed with scarring. Marked pigmentation in the upper keratin layer of the skin and diffuse hypertrichosis with focal areas of alopecia occurred in several cases. The urine contains increased amounts of uroporphyrin and coproporphyrin but no porphobilinogen or δ-aminolevulinic acid. Feeding of hexachlorobenzene to rats will result in a similar disorder[171] which can be ameliorated by the administration of adenosine monophosphate.[139]

Porphyrinurias

There are a number of conditions in which increased porphyrin excretion may occur.[2] The increased excretion of porphyrin in these varied disease states may reflect disordered hemoglobin or protein synthesis or disordered synthesis of heme compounds other than hemoglobin.

1. Lead Poisoning

Lead poisoning results in a marked disturbance in heme synthesis. Urinary excretion of δ-aminolevulinic acid, uroporphyrin, and coproporphyrin is increased and the concentration of free erythrocyte protoporphyrin is elevated.[13, 117, 212] A decrease in the activity of δ-aminolevulinic acid dehydrase is believed responsible for the accumulation of δ-aminolevulinic acid, and the increased excretion of porphyrins, despite a decrease in their synthesis, is postulated to be due to the interference by lead with the incorporation of iron into protoporphyrin.[65, 85]

 2. Rheumatic fever — coproporphyrin III[89]
 3. Poliomyelitis — coproporphyrin III[208]
 4. Liver disease[205]
  a. Alcoholic cirrhosis — coproporphyrin III
  b. Infectious hepatitis — coproporphyrin I
 5. Anemia[174, 204, 205]
  a. Refractory — coproporphyrin III
  b. Hemolytic anemia — coproporphyrin I
  c. Pernicious anemia — coproporphyrin I
 6. Idiopathic — coproporphyrin III[205]

Additional Factors Needed for Erythropoiesis

In addition to protein, metals and certain vitamins must be present if normal erythropoiesis is to continue.[21]

Iron. The various details of iron metabolism are discussed in Chapter V. Only a brief summary of this complex problem is presented at this time.

The daily diet of the average adult in the United States contains 12 to 15 mg. of iron, which is present mainly in the ferric form. Reduction to the ferrous form, the type of iron that is absorbed, is promoted by the acid reaction of the stomach and upper small intestine, by ascorbic acid, and by certain proteins. Iron is absorbed mainly in the upper portion of the small intestine and the amount of iron that gains entrance to the body is largely controlled by regulation of the absorption of iron through the mucosa. Normally, less than 10 per cent of the ingested iron is absorbed. Various factors, such as the amount and form of iron in the intestine, the iron-phosphate ratio and possibly other details of the diet, the status of the iron stores, the degree of erythropoietic activity, and perhaps other factors, influence this absorptive mechanism. After absorption, the iron is transported in the plasma in the ferric state in combination with a beta-1 globulin fraction to the reticuloendothelial cells of the liver, spleen, and bone marrow where it is stored in the form of ferritin and hemosiderin or used in the production of hemoglobin. From these stores, the iron is mobilized for hemoglobin production in the bone marrow. The body has no means of excreting significant amounts of iron and only minute amounts of iron, about 1 mg. per day, are lost by cell desquamation and other means. Reduction of the amount of iron in the body occurs mainly as the result of bleeding and pregnancy.

The metabolic pathways of iron are shown schematically in Figure 2–11.

Copper. Although anemia due to copper deficiency has not been produced in adult humans, in experimental animals a deficiency of copper leads to the development of an anemia that is similar to iron deficiency anemia. The adult human body contains 100 to 150 mg. of copper.[216] The plasma level has been found to be 105 ± 16 micrograms per cent in males and 116 ± 16 micrograms per cent in females. Ninety per cent of the copper in the plasma is bound to the alpha-2 globulin ceruloplasmin.[75] Copper appears to function in the absorption, mobilization, and utilization of iron in hemoglobin synthesis and in the formation and maintenance of the cytochromes.[177, 216] The metal may exert an effect on hematopoiesis through an effect on the function of respiratory enzymes.

Cobalt. Cobalt is known to play a role in animal nutrition and the administration of cobalt is known to stimulate erythropoiesis in man and in animals.[141] However, the mechanism by which cobalt effects an increase in red blood cell production is not understood.[105] It has not been established that cobalt has any role in normal erythropoiesis aside from its importance as a part of the vitamin B_{12} molecule.

Pyridoxine. For many years it was known that a deficiency of pyridoxine (vitamin B_6) in animals would produce a severe hypochromic microcytic anemia but only recently has a similar disorder been described in man.[70] The deficiency, which is corrected by the administration of pyridoxine, is characterized by splenomegaly, hepatomegaly, hypochromic microcytic anemia, elevation of serum iron level, and saturation of the iron binding capacity. The inability of these patients to metabolize iron normally is associated with disturbed tryptophan metabolism and the excretion of xanthurenic acid.

Vitamin B_{12} and folic acid. Both vitamin B_{12} and folic acid are necessary for the normal maturation of the red cells. A deficiency of either results in a defect in nucleic acid metabolism that is reflected by the development of the megaloblastic type of erythrocyte maturation. Vitamin B_{12} has now been identi-

METABOLIC PATHWAYS OF IRON

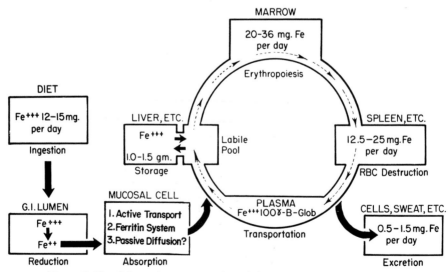

Figure 2–11.   Schematic representation of the metabolic pathways of iron.

fied as the *extrinsic factor* of Castle. An *intrinsic factor* in the stomach, a muco-protein, is necessary in order that the vitamin B_{12} ingested in the diet be absorbed.[8, 22] The chemical characteristics of the intrinsic factor have been worked out in considerable detail.[60, 191, 215] An absence or deficiency of the intrinsic factor is responsible for pernicious anemia. Folic acid, also present in the diet, does not require the intrinsic factor for its absorption. The functions of these two vitamins are not completely understood. Both are concerned with the formation of purine or pyrimidine bases which are constituent parts of the nucleic acids. There seems to be a reciprocal relationship between vitamin B_{12} and folic acid in the synthesis of nucleic acid in many tissues of the body, particularly those with rapid turnover, such as the hematopoietic and gastro-intestinal cells.[5, 130]

Ascorbic acid. Ascorbic acid appears to participate in metabolic activities which affect both vitamin B_{12} and folic acid. It is important in the conversion of folic acid to folinic acid, and there is some evidence that it stimulates the formation of folic acid. This vitamin has intense reducing properties and must play a significant role in oxidation-reduction reactions in the body.[51, 71]

Vitamin E (alpha-tocopherol). Deficiency of this vitamin has been shown to produce anemia in several animal species, mainly on the basis of ineffective erythropoiesis.[190a] Except for the possibility of a hemolytic anemia in premature infants,[141a, 141b] no deficiency has been clearly demonstrated in humans. The role of vitamin E deficiency in the anemia of protein-calorie malnutrition is still controversial.

Other vitamins may possibly play a role in erythropoiesis. Nicotinic acid

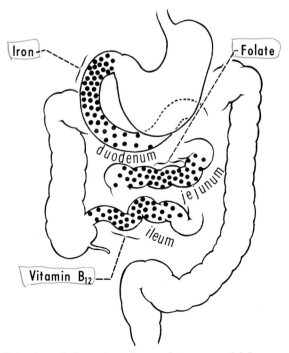

Figure 2–12. Main sites of absorption of some factors essential for normal erythropoiesis.

is thought to be essential for the synthesis of coenzymes in the developing erythrocyte but its role in hematopoiesis is not clearly established.[69] Riboflavin deficiency has been reported to be responsible for anemia in animals but no anemia of this type has been recognized in man. It is thought to exert its influence by taking part in cellular oxidations.[193]

References

1. Adair, G. C.: A comparison of the molecular weights of the proteins. Proc. Cambridge Phil. Soc., 2:75, 1924.
2. Aldrich, R. F., Labbe, F. F., and Talman, E. K.: A review of porphyrin metabolism with special reference to childhood. Am. J. M. Sc., 230:675, 1955.
3. Alexanian, R.: Erythropoietin and erythropoiesis in anemic man following androgens. Blood, 33:564, 1969.
4. Alpen, E. L., and Cranmore, D.: Observations on regulation of erythropoiesis and on cellular dynamics by Fe59 autoradiography. In Stohlman, F., Jr., Ed.: The Kinetics of Cellular Proliferation. Grune and Stratton, New York, 1959.
5. Angier, R. S., et al.: Synthesis of a compound identical with the L. casei factor isolated from liver. Science, 102:227, 1945.
6. Baart de la Faille-Kuyper, E. H., Rottier, P. B., and Baart de la Faille, H.: Epidermal changes in erythropoietic protoporphyria after irradiation with glass-filtered mercury light. Brit. J. Derm., 80:747, 1968.
7. Baker, H., and Turnbull, A.: Porphyria cutanea tarda treated by repeated venesection: clinical and biochemical response. Proc. Roy. Soc. Med., 62:590, 1969.
8. Berk, L., et al.: Observations on the etiologic relationship of achylia gastrica to pernicious anemia. New England J. Med., 239:911, 1948.
9. Bogorad, L.: The enzymatic synthesis of uroporphyrinogens from porphobilinogen. Conference on Hemoglobin. National Academy of Sciences, National Research Council Publ. 557, 1958, p. 74.
10. Bogorad, L., and Granick, S.: The enzymatic synthesis of porphyrins from porphobilinogen. Nat. Acad. Sc. Proc., 39:1176, 1953.
11. Bond, V. P., Fliedner, T. M., Cronkite, E. P., Rubins, J. R., and Robertson, J. S.: Cell turnover in blood and blood-forming tissues studied with tritiated thymidine. In Stohlman, F., Jr., Ed.: The Kinetics of Cellular Proliferation. Grune and Stratton, New York, 1959.
12. Borsook, H., Ratner, K., Tattrie, B., Teigler, D., and Lajtha, L. G.: Erythropoietin and the development of erythrocytes. Nature, 217:1024, 1968.
13. Boyett, J. D., and Butterworth, C. E.: Lead poisoning and hemoglobin synthesis. Am. J. Med., 32:884, 1962.
14. Brecher, G., and Cronkite, E. P.: Post-radiation parabiosis and survival in rats. Proc. Soc. Exper. Biol. & Med., 77:292, 1951.
15. Brown, A. K., and Zuelzer, W. W.: Studies on the neonatal development of the glucuronide conjugating system. J. Clin. Invest., 37:332, 1958.
16. Brown, E. G.: Evidence for the involvement of ferrous iron in the biosynthesis of δ-aminolaevulic acid by chicken erythrocyte preparations. Nature, 182:313, 1958.
16a. Bunn, H. F., and Jandl, J. H.: The renal handling of hemoglobin. Tr. A. Am. Physicians, 81:147, 1968.
17. Burnett, J. W., and Pathak, M. A.: Pathogenesis of cutaneous photosensitivity in porphyria. New England J. Med., 268:1203, 1963.
18. Burnham, B. F., and Lascelles, J.: Control of porphyrin biosynthesis through a negative-feedback mechanism. Biochem. J., 87:462, 1963.
19. Can. C., and Nigogosyan, G.: Acquired toxic porphyria cutanea tarda due to hexachlorobenzene (report of 348 cases caused by this fungicide). J.A.M.A., 183:88, 1963.
20. Carnot, P., and DeFlandre, C.: Sur l'activité du sérum hémopoiétique des differents organs au cours de la régénération du sang. Comp. Rend. Acad. Sc., 143:384, 1906.
21. Cartwright, G.: Dietary factors concerned in erythropoiesis. Blood, 2:111, 1947.
22. Castle, W. B.: The etiology of pernicious and related macrocytic anemias. Science, 82:159, 1935.
23. Comfort, A., Moore, H., and Weatherall, M.: Normal human urinary porphyrins. Biochem. J., 58:177, 1954.
24. Connon, J. J., and Turkington, V.: Hereditary coproporphyria. Lancet, 2:263, 1968.
25. Contopoulos, A. N., McCombs, R., Lawrence, J. H., and Simpson, M. E.: Erythropoietic

activity in the plasma of patients with polycythemia vera and secondary polycythemia. Blood, *12*:614, 1957.
26. Cookson, G. H., and Rimington, C.: Porphobilinogen. Biochem. J., *57*:476, 1954.
27. Crick, F. H. C., Barnett, L., Brenner, S., and Watts-Tobin, R. J.: General nature of the genetic code for proteins. Nature, *192*:1227, 1961.
28. Crosby, W. H., and Akeroyd, J. H.: The limit of hemoglobin synthesis in hereditary hemolytic anemia. Its relation to the excretion of bile pigment. Am. J. Med., *13*:273, 1952.
29. Cullis, A. C., Dintzis, H. M., and Perutz, M. F.: X-ray analysis of hemoglobin. Conference on Hemoglobin. National Academy of Sciences, National Research Council Publ. 557, 1958, p. 50.
30. Dacie, J. C.: The Hemolytic Anemias. 2nd Ed. Grune and Stratton, New York, 1960.
31. Dietrich, L. S., Nichol, C. A., Monson, W. J., and Elvehjem, C. A.: Observations on the interrelation of vitamin B_{12}, folic acid, and vitamin C in the chick. J. Biol. Chem., *181*:915, 1949.
32. Drabkin, D. L.: Metabolism of hemin chromoproteins. Physiol. Rev., *31*:345, 1951.
33. Duarte, L., Medal, L. S., Labardini, L., and Arriaga, L.: The erythropoietic effects of anabolic steroids. Proc. Soc. Exp. Biol. & Med., *125*:1030, 1967.
34. Epstein, J. H., and Pinski, J. B.: Porphyria cutanea tarda: Abnormal iron metabolism. Arch. Dermat., *92*:357, 1965.
35. Epstein, J. H., and Redeker, A. G.: Porphyria cutanea tarda: A study of the effect of phlebotomy. New England J. Med., *279*:1301, 1968.
36. Erslev, A. J.: Humoral regulation of red cell production. Blood, *8*:349, 1953.
37. Erslev, A. J.: Physiologic control of red cell production. Blood, *10*:954, 1955.
38. Erslev, A. J.: The effect of anemic anoxia on the cellular development of nucleated red cells. Blood, *14*:386, 1959.
39. Erslev, A. J.: Erythropoietin in vitro. II. Effect on "stem cells." Blood, *24*:331, 1964.
40. Falk, J. E., Dresel, E. I. B., and Rimington, C.: Porphobilinogen as a porphyrin precursor, and interconversion of porphyrins in a tissue system. Nature, *172*:292, 1953.
41. Field, E. O., Caughi, M. N., Blackett, N. M., and Smithers, D. W.: Marrow-suppressing factors in the blood in pure red cell aplasia, thymoma and Hodgkin's disease. Brit. J. Haem., *15*:101, 1968.
42. Finne. P. H.: Erythropoietin in concentrations of urine from healthy persons. Brit. M. J., *1*:697, 1965.
43. Fisher, J. W., Hatch, F. E., Roh, B. L., Allen, R. C., and Kelley, B. J.: Erythropoietin inhibitor in kidney extracts and plasma from anemic uremic human subjects. Blood, *31*:440, 1968.
44. Fried, W., Kilbridge, T., Krantz, S., McDonald, T. P., and Lange, R. D.: Studies on extrarenal erythropoietin. J. Lab. & Clin. Med., *73*:244, 1969.
45. Gajdos, A., and Gajdos-Török, M.: The therapeutic effect of adenosine-5-monophosphoric acid in porphyria. Lancet, *2*:175, 1961.
46. Gardner, F. H., Nathan, D. G., Piomelli, S., and Cummins, J. F.: The erythrocythaemic effects of androgen. Brit. J. Haem., *14*:611, 1968.
47. Giblett, E. R.: Haptoglobin: A review. Vox Sang., *6*:513, 1961.
48. Gibson, K. D., Laver, W. G., and Neuberger, A.: Initial stages in the biosynthesis of porphyrins. 2. The formation of δ-aminolevulinic acid from glycine and succinyl coenzyme A by particles from chicken erythrocytes. Biochem. J., *70*:71, 1958.
49. Gibson, K. D., Neuberger, A., and Scott, J. J.: The purification and properties of δ-aminolaevulinic acid dehydrase. Biochem. J., *61*:618, 1955.
50. Gibson, Q. H., and Antonini, E.: Rates of reaction of native human globin with some hemes. J. Biol. Chem., *238*:1384, 1963.
51. Goldberg, A., Rimington, C., and Lochhead, A. C.: Hereditary coproporphyria. Lancet, *1*:632, 1967.
52. Goldwasser, E., Jacobson, L. O., Fried, W., and Plzak, L. F.: Studies on erythropoiesis. V. The effect of cobalt on the production of erythropoietin. Blood, *13*:55, 1958.
54. Gordon, A. S.: Hemopoietine. Physiol. Rev., *39*:1, 1959.
55. Gordon, A. S., Piliero, S. J., Medici, P. T., Siegel, C. D., and Tannenbaum, M.: Attempts to identify the site of production of circulating erythropoietin. Proc. Soc. Exp. Biol. & Med., *92*:598, 1956.
56. Granick, S.: Direct evidence for iron insertion into protoporphyrin to form heme. Fed. Proc., *13*:219, 1954.
57. Granick, S.: Hepatic porphyria and drug-induced or chemical porphyria. Ann. N.Y. Acad. Sc., *123*:188, 1965.
58. Grant, W. C., and Root, W. S.: The relation of O_2 in bone marrow blood to post-hemorrhagic erythropoiesis. Am. J. Physiol., *150*:618, 1947.
59. Grant, W. C., and Root, W. S.: Fundamental stimulus for erythropoiesis. Physiol. Rev., *32*:449, 1952.

60. Grasbeck, R.: Studies on the vitamin B$_{12}$ binding principle and other biocolloids of human gastric juice. Acta med. scandinav., Suppl. 314, 1956.

61. Gray, C. H., and Neuberger, A.: Studies in congenital porphyria. 1. Incorporation of ^{15}N into coproporphyrin, uroporphyrin and hippuric acid. Biochem. J., 47:81, 1950.

62. Gross, S.: Hematologic studies on erythropoietic porphyria: A new case with severe hemolysis, chronic thrombocytopenia and folic acid deficiency. Blood, 23:762, 1964.

63. Gurney, C. W., and Fried, W.: Further studies on the erythropoietic effect of androgens. J. Lab. & Clin. Med., 65:775, 1965.

64. Haeger-Aronsen, B.: Erythropoietic protoporphyria. A new type of inborn error of metabolism. Am. J. Med., 35:450, 1963.

65. Haeger-Aronsen, B.: Studies on urinary excretion of δ-aminolevulinic acid and other haem precursors in lead workers and lead-intoxicated rabbits. Scandinav. J. Clin. & Lab. Invest., 12(Suppl. 47):1, 1960.

66. Haeger-Aronsen, B., Strathers, G., and Swahn, G.: Hereditary coproporphyria. Study of a Swedish family. Ann. Int. Med., 69:221, 1968.

67. Hahn, P. F., and Whipple, G. H.: Hemoglobin production in anemia limited by low protein intake. Influence of iron intake, protein supplements and fasting. J. Exper. Med., 69:315, 1939.

68. Haining, R. G., Cowger, M. L., Shurtleff, D. B., and Labbe, R. F.: Congenital erythropoietic porphyria. Am. J. Med., 45:624, 1968.

69. Handler, P., and Featherstone, W. P.: The biochemical defect in nicotinic acid deficiency. II. On the nature of the anemia. J. Biol. Chem., 151:395, 1943.

70. Harris, J. W., Whittington, R. M., Weisman, R., Jr., and Horrigan, D. L.: Pyridoxine responsive anemia in the human adult. Proc. Soc. Biol. & Med., 91:427, 1956.

71. Harris, L.: Vitamin C. Brit. M. Bull., 12:57, 1956.

72. Hellman, E. S., Tschudy, D. P., and Bartter, F. C.: Abnormal electrolyte and water metabolism in acute intermittent porphyria. Am. J. Med., 32:734, 1962.

73. Hodgkin, D. C., et al.: Structure of vitamin B$_{12}$. Nature, 176:325, 1955.

74. Hodgson, G.: Synthesis of RNA and DNA at various intervals after erythropoietin injection in transfused mice. Proc. Soc. Exp. Biol. & Med., 124:1045, 1967.

75. Holmberg, C. G., and Laurell, C. B.: Investigations in serum copper. I. Nature of serum and copper and its relation to the iron-binding protein in human serum. Acta chem. scandinav., 1:944, 1947.

76. Hunt, J. A., and Ingram, V. M.: Allelomorphism and the chemical differences of the human hemoglobins A, S and C. Nature, 181:1062, 1958.

77. Hurwitz, J., and Furth, J. J.: Messenger RNA. Scient. Am., 206:41, 1962.

78. Ingram, D. J. E., Gibson, J. F., and Perutz, M. F.: Orientation of the four haem groups in haemoglobin. Nature, 178:906, 1956.

79. Ingram, V. M.: A specific chemical difference between the globins of normal human and sickle-cell anaemia haemoglobin. Nature, 178:792, 1956.

80. Ingram, V. M.: Gene mutation in human hemoglobin: The chemical difference between normal and sickle cell hemoglobin. Nature, 180:326, 1957.

81. Ingram, V. M.: Constituents of human haemoglobin. Nature, 183:1795, 1959.

82. Itano, H.: The human hemoglobins: Their properties and genetic control. In Anfinsen, C. B., Jr., Anson, M. L., Bailey, K., and Edsall, J. T., Eds.: Advances in Protein Chemistry, vol. 12. Academic Press, New York, 1957, p. 215.

83. Jacobson, L. O.: Sites of formation of erythropoietin. In Jacobson, L. O., and Doyle, M. A., Eds.: Erythropoiesis. Grune and Stratton, New York, 1962.

84. Jacobson, L. O., Goldwasser, E., Fried, W., and Plzak, L.: The role of the kidney in erythropoiesis. Nature, 179:633, 1957.

85. Jandl, J. H., Inman, J. K., Simmons, R. L., and Allen, P. W.: Transfer of iron from serum iron-binding protein to human reticulocytes. J. Clin. Invest., 38:161, 1959.

86. Jayle, M. F., and Moretti, J.: Haptoglobin: Biochemical, genetic and physiopathological aspects. Progr. Hemat., 3:342, 1962.

87. Johns, W. H., and Bates, T. R.: Quantification of the binding tendencies of cholestyramine. J. Pharm. Sc., 58:179, 1969.

88. Kaplowitz, N., Javitt, N., and Harber, L. C.: Isolation of erythrocytes with normal protoporphyrin levels in erythropoietic protoporphyria. New England J. Med., 278:1077, 1968.

89. Kapp, E. M., and Coburn, A. F.: Studies on the excretion of urinary porphyrin in rheumatic fever. Brit. J. Exp. Path., 17:255, 1936.

90. Kendrew, J. C., and Perutz, M. F.: X-ray studies of compounds of biological interest. Ann. Rev. Biochem., 26:327, 1957.

91. Kilbridge, T. M., Fried, W., and Heller, P.: The mechanism by which plethora suppresses erythropoiesis. Blood, 33:104, 1969.

92. Kniffen, J. C.: Protoporphyrin removal in intrahepatic porphyrastasis. Clinical Res., *18*:77, 1970.

93. Kniffen, J. C., Noyes, W. D., and Porter, F. S.: Iron and cholestyramine in erythropoietic protoporphyria. Clin. Sc., *18*:38, 1970.

94. Kramer, S., Viljoen, E., Meyer, A. M., and Metz, J.: The anaemia of erythropoietic porphyria with the first description of the disease in an elderly patient. Brit. J. Haem., *11*:666, 1965.

95. Krantz, S. B., and Goldwasser, E.: On the mechanism of erythropoietin-induced differentiation. II. The effect on RNA synthesis. Biochem. et biophys. acta, *103*:325, 1965.

96. Krueger, R. C., Melnick, I., and Klein, J. R.: Formation of heme by broken-cell preparations of duck erythrocytes. Arch. Biochem., *64*:302, 1956.

97. Krumdieck, N.: Erythropoietic substance in the serum of anemic animals. Proc. Soc. Exper. Biol. & Med., *54*:14, 1943.

98. Kubanek, B., Tyler, W. S., Ferrari, L., Porcellini, A., Howard, D., and Stohlman, F., Jr.: Regulation of erythropoiesis. XXI. The effect of erythropoietin on the stem cell. Proc. Soc. Exp. Biol. & Med., *127*:770, 1968.

99. Kuehl, F. A., Shunk, C. H., and Folkers, K.: Vitamin B_{12}. J. Am. Chem. Soc., 77:251, 1955.

100. Kuratowska, Z., Lewartowski, B., and Lipinski, B.: Chemical and biologic properties of an erythropoietin generating substance obtained from perfusate of isolated anoxic kidneys. J. Lab. & Clin. Med., *64*:226, 1964.

101. Labbe, R. F.: An enzyme which catalyzes the insertion of iron into protoporphyrin. Biochem. et biophys. acta, *31*:589, 1959.

102. Labbe, R. F.: Metabolic anomalies in porphyria. The result of impaired biological oxidation. Lancet, *1*:1361, 1967.

103. Labbe, R. F., Talman, E. L., and Aldrich, R. A.: Porphyrin metabolism. II. Uric acid excretion in experimental porphyria. Biochem. et biophys. acta, *15*:590, 1954.

104. Labbe, R. F., Talman, E. L., and Aldrich, R. A.: Purine metabolism in porphyria. Fed. Proc., *14*:241, 1955.

105. Laforet, M. T., and Thomas, E. D.: The effect of cobalt on heme synthesis by bone marrow in vitro. J. Biol. Chem., *218*:595, 1956.

106. Lajtha, L. G.: Bone marrow cell metabolism. Physiol. Rev., *37*:50, 1957.

107. Lajtha, L. G.: Stem cell kinetics and erythropoietin. In Jacobson, L. O., and Doyle, M. A., Eds.: Erythropoiesis. Grune and Stratton, New York, 1962.

108. Lajtha, L. G.: Recent studies in erythroid differentiation and proliferation. Medicine, *43*:625, 1964.

109. Lajtha, L. G., Oliver, R., and Gurney, C. W.: Kinetic model of a bone-marrow stem-cell population. Brit. J. Haem., *8*:442, 1962.

110. Lajtha, L. G., and Suit, H. D.: Uptake of radioactive iron (^{59}Fe) by nucleated red cells. Brit. J. Haem., *1*:55, 1955.

111. Lathem, W., Davis, B. B., Zweig, P. H., and Dew, R.: Demonstration and localization of renal tubular reabsorption of hemoglobin by stop flow analysis. J. Clin. Invest., *39*:840, 1960.

112. Lathem, W., and Worley, W. E.: Distribution of extracorpuscular hemoglobin in circulating plasma. J. Clin. Invest., *38*:474, 1959.

113. Lathem, W., and Worley, W. E.: Renal excretion of hemoglobin: Regulatory mechanisms and differential excretion of free and protein-bound hemoglobin. J. Clin. Invest., *38*:652, 1959.

114. Laurell, C-B., and Nyman, M.: Studies on the serum haptoglobin level in hemoglobinemia and its influence on renal excretion of hemoglobin. Blood, *12*:493, 1957.

115. Leavell, B. S., Thorup, O. A., Jr., and McClellan, J. R.: Observations on the anemia in myxedema. Tr. Am. Clin. & Climat. Ass., *68*:137, 1957.

116. Lemberg, R., and Legge, J. W.: Hematin Compounds and Bile Pigments. Interscience Publishers, Inc., New York, 1949.

117. Lichtman, H. C., and Feldman, F.: In vitro pyrrole and porphyrin synthesis in lead poisoning and iron deficiency. J. Clin. Invest., *42*:830, 1963.

118. Lockwood, W. H., and Rimington, C.: Purification of an enzyme converting porphobilinogen to uroporphyrin. Biochem. J., *67*:8p, 1957.

119. London, I. M., and West, R.: The formation of bile pigment in pernicious anemia. J. Biol. Chem., *184*:359, 1950.

120. London, I. M., West, R., Shemin, D., and Rittenberg, D.: On the origin of bile pigment in normal man. J. Biol. Chem., *184*:351, 1950.

121. London, I. M., West, R., Shemin, D., and Rittenberg, D.: Porphyrin formation and hemoglobin metabolism in congenital porphyria. J. Biol. Chem., *184*:365, 1950.

122. London, I. M., Shemin, D., and Rittenberg, D.: Synthesis of heme in vitro by the immature non-nucleated mammalian erythrocyte. J. Biol. Chem., *183*:749, 1950.

123. Macalpine, I., and Hunter, R.: The "insanity" of King George III: A classic case of porphyria. Brit. Med. J., *5479*:65, 1966.

124. Macalpine, I., Hunter, R., and Rimington, C.: Porphyria in the royal house of Stuart, Hanover and Prussia: A follow-up study of George III's illness. Brit. Med. J., *1*:7, 1968.

125. Magnus, I. A., Jarrett, A., Prankerd, T. A. J., and Rimington, C.: Erythropoietic protoporphyria. A new porphyria syndrome with solar urticaria due to protoporphyrinemia. Lancet, *2*:448, 1961.

126. Marver, D., and Gurney, C.: Renal erythropoietin excretion as a function of acid-base balance. Ann. N.Y. Acad. Sc., *149*:570, 1968.

127. Matheweson, J. H., and Corwin, A. H.: Biosynthesis of pyrrole pigments: A mechanism for porphobilinogen polymerization. J. Am. Chem. Soc., *83*:135, 1961.

128. Mauzerell, D.: The condensation of porphobilinogen to uroporphyrinogen. J. Am. Chem. Soc., *82*:2605, 1960.

129. Mirand, E. A., Gordon, A. S., and Wenig, J.: Mechanism of testosterone action in erythropoiesis. Nature, *206*:270, 1965.

130. Moore, C. V., Bierbaum, O. S., Welch, A. D., and Wright, L. D.: The activity of synthetic Lactobacillus casei factor (folic acid) as an antipernicious anemia substance. J. Lab. & Clin. Med., *30*:1056, 1945.

131. Moores, R. R., Wright, C. S., Collins, L. R., Gardner, E., Jr., Lewis, J. P., and Smith, L. L.: Stimulation of erythropoietin by androgen in the human. Scand. J. Haem., *5*:6, 1968.

132. Morse, B. S., and Stohlman, F., Jr.: Regulation of erythropoiesis. XVIII. The effect of vincristine and erythropoietin on bone marrow. J. Clin. Invest., *45*:1241, 1966.

133. Naets, J. P., and Wittek, M.: Erythropoiesis in anephric man. Lancet, *1*:941, 1968.

134. Nathan, D. G., Schupak, E., Stohlman, F., Jr., and Merrill, J. P.: Erythropoiesis in anephric man. J. Clin. Invest., *43*:2158, 1964.

135. Neuberger, A., and Muir, H. M.: Biosynthesis of porphyrins and congenital porphyria. Nature, *165*:948, 1950.

136. Neve, R. A., and Aldrich, R. A.: Porphyrin metabolism III. Urinary and erythrocyte porphyrin in children with acute rheumatic fever. Pediatrics, *15*:553, 1955.

137. Nirenberg, M. W.: The genetic code: II. Scient. Am., *208*:80, 1963.

138. Nyman, M.: Serum haptoglobin: Methodological and clinical studies. Scand. J. Clin. & Lab. Invest., Suppl. 39, 1959.

139. Ockner, R. K., and Schmid, R.: Acquired porphyria in man and rat due to hexachlorobenzene intoxication. Nature, *189*:499, 1961.

140. Olesen, H., and Fogh, J.: Apparent molecular weight of erythropoietin determined by gel filtration. Scand. J. Haem., *5*:211, 1968.

141. Orten, J. M., Underhill, F. A., Mugrage, E. R., and Lewis, R. C.: Blood volume studies in cobalt polycythemia. J. Biol. Chem., *99*:457, 1932-33.

141a. Oski, F. A., and Barness, L. A.: Vitamin E deficiency: Previously unrecognized cause of hemolytic anemia in premature infants. J. Pediat., *70*:211, 1967.

141b. Oski, F. A., and Barness, L. A.: Hemolytic anemia in vitamin E deficiency. Am. J. Clin. Nutr., *21*:45, 1968.

142. Pauling, L.: The oxygen equilibrium of hemoglobin and its structural interpretation. Proc. Nat. Acad. Sc., *21*:186, 1935.

143. Pavlovic-Kentera, V., Hall, D. P., Bragassa, C., and Lange, R. D.: Unilateral renal hypoxia and production of erythropoietin. J. Lab. & Clin. Med., *65*:577, 1965.

144. Perutz, M. F.: Absorption spectra of single crystals of haemoglobin in polarized light. Nature, *143*:731, 1939.

145. Perutz, M. F., Liquori, A. M., and Eirich, F.: X-ray and solubility studies of the haemoglobin of sickle cell anaemia patients. Nature, *167*:929, 1951.

146. Perutz, M. F., Rossman, M. G., Cullis, A. F., Muirhead, H., Will, B., and North, A. C. T.: Structure of hemoglobin. Nature, *185*:416, 1960.

147. Peterka, E. S., Fusaro, R. M., and Goltz, R. W.: Erythropoietic protoporphyria. II. Histological and histochemical studies of cutaneous lesions. Arch. Dermat., *92*:357, 1965.

148. Peterka, E. S., Fusaro, R. M., Runge, W. J., Jaffe, M. D., and Watson, C. J.: Erythropoietic protoporphyria. J.A.M.A., *193*:120, 1965.

149. Porra, R. J., and Falk, J. E.: The enzymatic conversion of coproporphyrinogen III into protoporphyrin IX. Biochem. J., *90*:69, 1964.

150. Porra, R. J., and Jones, O. T. G.: An investigation of the role of ferrochelatase in the biosynthesis of various haem prosthetic groups. Biochem. J., *87*:186, 1963.

151. Porter, F. S., and Lowe, B. A.: Congenital erythropoietic protoporphyria. I. Case reports, clinical studies and porphyrin analysis in two brothers. Blood, *22*:521, 1963.

152. Price, D. C., Epstein, J. H., Winchell, S., Sargent, T. W., Pollycove, M., and Cavalieri, R. R.: Iron kinetics in porphyria cutanea tarda. Clin. Res., *16*:124, 1968.

153. Radin, N. S., Rittenberg, D., and Shemin, D.: The role of glycine in the biosynthesis of heme. J. Biol. Chem., *184*:745, 1950.
154. Radin, N. S., Rittenberg, D., and Shemin, D.: The role of acetic acid in the biosynthesis of heme. J. Biol. Chem., *184*:755, 1950.
155. Raine, D. N.: An ether-soluble precursor of coproporphyrin in urine. Biochem. J., *47*:xiv, 1950.
156. Ratner, A. C., and Dibson, R. L.: Hepatic cutaneous porphyria: Response of a patient to treatment with adenosine-5-monophosphate. Arch. Dermat., *89*:505, 1964.
157. Redeker, A. G., and Sterling, R. E.: The "glucose effect" in erythropoietic protoporphyria. Arch. Int. Med., *121*:446, 1968.
158. Reissmann, K. R.: Studies on the mechanism of erythropoietic stimulation in parabiotic rats during hypoxia. Blood, 5:372, 1950.
159. Rhinesmith, H. S., Schroeder, W. A., and Pauling, L.: A quantitative study of the hydrolysis of human dinitrophenyl (DNP) globin: The number and kind of polypeptide chains in normal adult human hemoglobin. J. Am. Chem. Soc., *79*:4682, 1957.
160. Ridley, A.: The neuropathy of acute intermittent porphyria. Quart. J. Med., *38*:307, 1969.
161. Rimington, C.: Haems and porphyrins in health and disease. II. Acta med. scandinav., *143*:177, 1952.
162. Rimington, C.: Biosynthesis of haemoglobin. Brit. M. Bull., *15*:19, 1959.
163. Rimington, C.: Porphyrin and haem biosynthesis and its control. Acta med. scandinav., *179*:11, 1966.
164. Rosse, W. F., and Waldmann, T. A.: The metabolism of erythropoietin in patients with anemia due to deficient erythropoiesis. J. Clin. Invest., *43*:1348, 1964.
165. Rudolph, W., Perretta, M.: Effects of erythropoietin on C14-formate uptake by spleen and bone marrow nucleic acids of erythrocyte-transfused mice. Proc. Soc. Exp. Biol. & Med., *124*:1041, 1967.
166. Ryan, E. A., and Madill, G. F.: Electron microscopy of the skin in erythropoietic protoporphyria. Brit. J. Derm., *80*:561, 1968.
167. Salomon, K., Richmond, J. E., and Altman, K. I.: Tetrapyrrole precursors of protoporphyrin IX. J. Biol. Chem., *196*:463, 1952.
168. Sano, S., and Granick, S.: Mitochondrial coproporphyrinogen oxidase and protoporphyrin formation. J. Biol. Chem., *236*:1173, 1961.
169. Schachter, D.: Nature of the glucuronide in direct-reacting bilirubin. Science, *126*:507, 1957.
170. Schmid, R.: Direct-reacting bilirubin, bilirubin glucuronide, in serum, bile, and urine. Science, *124*:76, 1956.
171. Schmid, R.: Cutaneous porphyria in Turkey. New England J. Med., *263*:397, 1960.
172. Schmid, R., and Schwartz, S.: Disturbance of catalase metabolism in experimental porphyria. J. Lab. & Clin. Med., *40*:939, 1952.
173. Schmid, R., Schwartz, S., and Sundberg, R. D.: Erythropoietic (congenital) porphyria: A rare abnormality of the normoblasts. Blood, *10*:416, 1955.
174. Schmid, R., Schwartz, S., and Watson, C. J.: Porphyrin content of bone marrow and liver in the various forms of porphyria. Arch. Int. Med., *93*:167, 1954.
175. Schmid, R., and Shemin, D.: The enzymatic formation of porphobilinogen from δ-aminolevulinic acid and its conversion to protoporphyrin. J. Am. Chem. Soc., 77:506, 1955.
176. Schulman, M. P., and Richert, D. A.: Utilization of glycine, succinate and δ-aminolevulinic acid for heme synthesis. Fed. Proc., *15*:349, 1956.
177. Schultze, M. O.: The relation of copper to cytochrome oxidase and hematopoietic activity of the bone marrow of rats. J. Biol. Chem., *138*:219, 1941.
178. Schwartz, H. C., Goudsmit, R., Hill, R. I., Cartwright, S. F., and Wintrobe, M. M.: The biosynthesis of hemoglobin from iron protoporphyrin and globin. J. Clin. Invest., *40*:188, 1961.
179. Schwartz, S., Gliekman, M., Hunter, R., and Wallace, J.: Plutonium project report. CH3720 AECD-2109 (1945) GC770, V.632.
180. Schwartz, S., and Wikoff, H. M.: The relation of erythrocyte coproporphyrin and protoporphyrin to erythropoiesis. J. Biol. Chem., *194*:563, 1952.
181. Shanley, B. C., Zail, S. S., and Joubert, S. M.: Effect of ethanol on liver delta-aminolaevulinate synthetase in rats. Lancet *1*:70, 1968.
182. Shemin, D.: The biosynthesis of porphyrins. Conference on Hemoglobin. National Academy of Sciences, National Research Council. Publ. 557, 1957, p. 66.
183. Shemin, D., Abramsky, T., and Russell, C. S.: The synthesis of protoporphyrin from δ-aminolevulinic acid in a cell-free extract. J. Am. Chem. Soc., 76:1204, 1954.
184. Shemin, D., Corcoran, J. W., Rosenblum, C., and Miller, I. M.: On the biosynthesis of the porphyrinlike moiety of vitamin B_{12}. Science, *124*:272, 1956.
185. Shemin, D., and Kumin, S. J.: The mechanism of porphyrin formation. The formation of a succinyl intermediate from succinate. J. Biol. Chem., *198*:827, 1952.

186. Shemin, D., and Rittenberg, D.: The utilization of glycine for the synthesis of a porphyrin. J. Biol. Chem., *159*:567, 1945.

187. Shemin, D., and Rittenberg, D.: The biological utilization of glycine for the synthesis of the protoporphyrin of hemoglobin. J. Biol. Chem., *166*:621, 1946.

188. Shemin, D., and Russell, C. S.: δ-Aminolevulinic acid, its role in the biosynthesis of porphyrins and purines. J. Am. Chem. Soc., *75*:4873, 1953.

189. Shemin, D., Russell, C. S., and Aramsky, T.: The surrinate-glycine cycle. I. The mechanism of pyrrole synthesis. J. Biol. Chem., *215*:613, 1955.

190. Shemin, D., and Wittenberg, J.: The mechanism of porphyrin formation. The role of the tricarboxylic acid cycle. J. Biol. Chem., *192*:315, 1951.

190a. Silber, R., and Goldstein, B. D.: Vitamin E and the hematopoietic system. Seminars Hemat., 7:40, 1970.

191. Smith, E. L.: Vitamin B_{12}. Brit. M. Bull., *12*:52, 1956.

192. Smithies, O.: Zone electrophoresis in starch gels; group variations in the serum proteins of normal human adults. Biochem. J., *61*:629, 1955.

193. Spector, H., Maass, A. R., Michaud, L., Elvehjem, C. A., and Hart, E. B.: The role of riboflavin in blood regeneration. J. Biol. Chem., *150*:75, 1943.

194. Stohlman, F., Jr.: Erythropoiesis. New England J. Med., *267*:342, 1962.

195. Stohlman, F., Jr.: The kidney and erythropoiesis. New England J. Med.,*279*:1437, 1968.

196. Stohlman, F., Jr., Lucarelli, G., Howard, D., Morse, B., and Leventhal, B.: Regulation of erythropoiesis. XVI. Cytokinetic patterns in disorders of erythropoiesis. Medicine, *43*:651, 1964.

196a. Terrhunen, R., Marver, H. S., and Schmid, R.: The enzymatic conversion of hemoglobin to bilirubin. Proc. Nat. Acad. Sc., *61*:748, 1968.

197. Thorell, B.: Studies on the formation of cellular substances during blood cell production. Acta med. scandinav., Suppl. 200, 1947.

198. Tschudy, D. P.: Biochemical lesions in porphyria. J.A.M.A., *191*:718, 1965.

199. Vogel, W., Richert, D. A., Pixley, B. Q., and Schulman, M. P.: Heme synthesis in iron deficient duck blood. J. Biol. Chem., *235*:1769, 1960.

200. Waldenstrom, J.: The porphyrias as inborn errors of metabolism. Am. J. Med., *22*:758, 1957.

201. Walsh, R. J., Thomas, E. D., Chow, S. K., Fluharty, R. G., and Finch, C. A.: Iron metabolism. Heme synthesis in vitro by immature erythrocytes. Science, *110*:396, 1949.

202. Ward, E., and Mason, H. L.: Free erythrocyte protoporphyrin. J. Clin. Invest., *29*:905, 1950.

203. Watson, C. J.: The erythrocyte coproporphyrin. Arch. Int. Med., *86*:797, 1950.

204. Watson, C. J.: Porphyrin metabolism in anemias. Arch. Int. Med., *99*:323, 1957.

205. Watson, C. J., and Larson, E. A.: The urinary coproporphyrins in health and disease. Physiol. Rev., *27*:478, 1947.

206. Watson, C. J., deMello, R. P., Schwartz, S., Hawkinson, V. E., and Bossenmaier, I.: Porphyrin chromogens or precursors in urine, blood, bile and feces. J. Lab. Clin. Med., *37*:831, 1951.

207. Watson, C. J., Runge, W., Taddeini, L., Bossenmaier, I., and Cardinal, R.: A suggested control gene mechanism for the excessive production of type I and III porphyrins in congenital erythropoietic porphyria. Proc. Nat. Acad. Sc., *52*:477, 1964.

208. Watson, C. J., Schulze, W., Hawkinson, V., and Baker, A. B.: Coproporphyrinuria (Type III) in acute poliomyelitis. Proc. Soc. Exper. Biol. & Med., *64*:73, 1947.

208a. Weatherall, J. D., and Clegg, J. B.: The control of human hemoglobin synthesis and function in health and disease. Prog. Hem., 6:261, 1969.

209. Whang, J., Frei, E., III, Tjio, J. H., Carbone, P. P., and Brecher, G.: The distribution of the Philadelphia chromosome in patients with chronic myelogenous leukemia. Blood, *22*:664, 1963.

210. Whipple, G. H., and Robscheit-Robbins, F. S.: Amino acids and hemoglobin production in anemia. J. Exper. Med., *71*:569, 1940.

211. Whipple, G. H., and Madden, S. C.: Hemoglobin, plasma protein and cell protein—their interchange and construction in emergencies. Medicine, *23*:215, 1944.

212. Whitaker, J. A., and Viett, T. J.: Fluorescence of the erythrocytes in lead poisoning in children: an aid to rapid diagnosis. Pediatrics, *24*:734, 1958.

213. Whitcomb, W. H., Moore, M., Dille, R., Hummer, L., and Bird, R. M.: Erythropoietin and erythropoiesis inhibitor activity in man. J. Clin. Invest., *44*:1110, 1965.

214. White, W. F., Gurney, C. W., Goldwasser, E., and Jacobson, L. O.: Studies on erthropoietin. Progr. Hormone Res., *16*:219, 1960.

215. Williams, R. T.: Biochemistry of vitamin B_{12}. Biochemical Society Symposia, 13, Cambridge University Press, London, 1955.

216. Wintrobe, M. M., Cartwright, G. E., and Gubler, C. J.: Studies on the function and metabolism of copper. J. Nutrition, *50*:395, 1953.

217. Wittenberg, J. B.: Formation of the porphyrin ring. Nature, *184*:876, 1959.

218. Wittenberg, J., and Shemin, D.: The location in protoporphyrin of the carbon atoms derived from the α-carbon atom of glycine. J. Biol. Chem., *185*:103, 1950.
219. Wong, K. K., Zanjani, E. S., Cooper, G. W., and Gordon, A. S.: The renal erythropoietic factor. V. Studies on its purification. Proc. Soc. Exp. Biol. & Med., *128*:67, 1968.
220. Wuepper, K. D., and Epstein, J. H.: Genetic study of erythropoietic protoporphyria (EPP). Clin. Res., *15*:256, 1969.
221. Yoneyama, Y., Okgama, H., Sugeta, Y., and Yoshikawa, H.: Formation in vitro of hemoglobin and myoglobin from iron protoporphyrin and globin in the presence of an iron chelating enzyme. Biochim. et biophys. acta, *74*:635, 1963.
222. Zail, S. S., and Joubert, S. M.: Hepatic delta-aminolaevulinic acid synthetase activity in symptomatic porphyria. Brit. J. Haem., *15*:123, 1968.
223. Zanjani, E. D., Contrera, J. F., Cooper, G. W., Gordon, A. S., and Wong, K. K.: Renal erythropoietic factor: Role of ions and vasoactive agents in erythropoietin formation. Science, *156*:1367, 1967.
224. Zanjani, E. D., Contrera, J. F., Gordon, A. S., Cooper, G. W., Wong, K. K., and Katz, R.: The renal erythropoietic factor (REF). III. Enzymatic role in the erythropoietin production. Proc. Soc. Exp. Biol. & Med., *125*:505, 1967.
225. Zieve, L., Hill, E., Schwartz, S., and Watson, C. J.: Normal limits of urinary coproporphyrin excretion determined by an improved method. J. Lab. Clin. Med., *41*:663, 1953.

III / Classification, Mechanisms, and Diagnosis of Anemia

The Classification of Anemia

Problems related to anemia constitute a large segment of investigative hematology and an appreciable part of any clinical practice. The present chapter is devoted to the classification of anemia and to brief discussions of the underlying mechanisms that are involved in each type of anemia. The different mechanisms are discussed briefly at this time to emphasize the importance of these fundamentals and to provide a basis for the development of a unifying, systematic approach to the various clinical syndromes. Discussions of the pathophysiology of anemia in the individual syndromes are given in more detail in Chapters IV through VIII.

Anemia may be defined as a reduction in the circulation of either hemoglobin or erythrocytes. It occurs whenever the hematopoietic equilibrium is disturbed and the loss of erythrocytes or hemoglobin from the circulation exceeds production.

Anemia is usually classified according to either causative factors or morphologic characteristics. Both classifications are important because neither is entirely satisfactory. Classification according to causative factors may be somewhat ambiguous because various details of a disease may be considered as "causes." Thus anemia may be "caused by" chronic blood loss; the blood loss may be due to several "causes," such as excessive vaginal bleeding and hemorrhoidal bleeding. Each of these types of bleeding may arise from one of several "causes," such as functional menorrhagia or uterine malignancy in one circumstance, and simple hemorrhoids or hemorrhoids associated with cirrhosis of the liver in the other. Difficulty in classification also arises if the mechanism is viewed as a "cause" when anemia results from more than one factor, such as increased destruction and diminished production of erythrocytes. Classification according to the morphologic characteristics of the erythrocytes is not entirely satisfactory either, because the same underlying disease may produce more than one type of anemia. "Aplastic" anemia may be normocytic or macrocytic; chronic bleeding may produce a simple microcytic type of anemia at one stage and a hypochromic microcytic type of anemia at another. Although each classification has shortcomings when used alone, all are very helpful in clinical hematology when they are used together. Determinations of the morphologic characteristics of the anemia and of the mechanism of its production are both important steps toward the identification of the underlying cause, which is the objective of diagnosis.

Morphologic classification. The morphologic classification of anemia is helpful in diagnosis because the characterization of the anemia according to the size and hemoglobin content of the erythrocytes directs the future investigation toward a definite group of possible causative factors or clinical syndromes and eliminates others from consideration. In order to classify anemia morphologically, it is necessary to determine the size and hemoglobin content of the erythrocytes. With the proper experience abnormalities in these details can be detected when a well prepared smear of the peripheral blood is examined carefully. In other circumstances the size and hemoglobin content of the erythrocytes can be determined most satisfactorily by the formulae devised by Wintrobe.[32]

$$\text{Mean Corpuscular Volume (MCV)} \atop \text{(in cubic microns, c.}\mu) = \frac{\text{Vol. packed red cells (in cc. per 1000 cc. blood)}}{\text{R.B.C. (in mil. per cu.mm.)}}$$

$$\text{Mean Corpuscular Hemoglobin (MCH)} \atop \text{(in micromicrograms, } \gamma\gamma) = \frac{\text{Hb. (in gm. per 1000 cc. blood)}}{\text{R.B.C. (in mil. per cu.mm.)}}$$

$$\text{Mean Corpuscular Hemoglobin Conc. (MCHC)} \atop \text{(in per cent, \%)} = \frac{\text{Hb. (in gm. per 100 cc.)} \times 100}{\text{Vol. packed R.B.C. (in cc. per 100 cc. blood)}}$$

Anemia may be classified according to cell size and hemoglobin content as shown in Table 3–1. When this method of determining cell size and hemo-

Table 3–1. Classification of Anemia According to Size and Hemoglobin Content of the Erythrocytes

Type	MCV (c.μ)	MCHC (%)
1. Macrocytic	> 94	> 30
2. Normocytic	80-94	> 30
3. Simple Microcytic	< 80	> 30
4. Hypochromic Microcytic	< 80	< 30

(From Wintrobe, M. M.: The size and hemoglobin content of the erythrocyte. J. Lab. & Clin. Med., *17*:899, 1932.)

globin content is employed it must be remembered that obtaining a result that is expressed numerically does not insure accuracy; an error in any of the determinations necessary for the calculations will lead to an erroneous result. Furthermore, the result is an average figure that does not reveal the differences that may exist among the individual cells.

Classification according to mechanism. If "cause" of the anemia is thought of in the restricted sense of the immediate cause or "mechanism," a workable classification of anemia can be devised. Such a classification helps the physician focus on this aspect of the problem and provides a sound basis for further systematic investigation or treatment. A classification of anemia according to causative mechanisms is presented in Table 3–2.

Mechanisms Responsible for Anemia

Diminished Erythropoiesis

When anemia results from diminished blood production, study of the peripheral blood usually reveals a normocytic or macrocytic anemia associated with a low or normal level of the reticulocytes. Leukopenia and thrombocytopenia are often present. If the diminished blood production is the result of vitamin B_{12} or folic acid deficiency, erythropoiesis is megaloblastic in type; if the anemia is due to other causes, erythropoiesis is normoblastic. Blood produc-

Table 3–2. *Classification of Anemia According to Mechanism of Production*

MECHANISM	CAUSE	DISEASE OR CLINICAL SYNDROME
I. DIMINISHED ERYTHROPOIESIS		
A. Nutritional Deficiency		
1. Diet	Inadequate intake	Multiple deficiencies
2. Defective absorption Stomach	Failure to secrete intrinsic factor	Vitamin B_{12} deficiency (Pernicious anemia)
	Total gastrectomy	
	Partial gastrectomy	Iron deficiency
Intestine	Diarrhea	Folic acid, vitamin B_{12}, or iron
	Diverticula	deficiency (Sprue, malabsorption
	Fistulae	syndrome, or pernicious
	Stricture	anemia)
3. Increased demand	Pregnancy	(Folic acid, vitamin B_{12}, or iron deficiency)
	Growth	Iron deficiency
B. Bone Marrow Failure	Associated disease	Primary disease
	Drugs	Aplastic anemia
	Chemicals	Aplastic anemia
	Irradiation	Aplastic anemia
	Endocrine	Myxedema, pituitary disease
	Idiopathic	Aplastic anemia
II. BLOOD LOSS		
A. Acute	Trauma or disease	Shock or anemia
B. Chronic	Lesion of gastrointestinal tract or gynecologic disturbance	Iron deficiency anemia or primary disease

Table 3-2. *Classification of Anemia According to Mechanism of Production (Continued)*

MECHANISM	CAUSE	DISEASE OR CLINICAL SYNDROME
III. INCREASED HEMOLYSIS A. Hereditary Hemolytic Disorders	Erythrocyte membrane defects	a. Hereditary spherocytosis b. Hereditary elliptocytosis c. Stomatocytosis d. Selective increase in membrane lecithin
	Pentose phosphate shunt–glutathione system enzyme deficiencies	a. Glucose-6-phosphate dehydrogenase b. Others: 6-phosphogluconate dehydrogenase, glutathione reductase, glutathione synthetase, glutathione peroxidase
	Glycolytic enzyme deficiencies	a. Pyruvate kinase deficiency b. Others: diphosphoglyceromutase, triosephosphate isomerase, phosphoglycerate kinase, glyceraldehyde-3-phosphate dehydrogenase, ATPase
	Hemoglobinopathy	a. Sickle cell anemia b. Hemoglobin C disease c. Thalassemia d. Combinations: sickle cell–hemoglobin C disease, sickle cell-thalassemia disease, and others e. Unstable hemoglobins: Zurich, Köln, Genova, Sydney, Hammersmith, Gun Hill, and others

B. Acquired Hemolytic Disorders	1. Antibody mediated
	  a. Isoantibodies
	
	  b. Drug-induced antibodies
	
	  c. Autoantibodies
		1a. Transfusion reactions; erythroblastosis fetalis
		1b. Quinidine sensitivity, penicillin sensitivity, alpha methyl dopa sensitivity
		1c. Idiopathic; secondary-malignancies, connective tissue disease, mycoplasma pneumonia, paroxysmal cold hemoglobinuria

	2. Mechanical hemolysis	2a. March hemoglobinuria 2b. Cardiac hemolytic anemia 2c. Microangiopathic hemolytic anemia
	3. Infections	3a. Malaria 3b. Pneumococcal pneumonia 3c. Septicemia 3d. Viral and bacterial infections
	4. Chemical agents	
	5. Physical agents	
	6. Hypersplenism	
	7. Uncertain	7a. Paroxysmal nocturnal hemoglobinuria

tion may be inadequate because of a deficiency of the factors that are essential for erythropoiesis or a failure of the bone marrow to utilize the essential substances although they are available.

Nutritional deficiency.   The factors essential for normal erythropoiesis are metals (cobalt, iron, copper), protein (certain amino acids), and vitamins (vitamin B_{12}, folic acid, ascorbic acid, pyridoxine, niacin and possibly riboflavin, pantothenic acid, and thiamine).[33] A deficiency of any one of these factors might be expected to produce anemia. In adults, only deficiencies of folic acid, vitamin B_{12}, iron, and ascorbic acid are important in the production of anemia.[33] A lack of amino acids appears to be an unlikely cause of anemia in man since amounts of these substances sufficient for erythropoiesis become available from some body source even when the serum protein levels and the protein intake are exceedingly low.[6] Nevertheless, kwashiorkor, a disease in infants characterized by severe protein deficiency and anemia, has been cited as evidence that protein deficiency can cause anemia, because iron, folic acid, and infection do not appear to be factors and protein feeding is followed by reticulocytosis and hematologic recovery. A deficiency of these essential factors may arise in various ways, such as faulty diet, defective absorption, or excessive demands for erythropoiesis.

Faulty diet is responsible for anemia in various parts of the world in usual or unusual circumstances; the intake of iron, folate, protein, or even vitamin B_{12} may be inadequate. In the United States dietary deficiency produces anemia in infants, but in adults, except in food faddists or alcoholics, nutritional deficiency rarely causes anemia unless other factors operate to produce a conditioned or secondary deficiency. When anemia occurs in adults because of faulty diet, the anemia is usually the result of folic acid deficiency, possibly because of the large body reserves of vitamin B_{12} and iron. Finch has concluded that protein malnutrition is associated with a mild normochromic anemia. There is good evidence that marrow function remains intact but that there is a decrease in stimulation of the erythroid marrow. This decrease in erythropoietin stimulus is a natural consequence of the reduction in oxygen requirements in the protein depleted individual.[16a]

Defective absorption is a common cause of nutritional anemia in adults. In pernicious anemia vitamin B_{12} deficiency arises in this manner as a result of defective gastric function and the failure to secrete the intrinsic factor that is essential for the normal absorption of vitamin B_{12}. A similar disorder is produced by total gastrectomy, a procedure that removes the tissue that secretes the intrinsic factor. In this circumstance the deficiency does not appear for several years after gastrectomy. Macrocytic anemia associated with a megaloblastic type of erythropoiesis that is characteristic of vitamin B_{12} or folic acid deficiency sometimes occurs in sprue or other diseases accompanied by severe diarrhea or other abnormalities which may lead to malabsorption. A similar anemia due to vitamin B_{12} deficiency that is refractory to oral treatment yet responsive to parenteral therapy has been reported in patients with diverticula, strictures, and fistulae of the small intestine. Iron deficiency anemia often occurs several years after partial gastrectomy. Investigation of such patients has shown that the iron deficiency in this circumstance is probably at least partly the result of an inability to absorb iron that is contained in food although the ability to absorb medicinal iron may be normal.[27]

Excessive demands for erythropoiesis may produce a deficiency of essential factors if the reserve stores of the body have been depleted, even though the normal dietary intake has been maintained. During pregnancy anemia sometimes occurs because of iron deficiency that is the result of the added demands of fetal erythropoiesis; a similar type of anemia is seen in some children because of the increased need for iron to meet the increase in blood volume that accompanies body growth. A deficiency of folic acid, or more rarely of vitamin B_{12}, develops in some women during pregnancy, particularly in those who have a poor diet or suffer from severe gastrointestinal upsets. Depletion of the body reserves of folic acid may lead to megaloblastic erythropoiesis in severe hemolytic anemia.

Bone marrow failure. Even if adequate amounts of all the substances required for erythropoiesis are ingested and absorbed normally, erythropoiesis may be inadequate because of defective function of the bone marrow. Inadequate erythropoiesis is responsible for the occurrence of anemia in a number of circumstances, in the presence of chronic disease, after the ingestion of drugs, after exposure to chemicals, after irradiation, or in endocrine diseases; in many patients the disease is "idiopathic."

Diseases of long duration such as chronic infections, particularly if accompanied by fever, and various metabolic disorders, such as the uremic state, often depress erythropoiesis. The decreased marrow activity is reflected by diminished iron utilization and reduced production of young red cells. Although all of the factors that are responsible for the depression of marrow activity are not known, some important details have been established. The plasma of uremic rabbits has been shown to contain a lower than normal quantity of the erythropoietic factor, and uremic rabbits have been shown to be less responsive than normal to injection of plasma rich in erythropoietin.[16] Bone marrow cultures from uremic patients have been shown to have lower iron utilization than cultures from normal individuals.[30] In other diseases, such as carcinomatosis, disseminated tuberculosis, and leukemia, actual mechanical encroachment on the erythropoietic tissue may be a factor in the anemia, although it is rarely the sole mechanism.

Drugs act to depress the bone marrow in various ways. Anemia may occur alone but more often it occurs in combination with leukopenia or thrombocytopenia. Some drugs depress the bone marrow, which is a tissue composed of rapidly dividing cells, by their pharmacologic action which interferes with nucleic acid metabolism and inhibits cell division or maturation. In this category are the various alkylating agents. Other drugs produce depression of hematopoiesis only in certain susceptible individuals. Marrow depression, which may be either temporary or permanent, may occur without warning. Reactions of this type have been reported to follow exposure to a variety of coal tar products, antibiotics, anticonvulsants, and heavy metals.

Chemicals that are employed in various industries and occupations may damage the bone marrow in the same manner as chemicals used as drugs. Usually an element of individual susceptibility is a factor. The chemicals that have been incriminated most often are organic solvents, particularly benzol and its derivatives. Exposure to chemicals often occurs through the use of cleaning agents, herbicides, or insecticide sprays.

Ionizing radiation from x-rays or radioactive materials causes anemia by depression of erythropoiesis if the bone marrow is exposed sufficiently. During roentgen ray therapy, or after the use of radioactive isotopes, the full hematologic effect may not be evident until several weeks after exposure. With the carefully calculated daily and total dosages that are used in irradiation therapy, permanent damage rarely results because therapy is rarely continued for more than several weeks at a time. Although the exact mechanism of action of irradiation is incompletely understood at present, it is known that cell multiplication is suppressed, possibly by inhibition of nucleic acid synthesis.[25]

Hormones. Both the pituitary gland and the thyroid gland are important in erythopoiesis. This is shown by the development of anemia after removal of either of the glands in animals and by the occurrence of anemia in patients with hypopituitarism and myxedema. The anemia in myxedema, which is rarely severe, probably represents an adjustment to the decreased body metabolism comparable to the effect produced by exposure to increased oxygen tension rather than a deficiency of the thyroid hormone per se.[4]

"Idiopathic" aplastic anemia. In some patients no explanation can be found for the bone marrow failure that is responsible for severe anemia. There is no history of unusual exposure to drugs, chemicals, or irradiation, and no evidence of an associated disease that might cause bone marrow depression. A congenital defect has been postulated for the disorder that occurs in infants and very young children, but aplastic anemia also develops in adults. The marrow hypoplasia is usually associated with pancytopenia, but in some patients anemia occurs alone; in others, the anemia is accompanied by either leukopenia or thrombocytopenia. Theoretically the marrow failure may be due either to the lack of some factor necessary for erythropoiesis or to the inability of the cells to respond to the factor or factors that normally stimulate erythropoiesis. Against the first possibility is the evidence that the plasma of adult patients with aplastic anemia contains large amounts of erythropoietin; such plasma induces an erythropoietic response when injected into hypophysectomized test animals.[17] These observations suggest that the hematopoietic cells have been damaged in some way and are unable to respond normally to stimuli. The observation that extramedullary hematopoiesis rarely occurs in aplastic anemia and occurs often when there is encroachment on the marrow by other tissue, such as carcinoma or fibrosis, also favors this interpretation.

Blood Loss

Acute blood loss usually results in a normocytic, normochromic type of anemia. Although the total blood volume falls immediately after hemorrhage, the hematocrit determination may not reflect the degree of blood loss until 48 hours have elapsed. In persons with a responsive bone marrow, acute hemorrhage, which affords a well known stimulus to erythropoiesis, is usually followed by an increase in platelets, leukocytes, and reticulocytes.

Chronic blood loss is a common cause of anemia. Bleeding of this type nearly always results in a deficiency of iron which, when severe, is characterized by a hypochromic microcytic anemia associated with normoblastic erythropoiesis in the bone marrow. In milder degrees of anemia due to deficiency of iron, hypochromia and microcystosis are absent.

Increased Hemolysis

The normal survival time of the circulating erythrocyte as determined by the Ashby, chromium[51], N[15]-glycine, and diisopropylfluorophosphate methods is about 120 days.[1a] Hemolytic anemia occurs whenever a decreased survival time of the erythrocytes is not balanced by increased erythropoiesis. A decrease in survival time of the erythrocytes to less than 20 days may be necessary to produce anemia if the bone marrow is functioning normally since the bone marrow has the capacity to increase its production of erythrocytes sixfold.[9] Unless erythropoiesis is depressed for some reason, hemolytic anemia is characterized by both increased hemolysis and increased erythropoiesis.

Several different pathogenic mechanisms may cause a diminution in the survival time of erythrocytes. These mechanisms can be conveniently classified as "intracorpuscular" or "extracorpuscular." "Intracorpuscular" defects, which are intrinsic in the erythrocytes produced by the patient, result in a diminished survival time of the patient's erythrocytes in his own circulation and also after transfusion into a normal compatible recipient. "Extracorpuscular" factors are different in that they are part of the environment that the erythrocytes encounter in the patient's circulation; normal erythrocytes have a diminished survival when transfused into the patient but the erythrocytes produced by the patient survive for the normal time when transfused into a normal recipient. Intracorpuscular defects are generally congenital, the result of some inherited disorder. Extracorpuscular defects are usually acquired as the result of some associated disease or disorder. In some patients the hemolytic anemia is the result of a combination of intracorpuscular and extracorpuscular abnormalities.

Hereditary defects (usually intracorpuscular). **Hereditary spherocytosis (congenital hemolytic jaundice).** Hereditary spherocytosis is inherited as a Mendelian dominant[35] and is characterized by erythrocytes that have a thickness/diameter ratio greater than normal. The cells are abnormally susceptible to hypotonic saline and the tendency of the cells to undergo lysis is increased by incubation. Studies have demonstrated that although there is an inherited "intrinsic" defect in the erythrocytes in hereditary spherocytosis, the decreased survival time of the red cells is the result of their sequestration and destruction by the spleen, and for this reason splenectomy cures the hemolytic anemia in nearly all patients even though the defect in the erythrocytes—spherocytosis—persists.

Thalassemia (Cooley's anemia, Mediterranean anemia). Thalassemia is a rare, inherited disorder that is found most often in families of Mediterranean origin. It may be manifested by different syndromes that vary in severity from mild hematologic abnormalities to severe anemia. A prominent feature of the disorder is the occurrence of hypochromic microcytes that are abnormally thin (leptocytes). These cells have the appearance of "target cells" on the stained blood smear and are abnormally resistant to hypotonic saline. The alterations that are responsible for the leptocytosis and the method of destruction of the cells in the patient, which occurs in the absence of the spleen, are unknown. Although the main defect in this disease is intracorpuscular, in some patients there is an additional extracorpuscular mechanism associated with the splenomegaly that leads to premature destruction of even normal cells that are transfused. Hemoglobin analysis has revealed an increase in fetal hemoglobin (HbF) and hemoglobin A_2 in some of the different thalassemic syndromes.

Hemoglobinopathies. Pauling, Itano, Singer, and Wells made the important discovery that the sickling phenomenon in sickle cell disease is due to a pathologic difference in the hemoglobin molecule that could be demonstrated by electrophoresis.[26] The difference between these hemoglobin molecules is in the globin portion and not in the heme fraction. The determination of the type of hemoglobin is genetically controlled. Normal adult hemoglobin contains two normal alpha chains and two normal beta chains and is written as alpha-2, beta-2 ($\alpha_2\beta_2$). Fetal hemoglobin is alpha-2, gamma-2 ($\alpha_2\gamma_2$) and A_2 hemoglobin is (alpha-2, delta-2) ($\alpha_2\delta_2$). Numerous abnormal hemoglobins have been reported, usually a result of a genetic defect in the synthesis of the alpha or beta chains. These, which can be identified by hemoglobin electrophoresis or other special tests, are discussed in Chapter VII. When the abnormal hemoglobin occurs in the heterozygous state along with normal adult hemoglobin, a non-symptomatic "trait" condition usually results. When the abnormal hemoglobin is present in the homozygous state, or when an individual is heterozygous for two abnormal hemoglobin types, a clinical disease characterized by a hemolytic disorder of the intracorpuscular type usually occurs (Fig. 3–1).

Glucose-6-phosphate dehydrogenase (G-6-PD) deficiency (primaquine sensitivity). Glucose-6-phosphate dehydrogenase (G-6-PD) deficiency in red cells has been studied extensively. It has been shown that the hemolytic anemia induced by primaquine is due to a metabolic defect that renders the cells susceptible to the drug.[14] This drug sensitivity, which has a familial distribution, is seen rarely in whites but occurs in about 10 per cent of the American blacks. Investigations have established that an inherited abnormality in cellular physiology is responsible not only for primaquine sensitivity, but also for the sensitivity that is concerned in the hemolytic anemia occurring in some individuals after the ingestion of sulfonamide drugs, fava beans, and other compounds, such as phenylhydrazine and naphthalene.[29] The clinical disease occurs as a result of the action of one of the extrinsic factors on erythrocytes that are susceptible because of an intrinsic hereditary defect.

Acquired hemolytic disorders. **Paroxysmal nocturnal hemoglobinuria (Marchiafava-Micheli syndrome).** Paroxysmal nocturnal hemoglobinuria is a rare acquired hemolytic disorder that is characterized by intravascular hemolysis and hemoglobinuria which is usually more marked during or immediately after sleep. The disease is an acquired one characterized by the production of erythrocytes with defective membranes; it sometimes appears in patients who have, or have had, aplastic anemia.

Auto-immune hemolytic anemias. Auto-immune hemolytic anemias are characterized by the production of antibodies that have the ability to act on the patient's own corpuscles. In most instances these "auto-antibodies" also act as iso-antibodies and react with other normal human erythrocytes to some degree. Hemolytic anemias of this type are acquired, and from a clinical standpoint

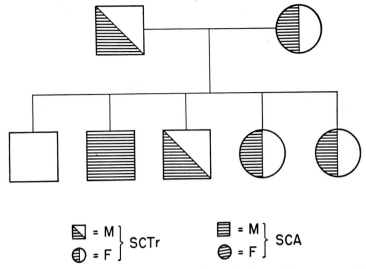

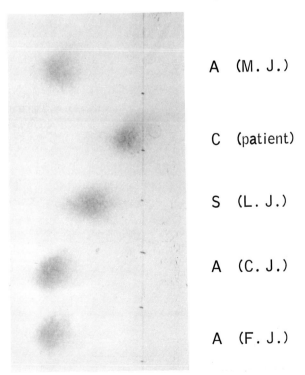

Figure 3–1. Heredity in sickle cell disease. Study of the hemoglobin types in a family which illustrates the results that occurred from the mating of parents who were heterozygous for hemoglobin S.

Figure 3–2. Example of hemoglobin electrophoresis showing characteristic mobilities of homozygous hemoglobins A, C, and S using filter paper as a supporting medium with a Veronal buffer at pH 8.6. Cathode to the right.

may be classified as (1) idiopathic (cause unknown), or (2) symptomatic (occurring in association with some other disease, such as malignant lymphoma, leukemia, virus pneumonia, or collagen disease). From a serologic standpoint the antibodies may be classified as "cold" antibodies, which are markedly potentiated by cold, or "warm" antibodies, which act in vitro at 37° at least as well as at lower temperatures.[12] The presence of the auto-antibodies of both the warm and cold types (which are absorbed on the patient's erythrocytes) is shown best by the antiglobulin (Coombs) test. During clinical remission the presence of auto-antibodies in the patient's serum can sometimes be demonstrated by testing with trypsinized cells when the indirect antiglobulin test is negative.[11]

Iso-immune hemolytic disease.   Iso-antibodies are the naturally occurring antibodies such as anti-A and anti-B, and those that develop in response to the stimulus afforded by exposure to erythrocytes of other blood groups. These antibodies do not affect the patient's own erythrocytes. Iso-immune hemolytic disease occurs as a result of the incompatibility of the blood group antigens. It occurs as a result of mismatched transfusions involving the ABO system, the Rh system, and other groups, when the individual's serum contains antibodies for the other blood group agglutinogens. A similar mechanism is responsible for the hemolytic disease of the newborn, erythroblastosis fetalis. The most severe disease occurs when the mother is Rh-negative (lacks the D antigen) and the fetus is Rh-positive (has the D antigen), but it also occurs in some instances of ABO incompatibility. The mother develops antibodies against the red cells of the fetus and the antibodies pass through the placenta to destroy erythrocytes in the fetal circulation.

Paroxysmal cold hemoglobinuria.   Paroxysmal cold hemoglobinuria is a very rare disease characterized by sudden attacks of intravascular hemolysis and hemoglobinuria. It has been considered to be a manifestation of syphilis, but its occurrence in patients in whom syphilis has been excluded has led to the suggestion that in some patients the positive serologic tests for syphilis are false-positive reactions that have occurred in the presence of the antibody of paroxysmal cold hematuria.[11]

Infectious agents.   Hemolytic anemia may occur as a result of a variety of infections. Among these are septicemia due to Cl. welchii, staphylococci, streptococci, and infections due to Vibrio cholerae. Hemolytic anemia has also been reported in various types of tuberculosis, bacterial endocarditis, and influenzal meningitis. In malaria, destruction of the erythrocytes occurs as a consequence of the localization of the parasites within the red cells. The severe fulminating hemolytic anemia, "blackwater fever," that sometimes occurs in infections with Plasmodium falciparum may be due in part to antibodies that are produced as a result of quinine ingestion.[13] A severe acute hemolytic anemia occurs in Oroya fever, which is caused by infection with the Bartonella bacillus. Viruses may produce hemolytic anemia either by a direct action on the erythrocytes or by the induction of antibodies that damage the cells.

Chemical agents.   Drugs and other chemicals may produce hemolytic anemia in a variety of ways. Some, such as penicillin, damage the red cells directly when large doses are given. Others, such as alpha-methyldopa, appear to cause an alteration in the red cell membrane that leads to its destruction by antibodies. Still others induce the formation of antibodies to the drug which become attached to the red cell, damage it, and cause its premature destruction. The degree of hemolysis that follows the ingestion of some compounds, such as phenylhydrazine and naphthalene (moth balls), is related to the amount consumed. Other compounds, such as sulfonamides, quinine, and primaquine, cause hemolytic anemia because of an inherited enzymatic defect in the erythrocyte.[1b, 29]

Physical agents. Hemolytic anemia, which is sometimes severe, occurs in extensive burns. As a result of damage to the erythrocytes by heat, the red corpuscles become more susceptible to trauma in the circulation and to stagnation in the tissues.[18] Increased hemolysis has been demonstrated during the first week in burns and is severe in third degree burns of more than 20 per cent.[21] In addition, N^{15}-glycine studies of hemoglobin production have shown that marked depression of erythropoiesis occurs about 10 days after the injury, at a time when the hemolytic anemia might be expected to lead to increased erythropoiesis.[20]

Hemolytic anemia develops in some patients who have had heart-valve prosthetic surgery and also in some patients with severe valvular disease who have not been operated upon. The anemia is the result of trauma, the turbulence and shearing forces that damage the red cells. The anemia is characterized by intravascular hemolysis and morphologic changes in the erythrocytes — burr cells, helmet cells, and schistocytes.

"Microangiopathic haemolytic anemia" is the name given to a type of severe hemolytic anemia seen in some patients with uremia, disseminated carcinoma, or thrombotic thrombocytopenic purpura.[5] The smear of the peripheral blood contains many poikilocytes — burr cells, helmet cells, and triangular cells; it has been suggested that these deformities and the shortened life span of the cells are the result of trauma sustained in the abnormal small blood vessels.

The inclusive term "impact hemolysis" has been suggested for the hemolytic anemia that occurs in valvular disease, small vessel disease, and march hemoglobinuria.

Vegetable poisons. A severe hemolytic anemia known as favism occurs in some individuals as the result of the ingestion of the bean Vicia fava. Most of the cases have occurred in Italy and Sardinia but cases have also been seen in other Mediterranean countries and the Middle East. Favism was formerly considered to be a manifestation of allergic sensitization.[11] Recent studies indicate that individuals who are susceptible to the fava bean have a constitutional anomaly of the erythrocytes, glucose-6-phosphate dehydrogenase deficiency, similar to that found in patients who are sensitive to primaquine and other drugs. Since some persons apparently do not develop the hemolytic anemia until after the second exposure to the offending drug or the fava bean, it has been postulated that at times both the enzyme deficiency and the sensitization to the noxious agent are necessary to produce hemolysis.[29]

Hypersplenism. Hemolytic anemia sometimes develops in patients who have splenomegaly when no auto-antibodies or other abnormal hemolytic mechanisms can be demonstrated by the usual tests. The usual features of hemolytic anemia may be present, but on occasions during the management of a patient with anemia by means of transfusions an increased demand for transfusions is the main clinical evidence of the hyperhemolysis. In some patients leukopenia and thrombocytopenia of considerable severity also occur. The reductions in the cellular elements of the circulating blood are associated with an apparently active bone marrow. Splenectomy is sometimes beneficial and the syndrome has been termed "hypersplenism." A primary disorder of this type appears to be extremely rare, if it exists. The syndrome is seen with spleno-megaly that occurs in many different diseases such as cirrhosis, portal vein thrombosis, diseases of the lymphoma group, collagen disorders, fungus dis-ease, tuberculosis, and other infections. The mechanism of the hyperhemolysis is unknown. The increased destruction of the erythrocytes may be related to the circulatory stasis in the enlarged spleen in some way. In some patients with tropical or non-tropical splenomegaly an increase in plasma volume rather than a decrease in the circulating red cell mass reduces hematocrit values in the peripheral blood.

Hemopathic hemolytic anemia.   The term hemopathic hemolytic anemia has been suggested for the hemolytic anemia that occurs in various disease states such as uremia, carcinoma, leukemia, and infections when no abnormal antibodies can be demonstrated.[31] The anemia is the result of a shortened sur-vival time of the erythrocytes associated with an inadequate marrow response. The presence of a hemolytic element has been established by cell survival studies and the subnormal response of the marrow has been shown by the absence of reticulocytosis or increased iron utilization.

Hemolytic anemia associated with liver disease.   An acute type of hemolytic anemia has been observed in acute hepatic necrosis without evidence of auto-immunization.[11] Chronic hemolytic anemia that is due to an extracor-puscular mechanism has been found to be the commonest type of anemia in chronic liver disease.[7, 22]

Diagnosis of the Patient with Anemia

The objectives in the management of the patient with anemia are, first, the discovery of the cause of the anemia, and, second, correction of the underlying defect. It is important to remember that the demonstration of "anemia" does not constitute a diagnosis but merely the recognition of a sign comparable to fever or edema. For this reason the seriousness of the anemia in any patient depends on the underlying cause of the anemia rather than the severity of the anemia. A mild degree of anemia caused by a carcinoma of the gastrointestinal tract is a serious affair for the patient but a severe degree of anemia from hemorrhoidal bleeding is not. Treatment of a patient with iron, or vitamins, or blood trans-fusions *without first making a diagnosis* other than "anemia" may jeopardize his chances of recovery. Anemia that is the result of iron deficiency secondary to blood loss from a carcinoma of the cecum may respond to iron salts orally or to blood transfusions while the carcinoma changes from a curable to an incurable lesion. In situations in which the underlying cause cannot be corrected, accurate diagnosis is still essential for proper management. Unless this fact is recognized a patient with a macrocytic anemia may be "cured" of his anemia by treatment with the folic acid present in many multivitamin preparations but the central nervous system lesions may progress and become irreversible if the patient is suffering from vitamin B_{12} deficiency.

A systematic investigation of the patient with suspected anemia nearly always provides the information necessary for the correct diagnosis and proper treatment. This investigation aims to provide answers to the following questions:

1. Does the patient have anemia?
2. What are the morphologic characteristics of the anemia?
3. What is the mechanism of the anemia?
4. What is the underlying cause or disease that is responsible for the abnormal mechanism?
5. What is the best form of treatment?

Although it is at times impossible to establish a complete diagnosis in a patient with anemia, in the vast majority of patients it is possible to classify the anemia according to the responsible mechanism, as due either to deficient production, blood loss, or increased hemolysis. This is usually possible by the use of relatively simple laboratory procedures that can be performed in the physician's office or the hospital laboratory. If the physician understands the mechanism that is responsible for the anemia, he is in a position to manage the patient intelligently by administering the proper treatment or by planning any further investigation that may be necessary to identify the disorder that is responsible for the abnormal mechanism.

The answer to the question "Does the patient have anemia?" often cannot be gained from the history or the physical examination. Anemia of moderate severity may not be detected even by careful inspection of the skin and mucous membranes. In another circumstance a neurasthenic individual with pallor of the skin and mucous membranes may report all of the symptoms of anemia even though the blood is entirely normal. The presence of anemia can be established only by laboratory procedures. The simplest and most reliable screening procedure is the hematocrit determination;[2] the normal range given for adult males is 40 to 54 per cent and for adult females 37 to 47 per cent. Other lower limits of normal of the hematocrit and hemoglobin are given in Table 3–3.[8] The hemoglobin determination, which has an accuracy comparable to that of the hematocrit if it is performed properly, is also advocated as a screen-

Table 3–3. Lower Limits of Normal Hematocrit and Hemoglobin at Sea Level

Years	Sex	Hemoglobin (gm 100 ml.)	Packed Cell Volume (%)
0.6–4	Both sexes	11	33
5–9	Both sexes	11.5	34.5
10–14	Both sexes	12	36
Adults	Men	14	42
	Women	12	36
	Pregnant women	11	33

(Reprinted from J.A.M.A., *203*:119, 1968.)

ing procedure by some authors.[3] In our experience the hematocrit determination has proved satisfactory, but even this procedure is far from infallible. Misleading values may be obtained if the blood is drawn from a vein subjected to too much stasis, if an improper amount of anticoagulant is used, or if centrifugation is faulty. The volume of packed cells is also influenced by the osmotic pressure in the plasma; low levels of serum electrolytes cause a rise in the hematocrit, and elevations cause a fall. Even if the techniques are not faulty, values in the normal range may be obtained occasionally in patients with either macrocytic anemia or iron deficiency anemia of mild degree. We have seen a patient with pernicious anemia and involvement of the central nervous system who had a hematocrit of 42 per cent, a hemoglobin of 14.3 gm. per 100 ml., and an erythrocyte count of 3.3 mil. per cu.mm. An analogous difficulty has been encountered in patients with iron deficiency when the hematocrit was 40 per cent, the red blood count 5.0 mil. per cu.mm., and the hemoglobin 8.0 gm. per 100 ml. Such unusual occurrences do not detract seriously from the usefulness of the hematocrit as a screening test because the use of either the hemoglobin determination or erythrocyte count alone as a screening procedure is subject to the same limitations. An increased plasma volume which occurs in some patients with splenomegaly and some with increased plasma proteins, produces subnormal values of the hematocrit. In this circumstance determinations of the plasma volume and the total circulating red cell mass are necessary for an accurate evaluation.

In order to answer the question "What is the mechanism responsible for the anemia?" a careful history, a physical examination, and certain laboratory tests that reveal the morphologic and other characteristics of the blood are necessary. Laboratory procedures have assumed the most prominent place in the diagnosis of hematologic problems but his does not mean that a carefully taken history is not important. Without the benefit of a complete history the laboratory results may be puzzling or even misleading.

The history.   When the history is obtained the patient should be allowed to give his account of his illness first and then he should be questioned about various details. A family history of anemia or splenectomy or a past history of recurrent episodes of anemia may be helpful, particularly if the patient has hemolytic anemia. The dietary history is important in children, in pregnancy, and in chronic illness for it is in these circumstances that a dietary deficiency is most likely to become manifest. The history of the use of "tonics" and vitamins may help clarify an anemia that is difficult to classify because the hematologic features characteristic of the underlying disease or syndrome have been altered by such preparations. Repeated exposures to drugs or chemicals encountered in the patient's occupation or in the pursuit of a hobby may be a factor in the causation of anemia. A careful review of the body systems should be part of the history taking because systematic questioning of this type may elicit important symptoms, such as paresthesias, mild ataxia, excessive menstrual bleeding, or even tarry stools, that have not been volunteered by the patient.

Physical examination.   Although the physical examination alone rarely if ever suffices for the complete diagnosis of anemia, nearly any part of the examination may contribute important information. The appearance of hemorrhages and exudates in the fundi may be the first indication that the patient has bacterial endocarditis, leukemia, uremia, or aplastic anemia. The presence of tumor masses, lymphadenopathy, hepatomegaly, or splenomegaly may bring the diseases of the reticuloendothelial system into consideration for the first time. Most hemolytic anemias, with the exception of sickle cell anemia, are associated with splenomegaly. Splenomegaly is unusual in untreated aplastic anemia and the detection of an enlarged spleen makes some other diagnosis more likely. An appraisal of the nutritional state of the patient, the color of the tongue, the appearance of the papillae, the presence of fissuring of the lips, and the texture of the fingernails may give clues to the presence of a deficiency of folic acid, vitamin B_{12}, or iron. The detection of telangiectases on the skin or mucous membranes may give the first clue to an explanation of gastrointestinal hemorrhage. Even the general appearance of the patient, the tone of his voice, and his manner of speaking may lead to the recognition of myxedema as the cause of an undiagnosed case of anemia that has proved refractory to the usual forms of "antianemic" therapy. The demonstration of mild ataxia or decreased vibratory sense in the extremities may be the first indication that the patient has pernicious anemia, particularly if the hematologic picture has been altered by inadequate specific therapy or by coexisting iron deficiency.

Laboratory studies. Examination of the peripheral blood by laboratory methods is a most important step in the identification of the mechanism that is responsible for the anemia. If the hematocrit value is low, the following procedures are indicated: determination of the hemoglobin; erythrocyte count; leukocyte count; and a study of the stained blood smear. Study of a well made and stained smear of the peripheral blood, once the main reliance of the hematologist, declined in popularity after determination of red cell indices, study of aspirated bone marrow, and other hematological examinations were introduced. Nevertheless, careful study of the leukocytes, erythrocytes, and platelets in the peripheral blood should be an important part of the examination of every patient suspected of having a hematologic disorder.

The leukocyte count can be estimated with considerable accuracy, and most cases of leukemia can be recognized by the number or immaturity of the leukocytes. In addition other abnormalities, although not diagnostic of a disease, give valuable information. Abnormalities of the lymphocytes suggest infectious mononucleosis or other viral infections. Multi-segmented polys or macropolycytes should make one suspect a deficiency of vitamin B_{12} or folate. Young cells of the granulocytic series accompanied by nucleated red cells and marked poikilocytosis, particularly the presence of teardrop forms, indicate myeloid metaplasia or leukemia.

The appearance of the erythrocytes also deserves careful scrutiny. Sickle cells and ovalocytes are practically diagnostic; large oval macrocytes are almost pathognomonic for vitamin B_{12} or folate deficiency, as is the appearance of megaloblasts in the circulating blood. Microspherocytes, helmet cells, schistocytes, polychromatophilic cells, and anisocytosis indicate the presence of a hemolytic anemia of some sort. Marked poikilocytosis is strong evidence against aplastic anemia. Hypochromic microcytes and anisocytosis suggest iron deficiency but are not diagnostic because they also occur in some patients with iron loading anemia and defective hemoglobin metabolism. Target cells occur in hemoglobinopathies and in some patients with liver disease. Rouleaux forma-

Table 3–4. *Laboratory Procedures Often Helpful in the Study of a Patient with Anemia*

USUAL INITIAL STUDIES
Hematocrit determination
Hemoglobin determination
Erythrocyte count
Reticulocyte count
Study of stained blood smear
Leukocyte count and differential count
Platelet count (or estimate from blood smear)

SUSPECTED IRON DEFICIENCY
Stool for occult blood
Serum iron and latent iron binding capacity
Stain of marrow preparations for iron
Roentgenographic study of the gastrointestinal tract

SUSPECTED VITAMIN B₁₂ OR FOLIC ACID DEFICIENCY
Bone marrow
Gastric analysis after histamine injection
Vitamin B₁₂ absorption test (radioactive cobalt) *schilling's test*
Serum vitamin B₁₂ level
Serum folate level
Roentgenographic study of the gastrointestinal tract

SUSPECTED HEMOLYTIC ANEMIA
Bone marrow
Serum bilirubin level
Fecal urobilinogen excretion
LDH determination
Test for sickling
Hemoglobin electrophoresis
Antiglobulin (Coombs) test
Hypotonic saline fragility test
Autohemolysis test
Alkali denaturation test
Hemoglobin determination, plasma and urine; urine hemosiderin
Cr⁵¹ tagging to determine erythrocyte survival and sequestration in the spleen
Screening tests for enzyme deficiencies

SUSPECTED APLASTIC ANEMIA
Bone marrow (aspiration or biopsy)
Skeletal roentgenograms
Serum iron and latent iron binding capacity
Mediastinal roentgenograms for thymoma
Radioiron to determine plasma iron clearance, iron utilization, and iron turnover

OTHER TESTS OFTEN USED ESPECIALLY TO DIAGNOSE THE PRIMARY DISEASE
"L.E." preparation
Blood urea
Tissue biopsy (skin, lymph node, liver)
Peroxidase stain
Plasma electrophoresis
Urine electrophoresis
Bone marrow

tion probably indicates hyperglobulinemia and should be investigated by a study for multiple myeloma or macroglobulinemia.

Thrombocytopenia can be recognized in a peripheral smear, and a study of the other cellular elements may help to identify the cause as aplastic anemia, leukemia, or viral infection. Thrombocytosis and large, bizarre-shaped platelets suggest a myeloproliferative disorder. A stain for reticulocytes affords a generally reliable indication of the erythropoietic activity of the bone marrow.

With the results of the hemoglobin, hematocrit, and erythrocyte determination the mean corpuscular volume (MCV), mean corpuscular hemoglobin (MCH), and mean corpuscular hemoglobin concentration (MCHC) can be determined and the anemia can be classified according to cell size and hemoglobin content as:

macrocytic (MCV > 94 c.μ) (MCHC > 30 per cent)
normocytic (MCV 80-94 c.μ) (MCHC > 30 per cent)
microcytic (MCV < 80 c.μ) (MCHC > 30 per cent)
hypochromic (MCV > 80 c.μ) (MCHC < 30 per cent)
hypochromic microcytic (MCV < 80 c.μ)[32] (MCHC < 30 per cent)

The method of calculating these values is given on page 57. The characterization of the anemia as macrocytic, normocytic, microcytic, or hypochromic microcytic provides a guide to other appropriate studies that are necessary to determine the mechanism and cause of the anemia. The determination of the cell size and hemoglobin content by such calculations does not mean that a careful study of the blood smear is unimportant; study of the smear gives valuable information that may not be apparent in the calculations. A list of the studies that are often helpful is presented in Table 3–4.

Macrocytic Anemia

If the patient is found to have macrocytic anemia of significant degree (MCV > 100 c.μ) it is unlikely that acute hemorrhage has occurred and for practical purposes chronic blood loss may be eliminated from consideration. A macrocytic anemia is usually due primarily to deficient blood production. Less often a hemolytic mechanism is responsible. Macrocytic anemia is most likely to be seen in the following circumstances: deficiency of vitamin B_{12} or folic acid; "aplastic" anemia; myxedema; and hemolytic anemia.

Deficiency of vitamin B_{12} and folic acid. If the macrocytosis is due to a deficiency of vitamin B_{12} there is usually leukopenia and thrombocytopenia, often of mild degree. If the anemia is moderate or severe in degree, the blood smear reveals considerable anisocytosis and poikilocytosis and shows oval macrocytes and large multisegmented neutrophils. In the untreated patient the normal or subnormal reticulocyte count reflects the failure of a normal response to anemia. The slightly elevated level of indirect reacting serum bilirubin and the increased fecal urobilinogen excretion reflect the increased destruction of erythrocytes in the peripheral circulation or in the bone marrow. The occurrence of the megaloblastic type of erythropoiesis in the bone marrow establishes the presence of a deficiency of vitamin B_{12} or folic acid almost unequivocally.

Since deficiencies of vitamin B_{12} and of folic acid can give identical hematologic pictures, further study is necessary to determine which is responsible. In this connection the gastric analysis is a very helpful procedure. With but rare exceptions, patients with pernicious anemia do not secrete hydrochloric acid after the administration of histamine and the presence of free HCl in the gastric analysis can be considered to almost exclude pernicious anemia from consideration. The other causes of vitamin B_{12} deficiency, such as total gastrectomy, intestinal shunts, fistulae, and malabsorption syndromes, are usually suggested by the history and confirmed by appropriate examinations. If the patient has evidence of posterolateral sclerosis associated with a normocytic or macrocytic anemia and histamine-fast achlorhydria, the diagnosis of pernicious anemia should be strongly suspected even though the marrow is not megaloblastic.

Folic acid administration can modify the appearance of the bone marrow and the peripheral blood in a patient with pernicious anemia while allowing the central nervous system lesions to progress. For this reason measurement of the level of vitamin B_{12} in the serum or use of one of the tests of vitamin B_{12} absorption such as the Schilling test, that utilize vitamin B_{12} labeled with radioactive cobalt may be necessary to establish the diagnosis. If subnormal amounts of B_{12} are absorbed and excreted, the test is repeated and intrinsic factor is administered with the oral vitamin B_{12}. The addition of the intrinsic factor leads to substantial improvement in absorption of vitamin B_{12} in patients with pernicious anemia but has little or no effect in those with malabsorption syndrome, shunts, and fistulae. If the patient has anemia and a megaloblastic bone marrow that are due to a deficiency of vitamin B_{12}, the administration of vitamin B_{12} parenterally produces a conversion of the megaloblastic erythropoiesis to the normoblastic type followed by a reticulocytosis and a rise of the hemoglobin and erythrocyte levels to normal.

When folic acid deficiency is responsible for the macrocytic anemia there is usually a history of inadequate diet or some disorder such as a malabsorption syndrome that produces a secondary deficiency. A dietary deficiency sufficient to produce this type of anemia is rare in the United States except in infancy, during pregnancy, in food faddists, and in alcoholics. Folic acid deficiency may produce the same hematologic picture as vitamin B_{12} deficiency but the neurologic lesions that are so common in vitamin B_{12} deficiency are usually absent or mild in folic acid deficiency. The occurrence of a macrocytic anemia and a megaloblastic marrow in an adult who has retained the ability to secrete free HCl strongly suggests the possibility of folic acid deficiency. In folate deficiency serum folate levels are reduced whereas levels of vitamin B_{12} are normal. Concurrent antibiotic administration usually vitiates the results of these tests if the microbiologic assay method is used.

Aplastic anemia.   Mild or moderate macrocytosis is slightly more common than normocytic anemia in aplastic anemia. Although anemia of this type is usually accompanied by definite leukopenia and thrombocytopenia, anemia may occur alone. The term "chronic erythrocytic hypoplasia" is used to distinguish patients of the latter type. The reticulocyte count and serum bilirubin level are usually normal or subnormal; in chronic erythrocytic hypoplasia the reticulocyte count is often 0 or 0.1 per cent. A slight increase in the percentage of reticulocytes is occasionally seen but when this occurs the absolute value (the number of reticulocytes per cu.mm.) is usually normal. The macrocytic anemia of aplastic anemia, even if severe, is rarely accompanied by a significant degree of poikilocytosis or anisocytosis. The bone marrow examination nearly always reveals the normoblastic type of erythropoiesis, but in rare cases a megaloblastic marrow occurs. Usually the marrow of patients with aplastic anemia is hypocellular, often markedly so, but a biopsy is necessary to determine cellularity and establish the diagnosis. At times, the history of exposure to irradiation, chemicals, or drugs is helpful. On occasion examination of the bone marrow in a patient with suspected aplastic anemia establishes a definite diagnosis of some other primary disease such as multiple myeloma, leukemia, carcinomatosis, or tuberculosis. In the majority of patients with aplastic anemia the cause remains obscure and the anemia is classified as "idiopathic."

Myxedema. A mild or moderately severe macrocytic anemia occurs commonly in patients with myxedema. The red blood count usually is over 3.0 mil. per cu.mm. The peripheral blood shows no appreciable poikilocytosis or anisocytosis and is generally normal in other respects. The erythropoiesis in the bone marow is normoblastic and the cellularity is either normal or slightly reduced. The diagnosis of myxedema is usually suggested by the clinical features of the disease and is confirmed by the appropriate laboratory tests, such as determinations of the serum cholesterol level, basal metabolic rate, radioactive iodine uptake, and measurement of the plasma bound iodine. When iron deficiency or vitamin B_{12} occurs in the patient with myxedema, the anemia is more severe than in mxyedema alone.

Hemolytic anemia. A macrocytic type of anemia is not uncommon in hemolytic disorders, particularly in the extracorpuscular or acquired type. The diagnosis of the patient with hemolytic anemia is considered in the discussion of hemolytic normocytic anemias.

Normocytic Anemia

If the patient is found to have a normocytic type of anemia (MCV 80 to 94 c.μ), hyperhemolysis, acute blood loss, and deficient blood production must be considered.

Hyperhemolysis. A reticulocyte count greater than 4 per cent in a patient who has neither had a recent hemorrhage nor received antianemic therapy should raise the suspicion of a hemolytic anemia. Often the reticulocyte count is over 10 per cent, and sometimes it is 30 per cent or more. Study of the stained smear often reveals suggestive evidence of a hemolytic process in the form of nucleated red cells, polychromatophilia, punctate basophilia, target cells, or spherocytes. Leukocytosis is often present. These abnormalities in the peripheral blood reflect the hyperplasia that is evident on examination of the bone marrow. At times the increase in erythropoiesis is so marked that a differential cell count of the marrow reveals that the myeloid-erythroid (M:E) ratio is 1:1 or less (normal 3:1 to 10:1). In some patients with hemolytic anemia striking hyperplasia occurs, and the early forms of normoblasts become so numerous that the normoblastic nature of the erythropoiesis may be misinterpreted as megaloblastic because of the morphologic similarities between the youngest cells of both series. Careful study of the cells at all different stages of development, particularly at the polychromatophilic stage, nearly always enables one to interpret the marrow properly; in some patients, however, the marrow actually becomes megaloblastic because of the development of folate deficiency.

Evidence of the hyperhemolysis is found in the moderate elevation of the indirect reacting bilirubin (1.0 to 4.0 mg. per 100 ml.) and in the increased fecal urobilinogen excretion. Measurement of the fecal urobilinogen may be a very useful test in suspected hemolytic disease even though the wide normal range of daily variations, from 40 to 280 mg., seriously limits the usefulness of the test as an accurate measure of hemoglobin destruction. When the mechanism of the anemia is not apparent, particularly in patients with mild degrees of anemia, the demonstration of an increase in the average 24 hour fecal urobilinogen excretion over a 3 or 4 day period may establish the presence of increased hemoglobin breakdown. In interpreting the values obtained for the 24 hour fecal urobilinogen excretion it is important to remember that the fecal urobilinogen excretion may be reduced by antibiotics that change the bacterial flora of the intestinal tract and may be increased by recent blood transfusions. The amount of urobilinogen excreted in the feces in 24 hours also depends on the total amount of circulating hemoglobin because a fixed percentage of the circulating hemoglobin is destroyed each day as a rule. The mass of the circulating hemoglobin can be approximated by determining the number of grams of hemoglobin per 100 ml. of blood and the body weight. The following formula suggested by Dameshek[13] is helpful in interpreting the significance of the average daily fecal urobilinogen excretion in patients with anemia:

$$\frac{\text{Normal Hb. (15 gm./100 ml.)}}{\text{Pt.'s Hb. (gm./100 ml.)}} \times \frac{\text{Normal weight (70 kg.)}}{\text{Pt.'s weight}} \times \text{daily f.u. output (mg.)} = \frac{\text{corrected daily}}{\text{fecal urobilinogen output (mg.)}}$$

The hemolytic index was also devised by Miller, Singer, and Dameshek[24] to relate the fecal urobilinogen excretion to the circulating mass of hemoglobin. It is calculated as follows:

$$\frac{\text{avg. (of 4 days) daily output of fecal urobilinogen (mg.)} \times 100}{\text{total Hb. (Hb. gm./100 ml.)} \times \text{total blood volume/100}}$$

The hemolytic index indicates the amount of urobilinogen derived daily from 100 grams of hemoglobin. The normal index is from 11 to 21.

Demonstration of a shortened erythrocyte survival time by means of tagged red cells is a useful way to establish the presence of hyperhemolysis in some circumstances. If a radioactive tag is employed, measurement of the accumulation of radioactivity in the spleen and liver gives some information from which inferences can be made about the site of destruction of the erythrocytes.

Although recognition of the hemolytic process is easy as a rule, it is sometimes difficult because all the signs of increased hemolysis and increased erythropoiesis may be absent or inconspicuous if the patient is seen during an "aplastic crisis." which occasionally develops during an intercurrent infection.

If the anemia is established as hemolytic in type, further tests are necessary to determine the nature of the hemolytic disorder. These include careful examination of the blood smear for erythrocyte abnormalities; Coombs test; a test for sickling; hemoglobin electrophoresis; determination of fetal hemoglobin; hypotonic saline fragility test with incubation; autohemolysis test; screening tests for enzyme deficiencies; and others listed in Table 3–4. At times study of parents or siblings is helpful in the diagnosis of a patient suspected of having hereditary spherocytosis, thalassemia, hemoglobinopathy, or an enzymatic defect.

Hemolytic anemia due to an extracorpuscular or acquired defect may be macrocytic or normocytic. In some patients the disease appears to be due to an auto-immune mechanism and in others to some other mechanism. If the antiglobulin (Coombs) test is positive, auto-immune hemolytic disease is likely even though the osmotic fragility test reveals abnormal susceptibility to hypotonic saline. In such circumstances further study is necessary to determine whether the hemolytic process is "idiopathic" or "secondary" to some underlying disease, such as one of the lymphoma group, carcinoma, sarcoidosis, or one of the collagen disorders. A careful diagnostic study that may include roentgenographic examinations, serum protein studies, a search for L.E. cells, and biopsy of a lymph node or other tissue is often necessary. A diagnosis of the idiopathic type of disease is reached by exclusion. At times the diagnosis of auto-immune hemolytic disease as either idiopathic or symptomatic can be established only after a prolonged period of observation and repeated examinations. The macrocytic anemia of chronic liver disease is usually due to an extracorpuscular type of hyperhemolysis, but the Coombs test is usually negative. When the hemolytic anemia is due to chronic liver disease abnormal liver function tests and clinical evidence of liver disease are usually present. In other disease states a hemolytic element may be present but demonstrable only by careful study; in these patients the hemolytic process is usually mild, and inadequate blood production is the most important mechanism.

Examination of the urine for hemosiderin and of the plasma for hemoglobin and measurement of the serum haptoglobin level are important if intravascular hemolysis and hemoglobinuria are suspected. If positive, other more definitive tests are performed.

Acute blood loss. The anemia that follows acute blood loss is nearly always normocytic. If the acute hemorrhage is external and results from trauma or disease its occurrence is generally recounted in the history. If the hemorrhage occurs from the gastrointestinal tract the event may not be noticed by the patient and the finding of anemia may be the first clue to its occurrence. In some patients hemorrhages from a duodenal ulcer or a lesion of the small intestine recur over a period of years and cause anemia that can be puzzling if the patient does not consult his physician until after the occult blood has disappeared from the feces. An elevated reticulocyte count in the absence of an increase in the serum bilirubin suggests recent hemorrhage if the patient has not recently been given specific therapeutic agents, such as iron or vitamin B_{12}. Leukocytosis and thrombocytosis in the peripheral blood and marked normoblastic hyperplasia in the bone marrow may also afford clues to a recent hemorrhage. The diagnosis of gastrointestinal bleeding is usually made from the history and by the detection of blood in the feces. The demonstration that a gastrointestinal lesion is the source of the bleeding is not always easy, and may not be possible without repeated roentgenographic study of the gastrointestinal tract or periodic observation of the patient. In the unusual circumstances in which the hemorrhage occurs into the muscles or other tissues as a result of trauma or ascorbic acid deficiency, reticulocytosis may occur in association with an elevation of the serum bilirubin and suggest the presence of hemolytic anemia.

Deficient blood production. Anemia that occurs in various chronic diseases is most often normocytic but sometimes is mildly microcytic or hypochromic. If the anemia is due to diminished erythropoiesis alone or to mild hyperhemolysis associated with depressed erythropoiesis, as sometimes occurs in patients with malignancies and other diseases, only the erythrocytes are reduced. The leukocytes and platelets are usually normal unless altered by the primary disease. It is unusual for anemia of this type to be the primary problem in diagnosis because the underlying disease such as chronic infection, arthritis, renal disease, malignancy, or endocrine disturbance is usually apparent. More important is the fact that anemia of this type is sometimes the first clinical indication of the underlying disease. Some ambulatory patients with renal disease present as problems of anemia because the slowly progressing renal insufficiency has not been recognized or suspected; uremia is probably not the explanation of anemia unless the renal disease is chronic and severe. (The diagnosis of aplastic anemia, which is often normocytic, is discussed with the macrocytic anemias.)

A normocytic anemia also occurs in some patients with mild anemia associated with iron deficiency. This may occur as an intermediate stage in the development of severe iron deficiency that is characterized by hypochromic microcytic anemia or it may occur during the stage of incomplete recovery. In patients with this type of anemia the history often suggests iron deficiency, but the demonstration of a low level of serum iron or an increased iron binding capacity or both, or the demonstration of reduced iron stores by examination of an appropriately stained specimen of marrow, or even a therapeutic trial with iron, may be necessary to establish the diagnosis.

Simple Microcytic Anemia

Simple microcytic anemia (MCV< 80 c.μ, MCHC > 30 per cent) is most often seen in association with various chronic diseases, circumstances in which a normocytic anemia is more common.

Hypochromic Microcytic Anemia

The finding of a hypochromic microcytic type of anemia (MCV < 80 c.μ, MCHC < 30 per cent) almost invariably means iron deficiency. The erythrocytes on a stained blood smear have an increase in central pallor and show considerable poikilocytosis and anisocytosis. Elongated "cigar" forms, racquet cells, and microcytes are often numerous. The leukocytes and platelets are usually normal. The cellularity of the bone marrow may be subnormal, normal, or increased; erythropoiesis is normoblastic in type. The existence of iron deficiency can be established definitely by finding a subnormal level of the serum iron associated with an increase in the latent iron binding capacity of the serum, or by the demonstration of reduced iron stores in the bone marrow.

The other diseases that may be confused with iron deficiency occur much less commonly and usually can be distinguished without difficulty. Pyridoxine deficiency and sideroachrestic anemia (iron loading anemia) are usually hypochromic and microcytic but the serum iron level is elevated and the storage iron is increased. In thalassemia the erythrocytes are hypochromic and microcytic but the condition can generally be distinguished from iron deficiency by the family history, reticulocytosis, marked splenomegaly, the presence of alkali resistant hemoglobin, the elevated level of the serum iron, and, if necessary, the failure to respond to therapy with iron preparations. When the serum iron level is low in thalassemia minor, as has been demonstrated in some cases, the differential diagnosis may be difficult and examination of the sternal marrow for stainable iron may be helpful.

When anemia is due to iron deficiency it is important to determine the cause. Except in infants and young children a dietary lack should not be accepted as an explanation of iron deficiency unless there are modifying factors. Among these are the increased need of iron during pregnancy and growth. However, iron deficiency may develop despite an adequate diet if absorption is impaired because of a malabsorption disorder or partial gastrectomy. In adult males, and in most postmenopausal women, unless there is some absorptive defect, iron deficiency anemia can be considered as practically synonymous with chronic blood loss. Blood loss usually occurs because of some ulcerated lesion in the gastrointestinal tract. Esophageal lesions, hiatus hernia, gastric carcinoma, benign gastric ulcer, duodenal ulcer, tumor of the small intestine, carcinoma of the colon, and hemorrhoids are all possible sources of chronic blood loss. Should the examination reveal no significant source of bleeding the patient should be reexamined periodically and the roentgenographic studies repeated, because any of the lesions, particularly carcinoma of the cecum and stomach and tumors of the small intestine, may be a source of bleeding even though they are not recognized on the initial roentgenographic study. A diaphragmatic hernia can be responsible for chronic blood loss, but this lesion is found so frequently in patients in the middle-aged and older groups that it should not be accepted as the explanation of the anemia unless careful study of the remainder of the gastrointestinal tract has disclosed no other lesion. Although iron deficiency can occur as the result of repeated bleeding from the genitourinary or respiratory tract, bleeding from these sites of sufficient degree to cause anemia is unusual. When bleeding of this type occurs it is readily apparent to the patient. Hemosiderinuria associated with intravascular hemolysis may be severe enough to produce iron deficiency and not be recognized by the patient.

In women menstruation and pregnancy afford added opportunities for the development of iron deficiency, since the increased need for iron in these circumstances may not be met by increased absorption of dietary iron. Even mildly excessive menstrual bleeding may lead to iron deficiency if the iron stores are low. If the individual has low iron stores early in life the iron reserves may not be restored to normal by the diet during growth and adolescence. In some premenopausal women it may be difficult to decide whether the number of pregnancies and the amount of menstrual bleeding can be accepted as a satisfactory explanation of the iron deficiency. If there is any reasonable doubt, repeated tests for occult blood in the feces and study of the gastrointestinal tract for a possible source of bleeding are indicated.

Examination of the Bone Marrow

Aspiration of the bone marrow, introduced by Arinkin in 1929, has become a widely used hematologic procedure. Details of different techniques for obtaining, preparing, and examining the marrow are described in monographs devoted to the subject.[10, 23]

Technique. Various sites are used for the aspiration. The most satisfactory areas for routine use are the upper portion of the body of the sternum at the level of the third costal cartilage, the area just distal to the iliac crest, and the spinous processes of the third and fourth lumbar vertebrae. The sternal puncture is the easiest to perform, but because of the proximity of the sternum to the vital structures in the mediastinum it is more dangerous than the other sites if the needle is inserted too deeply. Puncture in this region is also more likely to cause apprehension in anxious patients. For these reasons the iliac crest is preferred. In children less than 2 years of age the proximal end of the tibia is usually the most satisfactory site; however, the iliac crest and the spinous processes can generally be employed successfully.

The skin over the aspiration site is shaved if necessary and then cleansed with soap and water, followed by iodine or some other skin antiseptic and alcohol. Sterile drapes are placed around the area. Sterile gloves and instruments are used. The skin and periosteum are infiltrated with 0.5 to 1.0 per cent procaine solution by means of a hypodermic syringe and needle. Many different types of needles have been devised for the bone marrow puncture. A short needle that contains a stylet and has a guard set at 1.0 cm. from the tip of the needle (0.5 cm. for children) is usually satisfactory. The needle is pushed and rotated until a rather sudden decrease in resistance indicates that the marrow cavity has been entered. The stylet is then removed and a tightly fitting 10 ml. syringe is attached to the needle. The plunger is withdrawn slowly until marrow appears in the syringe. With the needle in the proper position in the marrow cavity some pain is usually experienced when the marrow is aspirated.

Thin preparations, made as a blood smear is made, from the first bit of marrow that is withdrawn are usually best because the specimen is largely undiluted with blood. Some hematologists prefer to withdraw a larger specimen from the marrow and eject the material from the syringe into a watch glass. Particles of marrow are then picked up on an applicator stick or some other instrument and touched to various areas of the clean slide. Such imprints give a better picture of the marrow architecture and of the fixed cells. However, preparations made in this manner usually contain a large number of damaged and unrecognizable cells. Bone marrow obtained by aspiration can be stained supravitally, with Wright's stain, with May-Grünwald-Giemsa stain, or by the peroxidase method. Marrow particles obtained by aspiration can also be fixed in paraffin and stained with hematoxylin and eosin.

A differential count is often performed on the nucleated cells in the marrow

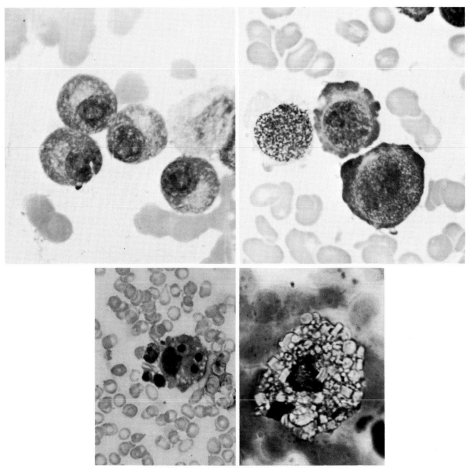

Figure 3–3. Bone marrow aspiration. *A*, Multiple myeloma. *B*, Megaloblastic erythropoiesis. *C*, Phagocytosis of cells by marrow histiocyte (reticulum cell sarcoma). *D*, Cystinosis. (F.S.: I, 34–38; II, 95; III, 102–107, 147.)

preparation. For a reproducible result it is usually necessary to count from 300 to 500 cells. The range of the different cells varies in normal marrows and the values given by different authors differ somewhat, as shown in Table 3–5. An accurate differential count is helpful in diagnosis on some occasions. It is also an excellent discipline for those in training because it forces a decision as to the identity of each cell. Nevertheless, it is time-consuming, and after a moderate amount of experience it is usually possible to gain the same information from a careful systematic study of the smear without actually doing a differential count.

In examining the bone marrow it is desirable to follow a definite plan. The slide is first examined with the low power objective. The cellularity of the specimen is noted, the number of megakaryocytes is estimated, and a search for sheets of malignant cells and other unusual cells is made, particularly near the edges of the preparation. The more suitably stained portions of the slide are examined under oil immersion. The erythrocyte precursors are studied and the type of erythropoiesis is noted as megaloblastic or normoblastic. Attention is also paid to the number and maturity of these cells. Next, the granulocytic series is studied with particular reference to number and any increase in the younger forms, particularly myeloblasts and progranulocytes. The presence of any macropolycytes or giant metamyelocytes is also noted. Megakaryocytes are studied for number, maturity, and evidence of platelet formation. The plasma cells, reticulum cells, histiocytes, and other cells are studied similarly for number and immaturity, and for cytoplasmic inclusions. The number of lymphocytes is estimated, and the presence of any tumor cells or other abnormal or unidentified cells is noted.

After the marrow preparation has been studied in this fashion the various observations can be noted in the report. The cellularity is classed as normal, increased, or decreased. Erythropoiesis is classified according to the type of maturation as normoblastic or megaloblastic, and according to activity as normal, hypoplastic, or hyperplastic. The granulocytic maturation is classed as normal or abnormal, and any abnormality is specified. The megakaryocytes and platelet formation are classed as normal, reduced, or increased. Similarly the number and maturity of the lymphocytes, plasma cells, and reticulum cells are recorded. These observations form the basis for the conclusions that can be drawn from the marrow examination.

The value of bone marrow examination. The bone marrow biopsy permits study of only a small, almost minute, piece of tissue from a large organ. It is not surprising that such a sample does not invariably reflect the status of the entire marrow, that localized lesions such as metastatic malignancy and

Table 3-5. *Normal Adult Differential Marrow Cell Counts by Various Authors*

CELL TYPE	WINTROBE[34] (%) (RANGE)	CUSTER[10] (%) (RANGE)	ISRAELS[19] (%) (RANGE)	LEITNER[23] (%)	YOUNG AND OSGOOD[36] (%) (RANGE)
Myeloblasts	0.3–5.0	0.0–3.5	0.3–2.0	1.2	0.0–1.2
Progranulocytes	1.0–8.0	0.5–5.0	1.0–8.0	2.2	0.0–7.8
Myelocytes:					
Neutrophils	5.0–18.0	7.0–34.6	5.0–20.0	12.6	0.0–2.6
Eosinophils	0.5–3.0	0.3–3.0	....	1.4	0.0–0.4
Basophils	0.0–0.5	0.0–0.5	....	0.02	....
Metamyelocytes	13.0–32.0	15.1–37.0	13.0–32.0	11.0	1.8–11.8
Band cells			....	24.0	15.8–33.0
Segmented:					
Neutrophils	7.0–30.0	3.0–19.8	7.0–30.0	28.4	7.4–25.2
Eosinophils	0.5–4.0	0.1–3.0	0.5–4.0	1.8	0.0–1.0
Basophils	0.0–0.7	0.0–1.0	0.0–1.0	0.02	0.0–0.2
Lymphocytes	3.0–17.0	0.0–6.8	3.0–20.0	7.6	4.8–16.0
Plasmacytes	0.0–2.0	0.0–1.2	0.0–2.0	1.0	0.0–1.0
Monocytes	0.5–5.0	0.1–3.2	0.5–5.0	1.4	0.0–4.2
Reticulum cells	0.1–2.0	0.3–2.6	....	2.0	....
Megakaryocytes	0.03–3.0	0.05–1.5	Occas.	0.8	0.0–0.2
Pronormoblasts	1.0–8.0	0.0–0.0	0.5–4.0	0.8	....
Normoblasts (basophilic, polychromatic and orthochromatic)	7.0–32.0	17.5–42.0	19.0–35.0	27.6	5.4–24.2
Myeloid: erythroid ratio	about 3:1–4:1	2:1–6:1	4:1–20:1	3:1	2:1–8:1

granulomas may not be seen. Nevertheless it usually gives a reliable picture of many disorders of the hematopoietic system and frequently discloses the nature of localized lesions as well. Examination of the bone marrow may establish a diagnosis of certain diseases with assurance, it may render some particular diagnosis very unlikely, or it may give helpful information that is of indirect or limited value. The ease with which bone marrow can be obtained for examination has led to the use of this procedure in circumstances when other, simpler procedures, such as a careful study of a smear of peripheral blood, would suffice for a diagnosis. The decision as to the desirability of a bone marrow examination is based on the circumstances in the individual case.

Although the marrow examination may not be necessary in order to establish the diagnosis, the following diagnoses can usually be made by this method:

1. Multiple myeloma.
2. Leukemia, all types.
3. Untreated or partially treated vitamin B_{12} or folic acid deficiency.
4. Storage disease, such as Gaucher's disease.
5. Metastatic malignancy (if "positive" cells are found).
6. Fungal disease (if "positive" cells are found).
7. Iron deficiency.
8. Iron overload.
9. Sideroblastic anemia.

In certain other diseases, when taken in conjunction with the peripheral blood, the bone marrow examination can often provide helpful information that is not diagnostic when taken alone. Among these are:

1. Aplastic anemia.
2. Idiopathic thrombocytopenic purpura.
3. Lymphosarcoma.
4. Hypersplenism.
5. Agranulocytosis.

It is sometimes difficult to exclude a diagnosis from further consideration because of the result of the bone marrow examination. "Myeloma cells" or a definite increase in plasma cells may not be found in multiple myeloma. Some patients with bone marrow failure have cellular specimens. Patients with pernicious anemia sometimes forget to relate that they have taken folic acid or received an injection of vitamin B_{12} from another physician. Aspiration occasionally yields a hypocellular or "aplastic" marrow in patients with leukemia. When the diagnosis remains in doubt, and when a hypocellular or acellular specimen is obtained by aspiration, a biopsy should be made with a Vim-Silverman or similar needle, or by an open operation. If abnormal bleeding is expected with operation, the iliac crest is the site of choice because bleeding can be more easily controlled than in the sternum or ribs. From the biopsy specimen both touch preparations for Wright's stain and paraffin sections for H and E and other stains can be made. A biopsy is necessary for staging the patient with lymphoma. Many pathologists and some hematologists prefer marrow sections to smears or imprints for routine study because sections give a better picture of the marrow architecture, cellularity, and iron content;[15] unfortunately identifying individual cells in such preparations is less accurate than in touch preparations. Often both types of marrow examination are needed.

Errors in Diagnosis

Some common errors in the diagnosis of anemia are:

In *adults:*

1. Errors in reporting laboratory values on chart.
2. Inadequate study of blood smear.
3. Incorrect determination of erythrocyte indices.
4. Failure to do reticulocyte count.
5. Failure to check stools for occult blood.
6. Failure to investigate patients for neoplasm or other sources of bleeding.
7. Failure to check blood urea or blood urea nitrogen for renal insufficiency.
8. Failure to palpate enlarged spleen or nodes.
9. Failure to consider multiple myeloma as a cause for anemia in middle-aged and elderly patients.
10. Failure to consider myxedema as a cause of anemia.

In *children:*

1. Failure to consider possibility of hemolytic anemias of various sorts.

Treatment in Relation to Diagnosis

The purpose of the diagnostic study is to enable the physician to decide what is the best form of treatment for the patient. The most desirable form of treatment is the removal or correction of the cause. When this cannot be accomplished therapy is directed toward the disordered mechanism. For either form of therapy it is important to establish an accurate diagnosis before treating the anemia unless the patient's condition demands immediate measures, such as transfusions. Premature treatment may be detrimental to the patient. The use of complex preparations that contain iron, vitamin B_{12}, folic acid, and other substances, under the impression that such therapy will afford adequate treatment for all types of anemia, may confuse the interpretation of the diagnostic studies without correcting the anemia. Even more important is the fact that treatment may produce a false sense of security when it corrects the anemia, which is but one aspect of the disorder, without affecting other more serious aspects of the disease. When no diagnosis has been established, often the best course is to withhold treatment until the nature of the anemia is better understood. It is rare that a delay in treatment until the necessary diagnostic studies are performed works to the disadvantage of the patient.

References

1. Adams, E. B.: Anemia associated with protein deficiency. Seminars Hemat., 7:55, 1970.
1a. Berlin, N. I., Waldmann, T. A., and Weissman, S. M.: Life span of red blood cell. Physiol. Rev., *39*:577, 1959.
1b. Beutler, E., Dern, R. J., and Alving, A. S.: The hemolytic effect of primaquine. IV. The relationship of cell age to hemolysis. J. Lab. & Clin. Med., *44*:439, 1954.
2. Biggs, R., and Macmillan, R. L.: The errors of some hematological methods as they are used in a routine laboratory. J. Clin. Path., *1*:269, 283, 1948.
3. Block, M.: Importance and interpretation of routine blood counts. Rocky Mountain M. J., *54*:894, 1957.

4. Bomford, R.: Anaemia in myxoedema: and the role of the thyroid gland in erythropoiesis. Quart. J. Med., 7:495, 1938.
5. Brain, M. C., Dacie, J. V., and Hourihane, D. O'B.: Microangiopathic haemolytic anemia: the possible role of vascular lesions in pathogenesis. Brit. J. Haemat., 8:358, 1962.
6. Castle, W. B.: Erythropoiesis: Normal and abnormal. Bull. N.Y. Acad. Med., 30:827, 1954.
7. Chaplin, H., Jr., and Mollison, P. L.: Red cell life-span in nephritis and hepatic cirrhosis. Clin. Sc., 12:351, 1953.
8. Committee on Iron Deficiency: Iron deficiency in the United States. J.A.M.A., 203:407, 1968.
9. Crosby, W. H., and Akeroyd, J. H.: Limit of hemoglobin synthesis in hereditary hemolytic anemia: Its relation to the excretion of bile pigment. Am. J. Med., 13:273, 1952.
10. Custer, R. P.: An Atlas of the Blood and Bone Marrow. W. B. Saunders Co., Philadelphia, 1949.
11. Dacie, J. V.: The Hemolytic Anemias, Congenital and Acquired. Grune and Stratton, New York, 1960, 1962.
12. Dacie, J. V.: The auto-immune hemolytic anemias. Am. J. Med., 18:810, 1955.
13. Dameshek, W.: Hemolytic anemia. Am. J. Med., 18:315, 1955.
14. Dern, R. J., Weinstein, I. M., LeRoy, G. V., Talmage, D. W., and Alving, A. S.: The hemolytic effect of primaquine. I. The localization of the drug-induced hemolytic defect in primaquine-sensitive individuals. J. Lab. & Clin. Med., 43:303, 1954.
15. Ellis, L. D., Jensen, W. N., and Westerman, M. P.: Needle biopsy of bone and marrow. Arch. Int. Med., 114:213, 1964.
16. Erslev, A. J.: Erythropoietic function in uremic rabbits. Clin. Res. Proc., 5:141, 1957.
16a. Finch, C. A.: Protein deficiency and anemia. Plenary session papers. International Society of Hematology, 1968, p. 154.
17. Gurney, C. W., Goldwasser, E., Jacobson, L. O., and Pan, C.: Demonstration of erythropoietin in human plasma. J. Clin. Invest., 36:896, 1957.
18. Ham, T. H., Shen, S. C., Fleming, E. M., and Castle, W. B.: Studies on the destruction of red blood cells in thermal injury. Blood, 3:373, 1948.
19. Israels, M. C. G.: An Atlas of Bone-Marrow Pathology. Grune and Stratton, New York, 1948.
20. James, G. W., III, Abbot, L. D., Jr., Brooks, J. W., and Evans, E. I.: Anemia of thermal injury. III. Erythropoiesis and hemoglobin metabolism studied with N¹⁵ glycine in dog and man. J. Clin. Invest., 33:150, 1954.
21. James, G. W., III, Purnell, O. J., and Evans, E. I.: The anemia of thermal injury. I. Studies of pigment excretion. J. Clin. Invest., 30:181, 1951.
22. Jandl, J.: The anemia of liver disease. Observations on its mechanism. J. Clin. Invest., 34:390, 1955.
23. Leitner, S. J.: Bone Marrow Biopsy. J. A. Churchill, Ltd., London, 1949.
24. Miller, E. B., Singer, K., and Dameshek, W.: Use of the daily fecal output of urobilinogen and the hemolytic index in the measurement of hemolysis. Arch. Int. Med., 70:722, 1942.
25. Mitchell, J. S.: Metabolic effects of therapeutic doses of X and gamma radiations. Brit. J. Radiol., 16:339, 1943.
26. Pauling, L., Itano, H. A., Singer, S. J., and Wells, I. C.: Sickle cell anemia: A molecular disease. Science, 110:543, 1949.
27. Pirzio-Biroli, G., Bothwell, T. H., and Finch, C. A.: Iron absorption. II. The absorption of radioiron administered with a standard meal in man. J. Lab. & Clin. Med., 51:37, 1958.
28. Schilling, R. F.: Intrinsic factor studies. II. The effect of gastric juice on the urinary excretion of radioactivity after the oral administration of radioactive B₁₂. J. Lab. & Clin. Med., 42:860, 1953.
29. Szeinberg, A., Asher, Y., and Sheba, C.: Studies on glutathione stability in erythrocytes of cases with past history of favism or sulfa-drug-induced hemolysis. Blood, 13:348, 1958.
30. Thorup, O. A., Strole, W. E., and Leavell, B. S.: The rate of removal of iron from culture medium by human bone marrow suspension. J. Lab. & Clin. Med., 52:266, 1958.
31. Wasserman, L. R., Stats, D., Schwartz, L., and Fudenberg, H.: Symptomatic and hemopathic hemolytic anemia. Am. J. Med., 18:961, 1955.
32. Wintrobe, M. M.: The size and hemoglobin content of the erythrocyte. J. Lab. & Clin. Med., 17:899, 1932.
33. Wintrobe, M. M.: Principles in the management of anemias. Bull. N.Y. Acad. Med., 30:6, 1954.
34. Wintrobe, M. M.: Clinical Hematology. 4th Ed. Lea and Febiger, Philadelphia, 1956.
35. Young, L. E.: Hereditary spherocytosis. Am. J. Med., 18:486, 1955.
36. Young, R. H., and Osgood, E. E.: Sternal marrow aspirated during life. Arch. Int. Med., 55:186, 1935.

IV / Disorders of
Vitamin B_{12} and
Folic Acid Metabolism

Both vitamin B_{12} and folic acid (pteroylglutamic acid) are essential for normal metabolic processes. A deficiency of either substance causes a megaloblastic type of anemia associated with abnormalities in the maturation of granulocytes and gives rise to macrocytosis in the mucosa of the mouth, stomach, intestine, and vagina; an inadequate amount of vitamin B_{12} also leads to serious derangements of the nervous system. A deficiency of either vitamin B_{12} or folic acid usually is most apparent in the cells involved in erythropoiesis. The delay in cell division and maturation is reflected in the appearance of the nuclei of the erythrocyte precursors; the chromatin pattern of the nucleus remains dispersed while the cytoplasm enlarges and hemoglobinization progresses. These morphologic abnormalities and the known importance of DNA and RNA metabolism in cell growth and division suggest that a main function of these vitamins is concerned with DNA and RNA metabolism. The unraveling of the biochemical functions of these two vitamins and their relationship to each other is incomplete, but various details of their natural occurrence, absorption, transport, and storage have been established. In addition, a number of different clinical disorders which have in common a functional deficiency of one or the other of these vitamins have been recognized.

Vitamin B_{12}

Vitamin B_{12}, which has molecular weight of 1355 and the formula C_{63} $H_{88}O_{14}N_{14}PCo$, is found in practically all animal tissue.[82] Beef liver has the high-

86

est concentration, 50 to 130 micrograms per 100 grams of fresh weight; beef kidney, 20 to 50 micrograms, and herring, 11 to 34 micrograms, are also rich sources. Beef muscle contains 2 to 8 micrograms; cheese (1.4 to 3.6 micrograms), egg yolk (1.2 micrograms), and milk (0.2 to 0.6 microgram) are relatively poor sources. In the United States the average daily diet probably contains over 5 micrograms. Vitamin B_{12} is synthesized exclusively by microorganisms and these are the source of the vitamin found in various foodstuffs.

Intrinsic factor secreted by the stomach is essential for the absorption of vitamin B_{12} in foodstuffs. In man the factor is secreted only by the glands of the body of the stomach, probably by the parietal cells, and not in the pyloric end of the stomach or the small intestine, as is the case in swine. The factor, which is water soluble but non-dialyzable, is destroyed by heat or boiling and can be precipitated by ammonium sulfate, characteristics which indicate that it is a protein; in addition to amino acids it contains hexoses, hexose amines, and sialic acid. Although the intrinsic factor has not been purified, intrinsic factor activity has been demonstrated in a mucoprotein isolated from the acid glandular protein of the stomach, and in stomach mucosal fractions which have molecular weights that range from 5000 to 100,000;[31] native intrinsic factor is thought to be a glycoprotein or mucopolysaccharide with a molecular weight of approximately 55,000.[36]

Vitamin B_{12} is absorbed in the small intestine, mainly in the distal portion of the ileum, at a roughly neutral pH; both intrinsic factor (IF) and calcium ions are necessary for the absorption of physiologic amounts, but the mechanism by which intrinsic factor promotes absorption is uncertain. The B_{12}-IF complex is resistant to digestion, a binding which may prevent utilization of the vitamin by the bacteria of the intestine before absorption occurs. The absorption of vitamin B_{12} is accomplished by some interaction between the mucosal cell and the complex of vitamin B_{12} and intrinsic fraction.[48] The role of calcium ions appears to be the attachment of intrinsic factor to mucosal cells; vitamin B_{12} first attaches to one of the active sites of the intrinsic factor and then the other active site of the IF attaches to the mucosal cell. As shown by studies in hamsters with vitamin $B_{12}{}^{57}Co$ and electron microscopy, the receptor is located on the microvilli of the ileal cells; the attachment appears to be by adsorption rather than by an energy requiring enzymatic reaction.[24] Although it has been suggested that the IF molecule enters the mucosal cell by pinocytosis or by other means, the evidence indicates that the intrinsic factor is not absorbed as vitamin B_{12} enters the cell. Intrinsic factor is necessary for the absorption of small quantities of vitamin B_{12}, but the vitamin can be absorbed in the absence of intrinsic factor when large amounts are ingested; when 30 micrograms is taken orally, 1 per cent appears in the urine,[36] and when 1000 micrograms is ingested, a prompt rise in the serum level occurs. It has been suggested that this occurs as a result of passive diffusion through the gut wall, but the size of the pores of the absorptive cell, 4Å, compared to the size of the molecule of vitamin B_{12}, 8Å, has been cited as an objection to this explanation.[97]

After absorption, vitamin B_{12} is transported in the plasma bound mainly to proteins which have different functions.[39] Intrinsic factor does not pass through the mucosal cells into the portal blood; studies which employed catheterization of the portal vein and the ingestion of $Co^{57}B_{12}$ disclose that the B_{12}-

binding material has a molecular weight of approximately 100,000 and none of the immunologic characteristics of IF.[22] Vitamin B_{12} in the plasma is taken up by transcobalamin II (TC II), a protein which has alpha$_2$-beta mobility.[36] The vitamin enters the blood from the intestine at a slow rate, first appearing 3 or 4 hours after a meal; absorption reaches a peak at from 8 to 12 hours and continues for 24 hours. Nevertheless, the combination of TC II and vitamin B_{12} is cleared rapidly from the plasma and the level of vitamin B_{12} bound in this way probably never exceeds 20 pg. per ml. of plasma; half an injected dose of TC II–vitamin B_{12} leaves the plasma in less than 5 minutes, the vitamin being taken up mainly by the liver but also by other tissues. The source of TC II in man is unknown, but the observations on patients in whom large amounts of small intestine have been removed indicate that the intestinal tissue is not the source; in the mouse, TC II is produced in the liver. The plasma content of TC II is thought to be about 25 micrograms per liter, an amount able to bind approximately 986 pg. of vitamin B_{12} per ml.; after oral absorption less than 2 per cent of the available TC II is bound to the vitamin B_{12} but once attached the protein is not reused.

Transcobalamin I (TC I) also has a role in transport of vitamin B_{12}. The level of TC I is approximately 60 micrograms per liter, an amount that can combine with 700 to 800 pg. of vitamin B_{12} per ml.: normally the binding capacity of TC I is about half saturated with vitamin B_{12} from endogenous sources. It has been postulated that the leukocytes are the source of TC I, which appears to be the mechanism for transport of covitamin B_{12}, methylcobalamin, in the plasma and in its passage from cells. The level of TC I is greatly increased in myeloproliferative states, particularly chronic granulocytic leukemia. Other abnormalities that have been noted are decreased levels of TC II in chronic myeloproliferative states and in some patients with pernicious anemia; in pernicious anemia usually there is a normal amount of TC I which carries subnormal amounts of vitamin B_{12}.

Although the binding capacity of the plasma for vitamin B_{12} is usually unimpaired, in at least one study five of ten patients with untreated pernicious anemia were found to have deficient binding of radioactive B_{12} to beta globulin; treatment with vitamin B_{12} resulted in a more normal binding capacity. In one of the five patients, who had virtually no beta globulin binding of B_{12} before treatment, the Schilling test gave a malabsorptive pattern; after treatment with vitamin B_{12}, both the beta globulin binding capacity and the ability to absorb oral vitamin B_{12} when given with intrinsic factor returned.[60]

The main storage site of vitamin B_{12} in man is the liver, which in an adult may contain several milligrams, possibly 4;[82] at birth the liver contains about 25 micrograms.[4] The urinary excretion of vitamin B_{12} by man on a normal diet is about 30 micromicrograms a day.[71] When vitamin B_{12} is injected, appreciable amounts are excreted in the urine within 8 hours; when 50 micrograms or more is given the quantity excreted in the urine increases with increasing doses. If 50 micrograms is injected, from 3 to 4 micrograms are excreted in 8 hours; with the injection of 1000 micrograms, from 330 to 470 micrograms is excreted in the same period. The formula $E = D - 1.2D^{0.89}$ has been proposed to calculate the urinary excretion; E is the amount of vitamin B_{12} excreted in 8 hours, D is the amount injected intramuscularly.[20]

Folic Acid

Folic acid and PGA are the terms most commonly used to designate pteroyl-glutamic acid; before the chemical identity of the compound was established, other names, such as vitamin M, vitamin B_c, and Lactobacillus casei factor, were used. Folic acid occurs in nature chiefly in conjugated forms; leafy vegetables, liver, and yeast are rich sources. Significant amounts of the compound are produced in the intestinal lumen by the action of the bacteria normally found there.

The average daily diet in the United States contains 184 ± 67 micrograms of total folic acid activity as measured by the S. fecalis assay method.[12] This consists of three fractions in the following proportions: N^{10}-formyl-pteroyl-glutamic acid, 101 micrograms; citrovorum factor, 63 micrograms; PGA, 20 micrograms. The folate activity of four daily diets measured by L. casei assay was found to be 688 micrograms; fractionation gave percentages similar to those observed with S. fecalis. Repeated boiling of food in large quantities of water reduces or destroys its folate activity; probably pH changes in the gastro-intestinal tract also affect the availability of ingested dietary folate.[11] Patients may have tropical sprue and megaloblastic anemia despite a daily diet containing well over 1000 micrograms of folic acid activity. Since the anemia may respond to the oral administration of as little as 25 micrograms of PGA, apparently very little of the native folate in the food is absorbed by patients with the disease.[80] It has been suggested that some folic acid compounds found in the diet are active in bacteriologic assay but not in man.[12] The minimal daily requirement of folate activity (as PGA) for adults is probably 50 micrograms per day.[43]

Absorption, which occurs in the small intestine, does not require intrinsic factor. Human intestinal juice contains a conjugase capable of liberating folates from the bound form that is present in food; synthetic pteroylglutamic acid, and probably methyl- and formyl-folates, can cross the intestinal mucosa intact.[11] Folic acid is transported in the plasma where the normal level is reported to be between 5.9 and 21.0 nanograms per ml. (ng. per ml.). In pernicious anemia the level is normal; in folic acid deficiency it is reported to be less than 4.0 ng. per ml.[89] and less than 7 ng. per ml.[43] The folic acid activity of serum is due largely to the monoglutamate form, N^5-methyl-tetrahydrofolic acid.[47] Microbiologic assay indicates that the total tissue store of the folate activity in man is 7.5 ± 2.5 mg.; the chief storage site of folic acid is the liver, which normally contains 3.5 to 7.5 mg.[43] Four and one-half months are required for a healthy adult to develop a megaloblastic anemia on a daily dietary intake of 5 micrograms of folate activity.

Metabolic Functions of Vitamin B_{12} and Folic Acid

The term "vitamin B_{12}" as used in the literature has two meanings.[35] It is used as a generic term for all the cobalamins active in man, but it is also used specifically for the commercially available cyanocobalamin, which is the form first isolated. The cobalamins are various derivatives of 5,6-dimethylimidazolyl-cobamide, and the coenzyme forms are therefore sometimes called "cobamide coenzymes." These coenzymes include a 5'-deoxyadenosylcobalamin and a methylcobalamin.

The cobalamins are among the most potent and important biological compounds known because they appear to be involved in nearly every known metabolic system in man.[35] They are essential for normal growth, hematopoiesis, the production of epithelial cells, and for maintaining the function of the cells of the nervous system. The function of vitamin B_{12} is intimately related to that of the folate compounds, particularly in DNA synthesis.

The term "folic acid" is also employed generically for a group of closely related compounds as well as for a particular compound. The more systematic name, pteroylglutamic acid, has been proposed for the particular form involved in human metabolism, but folic acid, or folate, is still widely used in that sense.[55a]

The active coenzyme form of pteroylglutamate, or folate, in the mammal is the reduced form, tetrahydrofolate, which is also known as "folinic acid" or "citrovorum factor." Tetrahydrofolate is commonly abbreviated as H_4 folate.

Tetrahydrofolate is involved in all the single-carbon transfer reactions except those utilizing CO_2 or methyl groups. Most of these reactions simply involve a transfer of one carbon unit from one compound to another via tetrahydrofolate, with one important exception. The transfer by which thymine is formed also involves the oxidation of the tetrahydrofolate to dihydrofolate. The various transfers are summarized in Table 4–1.

The conversion of dietary folate to H_4 folate involves two reductases, with the intermediate formation of H_2 folate. These enzymes are inhibited by folic acid antagonists, such as aminopterin and amethopterin (methotrexate), which therefore cause an effective deficiency of H_4 folate. It is in this connection that the concomitant formation of H_2 folate in thymine synthesis assumes especial importance, because the recovery of this product as H_4 folate will be inhibited by these antagonists. The antagonists are therefore more likely to affect dividing cells in which DNA synthesis, and therefore thymine synthesis, is proceeding.

Table 4–1. Metabolic Processes Dependent on Tetrahydrofolate

Process	Intermediate	Group Transferred
Methionine regeneration	5-Methyl-H_4folate	—CH_3
Thymine biosynthesis		
	5,10-Methylene-H_4folate	—CH_2—
Serine and glycine metabolism		
	5,10-Methylidyne-H_4folate	—CH=
Purine biosynthesis		
	10-Formyl-H_4folate	—CH=O
Histidine degradation	5-Formimino-H_4folate	—CH=NH

(Prepared by Dr. Robert W. McGilvery, Professor of Biochemistry, University of Virginia School of Medicine, Charlottesville, Virginia.)

The interrelationship of the action of vitamin B_{12} and folate has been the subject of numerous studies. Many pieces of evidence, such as the appearance of blood cells in the stained smear, measurement of chemical compounds, the action of the compounds in bacteria, and the results of numerous other studies have all pointed to some important role in DNA metabolism. It now appears that a vitamin B_{12} deficiency causes a secondary deficiency of folate because of the resultant accumulation of 5-methyl-H_4folate.[65b] This "methyl trap" hypothesis was proposed by Herbert and others.[7, 90]

The connection between the two vitamins comes from a requirement for methylcobalamin as a coenzyme in the reaction by which a methyl group is transferred from 5-methyl-H_4folate to homocysteine; this reaction is an important means of regenerating methionine. If the cobalamins are deficient, 5-methyl-H_4folate accumulates. The accumulation occurs because the compound is formed irreversibly from 5,10-methylene-H_4folate, and there is no way to dispose of it except by the cobalamin-dependent transfer of the methyl group. The reactions involved are summarized in Figure 4–1.

The evidence supporting this concept is as follows. De novo DNA synthesis, as measured by the incorporation of deoxyuridine into the thymine of DNA, is defective in the marrow of patients with vitamin B_{12} deficiency. In some patients with pernicious anemia the apparent serum folate level is elevated, and this has been shown to be due to accumulation of 5-methyl-H_4folate. Added vitamin B_{12} corrects the abnormality in vitamin B_{12} deficient marrows, but not in the folate deficient marrows, whereas folate (pteroylglutamate) corrects both types of deficiencies. Furthermore, a folate antagonist such as methotrexate blocks the corrective action of vitamin B_{12}. A series of experiments by Herbert and associates[91] led to the conclusion that inadequate synthesis of DNA in vitamin B_{12} deficiency is indeed due to a deficiency of tetrahydrofolate, because H_4folate must be continuously available to carry the one carbon unit necessary for de novo synthesis of thymine as its deoxynucleotide (Fig. 4–1). Thus, either folate deficiency, from inadequate intake or from the action of

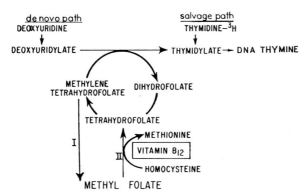

Figure 4–1. B_{12}, folic acid, methionine, and homocysteine interrelationships in thymidylate synthesis. I, 5,10-methylenetetrahydrofolic reductase; II, homocysteine transmethylase. (From Waxman, Metz, and Herbert: J. Clin. Invest., vol. 48, 1969, with permission of the authors and publisher.)

antagonists, or vitamin B$_{12}$ deficiency from whatever cause, may reduce H$_4$folate availability and impair or prevent de novo DNA synthesis.

The important action of vitamin B$_{12}$ in protecting the cells of the nervous system is not understood. The neurologic lesions do not respond to folate in the absence of vitamin B$_{12}$, and they may be the result of an impairment in other reactions requiring cobalamin coenzymes, such as the methylmalonyl coenzyme A isomerization that is involved in the metabolism of several amino acids and of fatty acids with odd-numbered chain lengths.

Classification of Megaloblastic Anemias

The most characteristic feature of deficiency of vitamin B$_{12}$ or folic acid is the occurrence of a megaloblastic anemia. A deficiency can arise in various ways, as shown in Table 4–2. Probably the commonest cause of vitamin B$_{12}$ deficiency is the deficiency of intrinsic factor that is found in pernicious anemia; folic acid deficiency is seen most often in persons with an inadequate intake associated with some other condition, such as pregnancy or cirrhosis of the liver, and in patients with a malabsorption syndrome. Very rarely a case of megaloblastic anemia is seen that cannot be fitted into one of the recognized causes; such cases are termed "idiopathic" for want of a better name. Vitamin B$_{12}$ deficiency that results from inability to utilize the vitamin must be extraordinarily rare if it occurs; most of the reported instances have been shown to be instances of folic acid deficiency or of some block in nucleic acid metabolism.

Table 4–2. *Classification of Megaloblastic Anemias*

I. Vitamin B$_{12}$ deficiency
  A. Inadequate intake
  B. Defective absorption
    1. Failure to secrete intrinsic factor
      a. Addisonian pernicious anemia
      b. Total gastrectomy
    2. Failure of absorption in the small intestine
      a. Malabsorption syndromes
      b. Blind loops and fistulas
      c. Fish tapeworm infestation

II. Folic acid deficiency
  A. Inadequate intake
  B. Defective absorption
    1. Malabsorption syndromes
    2. Blind loop syndrome
    3. Induced by drugs
  C. Inadequate utilization
    1. Ascorbic acid deficiency
    2. Therapy with folic acid antagonists
    3. Therapy with anticonvulsant drugs
    4. Therapy with pyrimethamine
  D. Excessive demands
    1. Pregnancy
    2. Infancy and growth
    3. Hyperhemolysis

Vitamin B_{12} Deficiency

Pernicious Anemia

Synonyms: Primary Anemia, Addison's Anemia, Biermer's Anemia

Pernicious anemia is a disease that has intrigued numerous investigators for many years. The history of pernicious anemia is an "illustrative case" of the development and progress of medicine. First, centuries of almost complete ignorance, then the slow accumulation of clinical information from many scattered sources over a period of about a hundred years, a period which was followed by the rapid progress in the past few decades. The disease affords an example of the successful combining of information gained from animal experiments with careful clinical observations to discover the clinical cure of a previously fatal disease. It is also an illustration of the way in which a significant contribution to clinical medicine stimulates further, more basic, investigation. This in turn leads to a better understanding of human physiology and chemistry that has a significance far beyond a particular disease.

History

The history of pernicious anemia has been reviewed by Haden[38] and by Castle.[13] Credit for reporting the first case of pernicious anemia is generally given to Combe for his report to the Medico-Chirurgical Society of Edinburgh on May 1, 1822. Thomas Addison of Guy's Hospital is given credit for recognizing the disease as a clinical entity. Addison described a progressive fatal type of anemia of unknown cause that occurred in both sexes, generally beyond the middle period of life. He observed the insidious onset, the increasing weakness, and pallor, and commented on the remarkable absence of wasting despite the fatal outcome of the extremely debilitating disease.[61] Biermer in 1871 independently described 15 cases of severe anemia, to which he gave the name "progressive pernicious anemia." Interest in the disease was stimulated and numerous papers followed. Ehrlich described the megaloblasts which he considered diagnostic of pernicious anemia[25] and provided a subject of interest and controversy for those interested in morphology that has continued to the present time. The importance of the gastric secretion of acid in various diseases was studied by Cahn and von Mering in 1886, and in 1921 Levine and Ladd demonstrated the almost constant occurrence of achlorhydria in pernicious anemia in a study of 107 patients with the disease. The relation of the gastric defect to the causation of pernicious anemia was demonstrated by Castle in 1929.[14, 16]

The studies of Whipple and Robscheit-Robbins demonstrated the importance of food factors, particularly liver, in correction of posthemorrhagic anemia in dogs, and suggested that such therapy deserved serious consideration in other more complex anemias, such as pernicious anemia.[93] Minot and Murphy's dramatic report on "The Treatment of Pernicious Anemia by a Special Diet" followed soon after.[64] The excellent results obtained with liver in this series of 45 patients with pernicious anemia were soon confirmed. The significance of this contribution has been emphasized by Haden: "There is nothing more dramatic in medicine than the effect of liver therapy on a patient with pernicious anemia. Only the use of sulfa drugs and other antibiotics such as penicillin afford such brilliant results."[38]

The use of whole liver by mouth led to the development of liver extracts of increasing potency that could be administered parenterally. The search for the active principle of liver extract culminated in the discovery of vitamin B_{12} by Smith[83] and by Rickes and colleagues in 1948.[72] The structural formula of vitamin B_{12} was determined by x-ray crystallographic analysis by Hodgkin in 1956.[51] Subsequent investigations by numerous workers have demonstrated important roles of vitamin B_{12} and folic acid in nucleic acid metabolism in the body.

Mechanism of Vitamin B_{12} Deficiency in Pernicious Anemia

The relationship between the abnormal gastric secretion and the effectiveness of the liver diet in pernicious anemia was shown by Castle and Townsend,[16] who utilized beef muscle, normal gastric juice, hydrochloric acid, and gastric juice from patients with pernicious anemia in their investigation. In a series of classic experiments they studied the hematologic effects of various combinations of these substances on patients with pernicious anemia in relapse. They demonstrated that patients with pernicious anemia lack a substance in the gastric juice that is necessary for the absorption of some factor present in meat that is essential for normal erythropoiesis. It was shown that this gastric factor, which could be destroyed by heat, is not hydrochloric acid. These studies thus established that the primary defect in pernicious anemia is the failure of the stomach to secrete a substance, probably an enzyme, that is necessary for the absorption of a dietary element essential to normal hematopoiesis. As a result of these observations it was postulated that an "extrinsic factor," present in the beef muscle, reacted with an "intrinsic factor," secreted in the normal gastric juice, to form an "erythrocyte maturation factor" which was the active principle that was stored in the liver. After vitamin B_{12} was isolated, Castle and co-workers repeated these experiments but substituted vitamin B_{12} for the beef muscle.[6] The results demonstrated that vitamin B_{12} is both an "extrinsic factor" and an "erythrocyte maturation factor." The function of the intrinsic factor is that of making possible the absorption of vitamin B_{12} from the diet for utilization in the bone marrow and for storage in the liver.

Pernicious anemia and intestinal malabsorption of some sort are the two most frequent causes of vitamin B_{12} deficiency. The Schilling test usually distinguishes between the two. In a few patients with pernicious anemia, however, the absorption of the radioactive vitamin B_{12} does not improve after intrinsic factor (IF) has been added to the test dose.[10, 33, 77, 92] Malabsorption of vitamin B_{12} in the small intestine may be produced by three different mechanisms. One is small bowel disease, a situation that usually can be recognized by demonstrating either abnormalities of the small bowel on x-ray or other evidences of small bowel disease. Another is vitamin B_{12} deficiency itself, which in some patients causes changes in the mucosal cells of the small bowel with impairment of their function; malabsorption of this type is usually corrected within 1 to 10 months by treatment with vitamin B$_{12}$. The third mechanism of malabsorption occurs in the presence of antibodies to the intrinsic factor; these block the action of IF, which is essential for the absorption of vitamin B$_{12}$ in physiological quantities. Pernicious anemia with coexisting malabsorption can be distinguished from vitamin B$_{12}$ deficiency which results from malabsorption by precise immunologic quantitation of the intrinsic factor; only in patients with pernicious anemia have antibodies against the intrinsic factor been demonstrated. Transient malabsorption of vitamin B$_{12}$ may result from reversible structural or functional changes in the parietal cells or ileal mucosa.[45]

The role of an auto-immune mechanism in pernicious anemia has attracted considerable attention.[26, 33, 34, 57, 58, 87] Auto-antibodies to parietal cells have been found in the serum of approximately 90 per cent of patients with pernicious anemia; similar antibodies have been found in from 5 to 8 per cent of the normal population between the ages of 30 and 60, in 14 per cent of women over 60 years of age, and in as high as 60 per cent of patients with thyroid disease, idiopathic gastritis, and other disorders. Clinical pernicious anemia occurs in 12 per cent of patients with primary myxedema or Hashimoto's goiter.[14a] Antibodies to intrinsic factor have been found in the serum of 60 per cent of patients with pernicious anemia and in either the serum or gastric juice in 90 per cent; more important, these antibodies are very rarely found in other disorders or in the general population. Antibodies toward the parietal cells indicate only that gastritis of some sort is present while the presence of antibodies to the intrinsic factor appears to be specific, or nearly so, for pernicious anemia. Up to the present time, however, neither antibody has been successfully incriminated in the production of the disease pernicious anemia. The occurrence of pernicious anemia in persons who have impaired antibody responsiveness and no demonstrable serum antibodies against parietal cells, intrinsic factor, or thyroid antigen indicates that these antibodies are not essential for the development of the disease.[21, 88] Because of these observations, the cellular immune mechanism would have to be involved in an immunological explanation.[45] It is of considerable interest that prednisolone therapy has produced reappearance of parietal cells associated with the secretion of hydrochloric acid and intrinsic factor, together with an increase in the absorption of vitamin B$_{12}$, in some patients with pernicious anemia; other changes found were a decrease in the antibody titer to intrinsic factor in the patient's serum; there was no change in the titer of the parietal cell antibodies. These results imply that the improvement noted in some patients with pernicious anemia after the administration of adrenocorticoid preparations is the result of stimulation of growth and function in the cells of the stomach rather than an interference with the action of antibodies,[2, 56] but the alternative explanation cannot be excluded.

Clinical Manifestations

Pernicious anemia affects individuals of either sex, occurs most often after the age of 40, and is rare before the age of 30. Although pernicious anemia is rare in Africans and in dark skinned white races,[94] the incidence in blacks in the United States approaches that in whites.[49]

The clinical picture of pernicious anemia is variable. Patients with untreated pernicious anemia usually complain of an insidious onset of weakness, anorexia, pallor, "indigestion," and numbness and tingling in the extremities. In older persons dyspnea, palpitation, dizziness, and angina of effort often develop because of the effect of anemia on the circulatory system. Soreness of the tongue and diarrhea may be present. Although it is seldom severe, some loss of weight usually occurs; in a series of patients seen by the authors the average weight loss before treatment was 25 pounds in blacks and 15 pounds in whites.[49]

In some patients with pernicious anemia, particularly since the advent of folic acid and the widespread use of multivitamin preparations, the hematologic abnormalities are mild or absent when neurologic manifestations are prominent. Subjective and objective neurologic findings have been reported in 80 per cent of patients, and were severe enough to cause some degree of incapacity in about 50 per cent.[76] The most common manifestations are paresthesias, incoordination, impairment of position and vibratory sense, and absence of reflexes. The symptoms range from subjective numbness and tingling of the extremities in the mildest form to an unsteady gait, difficulty in locomotion, and difficulty in buttoning the clothes in the more severely affected patients. In the most severe form of the disease the patient is unable to walk and voluntary control of the bladder and rectum is impaired or lost. Some patients undergo marked personality changes associated with memory loss, impaired judgment, disorientation, hallucinations, and delusions.

At times the diagnosis of pernicious anemia is suggested by aspects of the patient's appearance, such as gray hair, sallow skin, slight scleral icterus, and atrophy of the papillae of the tongue. The spleen is usually enlarged in hematologic relapse and is often palpable. In most patients neurologic examination reveals abnormalities of the peripheral nerves and posterolateral columns that are most marked in the lower extremities. The earliest signs are usually some loss of vibratory sense in the lower extremities and impairment of sensation to pin prick and touch that may be either spotty or of the "stocking" type. With more severe changes the Romberg test is positive, position sense is impaired, and the deep tendon reflexes are lost at the ankles and knees. Further progression of the disease in the spinal cord is associated with the development of hyperreflexia and the presence of pathologic reflexes, such as an extensor plantar response. Paraplegia and loss of sphincter control are late manifestations. The neurologic dysfunctions in pernicious anemia have been classified as (1) cerebral, (2) olfactory, (3) peripheral nerve and posterior column of the spinal cord, and (4) peripheral nerve, posterior and lateral columns of the spinal cord.[76] The distinction between peripheral neuropathy, posterior column disease, and combined system degeneration is useful as an indication of the severity of the disease, but classification in this way is not always easy.

Laboratory Examination

In nearly every patient with uncomplicated and untreated pernicious anemia macrocytic anemia occurs. Erythrocyte counts range from less than a million to near normal values. The MCV is nearly always over 100 cu. microns, and is often in the range of 120 to 130 cu. microns. The hemoglobin values are not reduced as much as the erythrocyte count and the MCH is usually increased (over 33 $\gamma\gamma$). The blood smear shows considerable anisocytosis and poikilocytosis of erythrocytes that appear to be well filled with hemoglobin; oval macrocytes are usually present. If the anemia is severe, stippled red cells and nucleated red cells of the megaloblastic series may be seen. In the untreated patient the reticulocyte count is either normal or subnormal.

Leukopenia and thrombocytopenia occur commonly in pernicious anemia. Leukocyte counts of 3000 to 4000 per cu.mm. are common, and levels of 1600 to 2000 per cu.mm. sometimes occur. The leukopenia is due mainly to a reduction in the granulocytes. Some of the granulocytes show abnormalities such as hypersegmentation and an increase in size; these cells are called "macropolycytes." In patients with severe anemia the platelets often number less than 100,000 per cu.mm.

The gastric secretion in pernicious anemia is abnormal in several respects. The total quantity of the gastric juice is greatly reduced and achlorhydria is an almost constant finding. These abnormalities persist after treatment. Because exceptions occur so rarely, failure to secrete free hydrochloric acid after the injection of histamine subcutaneously can be considered an almost essential feature for the diagnosis of pernicious anemia.

The bone marrow in relapse is usually hypercellular. The characteristic feature is the occurrence of the megaloblastic type of erythropoiesis (Fig. 4–2). If anemia is severe, promegaloblasts and basophilic megaloblasts are increased in number and mitotic figures are numerous. The polychromatophilic megaloblasts, which are the easiest cells to identify in this series, persist even after the anemia in the peripheral blood has been abolished by transfusion. The erythrocyte precursors in the marrow are extremely sensitive to specific therapy, and the parenteral administration of even a few micrograms of vitamin B₁₂ or the ingestion of a few milligrams of folic acid is sufficient to change the megaloblastic picture in the marrow to a normoblastic one within a day or two. In such circumstances the appearance of the bone marrow may not be diagnostic. However, the morphologic abnormalities in the marrow in pernicious anemia are not confined to cells of the erythrocytic series. Deficiency of vitamin B₁₂ or folic acid also leads to the production of giant metamyelocytes and multisegmented macropolycytes. These abnormalities in the granulocytic series do not disappear as promptly as the megaloblasts do after specific therapy and their presence may be helpful in diagnosis when the patient is seen for the first time soon after specific therapy has been started. The finding of multisegmented granulocytes in the smear of the peripheral blood is also one of the best screening procedures for a deficiency of vitamin B₁₂ or folate.

Other laboratory tests in the untreated patient generally reveal an increased level of the indirect reacting bilirubin in the plasma (1.0 to 1.5 mg.), an elevation of the serum iron, an increase in fecal urobilinogen excretion, a decreased blood volume, and an increase in the plasma lactic acid dehydrogenase (400 to 4000 units). The levels of the serum iron and folate are often elevated in the untreated patient but fall rapidly during the response to treatment with vitamin B₁₂. A diminution of the plasma protein is not unusual. The serum vitamin B₁₂ level is subnormal, less than 200 pg. per ml., usually less than 100 pg. per ml.

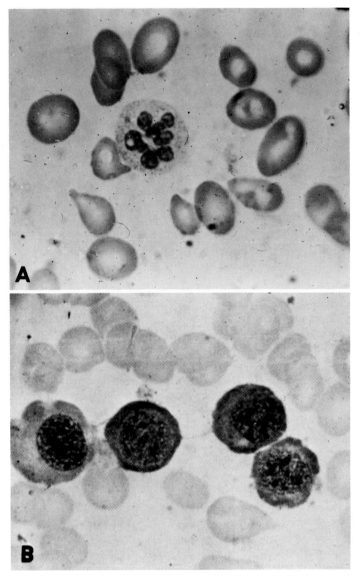

Figure 4–2. *A,* Peripheral blood and *B,* bone marrow from a patient with untreated pernicious anemia. The peripheral blood smear shows macrocytosis, anisocytosis, poikilocytosis, oval macrocytes, and a macropolycyte. The bone marrow shows the megaloblastic type of maturation. (F.S.: I, 34–38.)

Elevated serum muramidase activity occurs in patients with untreated megaloblastic anemia, presumably a reflection of the increased destruction of granulocytes in the marrow or circulation.[68]

Differential Diagnosis

The diagnosis of pernicious anemia in the untreated patient is usually made without difficulty. The presence of macrocytic anemia associated with histamine-fast achlorhydria and a megaloblastic bone marrow practically establishes the diagnosis. The diagnosis is proved when the parenteral administration of vitamin B_{12} produces the characteristic hematologic changes. These are the conversion of the megaloblastic type of erythropoiesis to the normoblastic type within a day or two, a rise in reticulocytes during the first week, and a return of the hemoglobin and red count to normal levels in succeeding weeks. The magnitude of the reticulocyte response depends on the degree of anemia and varies inversely with the erythrocyte count. The maximal reticulocyte count (R) that is expected to follow the intramuscular injection of liver extract or vitamin B_{12} in adequate amounts can be calculated from the formula;

$$R = \frac{82 - 22Eo}{1 + 0.5Eo}$$

where R represents the reticulocyte count in per cent and Eo represents the initial erythrocyte count in million per cu.mm.[53] For example, if the initial erythrocyte count is 1.5 mil. per cu.mm.:

$$R = \frac{82 - (22 \times 1.5)}{1 + (0.5 \times 1.5)} = \frac{82 - 33}{1 + 0.75} = \frac{49}{1.75} = 28 \text{ per cent}$$

In our experience it is not uncommon for the maximal reticulocyte count to fall slightly short of the expected maximum, even when the reticulocytes are counted twice a day (Fig. 4–3).

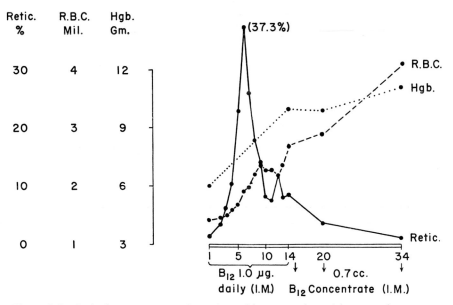

Figure 4–3. Reticulocyte response of a patient with untreated pernicious anemia to treatment with vitamin B_{12}. The maximal reticulocyte response, which was reached about the end of the first week in this patient, depends on the level of the erythrocytes before treatment.

At times pernicious anemia must be differentiated from other conditions characterized by the megaloblastic type of erythropoiesis. The most common disorders in this category are folic acid deficiency of sprue and other dietary deficiencies, and vitamin B_{12} deficiency secondary to intestinal fistulae, shunts, and diverticula. The fact that most conditions associated with folic acid deficiency do not produce histamine-fast achlorhydria often helps to distinguish pernicious anemia from folic acid deficiency. In addition, the disorders associated with folic acid deficiency are often manifested by rather severe gastrointestinal disturbance accompanied by only minor neurologic symptoms; the reverse is more likely to be the case in pernicious anemia. In doubtful cases the determination of the serum B_{12} level or the use of some test of vitamin B_{12} absorption, such as the Schilling test, may be necessary in order to establish the diagnosis.[78, 81]

The Schilling test is performed by giving the patient a measured amount, usually 0.5 microcuries, of cyanocobalamin ^{57}Co orally; 2 hours later the patient is given an intramuscular injection of 1 mg. of non-radioactive cyanocobalamin; urine is collected for 24 hours and the amount of radioactive cyanocobalamin is determined. Normally more than 7 per cent of the ingested dose is excreted within 24 hours. Should the result be subnormal, the test is repeated with oral porcine intrinsic factor, 60 mg.; if excretion is then normal it is concluded that the patient has deficiency of intrinsic factor, in all probability pernicious anemia. If the absorption and excretion do not return to normal after the addition of intrinsic factor it is possible that the patient has a blind loop syndrome or some other disturbance in the bacterial flora of the intestine which leads to malabsorption of vitamin B_{12}. At times this can be established by repeating the test 10 days after giving the patient tetracyline, 250 mg. four times a day. Other causes for low excretion of vitamin B_{12} are incomplete urine collection and renal disease.[81]

The term "achrestic anemia" was proposed for the group of patients with a megaloblastic bone marrow and a peripheral blood picture identical with that of pernicious anemia who responded poorly or not at all to parenteral therapy with liver extract of known potency.[54, 55] The patients that were reported had free HCl in the gastric secretion. The morbid anatomy closely resembled that of pernicious anemia. Known causes of macrocytic anemia such as dietary deficiency, pregnancy, sprue, intestinal parasites, and gastric operations were excluded in the reported cases. Because extracts made from the livers of fatal cases were shown to give excellent hematopoietic responses when administered parenterally to patients with pernicious anemia in relapse, it was suggested that the disease in these patients was due to a failure to utilize or mobilize the antianemic principle that was present in the tissue stores.[55] Sternal marrow biopsies showed various degrees of conversion from the megaloblastic to the normoblastic type of erythropoiesis after treatment with liver extract but usually resembled the marrow from an inadequately treated patient. In our experience cases that fit this description are even rarer than the reported incidence of one per 100 patients with pernicious anemia.[54] The report of Davidson suggests that at least some patients whose symptoms fit the description of achrestic anemia may well represent instances of folic acid deficiency. In a group of 375 patients with macrocytic anemia associated with a megaloblastic bone marrow, 25 with unexplained megaloblastic anemia (15 with achlorhydria) were refractory to therapy with potent extract.[23] The 15 who were treated orally with folic acid or proteolyzed liver responded to the treatment.

When the patient with pernicious anemia has the neurologic features of the disease without the characteristic hematologic abnormalities the diagnosis may be difficult. In such circumstances the patient usually has received vitamin B_{12} or folic acid in an amount that is sufficient to convert the megaloblastic type of erythropoiesis to the normoblastic type and raise the erythrocyte count to near normal levels. If examination of the peripheral blood and bone marrow does not suffice for the diagnosis, a gastric analysis should be done. If free hydrochloric acid is secreted after the histamine injection, the diagnosis of pernicious anemia can be discarded with considerable assurance. If histamine-fast achlorhydria is present, the Schilling test for vitamin B_{12} absorption or some other similar test should be performed since it will often clarify the diagnosis.

The tests of vitamin B_{12} absorption are also helpful in the evaluation of patients without neurologic disease who have received treatment with vitamin B_{12} or liver extract before the diagnosis was established. By such means the diagnosis can be verified or corrected without waiting months or years after specific therapy is withheld to see whether hematologic relapse occurs.

Both megaloblasts and sideroblasts appear in the marrow of some alcoholic patients; the abnormalities disappear rapidly when alcohol is withheld.[50]

Treatment

Prior to the report of Minot and Murphy in 1926 on the efficacy of liver, the treatment of pernicious anemia was unsatisfactory and the disease was invariably fatal.[64] Since that time more efficient preparations have been developed but all are forms of substitution therapy that must be continued for the life of the patient. Vitamin B_{12} is the essential factor, and the parenteral administration of as little as 1 microgram each day to a patient in relapse is sufficient to restore the blood to normal and prevent the development of neurologic lesions if these are not already present. In practice it is customary to administer larger amounts at longer intervals and to err toward an excessive dose rather than risk an amount that may be suboptimal.

Although the selection of the details of the schedule may be somewhat arbitrary, some definite program of treatment should be followed. The following schedule has been found satisfactory for patients in relapse in our experience: vitamin B_{12} 30 micrograms intramuscularly three times during the first week, then 30 micrograms once a week until the blood returns to normal. This schedule produces the expected reticulocyte response within the first week or 10 days and a return of the erythrocyte level to normal within 6 to 10 weeks. Thereafter the patient receives injections of 60 micrograms every 4 weeks. A program of 30 micrograms every 4 weeks has maintained patients in hematologic remission and prevented the development of neurologic lesions, but in one reported series of 51 patients treated with 30 micrograms of vitamin B_{12} parenterally each month, definite neurologic relapse occurred in the absence of hematologic relapse; three of these patients improved when the amount of vitamin B$_{12}$ was increased and one responded to liver extract.[79] Monthly injections of 250 or 500 micrograms have been recommended to sustain complete normality.[42] Such reports appear to confirm the clinical impression that not all patients with pernicious anemia require the same maintenance dosage. For this reason it is advisable to check the hematocrit levels every few months and the neurologic status at regular intervals so that the dosage of vitamin B$_{12}$ can be adjusted if the therapy is not adequate. Although effective oral preparations are available, parenteral therapy is preferred because of greater reliability, less expense, and better supervision of the patient. Unless careful supervision is maintained some patients will develop hematologic or, more important, neurologic relapse as a consequence of inadequate therapy. In one report of 41 patients treated orally with vitamin B$_{12}$ and folic acid, 5 failed to return and in 14 others oral therapy was discontinued because of neurologic or hematologic relapse.[79]

When an elderly patient is severely anemic, the circulation is sometimes compromised by the low levels of the circulating hemoglobin. When this occurs, transfusions may be administered if it is considered inadvisable to wait for the erythropoietic effect of the vitamin B$_{12}$. The use of packed cells is preferred to whole blood because the former gives the desired increase in circulating hemoglobin without as great an increase in blood volume.

When severe neurologic complications are present vitamin B$_{12}$ is often administered in amounts larger than those that are usually given to the patient with uncomplicated anemia. This practice is based on clinical observations which led to the belief that the optimal therapeutic dose of vitamin B$_{12}$ may not be the same for both the hematopoietic and nervous systems. It has been recognized that there is little or no correlation between the severity of the anemia and the extent of the neurologic lesion because some patients present with severe anemia and little or no neurologic involvement, and others have severe neurologic disease and only mild anemia. Although neurologic complications rarely if ever develop if a a normal hematologic status is maintained with parenteral vitamin B$_{12}$, it has not been established that 1 microgram a day is the optimal initial treatment for the patient with existing neurologic involvement of significant degree. The neurologic response to therapy is much slower than the hematologic and improvement may continue for several months after the blood has returned to normal. Some patients who show little neurologic improvement during the first month or two of therapy show gratifying improvement between the third and sixth months. Apparently little or no improvement can be anticipated after 10 to 12 months of therapy.

Because of these considerations we employ a larger dose of vitamin B$_{12}$ in patients with neurologic involvement (100 micrograms three times a week for 3 months, then 100 micrograms weekly for 3 months), although it is recognized that the value of a dose larger than that necessary to produce hematologic remission has not been established. Although parenteral vitamin B$_{12}$ is the most important treatment for patients with neurologic disease, physiotherapy is often very helpful in patients who are severely affected. It has been shown clearly that although folic acid therapy may maintain the patient in a normal hematologic status, it does not prevent the development of neurologic lesions.[8, 75]

Vitamin B$_{12}$ appears to be a complete therapy in pernicious anemia. Dilute hydrochloric acid, folic acid, and liver extract are unnecessary. Likewise iron is not indicated unless there is an associated iron deficiency from some other cause.

Failure to respond to therapy or the occurrence of a hematologic relapse while the patient is receiving adequate amounts of vitamin B₁₂ should raise the suspicion of the development of some infection, renal insufficiency, gastrointestinal bleeding, or the appearance of a carcinoma of the stomach. In former years the presence on the market of ineffective liver preparations was responsible for some therapeutic "failures."

Course and Prognosis

If the patient does not have significant neurologic involvement when he is first seen the prognosis is excellent. He should be restored to his previous status and with proper maintenance therapy his outlook should be that of his age group, with the possible exception of a greater likelihood of developing carcinoma of the stomach. The reported incidence of carcinoma of the stomach in patients with pernicious anemia varies considerably. One report placed the incidence in living patients at 1.7 per cent;[66] another roentgen study of 211 patients found gastric carcinoma in 8 per cent and benign polyps in 7.1 per cent.[73] Several reports place the frequency of carcinoma of the stomach at autopsy at from 8.4 per cent to 12.3 per cent,[59, 98] figures that are three to four times the incidence in individuals of the same age group who do not have pernicious anemia. The increased frequency of carcinoma suggests the desirability of periodic examinations in an effort to detect the carcinoma in an early stage. It has been recommended that the stool be examined for occult blood each month, that gastric cytology be studied every 3 to 6 months, and that suspicious cases have gastroscopy and roentgenographic study of the upper gastrointestinal tract.[98] In our experience these procedures have proved impractical as routine measures and the problem of early recognition of the development of carcinoma remains a perplexing one.

If neurologic complications are present the prognosis is related to the extent and duration of the manifestations. If symptoms have been present for only a few months the outlook is excellent, particularly if the individual is less than 50 years old. Signs of an upper motor neuron lesion, such as the Babinski sign, usually persist despite treatment but sometimes disappear. Absent deep tendon reflexes usually return. Marked improvement may occur promptly and maximal improvement occurs within 10 or 12 months. If paraplegia and loss of sphincter control have developed the outlook for recovery is poor. However, many patients who are severely ataxic and unable to walk improve after months of treatment and eventually recover sufficiently to resume most of their previous activities even though subjective and objective neurologic abnormalities persist.

JUVENILE PERNICIOUS ANEMIA

Although pernicious anemia characteristically occurs in persons who are middle-aged or older, the clinical picture has been observed in children from a few months to 18 years of age. The most common symptoms are pallor, weakness, listlessness, and irritability; fever, anorexia, vomiting, diarrhea, glossitis, and weight loss also occur. Hepatosplenomegaly, jaundice, mental retardation, and neurologic abnormalities have been reported but are unusual. The hematologic features are the same as those seen in adult pernicious anemia; these are corrected by treatment with vitamin B$_{12}$ or liver extract and recur if treatment is discontinued. The disorder usually responds to the intramuscular injection of from 15 to 30 micrograms of vitamin B$_{12}$ every 2 to 4 weeks.

The reported cases may be divided into several groups.[63] In one group of 20 patients, in 16 of whom the onset occurred before 2½ years of age, histology of the gastric mucosa and secretion of acid were normal but secretion of the intrinsic factor was lacking; antibodies to intrinsic factor were not demonstrated in the serum. In the second group of 6 patients, the disease became manifest later in childhood and was characterized by failure of secretion of the intrinsic factor associated with histamine-fast achlorhydria and atrophic gastritis; antibodies against intrinsic factor were demonstrated in 4 patients, all of whom had associated hypofunction of one or more endocrine glands. It has been suggested that the first group may represent a disease that results from a metabolic error with selective failure of intrinsic factor secretion; it may be distinct from and not genetically related to adult pernicious anemia. The second group more closely resembles the adult form of the disease.

Another group of patients with deficiency of vitamin B$_{12}$ has been considered by some authors to be a form of "juvenile pernicious anemia."[84] In 18 patients no abnormality was found in the secretion of acid or intrinsic factor and biopsy of the gastric mucosa was normal; all had proteinuria. These patients apparently had a specific defect in the absorption of vitamin B$_{12}$. Since the absorption defect in these patients does not appear to be related to any lack of the intrinsic factor, use of the term "pernicious anemia" for this type of vitamin B$_{12}$ deficiency appears incorrect. The eponym Imerslund's syndrome has been applied to this disorder, reported in at least 28 patients; it has been postulated that the malabsorption of vitamin B$_{12}$ is the result of an anomaly in the small intestine, a defect in the mechanism which releases vitamin B$_{12}$ from intrinsic factor.[28]

Illustrative Cases

CASE 1

A 56 year old white housewife was admitted to the hospital for the evaluation of progressive numbness and pain in her hands and feet of 2 years' duration. In the last few weeks before admission her gait had become unsteady. She had been taking "vitamin pills" as a tonic for many months. On an admission 13 years previously she was found to have histamine-fast achlorhydria and hypochromic anemia; the anemia responded to treatment with iron.

Physical examination.   The patient was an obese white woman in no apparent distress. Pertinent abnormalities were found only on the neurologic examination. These were: absent gag reflex; moderate spastic paraparesis and increased tendon reflexes in the lower extremities; abnormal Babinski signs bilaterally; impairment of position sense in the hands and feet; and absence of vibratory sense in the feet and legs.

Laboratory examination. Admission blood studies disclosed the following: Hct. 42 per cent, Hb. 14.3 gm. per 100 ml., R.B.C. 4.3 mil. per cu.mm. There was moderate anisocytosis of the red cells; both microcytic and macrocytic forms were present. Examination of the urine, stool, and spinal fluid was normal. Gastric analysis on two occasions revealed the absence of free hydrochloric acid after the injection of histamine. Examination of the bone marrow showed a normoblastic type of erythropoiesis. A Schilling test for radioactive vitamin B$_{12}$ (B$_{12}$Co^{60}) absorption was performed. No significant absorption of vitamin B$_{12}$ occurred (0 per cent excretion). When the test was repeated with the addition of intrinsic factor, absorption of the orally administered vitamin B$_{12}$ occurred (9 per cent excretion).

Diagnosis and treatment. A diagnosis of pernicious anemia with subacute combined degeneration of the spinal cord was made. The patient was treated with vitamin B$_{12}$ intramuscularly. During the next 10 months her gait improved gradually and returned to normal. Impaired vibratory sense and paresthesias persisted.

Comment. The neurologic manifestations of pernicious anemia occurred in this patient in the absence of anemia. The diagnosis was suggested by the clinical features of neurologic disease associated with histamine-fast achlorhydria and was established by the demonstration of faulty vitamin B$_{12}$ absorption. It is probable that the essentially normal blood values and the normoblastic bone marrow were the results of folic acid contained in the multivitamin tablets which the patient had taken. This case also illustrates the well recognized occurrence of histamine-fast achlorhydria some years before the onset of clinical pernicious anemia.

CASE 2

A 67 year old white farmer was admitted to the hospital in August 1947 because of weakness, dizziness, exertional dyspnea, ataxia, and numbness of the hands of 6 months' duration.

Physical examination. The skin and mucous membranes were pale and the tongue was smooth. Vibratory sense was diminished in the legs, the knee jerks were diminished, and ankle jerks were absent. No pathologic reflexes were present.

Laboratory examination. Admission blood studies disclosed the following: Hb. 9.0 gm. per 100 ml.; R.B.C. 1.58 mil. per cu.mm.; Hct. 24 per cent (MCV 150 cu.μ, MCH 56 $\gamma\gamma$, MCHC 36 per cent); W.B.C. 2500 per cu.mm.; platelets 70,000 per cu.mm.; reticulocytes 0.6 per cent; differential count (per cent), granulocytes 36, lymphocytes 63. Examination of a smear of the peripheral blood revealed considerable anisocytosis and poikilocytosis; many macrocytes that were well filled with hemoglobin were seen. Roentgenographic studies of the upper gastrointestinal tract and colon were normal. Gastric analysis revealed the absence of free HCl after the injection of histamine. Examination of the bone marrow disclosed that erythropoiesis was megaloblastic in

character; giant band forms, large metamyelocytes, and macropolycytes were also present.

Diagnosis and treatment.   A diagnosis of pernicious anemia was
made and the patient was treated with daily intramuscular injections
of 15 units of liver extract. After the first week, the dose was reduced
to 15 units a week. Although the peak reticulocyte response of 7.8
per cent was well below the predicted maximum, the hemoglobin,
red count, and hematocrit returned to normal within 10 weeks. During
the next 7 years the patient got along well on treatment with parenteral
liver extract, 30 units each month, and later with vitamin B$_{12}$, 30
micrograms each month.

Course.   In March 1954 a barium study of the stomach was done
with normal results. In February 1955 when the patient was 75 years
of age, he developed vague epigastric discomfort. A barium study
about one month after the onset of symptoms revealed a filling defect
in the antral portion of the stomach. Operation disclosed the presence
of a carcinoma of the stomach that had already penetrated the serosal
surface. A partial gastrectomy was performed and the patient was
largely asymptomatic for about a year. After this time his health
declined steadily until he died of his carcinoma in late 1956, one and
a half years after its discovery.

Comment.   This case illustrates many interesting points that are
considered typical of pernicious anemia. When first seen, the patient
was an elderly man with a severe anemia without significant weight
loss. The anemia was macrocytic, and was associated with leukopenia,
thrombocytopenia, a megaloblastic bone marrow, and histamine-fast
achlorhydria. The diagnosis of pernicious anemia was established by
the response to specific therapy. Neurologic disease was never a problem. After being well for nearly 8 years, the patient developed a
carcinoma of the stomach which proved fatal in less than 2 years. The
incidence of carcinoma of the stomach in patients with pernicious
anemia has been reported to be several times that in the general
population. The difficulty in dealing with the problem is shown by
this patient. Radiographic study of the upper gastrointestinal tract
was performed every 12 to 18 months, and yet the patient had an
incurable carcinoma when it was recognized only one month after
the onset of vague gastrointestinal complaints.

Less Common Causes of Vitamin B$_{12}$ Deficiency

Dietary deficiency.   Vitamin B$_{12}$ deficiency that results solely from an
inadequate intake is extremely rare in the Western world. The absorption of
only a minute amount, about 1 microgram a day, is required by an adult.
Very strict vegetarians are candidates for a deficiency of vitamin B$_{12}$ but rarely
develop it.

Postgastrectomy.   Total gastrectomy, which removes the organ of secretion of the intrinsic factor, produces the clinical picture of pernicious anemia
if the patient survives until the body stores of vitamin B$_{12}$ have been depleted.
This usually requires 3 or 4 years. Patients who have had a total gastrectomy

require the regular administration of vitamin B_{12} just as patients with pernicious anemia do. Partial gastrectomy sometimes interferes with vitamin B_{12} absorption, but rarely produces a clinical deficiency because the intrinsic factor is secreted in the cardiac portion of the stomach. Nevertheless, some patients, possibly because of partial atrophy of the gastric remnant, have suboptimal vitamin B_{12} serum levels and should receive supplements of this factor.

Malabsorption, blind loops, and fistula. Impaired absorption of vitamin B_{12} sometimes occurs in patients with ileitis and those who have had extensive surgical resections of the small bowel but this malabsorption is rarely severe enough to produce megaloblastic anemia. A more severe deficiency occurs in certain patients with fistulae, diverticula, blind loops, and strictures of the small intestine; in such patients the defective absorption appears to be related in some way to the bacterial flora of the intestine because the ability to absorb vitamin B_{12} is restored by treatment with antibiotics administered by the oral route but is not corrected by supplements of intrinsic factor.[40] Severe prolonged diarrhea, sprue, and other malabsorption syndromes are much more likely to produce severe folic acid deficiency accompanied by only mild and often insignificant vitamin B_{12} deficiency.

Other uncommon causes of malabsorption of vitamin B_{12} are folate deficiency and the ingestion of ethanol, neomycin, colchicine or para-amino salicylic acid.[22a]

Fish tapeworm infestation. A disease found mainly in Finland, Norway, and Sweden with the hematologic and neurologic manifestations identical to those seen in pernicious anemia occurs in some of the individuals who are infected with the fish tapeworm, Diphyllobothrium latum.[9] Approximately 2 per cent of those infested have anemia; in 50 per cent the serum B_{12} level is low.[66a] Apparently the tapeworms produce the deficiency by competing successfully for the available vitamin B_{12} or by interfering with its absorption, because elimination of the parasites without other treatment is followed by recovery.

Folate Deficiency

Dietary Deficiency

Folate deficiency associated with a megaloblastic anemia may be the result of an inadequate diet. Tropical macrocytic anemia is perhaps the best known example, but a similar type of anemia occurs in other parts of the world where the diet is suboptimal, particularly when it is deficient in meat and leafy vegetables. Poverty and ignorance are probably the most important causes. At times a dietary deficiency may be produced by improper cooking of food that contains folate. In the Western world, even in vegetarians, dietary deficiency of folic acid is rarely a cause of anemia; anemia of this type occurs in pregnancy because the demands of folic acid are increased; megaloblastic anemia of folate deficiency is also seen in patients with portal cirrhosis who have a grossly deficient diet that consists mainly of carbohydrate in the form of alcohol. Treatment with a small amount of folic acid, 100 micrograms by mouth, has been recommended because a larger dose may obscure a coexisting deficiency of vitamin B_{12}.[42] Treatment with this dose of folic acid while the patient follows a diet low in folate (avoidance of liver, fresh fruits, fruit juices, and green vegetables) may be a diagnostic procedure; a reticulocyte response that peaks in 10 days is a positive result.

Malabsorption Syndromes

Although some authors believe that idiopathic sprue (adult celiac disease, non-tropical sprue), childhood celiac disease, and tropical sprue are but variants of the same disease, most writers distinguish tropical sprue from idiopathic sprue, and consider that the latter disorder may become manifest either in childhood as "celiac disease" or in adult life as "non-tropical" sprue. In addition, the malabsorption syndrome may arise secondary to diseases of the small bowel. A classification is presented in Table 4–3.

If the absorption of vitamin B_{12} or folic acid is impaired sufficiently, a hematologic picture identical to that seen in untreated pernicious anemia occurs. When megaloblastic anemia occurs in patients with the malabsorption syndrome, a deficiency of folate usually is responsible; megaloblastic anemia rarely develops in the secondary malabsorption disorders. Iron deficiency anemia occurs in some patients with the malabsorption syndrome as a result of blood loss from the gastrointestinal tract or from impaired absorption of iron.

In order to establish a diagnosis in a patient with suspected malabsorption syndrome, various examinations may be necessary. These include the following: measure of the amount of fat in the stools; determination of the levels of serum calcium, iron, cholesterol, and carotene; the d-xylose and vitamin A absorption tests; and roentgenographic study of the small intestine. Jejunal biopsy often provides very valuable information.

Non-Tropical Sprue

An increasing amount of evidence indicates that celiac disease in childhood and adult idiopathic steatorrhea or non-tropical sprue are the same disease. The disorder is probably an inherited defect in absorption. In most

Table 4–3. *Malabsorption in the Small Bowel*

A. Primary malabsorption
  1. Non-tropical sprue (idiopathic sprue, celiac disease, adult celiac disease, idiopathic steatorrhea)
  2. Tropical sprue

B. Secondary syndromes
  1. Lymphoma
  2. Whipple's disease
  3. Collagen disease
  4. Operative resection of the small bowel
  5. Others

patients improvement follows the exclusion of gluten-containing foods, wheat, rye, and barley, from the diet.

Non-tropical sprue is usually a chronic disorder. Persistent or recurrent diarrhea occurs in the vast majority of patients but malabsorption sometimes occurs in the absence of diarrhea. In one series of 94 patients with idiopathic sprue seen at the Mt. Sinai Hospital in New York[1] diarrhea, weakness, and weight loss each occurred in 80 per cent; about one-half had glossitis; flatulence, abdominal discomfort, anorexia, nausea, and vomiting were found in 20 to 30 per cent. In the same series about 25 per cent of the patients had tetany and abnormal bleeding (ecchymoses, epistaxis, melena, hematuria, menorrhagia, gingival bleeding) secondary to prothrombin deficiency; less than 20 per cent of the patients had paresthesias, bone pain, mental symptoms, and fever. The commonest abnormality seen on the physical examination was emaciation which occurred in 65 per cent. Abdominal distention, edema, hepatomegaly, hypotension, tetany, and bleeding each had an incidence of from 20 to 35 per cent. Other abnormalities which had a frequency of about 10 per cent or less were pigmentation, lymphadenopathy, dry skin, splenomegaly, abdominal tenderness, absent reflexes, paresthesias, and sensory disturbances. Rarely, patients with long-standing disease develop signs of severe posterior column involvement that does not respond to treatment with vitamin B_{12}, folic acid, or liver extract.

Various types of anemia develop as the result of blood loss or defective absorption of factors essential for normal erythropoiesis. The reported incidence of macrocytic anemia in idiopathic sprue varies from 14 to 95 per cent and the incidence of iron deficiency from 6 to 17 per cent.[1] In one series macrocytosis was present in 57.6 per cent, normal erythrocytes in 33 per cent, and hypochromic cells in 9.4 per cent. Hemoglobin levels of less than 10 grams per 100 ml. occurred in 51 per cent. In children the anemia is usually hypochromic and microcytic. Adults sometimes develop iron deficiency anemia in the absence of diarrhea, a circumstance in which malabsorption may not be suspected.

Although a deficiency of folate is usually responsible for megaloblastic anemia, abnormalities in vitamin B_{12} absorption occur often and are sometimes of clinical importance. In a group of 25 patients with idiopathic sprue, 20 were found to have impaired absorption of vitamin B_{12} that did not improve when intrinsic factor was administered.[67] In another study, lowered serum vitamin B_{12} levels were found in about one-third of the patients with steatorrhea.[65] The absorption of vitamin B_{12} in the presence of added intrinsic factor has been found to improve after administration of corticosteroids.[32] Impaired absorption of folic acid has been shown to occur commonly in idiopathic steatorrhea.[29]

Treatment of the patient with non-tropical sprue generally entails use of a gluten-free diet for at least 6 months plus treatment for specific deficiencies. The administration of folic acid orally or intramuscularly in doses of 5 to 15 mg. a day usually produces a good hematologic response; smaller amounts, 0.5 to 1.0 mg. by mouth, are probably adequate.[42] Most patients are refractory to treatment with vitamin B_{12} parenterally[44] but some respond at least partially. The response of the individual patient probably depends on the state of the vitamin B_{12} stores and the degree of folate deficiency; when both substances are deficient both folic acid and parenteral vitamin B_{12} are necessary. Gastrointestinal symptoms usually persist or recur despite improvement in the blood if treatment consists only of administration of both folic acid and vitamin B_{12}. The majority of patients become symptom-free on the gluten-free diet but even in these patients the persistence of some malabsorptive defect has been demonstrated. The inability of the intestinal tract to absorb vitamin B_{12} and folic acid sometimes persists whether the patient is in remission or relapse;[1] continued treatment with these vitamins and also iron may be necessary. Acutely ill patients and those with the more severe or resistant forms of the disease are usually treated with prednisone, or a related compound, which produces striking improvement in all the manifestations of the disease. The initial dose of prednisone, 50 to 60 mg. a day, is usually necessary for a week or two; the amount is then reduced to a maintenance dosage, often no more than 5 mg. a day, which may be necessary for years.

Tropical Sprue

Tropical sprue is seen most frequently in people living in the Caribbean region and in parts of Asia. The nature of the disorder is puzzling because folate deficiency develops despite a diet that may be high in folate activity. The onset of tropical sprue may be sudden, but if the disorder has persisted for some time, the clinical manifestations may closely resemble those usually seen in non-tropical sprue; however, the disorders differ in some important details. In tropical sprue, the usual hematologic picture is one that is indistinguishable from pernicious anemia and responds to treatment with folic acid or vitamin B_{12} or both. In addition there are often striking improvement in appetite, weight, sense of well being, and the gastrointestinal symptoms, a return of folate absorption to normal, and renewal of intestinal villi, changes that are rarely if ever seen in non-tropical sprue. Although the appearance of the small intestinal mucosa improves in a prompt and striking manner after treatment with folic acid or vitamin B_{12}, it is incomplete; both the morphologic abnormalities in the villi and some degree of malabsorption persist.[86] These observations suggest that the deficiencies of folate and vitamin B_{12} found in patients with tropical sprue are the result of malabsorption rather than the cause; the nature of the basic lesion responsible for the malabsorption has not been determined. It has also been demonstrated that treatment with tetracycline and other antibiotics is often effective in tropical sprue but ineffective in non-tropical sprue.[37] The gluten-free diet which has been shown to be effective in the majority of patients with non-tropical sprue has not been shown to be effective in tropical sprue.

Other Causes of Malabsorption

Malabsorption of folate has been reported after oral contraceptive therapy[65a] and after ingestion of anticonvulsant drugs.[52, 74] A study of patients taking orally administered contraceptives for at least a year indicated that their serum folate level was lower than that in the controls, although the absorption of monoglutamic folate was equal in the two groups. The results suggest that orally administered contraceptives interfere with the absorption of polyglutamic folate. Whether this effect is through enzyme inhibition or through some other mechanism is uncertain.[84a] The malabsorption is rarely severe enough to produce clinical disease.

Inadequate Utilization of Folic Acid

Associated Ascorbic Acid Deficiency

Megaloblastic anemia with the blood picture characteristic of vitamin B_{12} or folate deficiency sometimes is seen in infants between the ages of 2 and 17 months.[99] The onset is insidious, with increasing pallor, failure to gain weight, recurrent fever, inconstant diarrhea, and, occasionally, episodes of abnormal bleeding. Premature infants are more liable to the disorder, which develops if the milk used for infant feeding has a low folate content; added factors of rapid growth and diarrhea may be contributory. A deficiency of ascorbic acid is also apparently a factor in the development of this syndrome; the powdered milk preparations used by patients with this disorder had a low content of ascorbic acid, and the disorder has almost disappeared since the foods have been fortified with ascorbic acid. The anemia responds to treatment with folic acid in doses of 10 to 30 mg. orally or parenterally but at times simultaneous administration of ascorbic acid is necessary.

Therapy with Folate Antagonists

Megaloblastic anemia may be produced in patients with leukemia or other forms of lymphoma who are treated with anti-folic compounds such as aminopterin, amethopterin, 6MP, 5-fluorouracil, and cytosine arabinoside; such patients may develop macrocytic anemia, megaloblastic bone marrow, and the other changes associated with folic acid deficiency as well as gastrointestinal symptoms of glossitis and diarrhea.

Megaloblastosis has occurred during the administration of pyrimethamine; apparently the drug acts as an antifolate.[90]

Therapy with Anticonvulsant Drugs

Over 50 cases of megaloblastic anemia associated with anticonvulsant drug therapy have been reported since Badenoch called attention to the entity in the English literature in 1954.[3, 27, 30, 41] Diphenylhydantoin sodium, primidone, phenobarbital derivatives and more recently a preparation containing aspirin, salicylamide, and caffeine have been the associated drugs.[95] Nearly all the patients who developed the anemia had been taking the drugs for long periods, usually for years, but it has been reported after only 6 months of treatment. The peripheral blood is characterized by a macrocytic anemia, leukopenia with multisegmented granulocytes, and thrombocytopenia. Although the pathogenesis of the syndrome is not entirely understood, several explanations have been suggested. One postulates that the anemia is a manifestation of folate deficiency produced by the drug's acting as a competitive inhibitor of some enzyme system normally involving folic acid as a cofactor, another that the drug displaces folate from its plasma carrier; a third suggestion is that the drug by inhibiting intestinal conjugases in some way interferes with absorption of folate.[52, 74] In any event an inadequate dietary intake, particularly of folic acid and ascorbic acid, may be a contributing factor.

Recovery from the anemia has followed withdrawal of the drug; recovery also has followed treatment with even small amounts of folic acid, vitamin B_{12}, or a combination of the two vitamins. The anemia nearly always responds to the administration of folic acid, even if the anticonvulsant drug is continued. Mild or moderate deficiency of vitamin B_{12} may occur in this group of patients but significant vitamin B_{12} deficiency is unusual.

Excessive Demands

Megaloblastic anemia develops when the demand for folate exceeds the supply. In pregnancy the daily requirement of folate is probably 400 micrograms, more than the usual American or European diet contains.[85, 96] The appearance of increased numbers of hypersegmented neutrophils in the peripheral blood is often the first evidence of folate deficiency.[19] When a physician prescribes a vitamin supplement to correct or prevent this deficiency during pregnancy he must be careful to select a preparation that contains adequate folate because many multivitamin preparations contain no folate.

Severe hemolytic anemia may produce megaloblastic anemia because of the large amounts of folate required for the dividing marrow cells.

Folate deficiency and megaloblastic hematopoiesis have been observed in patients with chronic renal disease, particularly those who are receiving long term hemodialysis. Serum vitamin B_{12} levels were normal and serum folate levels were low; it appeared that folate was removed by dialysis whereas vitamin B_{12} was not.[40a]

References

1. Adlersberg, D.: The Malabsorption Syndrome. Grune and Stratton, New York, 1957.
2. Ardeman, S., and Chanarin, I.: Steroids and addisonian pernicious anemia. New England J. Med., *273*:1352, 1965.
3. Badenoch, J.: The use of labelled vitamin B_{12} and gastric biopsy in the investigation of anaemia. Proc. Roy. Soc. Med., *47*:426, 1954.
4. Baker, S. J., Jacob, E., Rajan, K. T., and Swaminathan, S. P.: Vitamin B_{12} deficiency in pregnancy and the puerperium. Brit. M. J., *1*:1658, 1962.
5. Baugh, C. M., and Krumdieck, C. L.: Effects of phenytoin on folic-acid conjugases in man. Lancet, 2:519, 1969.
6. Berk, L., et al.: Observations on the etiologic relationship of achylia gastrica to pernicious anemia. X. Activity of vitamin B_{12} as food (extrinsic) factor. New England J. Med., *239*:911, 1948.
7. Bertino, J. R., and Johns, D. G.: Folate metabolism in man. Plenary session papers. International Society of Hematology, 1968, p. 133.
8. Bethell, F. H., and Sturgis, C. C.: The relation of therapy in pernicious anemia to changes in the nervous system. Early and late results in a series of cases observed for periods of not less than 10 years, and early results of treatment with folic acid. Blood, *3*:57, 1948.
9. Björkenheim, G.: Neurological changes in pernicious tapeworm anaemia. Acta med. scand., Suppl. 260, *140*:1, 1951.

10. Brody, E. A., Estren, S., and Herbert, V.: Coexistent pernicious anemia and malabsorption in four patients, including one whose malabsorption disappeared with vitamin B_{12} therapy. Ann. Int. Med., *64*:1246, 1966.

11. Butterworth, C. E., Jr.: The availability of food folate. Annotation. Brit. J. Haemat., *14*:339, 1968.

12. Butterworth, C. E., Santini, R., and Frommeyer, W. B.: The pteroylglutamate components of American diets as determined by chromatographic fractionation. J. Clin. Invest.,*42*:1929, 1963.

13. Castle, W. B.: A century of curiosity about pernicious anemia. Tr. Am. Clin. & Climatol. A., *73*:54, 1961.

14. Castle, W. B.: Observations on the etiologic relationship of achylia gastrica to pernicious anemia. I. The effect of the administration to patients with pernicious anemia of the contents of the normal human stomach recovered after the ingestion of beef muscle. Am. J. M. Sc., *178*:748, 1929.

14a. Castle, W. B.: Current concepts of pernicious anemia. Am. J. Med., *48*:541, 1970.

15. Castle, W. B., Rhoads, C. P., Lawson, H. A., and Payne, G. C.: Etiology and treatment of sprue—observations on patients in Puerto Rico and subsequent experiments on animals. Arch. Int. Med., *56*:627, 1935.

16. Castle, W. B., and Townsend, W. C.: Observations on the etiologic relationship of achylia gastrica to pernicious anemia. II. Effect of the administration to patients with pernicious anemia of beef muscle after incubation with normal human gastric juice. Am. J. M. Sc., *178*:764, 1929.

17. Chanarin, I., Anderson, B. B., and Mollin, D. L.: The absorption of folic acid. Brit. J. Haem., *4*:156, 1958.

18. Chanarin, I., Dacie, J. V., and Mollin, D. L.: Folic acid deficiency in haemolytic anaemia. Brit. J. Haemat., *5*:245, 1959.

19. Chanarin, I., Rothman, D., Ardeman, S., and Berry, V.: Some observations on the changes preceding the development of megaloblastic anaemia in pregnancy with particular reference to the neutrophil leucocytes. Brit. J. Haemat., *11*:557, 1965.

20. Chesterman, D. C., Cuthbertson, W. F., Jr., and Pegler, H. F.: Vitamin B_{12}. Excretion studies. Biochem. J., *48*:li, 1951.

21. Clark, R., Tornyos, K., Herbert, V., and Twomey, J. J.: Studies on two patients with concomitant pernicious anemia and immunoglobulin deficiency. Ann. Int. Med., *67*:403, 1967.

22. Cooper, B. A., and White, J. J.: Absence of intrinsic factor from human portal plasma during $Co^{57}B_{12}$ absorption in man. Brit. J. Haemat., *14*:73, 1968.

22a. Corcino, J. J., Waxsman, S., and Herbert, V.: Absorption and malabsorption of vitamin B_{12}. Am. J. Med., *48*:562, 1970.

23. Davidson, L. S. P.: Refractory megaloblastic anemia. Blood, *3*:107, 1948.

24. Donaldson, R. M., Mackenzie, I. L., and Trier, J. S.: Intrinsic factor mediated attachment of vitamin B_{12} to brush borders and microvillous membranes of hamster intestine. J. Clin. Invest., *46*:1215, 1967.

25. Ehrlich, P., and Lazarus, A.: Anemia. Rebman, Ltd., London, 1910, p. 69.

26. Fisher, J. M., and Taylor, K. B.: A comparison of autoimmune phenomena in pernicious anemia and chronic atrophic gastritis. New England J. Med., *272*:499, 1965.

27. Flexner, J. M., and Hartmann, R. C.: Megaloblastic anemia associated with anticonvulsant drugs. Am. J. Med., *28*:386, 1960.

28. Francois, R., Revol, L., Germain, D., Bourlier, V., Karlin, Mme., Coeur, P., Pellet, H., and Manuel, Y.: Imerslund's syndrome. Ann. pédiat., *43*:490, 1967.

29. Girdwood, R. H.: A folic excretion test in the investigation of intestinal absorption. Lancet, *2*:53, 1953.

30. Girdwood, R. H., and Lenman, J. A. R.: Megaloblastic anemia occurring during primidone therapy. Brit. M. J., *1*:146, 1956.

31. Glass, G. B. J.: Gastric intrinsic factor and its function in the metabolism of vitamin B_{12}. Physiol. Rev., *43*:529, 1963.

32. Glass, G. B. J.: Intestinal absorption and hepatic uptake of vitamin B_{12} in diseases of the gastro-intestinal tract. Gastroenterology, *30*:37, 1956.

33. Goldberg, L. S., Bickel, Y. B., and Fudenberg, H. H.: Immunologic approaches to malabsorption of vitamin B_{12}. Arch. Int. Med., *123*:397, 1969.

34. Goldberg, L. S., and Fudenberg, H. H.: The autoimmune aspects of pernicious anemia. Am. J. Med., *46*:489, 1969.

35. Goodman, L. S., and Gilman, A.: The Pharmacological Basis of Therapeutics. 3rd Ed. The Macmillan Co., New York, 1965.

36. Grasbeck, R.: Nature and action of intrinsic factor. Plenary session papers. International Society of Hematology. 1968, p. 124.

37. Guerra, R., Wheby, M. S., and Bayless, T. M.: Long-term antibiotic therapy in tropical sprue. Ann. Int. Med., *63*:619, 1965.
38. Haden, R. L.: Pernicious anemia from Addison to folic acid. Blood, *3*:22, 1948.
39. Hall, C. A.: Annotation. Transport of vitamin B_{12} in man. Brit. J. Haemat., *16*:429, 1969.
40. Halsted, J. A., Lewis, P. M., and Gasster, M.: Absorption of radioactive vitamin B_{12} in the syndrome of megaloblastic anemia associated with intestinal stricture or anastomosis. Am. J. Med., *20*:42, 1956.
40a. Hampers, C. L., Streiff, R., Nathan, D. G., Snyder, D., and Merrill, J. P.: Megaloblastic hematopoiesis in uremia and in patients on long-term hemodialysis. New England J. Med., *276*:551, 1967.
41. Hawkins, C. F., and Meynell, M. J.: Macrocytosis and macrocytic anemia caused by anticonvulsant drugs. Quart. J. Med., *27*:45, 1958.
42. Herbert, V.: Current concepts in therapy. Megaloblastic anemia. New England J. Med., *268*:368, 1963.
43. Herbert, V.: Minimal daily adult folate requirement. Arch. Int. Med., *110*:649, 1962.
44. Herbert, V.: The Megaloblastic Anemias. Grune and Stratton, New York, 1959.
45. Herbert, V.: Annotation. Transient (reversible) malabsorption of vitamin B_{12}. Brit. J. Haemat., *17*:213, 1969.
46. Herbert, V., and Castle, W. B.: Intrinsic factor. New England J. Med., *270*:1181, 1964.
47. Herbert, V., Larrabee, A. R., and Buchanan, J. M.: Studies on the identification of a folate compound of human serum. J. Clin. Invest., *41*:1134, 1962.
48. Herbert, V., Streiff, R. B., and Sullivan, L. W.: Notes on vitamin B_{12} absorption, auto-immunity and childhood pernicious anemia. Medicine, *43*:679, 1964.
49. Hicks, M., and Leavell, B. S.: Pernicious anemia in the American Negro. Ann. Int. Med., *33*:1438, 1950.
50. Hines, J. D.: Reversible megaloblastic and sideroblastic marrow abnormalities in alcoholic patients. Brit. J. Haemat., *16*:87, 1969.
51. Hodgkin, D., et al.: Structure of vitamin B_{12}. Nature, *178*:64, 1956.
52. Huffbrand, A. V., and Necheles, T. F.: Mechanism of folate deficiency in patients receiving phenytoin. Lancet, *2*:528, 1968.
53. Isaacs, R., and Friedman, A.: Standards for maximum reticulocyte percentage after intramuscular liver therapy in pernicious anemia. Am. J. M. Sc., *196*:718, 1938.
54. Israels, M. C. G., and Wilkinson, J. F.: New observations on the aetiology and prognosis of achrestic anaemia. Quart. J. Med., *9*:163, 1940.
55. Israels, M. C. G., and Wilkinson, J. F.: Achrestic anaemia. Quart. J. Med., *5*:69, 1936.
55a. IUPAC-IUB Commission on Biochemical Nomenclature: Tentative rules. Jour. Biol. Chem., *241*:2987, 1966.
56. Jeffries, G. H.: Recovery of gastric mucosal structures and function in pernicious anemia during prednisone therapy. Gastroenterology, *45*:371, 1965.
57. Jeffries, G. H.: Parietal cell antibodies. Editorial. Ann. Int. Med., *63*:717, 1965.
58. Jeffries, G. H., Hoskins, D. W., and Sleisenger, M. H.: Antibody to intrinsic factor in serum from patients with pernicious anemia. J. Clin. Invest., *41*:1106, 1962.
59. Kaplan, H. S., and Rigler, L. G.: Pernicious anemia and carcinoma of the stomach—autopsy studies concerning their interrelationship. Am. J. M. Sc., *209*:339, 1945.
60. Lawrence, C.: B_{12}-binding protein deficiency in pernicious anemia. Blood, *27*:389, 1966.
61. Major, R. H.: Classic Descriptions of Disease. 3rd Ed. Charles C Thomas, Springfield, Ill., 1955, p. 291.
62. Mason, J. D., and Leavell, B. S.: The effect of transfusions of erythrocytes on untreated pernicious anemia. Blood, *11*:632, 1956.
63. McIntyre, O. R., Sullivan, L. W., Jeffries, G. H., and Silver, R. H.: Pernicious anemia in childhood. New England J. Med., *272*:981, 1965.
64. Minot, G. R., and Murphy, W. P.: Treatment of pernicious anemia by special diet. J.A.M.A., *87*:470, 1926.
65. Mollin, D. L., and Ross, G. I. M.: Vitamin B_{12} deficiency in the megaloblastic anemias. Proc. Roy. Soc. Med., *47*:428, 1954.
65a. Necheles, T. F., and Synder, L. M.: Malabsorption of folate associated with oral contraceptive therapy. New England J. Med., *282*:858, 1970.
65b. Nixon, R. F., and Bertino, J. R.: Interrelationships of vitamin B_{12} and folate in man. Am. J. Med., *48*:555, 1970.
66. Norcross, J. W., Monroe, S. E., and Griffin, B. G.: The development of gastric carcinoma in pernicious anemia. Ann. Int. Med., *37*:338, 1952.
66a. Nyberg, W., Gräsbeck, R., Saarni, M., and Von Bonsdorff, B.: Serum vitamin B_{12} levels and incidence of tapeworm anemia in a population heavily infected with *Diphyllobothrium latum*. Amer. J. Clin. Nutr., *9*:606, 1961.
67. Oxenhorn, S., Estren, S., Wasserman, L. R., and Adlersberg, D.: Malabsorption syndrome: Intestinal absorption of vitamin B_{12}. Ann. Int. Med., *48*:30, 1958.

68. Perillie, P. E., Kaplan, S. S., and Finch, S. C.: Significance of changes in serum muramidase activity in megaloblastic anemia. New England J. Med., *277*:10, 1967.

69. Pritchard, J. A., Scott, D. E., and Whalley, P. J.: Folic acid requirements in pregnancy-induced megaloblastic anemia. J.A.M.A., *208*:1163, 1969.

70. Rabinowitz, J. C., and Himes, R. H.: Folic acid coenzymes. Fed. Proc., *19*:963, 1960.

71. Register, U. D., and Sarett, H. P.: Urinary excretion of vitamin B_{12}, folic acid, and citrovorum factor in human subjects on various diets. Proc. Soc. Exper. Biol. & Med., 77:837, 1951.

72. Rickes, E. L., Brink, N. G., Koniuszy, F. R., Wood, T. R., and Folkers, K.: Crystalline vitamin B_{12}. Science, *107*:396, 1948.

73. Rigler, L. G., Kaplan, H. S., and Fink, D. L.: Pernicious anemia and the early diagnosis of tumors of the stomach. J.A.M.A., *128*:426, 1945.

74. Rosenberg, I. H., Streiff, R. R., Godwin, H. A., and Castle, W. B.: Absorption of polyglutamic folate: participation of deconjugating enzymes of the intestinal mucosa. New England J. Med., *280*:985, 1969.

75. Ross, J. F., Belding, H., and Paegel, B. L.: The development and progression of subacute combined degeneration of the spinal cord in patients with pernicious anemia treated with synthetic pteroylglutamic (folic) acid. Blood, *3*:68, 1948.

76. Rundles, R. W.: Prognosis in neurologic manifestations of pernicious anemia. Blood, *1*:209, 1946.

77. Schade, S. G., et al.: Occurrence in gastric juices of antibody to a complex of intrinsic factor and vitamin B_{12}. New England J. Med., *275*:528, 1966.

78. Schilling, R. F.: Intrinsic factor studies. II. The effect of gastric juice on the urinary excretion of radioactivity after the oral administration of radioactive vitamin B_{12}. J. Lab. & Clin. Med., *42*:860, 1953.

79. Schwartz, S. O., Friedman, I. A., and Gant, H. L.: Long-term evaluation of vitamin B_{12} in treatment of pernicious anemia. J.A.M.A., *157*:229, 1955.

80. Sheehy, T. W., Rubini, M. E., Perez-Santiago, E., Santini, R. J., and Haddock, J.: The effect of "minute" and "titrated" amounts of folic acid on the megaloblastic anemia of tropical sprue. Blood, *18*:623, 1961.

81. Silberstein, E. B.: The Schilling test. J.A.M.A., *208*:2325, 1969.

82. Smith, E. L.: Vitamin B_{12}. Methuen & Co., London, 1960.

83. Smith, E. L.: Purification of antipernicious anemia factors from liver. Nature, *161*:638, 1948.

84. Spurling, C. L., Sacks, M. S., and Jiji, R. M.: Juvenile pernicious anemia. New England J. Med., *271*:995, 1964.

84a. Streiff, R. F.: Folate deficiency and oral contraceptives. J.A.M.A., *214*:105, 1970.

85. Strieff, R. R., and Little, A. B.: Folic acid deficiency in pregnancy. New England J. Med., *276*:776, 1967.

86. Swanson, V. L., Wheby, M. S., and Bayless, T. M.: Morphologic effects of folic acid and vitamin B_{12} on the jejunal lesion of tropical sprue. Amer. J. Path., *49*:167, 1966.

87. Taylor, K. B., Roitt, I. M., Doniach, D., Couchman, K. G., and Shapland, C.: Autoimmune phenomena in pernicious anaemia: gastric antibodies. Brit. M. J., *2*:1347, 1962.

88. Twomey, J. J., Jordan, P. H., Jarrold, T., Trubowitz, S., Ritz, N. D., and Conn, H. O.: The syndrome of immunoglobulin deficiency and pernicious anemia: a study of ten cases. Am. J. Med., *47*:340, 1969.

89. Waters, A. H., and Mollin, D. L.: Studies on folic acid activity of human serum. J. Clin. Path., *14*:335, 1961.

90. Waxman, S., and Herbert, V.: Mechanism of pyrimethamine-induced megaloblastosis in human bone marrow. New England J. Med., *280*:1316, 1969.

91. Waxman, S., Metz, J., and Herbert, V.: Defective DNA synthesis in human megaloblastic bone marrow: effects of homocysteine and methionine. J. Clin. Invest., *48*:284, 1969.

92. Wheby, M. S., and Bayles, T. M.: Intrinsic factor in tropical sprue. Blood, *31*:817, 1968.

93. Whipple, G. N., and Robscheit-Robbins, F. S.: Favorable influence of liver, heart, and skeletal muscle in diet on blood regeneration in anemia. Am. J. Physiol., *72*:408, 1925.

94. Whitby, L. E. H., and Britton, C. J. C.: Disorders of the Blood. 5th Ed. The Blakiston Co., Philadelphia, 1946.

95. Williams, J. O., Mengel, C. E., Sullivan, L. W., and Hag, A. S.: Megaloblastic anemia associated with chronic ingestion of an analgesic. New England J. Med., *280*:312, 1969.

96. Willoughby, M. L. N.: An investigation of folic acid requirements in pregnancy. Brit. J. Haemat., *13*:503, 1967.

97. Wilson, T. H.: Membrane transport of vitamin B_{12}. Medicine, *43*:669, 1964.

98. Zamcheck, N., Grable, E., Ley, A. B., and Norman, L.: Occurrence of gastric cancer among patients with pernicious anemia at the Boston City Hospital. New England J. Med., *252*:1103, 1955.

99. Zuelzer, W. W., and Ogden, F. N.: Megaloblastic anemia of infancy. Am. J. Dis. Child., *71*:211, 1946.

V / Disorders of Iron Metabolism

Iron Metabolism

Iron is an essential element in many of the physiological processes in the body. It combines with protoporphyrin to form heme and with various proteins to form many important enzymes, such as catalase, cytochrome, and peroxidase. Since iron plays an essential role in hemoglobin metabolism, some knowledge of iron metabolism is necessary for the understanding and proper management of many of the problems of anemia seen in clinical practice. The history of iron in medicine has been reviewed by Fowler[41] and excellent summaries and monographs have been published.

The total quantity of iron in the body of an adult is determined largely by the size of the subject and the level of the circulating hemoglobin (Table 5–1). The normal range is from 3.0 to 5.0 gm. The iron is distributed as follows: hemoglobin, from 1.5 to 3.0 gm.; myoglobin, catalase, and cytochrome, about

Table 5–1. *Iron Values in the Human Adult, According to Various Authors*[33, 35, 45, 50, 94]

Daily dietary intake	12–15 mg.
Daily absorption	0.6–1.5 mg.
Total body iron	3.0–5.0 gm.
Hemoglobin iron	1.5–3.0 gm.
Storage iron	1.0–1.5 gm.
Parenchymatous iron	0.1–0.3 gm.
Daily loss, males	0.5–1.5 mg.
Daily loss, females	1.0–2.5 mg.
Daily loss, pregnant females	1.0 mg.

Table 5-2. *Estimated Dietary Iron Requirements*

	ABSORBED IRON REQUIREMENT (mg./day)	DAILY FOOD REQUIREMENT* (mg./day)
Normal men and non-menstruating women	0.5–1	5–10
Menstruating women	0.7–2	7–20
Pregnant women	2–4.8	20–48†
Adolescents	1–2	10–20
Children	0.4–1	4–10
Infants	0.5–1.5	5–15‡

*Assuming 10 per cent absorption.

†This amount of iron cannot be derived from diet and should be met by iron supplementation in the latter half of pregnancy.

‡15 mg. is the maximum.

(Reprinted from J.A.M.A., *203*:407, 1968.)

300 mg.; plasma, 3 to 4 mg.; storage iron, 600 to 1600 mg.[33, 35, 50, 94, 136] A Committee on Iron Deficiency of the Council on Food and Nutrition in the United States considered the following values to be normal: Total—70 kg. man, approximately 3.5 gm.; woman, 2.3 gm. Storage iron—men, 1000 mg.; women, 200 to 400 mg.[23] The daily iron requirement for members of both sexes of different ages has recently been estimated as shown in Table 5-2.[23]

The quantity of iron in the body is regulated by the amount of iron that is absorbed. There is no balanced mechanism of absorption and excretion like that which exists for many metals, such as calcium and sodium. This was first shown in 1937 by Widdowson and McCance.[135] They studied the urinary and fecal excretion of iron by two men and two women on a low iron intake, on a very high iron intake of 1000 mg. a day, and when they were again placed on a low iron intake. It was observed that on the low iron intake practically all of the ingested iron was recovered in the feces and the subjects were considered to be "in balance." During the high iron intake period, when each subject ingested 1000 mg. per day for 36 to 40 days, it was calculated that each individual absorbed from 2000 to 5000 mg. of iron without any significant increase in the hemoglobin levels. When the subjects were again placed on a low iron intake of 7 to 10 mg. a day for a period of 8 to 10 days, they excreted all of the iron ingested during that time but none of the iron that was absorbed during the preceding period of high iron intake. From these studies it was concluded that the intestine cannot significantly alter the iron stores by varying the amount excreted in the feces; except in pregnancy and when bleeding occurs, the quantity of iron in the body is determined by the amount that is absorbed.

Dietary Sources of Iron

The amount of iron in the diet is only one factor that determines its usefulness; even more important is the facility with which it can be absorbed. The average daily diet of adults in the Western world contains from 10 to 30 mg. of iron. Muscle meats, eggs, legumes, wheat, and leafy vegetables contain more iron than fruit, potatoes, or rice; milk contains very little iron and refined sugar has none. Information about the availability of dietary iron has been provided by studies that utilized the incorporation of tracer iron into various food-stuffs.[21, 95, 112] These studies have shown that hemoglobin and liver are rich sources of iron; eggs and greens are relatively poor. Normal adults absorb from 5 to 10 per cent of the dietary iron and adults with iron deficiency absorb from 10 to 20 per cent.[95, 100] About 1 mg. of iron is absorbed from an average daily diet by a normal adult; adults with severe iron deficiency anemia are unable to absorb more than 4 or 5 mg. of iron from a normal diet.[40] Comparable values have been found in children. In a group of normal children less than 5 years of age the mean absorption of tracer iron incorporated in eggs, cereal, rice, chicken liver, and whole milk was between 8 and 12 per cent. An average of 18 per cent was absorbed from eggs by children with iron deficiency. Neither children 5 to 15 years of age nor adults absorbed iron from eggs and whole milk as well as the younger children did. Absorption of 10 per cent of the iron contained in an optimal diet should meet the need for iron during the period of maximal growth.[112]

Iron absorption in humans has been difficult to measure accurately because of variations that exist between one normal person and another and from day to day in the same person. Studies of absorption of food iron in 131 individuals carried out in a way designed to minimize these variations showed relatively low absorption of the iron (1.7 to 7.9 per cent) in wheat, corn, black beans, lettuce, and spinach, compared to the absorption from soy beans, fish, veal, and hemoglobin (15 to 20 per cent).[25]

Absorption of Iron

The quantity of iron that is absorbed after ingestion is determined by factors such as the amount and type of iron in the lumen of the intestine, the presence or absence of food, the nature of the food, the state of the iron stores in the body, the activity of the bone marrow, the secretions of the pancreas, and the function of the intestinal mucosa.

Both the quantity and the chemical state of the iron in the gastrointestinal tract influence absorption. Whipple[134a] and others[12] have demonstrated that increasing the amount of iron ingested increases the amount that is absorbed, even though the percentage of absorption is smaller with larger amounts. Ferrous iron is absorbed better than ferric iron; in man and in most animals iron is absorbed mainly in the ferrous form.[94, 120]

The absorption of dietary iron has been studied by chemical analysis of the diet and feces,[70] by measuring the absorption of radioisotopic iron incorporated in foods such as eggs, muscle meat, vegetables, and bread during their production,[95] and by measuring the absorption of radioactive iron that has been mixed with food.[21, 100] Many factors influence the absorptive process. The presence of food affects the absorption of iron significantly; merely mixing ferrous salt with food before ingestion reduces the absorption of the iron by approximately 50 per cent,[21, 100, 118] possibly by the mechanical effect of the food. The iron-phosphorus ratio of the meal may be a factor; higher ratios favor absorption at certain levels of phosphorus in the diet. Large amounts of ascorbic acid and probably other reducing substances promote absorption.[95] Phytates inhibit movement of inorganic iron from the lumen because they bind the iron, but they are not an important factor in the absorption of food iron. Pancreatic secretions apparently inhibit iron absorption, and a deficiency may enhance absorption in certain disorders such as cirrhosis of the liver or chronic pancreatitis.[18]

Although iron probably can be absorbed from any part of the gastrointestinal tract, absorption is greatest in the duodenum and diminishes progressively in the more distal portion of the bowel; the absorption of food iron occurs mainly if not exclusively in the duodenum.[16] The molecule of hemoglobin iron, an important dietary source of iron in meat, apparently enters the mucosal cell where a substance that is presumably an enzyme, possibly xanthine oxidase, effects the release of iron and permits its passage from the mucosal cell into the plasma.[31]

The factors that control or influence the absorption of iron from the gut have been studied extensively. Iron deficiency, increased erythropoiesis, anoxia of high altitude, and ingestion of excessive amounts of iron all lead to increased iron absorption; increased iron stores, diminished erythropoiesis, and oxygen excess are associated with decreased absorption. An essential role in the absorptive process is played by the mucosal cell in the small intestine. The level of hemoglobin, the level of serum iron, the amount of unsaturated transferrin in the plasma, and the oxygen tension of the blood have been investigated as possible humoral factors that act as signals to the mucosal cell.

Several studies[118, 137] indicated that the relative saturation of transferrin exerts little or no control over iron absorption; another, which utilized the double isotope technique, supported the concept that the saturation of transferrin in the general circulation regulates the absorption of iron from the gastrointestinal tract.[47] The dilemma was resolved when still another study demonstrated that saturation or near saturation of plasma transferrin in rats, dogs, and man did not significantly influence the amount of iron absorbed; the absorbed iron was deposited in the liver during the first circulation through the portal system and did not appear in the general circulation; this absorption was missed when only plasma iron in the peripheral circulation was studied.[133]

Other investigations have failed to demonstrate that the erythropoietin levels of the plasma,[75] the amount of iron stored in the liver, or the quantity excreted in the bile[132] exert any influence on iron absorption. Conflicting data have been presented concerning the influence of anemia and anoxia; observations on anemic patients with hypocellular marrows indicate that anemia per se does not lead to increased iron absorption,[100] but experiments on mice with marrow hypoplasia have shown that iron absorption increased after different types of anemia were produced, even when erythropoiesis was practically nil and adequate iron stores were maintained. Anoxia was also found to be a stimulus to iron absorption even though there was no demonstrable increase in erythropoiesis.[91] The balance of the evidence, however, seems to indicate that in man anemia and anoxia do not exert a direct effect, but may act indirectly.

The complexity of the absorptive process is also shown by studies on the influence of iron deficiency and achlorhydria. Iron deficiency is nearly always associated with an increased absorption of food iron and inorganic iron. Nevertheless the production of iron deficiency in rats has been followed by a significant change in the total acid secretion and acid concentration as compared to the normal animals.[97] Impaired iron absorption from labeled hemoglobin has been demonstrated in children with severe iron deficiency anemia, a defect that disappeared when the iron stores were replenished;[74] a similar defect was demonstrated in puppies, and the authors suggested that a decrease in the iron containing or iron dependent enzymes in the mucosa might produce secondary malabsorption. Although hydrochloric acid is not necessary for the absorption of inorganic ferrous iron, the acid apparently is important in the absorption of ferric iron, the type present in food. Studies on normal subjects and patients with pernicious anemia indicate that hydrochloric acid may facilitate the chelation of the ferric salts of ascorbate and other agents. Thus a deficiency in acid secretion may lead to faulty absorption of food iron by patients with achlorhydria as well as those who have had a partial or total gastrectomy. Over a period of years such a defect may produce or contribute to iron deficiency.[111]

One concept that has been proposed to explain the regulation of iron absorption is the "mucosal block" theory, which assigns an important role to the ferritin mechanism. This theory was based mainly on two observations: first, the demonstration by Hahn et al.[46] that in dogs the oral administration of iron partially blocked the absorption of a second dose given several hours later; and second, Granick's observation that in guinea pigs oral iron stimulated the mucosal cells to produce a protein, apoferritin, which combines with iron to form ferritin.[44] According to this concept, ferritin acted as a blocking agent. When the ferrous iron in the lumen of the intestine was in equilibrium with the ferric iron of the mucosal cells, no ferrous iron would be absorbed; after the ferric iron content of the cells was diminished by passage of iron from the mucosal ferritin into the blood stream, iron would pass from the lumen into the mucosa. At the time the theory was proposed it was known that any blocking mechanism which might exist was not completely effective, either in normal individuals or in patients with certain diseases, particularly hemochromatosis.[52, 134a] Evidence against the existence of mucosal block as a physiologic mechanism was reported by Brown et al. in 1958.[16] Their studies confirmed the observation of Hahn et al. that in man a large dose of iron salt administered orally produces a partial and transient block to the absorption of a second dose of iron; however, they found that the amount of iron in the diet is too small to produce this effect. Other evidence against the mucosal block concept has been provided by animal experiments.[53] Heilmeyer gave guinea pigs 15 mg. of iron daily for 28 days and found that the amount of iron in the liver continued to increase over a period of 14 days, a time when the content of the ferritin in the stomach and small intestine was maximal. After the fourteenth day there was no further absorption, even though the ferritin in the mucosa of the stomach and small intestine diminished.

The function that is served by the build-up of ferritin in the mucosal cells is uncertain. Crosby and associates have reported that the ferritin iron in the epithelial cells is not absorbed but instead is sequestered and prevented from entering the circulation;[26] the iron is lost when the ferritin-containing cells are shed into the intestinal lumen. Conrad et al.[24] studied the effect of intravenously injected iron on the intestinal absorption of iron and observed that radioactive iron injected in this way was incorporated into the epithelial cells of the mucosa at the time the cells were formed in the crypts of Lieberkühn in normal and iron loaded rats but not in iron deficient animals. They considered that the amount of this "messenger iron" in the cells might be the basis of control of iron absorption because the "messenger iron" seemed to reflect the status of the body stores; their studies indicated a correlation among the size of the dose of iron injected intravenously, the amount sequestered by the mucosal cells, and the amount of oral iron absorbed. The iron remained in the mucosal cells as they migrated toward the villous tip where they were shed. The authors concluded that the iron content of the intestinal epithelium plays an important role in the regulation of iron equilibrium in the body.

Many experiments indicate that the mucosal cell has a mechanism for transporting iron across the cell into the plasma and a mechanism for trapping iron in the mucosal cell. Although the importance of ferritin in these functions has not been defined, the model proposed by Wheby shown in Figure 5–1 provides a useful concept of the functioning of the mucosal cell. In iron deficiency the cell permits the rapid passage of dietary iron through the mucosal cell into the circulation. In iron storage disease the cell resists iron absorption but is not completely effective. In iron overload other cells, such as glandular epithelial cells and macrophages, also accumulate iron, and their subsequent desquamation increases the excretion of iron from the body.

The relationship between erythropoietic activity and absorption of iron from the gut has been studied in rats.[128] During 8 days of low atmospheric pres-

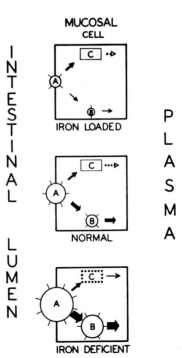

Figure 5–1. Proposed model· of iron absorption. Each *square* represents a small intestinal epithelial mucosal cell. State of body iron is indicated. *A* represents the active transport mechanism for mucosal uptake of iron from intestinal lumen. *B* represents the active transport mechanism for mucosal transfer of iron to plasma. *C* represents the mechanism for temporary storage of iron. The sizes of *A* and *B* illustrate the relative transport rates. Both *A* and *B* are related to body iron requirements, but *A* is always greater than *B*. Iron is preferentially moved from *A* to *B* to plasma, but depending on the amount of iron available to *A* and the relationship of *A* to *B*, a variable portion of the iron transported by *A* moves to *C* for temporary storage. As indicated by the *dotted arrow* in normal and iron-loaded states, subsequent transfer of iron from *C* to plasma is very slow and may not occur before the cell is sloughed. *C* is *dotted* in the iron-deficient mucosal cell to indicate that the efficiency of *B* is such that storage may not occur unless large doses of iron are used. Within limits, these transport and storage mechanisms regulate the amount of iron absorbed. (From Wheby: Gastroenterology, vol. 50, 1966. Reprinted with permission of the author and the Williams and Wilkins Co.)

sure both erythropoiesis and iron absorption increased significantly; when the rats were restored to normal atmospheric pressure in a state of relative polycythemia, bone marrow activity and iron utilization immediately diminished, whereas deposition of iron in the mucosa of the intestine was elevated. Crosby has proposed the following sequence to explain the function of the intestinal mucosal cell in these circumstances.[27] When erythropoiesis increases because of hemorrhage or some other stimulus, more iron is utilized, plasma iron turnover accelerates, iron leaves the intestinal mucosal cells at a faster rate, and the iron content of the mucosa falls. The new epithelial cells that form in the crypts contain little iron and permit the passage of iron from the lumen; since such cells constitute practically the entire lining of the small intestine within 2 or 3 days, absorption increases until equilibrium is re-established. This hypothesis would explain the 3 or 4 day lag in increased iron absorption that follows bleeding, as well as the increase that occurs after bleeding and during hemolysis despite adequate or even excessive iron stores in the liver.

Although the exact mechanisms involved in the transfer of iron across the mucosal cell are unknown, iron transfer has been shown to be an active metabolic process. Dowdle et al.,[34] who utilized segments of small intestine from rats, have shown that the transport of iron across the mucosal cell can take place against a concentration gradient, is limited in capacity, and requires oxidative metabolism and the generation of phosphate bond energy. Other evidence indicates that the active transfer across the cell involves two steps, mucosal uptake and transfer to the serosal surface (or into the blood stream);[88, 89] both require oxidative metabolism. It was also observed that both divalent and trivalent iron are taken up at the mucosal surface, but that net transfer to the serosal surface (or blood stream), which is the slower step, is relatively specific for divalent iron (85 per cent). Wheby et al.[134] confirmed these findings; they injected radioiron salts into closed loops of the small intestine created in otherwise intact rats and measured both the amount of radioactive iron in the intestinal wall after careful washing and that present in the whole carcass. They found two stages of mucosal absorption, a rapid uptake of iron from the lumen and a slower transfer of iron to the carcass; the second stage was restricted largely to the duodenal mucosa. Both steps varied inversely with the state of the body stores of iron. Absorption can be extremely rapid, as shown by the passage of radioiron through the mucosal cells within 15 seconds after injection in blind loops of iron deficient rats; in other circumstances the mucosal cells act as temporary storage areas for the iron.

Transferrin and the Transport of Iron

When it leaves the mucosal cells, iron in the ferric form is transported in the plasma attached to a beta-1-globulin, variously termed transferrin, siderophilin, iron binding protein, or metal binding globulin. The existence of a binding component in the serum was reported in 1945 by Holmberg and Laurell;[61] they concluded that the toxic effects of intravenously administered iron occurred when the saturation limit of the plasma, about 300 micrograms per 100 ml., was exceeded and the surplus iron left the blood stream. In 1946, Schade and Caroline identified the protein fraction in human plasma that possessed the capacity to bind iron at physiologic pH as being a beta-1-globulin.[110] The protective effect of the protein binding of the iron in the blood has been demonstrated by means of intravenous injections of iron preparations. Poorly dissociated iron compounds, such as iron saccharide, can be given intravenously in large amounts, but easily dissociated iron compounds can be given only in small amounts, 5 to 10 mg. Larger amounts of easily dissociated iron compounds quickly saturate the total iron binding capacity of the plasma and the excess iron causes flushing, nausea, vomiting, shock, and even death.

Transferrin has a molecular weight of about 90,000. Each molecule combines with two molecules of ferric iron.[94] The biologic half-life of radioiodinated transferrin has been reported to be 12 days in a normal child and from 6.7 to 8.4 days in adults.[42, 71] The existence of variants in human transferrin that are under genetic control was first demonstrated by Smithies in 1957.[116] Since then at least 15 transferrins have been identified by starch gel electrophoresis.[2, 120] Only transferrin C is found in the majority of persons. The transferrin variants apparently do not differ in their ability to transport iron and deliver it to the tissues. Normally the transferrin in the plasma is about one-third saturated; the total iron binding capacity is usually in the range of 300 to 359 micrograms per 100 ml., but the upper limit has been reported as high as 420.[94]

Transferrin functions not only for the transport of iron in the plasma, but also in the transfer of iron from the plasma to the developing erythrocytes. Jandl and Katz have shown that transferrin plays an important role in iron utilization by the developing normoblasts and reticulocytes, a process which involves the attachment of the transferrin molecule to the cell membrane.[67, 71, 73] The iron, which is tightly bound to the transferrin molecule, is transferred into

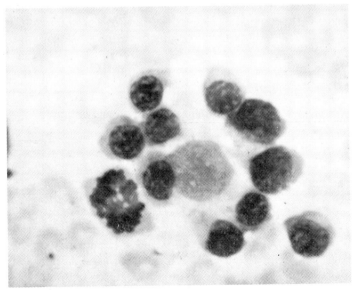

Figure 5–2. Reticulum cell surrounded by normoblasts in iron deficiency anemia; bone marrow aspiration. (Courtesy of Dr. S. G. Tan.)

the cell from the transferrin attached to the cell membrane in about 1 minute. The mechanism is energy dependent. The rate of entry of transferrin bound iron into erythroid cells is affected by several factors. A probable one is the age of the cells; younger cells have a larger number of binding sites for transferrin molecules than older cells do. Another is the concentration of transferrin bound iron in the surrounding medium; uptake increases as the absolute concentration of the transferrin-iron complex increases and is more important than its relative saturation. In addition, it has been proposed that the amount of heme in reticulocytes, and presumably earlier cells, also regulates the entrance of iron into the cells by a feedback mechanism.[102] This interpretation is supported by the observation that the uptake of radioiron is decreased in reticulocytes incubated with heme and by the observation that in the sideroblastic anemias, where heme synthesis is inhibited, excessive amounts of non-hemoglobin iron are found in the normoblasts and in the erythrocytes. Most of the iron is taken up by the pronormoblasts and basophilic normoblasts, less by older nucleated cells, but some is taken up by reticulocytes.[78]

Electron microscopy has shown that early erythroid cells contain ferritin, and Bessis and Breton-Gorius have demonstrated by electron microscopy that some ferritin is transferred directly from reticulum "nurse" cells to surrounding normoblasts; they termed the process ropheocytosis to indicate that the nutrient material is transferred by aspiration rather than by micropinocytosis.[3] The authors postulate that the iron in the marrow reticulum cells is largely that transported by transferrin and to a lesser extent is derived from erythrophagocytosis in the marrow. Although the importance of these observations and their interpretation cannot be fully evaluated at present, the studies of Jandl and Katz,[68] and the demonstration that immature red cells assimilate iron from transferrin in vitro much more readily than reticulum cells do[77, 78] both favor the concept that the direct transfer of iron from the plasma to the young red cell is the normal mechanism. Also, it has been suggested that ferritin is being transferred from the normoblasts to the reticulum cells, rather than the reverse.[77] The non-essential role of the transferrin level in iron absorption and the apparent importance of transferrin for iron utilization in erythropoiesis were evident in studies of a patient reported by Heilmeyer et al.; this patient, who had no demonstrable plasma transferrin, had a hypochromic anemia associated with greatly increased storage iron.[55]

The normal plasma iron level in micrograms per 100 ml. has been reported to be 50 to 180, 80 to 160, and 43 to 210.[12, 19, 94] In the latter study the mean was 104.7 ± 3.4. In some series, the plasma iron values for males have been higher than those for females but in others there has been no significant difference. In one series the mean for men was 119.6 ± 6.7 micrograms per 100 ml. (range 61 to 228) and for women, 101.9 ± 5.5 micrograms per 100 ml. (range 35 to 246);[108] in another, the ranges were 81 to 162 micrograms per 100 ml. in men and 64 to 128 micrograms per 100 ml. in women.[56] Usually the level is highest in the morning and falls in the evening; in one study mean changes were −35.3 ± 6.0 in men and −16.1 ± 3.6 micrograms per 100 ml. in women. A mean serum level of 107.6 micrograms per 100 ml. has been reported in a group of boys and girls 4.5 to 8 years of age.[108] In children from 2 to 4.5 years of age the mean in boys was 95.9 micrograms per 100 ml. and in girls, 59.7 micrograms per 100 ml.

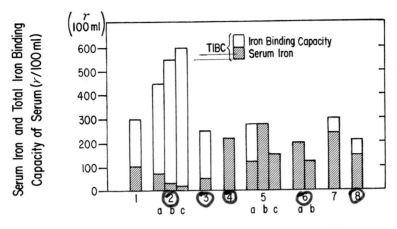

**Levels of Serum Iron and Total Iron Binding
Capacity Observed in Patients with Various Disorders**

Figure 5–3. 1, Normal. 2, Iron deficiency (a, mild; b, moderate; c, severe). 3, Infection.
4, Viral hepatitis. 5, Bone marrow failure (a, untreated idiopathic; b, untreated drug induced;
c, idiopathic, over 300 blood transfusions). 6, Idiopathic hemochromatosis (a, untreated; b, treated).
7, Hereditary iron loading anemia. 8, Untreated pernicious anemia.

Levels of iron and transferrin in the plasma vary in certain circumstances
(Fig. 5–3). A rise in the plasma iron usually occurs in less than an hour after the
ingestion of ferrous sulfate. The level is usually higher than normal in hemolytic
anemia, untreated pernicious anemia, aplastic anemia, hemochromatosis, and
hemosiderosis; in these disorders the total iron binding capacity of the serum is
not elevated but the percentage of saturation is increased. The serum iron level
is also elevated in infectious hepatitis and the rise appears to be correlated with
the degree of parenchymal necrosis. In iron deficiency anemia the characteristic finding is a subnormal level of the plasma iron associated with an increase
in the total iron binding capacity. Similar changes usually occur during the latter part of pregnancy. The transferrin level is lower than normal in some
patients with disturbed protein metabolism that occurs in certain disease states,
such as nephrosis, uremia, liver disease, and starvation. In infections both the
plasma iron and total iron binding capacity are usually lower than normal; a
decrease in the plasma iron has been observed within 24 hours after the production of fever.[19, 20] The low serum iron values seen in infection and malignancy
are probably due to a reduced movement of iron from reticuloendothelial cells
into plasma rather than an acceleration of outflow of iron from the plasma to
these storage cells; the utilization of iron that has gained access to the plasma
appears unimpaired.[72] Moderately lowered serum iron levels also occur in
many patients with uremia or rheumatoid arthritis.

Storage of Iron

The storage iron, usually from 600 to 1600 mg., constitutes from 16 to 23
per cent of the total in the body.[50, 94] This iron is stored as ferritin or hemo-

siderin chiefly in the phagocytic cells of the reticuloendothelial system in the liver, spleen, and bone marrow. The iron in both ferritin and hemosiderin can be utilized for hemoglobin formation.

Ferritin is a protein that has a molecular weight of about 560,000 and contains about 23 per cent iron in the form of ferric-hydroxy-phosphate,[3] the protein part of the complex is apoferritin. Studies of ferritin with the electron microscope have shown that the molecule is polygonal in shape, usually a regular hexagon, with a diameter of 100 to 110Å and sides measuring 70 to 80Å. The iron forms a central core of the protein shell. The apoferritin molecule is identical to the ferritin molecule except iron is absent. Bessis and Breton-Gorius report that hemosiderin, which has been reported to contain from 1.5 to 37 per cent iron, is not a specific compound but a substance that contains a variable mixture of ferritin, apoferritin, and other material.[3]

Iron recently deposited in the tissues is utilized for erythropoiesis in preference to the older stores. When erythrocytes which have been tagged with radio-iron and damaged by storage are injected into the circulation they are removed by the reticuloendothelial system at 20 to 40 times the normal rate; the tagged iron is promptly utilized for erythropoiesis, 85 per cent being used in 12 days.[99]

The incorporation of the plasma iron into the ferritin in the storage areas is an energy dependent reaction involving ATP and ascorbic acid. Mazur et al. have used radioactive iron and slices of liver from rats to study the mechanism of the incorporation of plasma iron into hepatic ferritin.[90] They suggested that a complex is formed which involves 2 mols of ATP, 1 mol of ascorbic acid, and the iron bound transferrin of the plasma. It was postulated that on stimulation of the oxidation of ascorbic acid by ATP the ferric iron bound to transferrin is reduced to ferrous iron and thus released from its bond to the protein for incorporation into ferritin.

The iron stores, which are estimated for clinical purposes by iron stains of marrow tissue and determinations of serum iron and transferrin levels, may be normal, subnormal, or increased. Subnormal stores occur most often in infants 12 to 24 months of age, and in situations in which there is uncompensated iron loss. Iron excess arises in two ways, either from excessive intestinal absorption or from hyperhemolysis. Excessive intestinal absorption of iron, which may occur as the result of either an intestinal defect (idiopathic hemochromatosis) or a diet high in iron (African Bantu), leads to the deposition of iron in the parenchymal cells. Excessive destruction of the red cells leads to the accumulation of excess iron in the reticuloendothelial cells, the clinical entity hemosiderosis. Iron overload also occurs in sickle cell anemia, thalassemia, "iron loading" anemia, and refractory anemia associated with ineffective erythroid hyperplasia; in these patients the iron accumulation, which is augmented by increased intestinal absorption, may involve both epithelial cells and the reticuloendothelial cells.

The transfer of iron to the fetus takes place across the placenta, where the blood in the fetal circulation is separated from that of the mother only by the thin-walled villi that are in contact with a pool of maternal blood. The total amount of iron in the infant is approximately 300 mg.[103] The fetus acts as a parasite and is able to assimilate the required amount of iron even when the mother is deficient in iron. It accomplishes this in some manner other than simple diffusion because iron from the maternal plasma is transferred to the fetal plasma even though the plasma level of the iron there is higher than in the maternal plasma; iron that enters the fetal circulation does not reenter the maternal circulation. In the fetus the transferrin level is lower and the degree of saturation greater than in the mother.

Excretion of Iron

The body normally conserves iron in a tenacious fashion. Only a very small amount is lost daily as a result of desquamation of cells of the skin and gastrointestinal tract, through the migration of leukocytes into the gastrointestinal tract, by the shedding of hair, and in the excretion of minute amounts of iron in the bile, urine, and sweat. Moore and Dubach found the fecal excretion of normal persons to be 0.3 to 0.5 mg. daily; in iron deficiency the amount may be only one-tenth as much.[94] The average man and the postmenopausal woman each lose about 0.5 to 1.5 mg. per day by various routes; menstruating women lose an average of about 1.0 to 2.5 mg. per day. During pregnancy an additional 1 mg. per day is lost, because the developing fetus is furnished a total of 0.3 to 0.5 gm. and other iron is lost as blood at the time of delivery. The normal loss of only 1.0 mg. per day means that years are required for a man or a post- menopausal woman with normal stores to develop iron deficiency solely because of a deficient diet. Iron deficiency in men and postmenopausal women is nearly always an indication of chronic blood loss. The conservation of iron is generally advantageous but the inability of the physiologic mechanisms to rid the body of more than a small amount each day allows the accumulation of iron when excessive amounts gain access to the body as a result of blood transfusions, parenteral injection of iron, or abnormal absorption from the intestine. Crosby has placed the maximal limit of iron excretion through shedding iron laden cells from the gastrointestinal tract at 5 mg. per day.[26]

Ferrokinetics

The availability of radioactive iron has made it possible to trace the pathways of iron in the body. Plasma iron can be labeled by the injection of a tracer amount of radioiron and its clearance from the plasma can be followed by counting that which remains in the plasma at various intervals. From this determination, if the level of the serum iron is known, the plasma iron turnover can be calculated. The amount of iron that is utilized for effective hemoglobin synthesis can be measured by determining the amount that is incorporated in the circulating erythrocytes at various intervals of time. Normally, the half-time disappearance rate of iron injected intravenously is 90 to 100 minutes; 85 to 100 per cent of the injected iron can be accounted for in the circulating erythrocytes within a period of 7 to 10 days in normal subjects. The quantity of labeled iron in the sacral marrow, liver, and spleen can be ascertained by counting the gamma ray emission over these areas. Studies of this type by Huff,[64] Pollycove,[101] and Finch[11] and their associates form the main basis of our present concepts of internal iron metabolism.

The daily requirements of hemoglobin production of a normal adult human being can be calculated. If the hemoglobin level is 15 gm. per 100 ml., the total blood volume is 5000 ml., and the life span of the erythrocyte is 120 days, then the daily production of hemoglobin is 6.25 gm. $\left(\dfrac{15 \times 50}{120} = 6.25\right)$. Since each gram of hemoglobin contains 3.3 mg. of iron, the daily requirement of iron for hemoglobin production is about 21 mg. The average daily iron absorption, approximately 1 mg., just balances the daily loss from the body. The daily iron need for hemoglobin production is provided by the hemoglobin contained in the erythrocytes destroyed each day. This iron is mainly that transported from the reticuloendothelial cells to the erythropoietic tissue by the plasma, bound to transferrin. Since the total plasma iron amounts to 3 or 4 mg. it is evident that the total iron in the plasma must be renewed six or eight times in 24 hours.

The plasma iron turnover rate can be measured by the use of radioactive iron. A known amount of tagged iron is injected intravenously and the disappearance of the iron from the circulation is followed. If the level of the plasma iron and the blood volume are known, the turnover can be calculated. A simplified formula, which obviates determination of the blood volume, has been introduced by Bothwell and Finch:[11]

$$\frac{\text{Plasma iron turnover}}{\text{(mg./day/100 ml. whole blood)}} = \frac{\text{plasma iron (micrograms/100 ml.)}}{\text{T}\frac{1}{2}\text{ (minutes)}} \times \frac{100 - \text{Hct.}}{100}$$

($\text{T}\frac{1}{2}$ = time of clearance of 50 per cent of radioactivity from the plasma.) The authors point out that significant error may be introduced if the plasma volume or red cell mass is significantly abnormal. The presence of anemia does not lead to appreciable error, since the blood volume changes are in the range of 10 to 15 per cent. The formula is not suitable for use in patients with acute hemorrhage, burns, or salt depletion. Bothwell and Finch prefer to express the results in mg. per 100 ml. of whole blood per day because it obviates the differences that result from body size as well as errors that may be introduced in measuring or assuming a figure for the blood volume. By this method the plasma iron turnover has been found to be about 0.6 mg. per 100 ml. of whole blood per day. With a blood volume of 5 liters the normal turnover is 30 mg. per day; if the total plasma iron is 3 or 4 mg., the complete turnover is at a rate of once every $2\frac{1}{2}$ to 3 hours.

The measured figure for plasma turnover of 0.6 mg. per 100 ml. of whole blood per day (30 mg. per day) is appreciably above the theoretical value calculated for hemoglobin production, 0.42 mg. per 100 ml. of whole blood per day (21 mg. per day). The figures indicate that about 30 per cent of the iron entering and leaving the plasma each day is not utilized for effective hemoglobin production. This means that there is appreciable movement of iron which apparently is not immediately involved in erythropoiesis. Efforts to interpret the results obtained by this type of study have led to the conclusion that the plasma iron is in equilibrium with one or more functional pools or compartments.[11, 65, 101, 114] Pollycove has suggested that the labile pool is in the marrow, but the anatomic site of the pool has not been established conclusively. Bothwell and Finch point out that the change in the slope of the iron disappearance curve to a less steep one after 8 hours indicates that there are multiple components to the curve.[11] They also find good evidence of tissue exchange with a significant return of radioiron to the plasma. It is suggested that an appreciable portion of the plasma iron, 25 to 30 per cent, initially goes to tissue other than the marrow, mainly to the liver, while 10 per cent of the iron that goes to the marrow is involved in ineffective erythropoiesis, the erythrocytes being destroyed in the marrow without reaching the general circulation.

In addition to clarifying many aspects of normal iron metabolism, techniques that employ radioiron have led to a better understanding of the derangements that occur in certain diseases. By measuring the rate of clearance of iron from the plasma, the plasma iron turnover, and incorporation of iron into circulating erythrocytes, one can estimate the erythropoietic activity of the marrow and determine its effectiveness. In patients with hypocellular inactive marrows, and in some with cellular marrows, both the clearance of iron from the plasma and its incorporation into circulating erythrocytes are diminished and the iron going to storage is increased. In other patients with refractory anemia who have cellular marrows, and also in patients with pernicious anemia, the clearance of iron from the plasma is normal or increased but the incorporation into circulating erythrocytes is greatly diminished; such results indicate ineffective erythropoiesis, either a diversion of iron to storage because of defective maturation or a premature destruction of the erythrocytes before they are released from the marrow.

Anemia of Iron Deficiency

Anemia that is due to iron deficiency has been described under various names. Many of the terms that at present appear to be no more than different names for iron deficiency in special circumstances were used to indicate the various syndromes before the nature of the mechanism responsible for the anemia was appreciated. The following terms have been used: secondary anemia, idiopathic hypochromic anemia, chlorosis, chlorotic anemia, hypochromic anemia of pregnancy, hypochromic anemia of prematurity and adolescence, and iron deficiency anemia.

An interesting account of the history of iron in medicine has been published by Fowler.[41] According to this account the presence of iron in the blood was first discovered by Lemery and Geoffrey in 1713. This discovery did not come until sometime after iron deficiency had been described and iron had been used as a therapeutic agent. Iron deficiency anemia was first described by Johannes Lange of Basle in 1554 as "De Morbo Virgineo."[79] In this description of the syndrome that was later called "chlorosis," Lange noted that the disease was peculiar to virgins and described the change from rosiness of the cheeks to pallor, the pulsation of the temporal vessels, and the dyspnea on dancing and climbing stairs. Iron was first used to treat the anemia of chlorosis in the 1600's by Thomas Sydenham, one of the great English clinicians. In 1889 Hayem recognized that the anemia of iron deficiency is characterized by erythrocytes that are smaller than normal and contain a smaller than normal amount of hemoglobin.[51]

Mechanism of Disease

Iron deficiency, which is probably the commonest type of anemia in the world, occurs in a number of clinical conditions and various mechanisms may be involved. An improper diet is rarely the sole cause of iron deficiency except in infancy. Nevertheless, an inadequate intake may be an important factor in certain situations, particularly in infancy, during early childhood, in adolescence, and during pregnancy.

The anemia in infancy and childhood is mainly the result of a dietary iron deficiency; the amount of iron ingested is not adequate to provide for the increase in blood volume that is part of growth of the child. The state of the maternal iron stores has little or no effect on the development of anemia in the child because the fetus can obtain the needed iron, about 80 mg. per kg., even if the mother has iron deficiency. An unusual type of hypochromic microcytic anemia associated with virtual absence of marrow iron and excessive iron accumulation in the liver has been reported in two young children who had no defect in transferrin;[113] the mechanism is uncertain.

Mild or moderate anemia of iron deficiency is not uncommon in adolescence but severe anemia ("chlorosis" of earlier times) is a rarity. The anemia, which is seen almost exclusively in girls, is usually explained by an iron intake that is insufficient to meet the requirements of rapid growth and the onset of menstruation.

Pregnancy is a common cause of iron deficiency anemia; the incidence varies in different parts of the world but is probably about 25 per cent even in areas where nutritional problems are rare or minor. The development of the iron deficiency depends on several factors. One is the state of iron stores of the mother at the beginning of pregnancy; this is related to the economic status of the mother, the number of previous pregnancies, and the presence or absence of various diseases, particularly those associated with blood loss. Another factor is the iron intake of the mother, which is most important during the last half of pregnancy.

The commonest cause of iron deficiency anemia in both men and women is chronic blood loss. In adult males iron deficiency anemia is nearly always the result of chronic blood loss from the gastrointestinal tract. Any ulcerating lesion may be responsible—esophageal ulceration, hiatus hernia, gastric or duodenal ulcer, benign and malignant lesions of the stomach, small bowel, or colon, or hemorrhoids. Blood loss from hookworm infestation is a major factor in iron deficiency in many parts of the world. In women, in addition to gastrointestinal bleeding, excessive vaginal bleeding and pregnancy are common causes of iron deficiency. The state of the iron stores is important in the development of anemia from vaginal bleeding or pregnancy; the loss of small quantities of blood in normal menstruation may produce severe anemia in women whose iron stores are low, yet much more severe bleeding may produce only transient anemia if the reserves of iron are normal.

A less common cause of iron deficiency is impairment of the absorption of iron. This is seen most often in the United States in patients who have undergone partial gastrectomy. Such patients can absorb iron salts but the absorption of dietary iron is markedly reduced and as a consequence the iron stores may become depleted over a period of years.[100] Iron deficiency anemia usually develops in patients who have had total gastrectomy if they survive long enough. Poor absorption of iron also occurs in prolonged severe diarrhea and in the malabsorption syndromes.

Although probably not an important factor in the production of anemia, the life span of the red cell in patients with iron deficiency anemia was found to be shortened, 46 to 85 days, when studied by the Ashby technique; erythrocytes from normal individuals survived normally when transfused into patients with iron deficiency anemia.[83]

Different morphological varieties of anemia have been reported in kwashiorkor. A study of 22 African children indicates that although hypochromia is common, there usually is stainable iron in the bone marrow; both plasma iron and iron binding capacity are generally reduced.[1] The bone marrow in many patients shows some degree of megaloblastic change. On recovery from the disease with improvement in the plasma proteins the picture typical of iron deficiency develops in about half the infants. It still remains uncertain how important infection, iron deficiency, and other dietary deficiencies are in the occurrence of anemia in this disease.

Clinical Manifestations

The symptoms that occur in the patient with iron deficiency anemia may be related to the primary disease or to anemia. Some patients consult a physician because they have noticed abnormal blood loss such as menorrhagia or rectal bleeding. Other patients, who have not noted any abnormal blood loss, visit a physician because of symptoms that are related to the anemia per se, such as weakness, easy fatigue, dyspnea on exertion, and palpation. In addition to the usual symptoms of anemia, patients with iron deficiency sometimes complain of dysphagia, sore tongue, sore mouth, and brittle nails. Still other patients seek help because of symptoms that are caused by a lesion of the gastrointestinal tract, such as a duodenal ulcer or carcinoma of the bowel, and the presence of anemia is not suspected until a blood count is done. Some patients with iron deficiency anemia develop an extreme hunger for ice and eat more than one or two trays of ice cubes a day; at times the symptom disappears on administration of iron before the anemia has been corrected. The eating of clay (pica) is sometimes considered to be a sign of iron deficiency, particularly in children. In addition, the ingestion of laundry starch may be at least a contributing factor to the production of iron deficiency.[106a]

Physical examination in some patients reveals no abnormality and in others simply pallor of the skin and mucous membranes. At times fissuring at the angles of the mouth, atrophy of the papillae of the tongue, and glossitis are evident. In severe, long-standing iron deficiency the nails may be "spoon-shaped" and abnormally brittle. The spleen is often palpable in children and adults with iron deficiency but does not extend more than a few centimeters below the left costal margin in the uncomplicated case. Throbbing headaches sometimes occur when the hemoglobin is greatly reduced and disappear when the anemia is corrected. When the anemia is moderately severe an apical or precordial systolic murmur is usually present. Other cardiovascular abnormalities, such as cardiac dilatation and congestive failure, occur most often in younger children and in older persons with some coexisting heart disease.

Abnormalities other than anemia occur at times in patients with iron deficiency. Most common among these are fissuring about the mouth, trophic changes in the fingernails, koiloncyhia, and dysfunction of the esophagus. These abnormalities have been reported as manifestations of iron deficiency in the absence of anemia because these lesions have been found in non-anemic patients and improvement in the lesions has followed promptly after the administration of iron salts. A similar response to treatment with iron has been reported in non-anemic patients who had normal levels of serum iron. Correction of achlorhydria, which is present in about 50 per cent of patients with iron deficiency anemia, has been reported after iron therapy[48] but was not confirmed in a more recent study.[81] No improvement in the histologic appearance of the gastric mucosa or in the acid secretion occurred after a year of treatment with iron. Further evidence of a discrepancy between the iron content of the blood and the iron content of the tissues, particularly iron-containing enzymes, is afforded by the work of Beutler, who found that in rats that were made iron deficient by bleeding and special diets the decrease in the cytochrome C of the liver and kidney greatly exceeded the decrease in hemoglobin.[5, 6] Other studies have shown that not all iron-containing enzymes are so dependent on adequate supplies of iron. The concentration of catalase has been found to be normal in human red cells even under conditions of severe iron need.

Laboratory Examination

The anemia of severe iron deficiency is characteristically hypochromic and microcytic (MCV is less than 80 cu. microns, MCH less than 30 micromicrograms, and MCHC less than 30 per cent). Very low values are often found. In the majority of patients with iron deficiency study of a stained smear of the peripheral blood reveals that most of the erythrocytes are smaller than normal and show an increase in the central pallor that may be extreme (hypochromic microcytes); other erythrocytes appear normal in color and some show polychromatophilia if erythropoiesis is active. Poikilocytosis is often evident and elongated "cigar forms" are seen frequently. Occasionally nucleated red cells are present. The leukocyte count, platelet count, and reticulocyte counts are usually normal; thrombocytopenia sometimes occurs in severe iron deficiency. Erythropoiesis is normoblastic in type but the cellularity of the marrow may appear normal, reduced, or increased.

In patients with less severe iron deficiency the anemia is not always hypochromic and microcytic; it may be hypochromic and normocytic, or normochromic and normocytic. In such patients other laboratory procedures may be helpful in establishing a diagnosis of iron deficiency. The presence of iron deficiency usually is accompanied by a reduction in the level of the serum iron, generally to less than 40 μg. per 100 ml. (normal 50 to 150), and an increase in the latent iron binding capacity of the serum to two or three times the normal value (normal 200 to 300 μg. per cent).

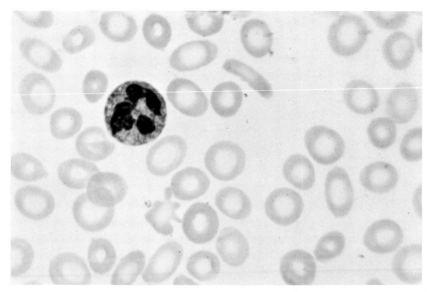

Figure 5-4. Smear of peripheral blood of patient with iron deficiency anemia. (F.S.: I, 25–27.)

In iron deficiency the saturation of transferrin is often but not invariably less than 10 per cent; low saturations, 10 to 16 per cent, also occur in infections. Study of bone marrow that is obtained by aspiration and stained for iron may also provide a reliable index of the state of the iron stores, particularly if the stores are low.[37]

Sections of bone marrow tissue are more satisfactory than smears for estimation of iron stores; preparations can be studied in the unstained state or after staining with Prussian blue.[98] The amount of iron in the storage cells is probably the most reliable index of the body stores of iron; nevertheless all the iron in the cells may not be used for hemoglobin production. The major portion of injected iron dextran is available for hemoglobin synthesis only after it has been processed by the reticuloendothelial system. Several weeks after injection, iron may be seen in the marrow reticuloendothelial cells, even though it has become progressively unavailable for hemoglobin synthesis.[57] The number and appearance of iron granules in the nucleated red cells give some indication of iron utilization. Normally one-third of the marrow normoblasts contain siderotic granules; these become small and virtually disappear in iron deficiency and increase in some situations in which iron utilization is defective. These non-hemoglobin granules are thought to be aggregates of ferritin molecules. When anemia is due to iron deficiency the serum bilirubin is not elevated and the 24 hour fecal urobilinogen excretion is usually lower than normal because the mass of the circulating hemoglobin is reduced. The free erythrocyte protoporphyrin is increased in iron deficiency.[19] Achlorhydria occurs commonly in patients with this disorder.

The development of iron deficiency produces the following sequence of changes: (1) depletion of iron stores, which is usually evident in the bone marrow; (2) elevation of the iron binding capacity of the serum; (3) fall in serum iron level; (4) development of normochromic or slightly hypochromic anemia;

and (5) development of hypochromic microcytic anemia. The reverse sequence occurs when the deficiency is treated with oral iron.

Differential Diagnosis

The first step in making a diagnosis of this type of anemia is to establish the presence of iron deficiency and the next is to determine the cause. If the anemia is hypochromic and microcytic, the commonly seen iron deficiency must be distinguished from the uncommon thalassemia and the rare pyridoxine deficiency and other "iron loading" disorders. Thalassemia is characterized by a family history of anemia, the occurrence of many target cells on the stained smear, and an elevated reticulocyte count; the spleen is usually enlarged and may extend below the level of the umbilicus. Determination of the serum iron level and examination of properly stained marrow preparations fail to reveal any iron deficiency. Fetal hemoglobin and hemoglobin A_2 are usually increased. Pyridoxine deficiency and "iron loading anemia," which are rare in man, are characterized by a hypochromic microcytic anemia but, even though the erythrocytes appear hypochromic, the level of the serum iron is elevated and administration of iron produces no improvement in the anemia. The demonstration of a lack or an excess of iron in the bone marrow preparations probably is the most reliable and simplest means of distinguishing between iron deficiency anemia and other conditions associated with hypochromic cells. In the milder degrees of iron deficiency the anemia may be hypochromic, normochromic, normocytic, or slightly microcytic rather than hypochromic microcytic. This is most likely to occur when severe deficiency has not developed or when the severe deficiency has been only partly corrected. In such circumstances the demonstration of a low serum iron level or an increase in the latent iron binding capacity, or a histologic demonstration of low iron stores in the tissue, often establishes the presence of iron deficiency.

If the presence of iron deficiency has been established, an effort is made to find the cause of the deficiency. Faulty diet may be an acceptable explanation in infants and very young children but in adults a search must be made for the cause of the blood loss. The absence of occult blood from a single specimen of feces does not exclude chronic or recurrent gastrointestinal bleeding from consideration. Unless the cause of the iron deficiency is clear-cut, most patients, particularly those who are middle-aged or older, will need a roentgenographic study of the upper and lower gastrointestinal tract. Almost any ulcerative lesion in the esophagus, stomach, small intestine, or large bowel can be responsible for chronic bleeding and iron deficiency. Although hiatus hernia with ulceration often causes gastrointestinal bleeding and anemia, one should not conclude that the demonstration of a hiatus hernia in a patient with anemia has disclosed the source of the bleeding. Many middle-aged and older patients have an asymptomatic hiatus hernia. Examination of the small intestine and large bowel should be performed and the hernia accepted as the cause of the bleeding only when no other likely site can be demonstated. If a lesion of the gastrointestinal tract is suspected but not demonstrated at the time of the initial examination, the appropriate studies should be repeated because of the importance of demonstrating any lesion, particularly a neoplasm, that might require surgical correction. In women, particularly those of child-bearing age, the decision must be made whether or not the history of vaginal bleeding and pregnancies gives an adequate explanation of the anemia. Roentgeno-graphic investigation of the gastrointestinal tract is often indicated but the risk of irradiation to the ovaries or to an unsuspected early pregnancy should not be ignored. The ingestion of aspirin is a fairly common cause of bleeding, either from local irritation or through an effect on platelet aggregation.

Treatment, Course, and Prognosis

The most important aspect of the treatment of iron deficiency anemia is the correction of the cause. This is much more important than the correction of the anemia unless the patient is critically ill. The prognosis is related more to the underlying disease than to the severity of the anemia, which may have little or no influence on the outcome.

In patients with anemia that is due to iron deficiency the administration of ferrous salts is followed by a reticulocytosis during the first week (Fig. 5-5). The magnitude of reticulocyte response, which is usually in the range of 4 to 10 per cent, depends on the initial hemoglobin level and not on the level of the erythrocyte count. Unless complicating factors are present the reticulo-cytosis is followed by the return of the hemoglobin and red cells to normal

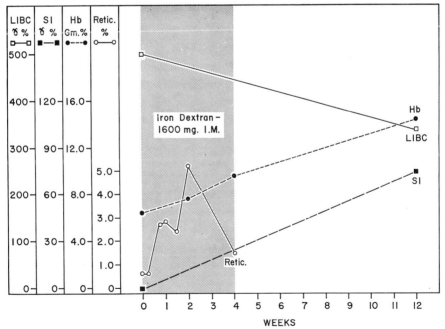

Figure 5-5. Chart showing hematologic response of a patient with iron deficiency anemia to treatment with iron. The reticulocyte peak, which is not as great as that seen after specific treatment in pernicious anemia, occurs before there is an increase in the levels of hemoglobin and serum iron and a decrease in the latent iron binding capacity.

levels within a period of 6 to 10 weeks. If the therapy with iron is successful the hemoglobin level should increase 2.0 gm. per 100 ml. in the first 3 weeks of treatment. The levels of iron and latent iron binding capacity, and the storage iron in the marrow, which probably reflect the state of the stores of iron, return to normal much more slowly. Treatment probably should be continued until this occurs, but such complete therapy may require small amounts of iron salts orally for a long period, particularly if the patient is either a premenopausal woman or has had a partial gastrectomy. Prolonged treatment of this type is considered impractical by some.

The anemia of iron deficiency is usually corrected by the oral administration of 0.2 or 0.3 gm. of ferrous sulfate or ferrous gluconate three times a day. Various preparations contain between 35 and 70 mg. of iron per tablet; of the total dose of between 100 and 200 mg. of iron, probably no more than 20 or 30 mg. is absorbed. If a small amount of the drug is given initially and the dosage is increased gradually, gastrointestinal upsets rarely occur. Some patients tolerate one preparation better than another, and if one preparation is causing undesirable griping, diarrhea, or other symptoms, another compound should be substituted. Iron is less likely to cause gastrointestinal symptoms if it is given after meals. Although this is not an optimal time for iron absorption, adequate absorption usually occurs if the medication is given at this time. A single tablet of ferrous gluconate or ferrous sulfate at bedtime generally produces a satisfactory response and many patients find it simpler and more convenient to follow this schedule. The use of "sustained-release" preparations is not recommended; in one study no sustained release could be demonstrated and indeed less iron was available than in usual preparations.[92]

Although iron salts administered orally correct the anemia in most patients, the method of treatment is not an efficient means of correcting the iron stores because iron absorption decreases when the blood returns to normal. In order to replenish the iron stores by the oral route it is often necessary to continue treatment for months or years. For this reason parenteral preparations are sometimes employed. Saccharated iron oxide given intravenously in an initial dose of 20 to 50 mg. and in subsequent daily doses of 100 to 200 mg. produces excellent therapeutic results. Intramuscular therapy with iron dextran is also effective. Injections of 100 to 500 mg. may be given weekly or several times a week. The total amount given in a course of intramuscular treatment is usually between 1500 and 5000 mg., an amount sufficient to correct the anemia and replenish the iron stores. Reactions such as fever and even vasomotor collapse may occur but are infrequent. The risk of late complications of the intramuscular injections has not been determined precisely but probably is slight.

Illustrative Cases

CASE 1

A 74 year old white housewife was admitted to the hospital for evaluation of anemia and weight loss of 20 pounds during the preceding year. About 1½ years prior to admission she had an episode of constipation, cramping midabdominal pain, and vomiting. Roentgenographic examinations of the gallbladder and upper gastrointestinal tract were negative. Her attacks recurred with increasing frequency and about 6 weeks before admission were occurring once or twice a week. At this time the patient was found to be anemic and was treated with iron.

Physical examination. The skin and mucous membranes were pale. The right side of the abdomen was moderately tender and a firm, movable 6 by 10 cm. mass was felt in the right lower quadrant. The liver edge was palpable 2 cm. below the right costal margin.

Laboratory studies. Admission blood studies disclosed the following: Hct. 26 per cent, Hb. 6.7 gm. per 100 ml., R.B.C. 3.4 mil. per cu.mm., W.B.C. 4900 per cu.mm.; serum iron 11.5 μg. per 100 ml.; unsaturated iron binding protein 455 μg. per 100 ml. The feces gave a strongly positive benzidine reaction.

Barium enema examination revealed a 5 or 6 cm. constricted area in the ascending colon and another filling defect in the sigmoid colon. After blood transfusions operation was performed. A carcinoma of the ascending colon and a carcinomatous polyp in the descending colon were found. Both lesions were resected and convalescence was uneventful.

Three months later the Hct. was 43 per cent, Hb. 12.6 gm. per 100 ml., R.B.C. 4.4 mil. per cu.mm., plasma iron 99 μg. per 100 ml., and unsaturated iron binding protein 270 μg. per 100 ml.

Comment. At the time of admission this patient had evidence of severe iron deficiency in the form of hypochromic microcytic anemia associated with a decrease in the level of serum iron and an increase in the unsaturated iron binding capacity. The most important aspect of the diagnosis in a patient with anemia of this type is the demonstration of the cause of the anemia. Usually, as was the case in this patient, the iron deficiency is the result of chronic blood loss. In adult males and elderly women chronic unrecognized blood loss is nearly always the result of a lesion in the gastrointestinal tract. This patient had two primary malignant lesions in the colon. It appears likely that the lesion in the ascending colon was responsible for the blood loss and the tumor in the sigmoid colon was responsible for the symptoms of partial intestinal obstruction. In all probability a more thorough examination at the time her symptoms began, a year and a half before admission, would have revealed a lesion in the colon. Fortunately this patient appeared to have no metastases when her bowel resections were performed, despite a delay in diagnosis that might well have been fatal.

CASE 2

This 69 year old white housewife was admitted with the chief complaint of "anemia" of 2 years' duration. She related that for 2 years she had felt weak, nervous, and slightly dizzy. She had been treated irregularly for 2 years with liver extract and iron. Despite this therapy some degree of anemia persisted and she was referred for further study. Careful questioning elicited no history of weight loss, gastrointestinal symptoms, or abnormal bleeding.

Physical examination. The patient was well developed, well nourished, and somewhat obese. General examination revealed no specific abnormalities but the pelvic examination revealed an erosion of the cervix.

Laboratory examination. Admission blood studies: Hb. 9.1 gm. per 100 ml.; R.B.C. 3.8 mil, per cu.mm.; Hct. 31 per cent; retics. 1.9 per cent. The leukocyte count, platelet count, and differential count were normal. Bone marrow examination disclosed a hypercellular marrow with a normoblastic type of erythropoiesis. Repeated stool examinations were consistently positive for occult blood.

Gastrointestinal x-ray study revealed a hiatus hernia that was about 10 cm. in the greatest diameter. Barium enema examination revealed a lesion at the hepatic flexure which was associated with some narrowing over an area of 2 or 3 cm. Proctoscopic examination disclosed no lesion. Biopsy of the cervix was reported as showing an epidermoid carcinoma.

Treatment and course. The patient was transfused with 3 units of blood and was operated upon 9 days after admission. A right colectomy was performed and the patient stood the procedure well. At the time of operation there was no evidence of metastases from the lesions in bowel or cervix. Histologic study of the bowel tumor revealed mucinous adenocarcinoma grade III extending through the thickness of the wall. The regional lymph nodes were free of tumor. The patient's convalescence from the laparotomy was uneventful, and 16 days after her right colectomy radium was applied to the cervix. She received 6000 mg. hours using six sources and the following month she received 6000 r of external radiation.

Comment. This patient illustrates many instructive points. She was treated for 2 years for anemia with iron and liver extract without any effort being made to discover the cause of the anemia. This treatment altered the morphologic characteristics of the red blood cells without correcting the anemia. This case illustrates the importance of determining the cause of the anemia before treatment. When the gastrointestinal tract was investigated two possible bleeding sites were found. The hiatus hernia was found first, but this lesion occurs so frequently in this age group that it was thought important to study the lower gastrointestinal tract. This was done and the carcinoma of the colon was discovered. Fortunately the lesion was operable despite the duration of the illness. The finding of a carcinoma of the cervix on the routine examination emphasizes the importance of a complete examination in all patients.

Anemias Associated with Abnormal Utilization of Iron

"Iron loading anemia," "sideroblastic anemia," and "sideroachrestic anemia" are diagnostic terms that have been applied to patients who have anemia associated with an abnormality in iron metabolism. These patients seem to be different from patients with thalassemia and the other known hemoglobinopathies.

Knowledge of the pathologic physiology in these patients is incomplete; in some even the natural history of disease is unknown. Because of these inadequacies, many questions remain and the anemias cannot be classified in a satisfactory manner. Some patients appear to fit into a well-defined syndrome, but others manifest features found in several different syndromes. An example is the patient who appears to have a hereditary form of the disorder yet responds partially to treatment with pyridoxine. The bone marrow of patients with these disorders contains many sideroblasts, but whether the presence of "ringed sideroblasts" is a sine qua non for the inclusion in this group of diseases is uncertain; some patients have iron overload and anemia but a careful search of the marrow does not reveal any typical ringed sideroblasts.

The so-called "sideroblastic" anemias have the following characteristics: (1) hypochromic and microcytic or normocytic anemia with marked anisocytosis and poikilocytosis of the red cells; (2) normal or elevated serum iron levels; (3) refractoriness to iron therapy; (4) erythroid hyperplasia of the bone marrow; (5) increased sideroblasts in the marrow; (6) markedly reduced iron incorporation in the cells; (7) normal or slightly reduced red cell survival time; and (8) marked hemosiderosis that can lead to hemochromatosis. A characteristic feature of these disorders is an increase in the number and size of the non-hemoglobin iron-containing granules in the normoblasts; when these siderotic granules accumulate in the perinuclear area they produce the cell termed the "ringed sideroblast."

The increase in size and amount of non-hemoglobin iron in the perinuclear area has been explained by studies with electron microscopy which have disclosed the accumulation of excessive amounts of iron in the mitochondria.[4] The accumulation of iron in the mitochondria is related to the defect in heme synthesis which exists in these disorders. Mitochondria are concerned in the first step in porphyrin synthesis and also in the last step (Fig. 5–6). In the first step, which requires pyridoxal-5-phosphate and the Kreb's cycle, glycine combines with succinyl CoA to form delta-aminolevulinic acid. The last step, coupling of protoporphyrin and iron to form heme, requires heme synthetase and also pyridoxal phosphate, which probably is necessary for the release of iron from the mitochondria. Iron may accumulate in excess because of some defect in the control of the entrance of iron into the cell or as a result of defective utilization because of some metabolic block. Excessive amounts of iron from whatever cause might damage the mitochrondria or other organelles in the cell. (F.S.: I, 28–31.)

The mitochondrial accumulation of particles of iron, usually small and few in number, has also been reported in patients with thalassemia, mechanical hemolytic anemia, and porphyria cutanea tarda, and in those receiving chloramphenicol.[43] It is possible that both a metabolic block and deranged ingress of iron into the cell are factors.

The studies of patients with iron loading[54] have shown enzymatic defects located at different steps in the synthesis of heme; the different defects can produce identical or similar clinical pictures. In pyridoxine responsive anemia there is iron loading and, in addition, a diminution in the free erythrocyte portoporphyrin and coproporphyrin; this can be explained if there is a block in the first stage of porphyrin metabolism, the union of glycine and succinyl-

SYNTHESIS OF HEME

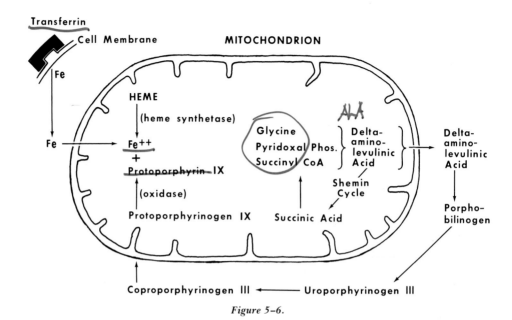

Figure 5–6.

CoA to form delta-aminolevulinic acid, a reaction that requires pyridoxal phosphate. The existence of such a block or blocks appears to be confirmed by Vogler and Mingioli, who studied hemoglobin synthesis in reticulocytes of patients with pyridoxine responsive anemia with the use of labeled glycine and delta-aminolevulinic acid; when labeled glycine was added no increase in heme was found, but when labeled delta-aminolevulinic was added, increased heme production followed.[126, 127] Their later studies disclosed a defect in the incorporation of glycine into heme, the rate being only from 11 to 25 per cent of normal. The incorporation of delta-aminolevulinic acid into heme was only 46 to 81 per cent of normal. These observations suggested two defects in the synthesis of heme, the major one occurring prior to the formation of ALA and the minor one occurring somewhere between the synthesis of ALA and heme. Studies after repeated phlebotomies disclosed that when the iron stores were reduced to normal, incorporation of delta-aminolevulinic acid by the patient's reticulocytes equaled the normal rate, although glycine incorporation was still reduced. These results indicated that excess of iron was a significant factor in reduced heme synthesis activity in patients whose primary defect was probably defective ALA synthetase activity.[127]

According to Heilmeyer,[54] in the congenital form of sideroachrestic anemia there are iron loading and an increase in erythrocyte coproporphyrin associated with a normal or reduced level of erythrocyte protoporphyrin, a combination which suggests a block in heme synthesis at the step between the formation of coproporphyrinogen and protoporphyrin IX, probably a failure of the oxidase enzyme. In the acquired type of sideroachrestic anemia, characterized by the

Table 5–3. *Classification of Siderolastic Anemia*

A. Primary
  1. Hereditary
  2. Acquired

B. Secondary
  1. Associated with chemicals (isoniazid, cycloserine, lead, possibly others)
  2. Associated with other diseases (rheumatoid arthritis, polyarteritis nodosa, leukemia and other myeloproliferative disorders, myeloma, carcinoma, alcoholism, hemolytic anemia)

C. Unclassified
  1. Pyridoxine responsive anemia
  2. Anemia responsive to crude liver extract

(Modified from Mollin, D. L.: Brit. J. Haemat., *11*:41, 1965.)

increase in the iron associated with increase in coproporphyrin and protoporphyrin, there appears to be a defect in the union of iron and protoporphyrin IX, probably a deficiency in the enzyme heme synthetase. In lead intoxication, and in anemia associated with therapy with INH, there are increases in coproporphyrin and protoporphyrin which suggest a block in the combining of iron with protoporphyrin to form heme; in addition, there probably are defects or partial blocks earlier in the metabolic pathway.

There may well be blocks at other steps in the metabolic pathway in other patients who fit into this syndrome. Heilmeyer, London, and others have produced evidence to indicate that heme, protoporphyrin, and coproporphyrin all may act by feedback mechanisms to slow down the first stage of porphyrin metabolism when the other substances are present in increased amounts. The production of globin and heme ordinarily proceed at approximately the same rate. An imbalance in these reactions is a possible explanation for the defect in iron metabolism found in beta thalassemia: with the slow production of the beta chain, globin production lags, and consequently, iron plus the other compounds, protoporphyrin, and coproporphyrin accumulate.

A clinical classification of the sideroblastic anemias is presented in Table 5–3. Pyridoxine responsive anemia and the anemia responsive to crude liver extract are placed in separate catagories because of the unpredictable response to treatment with pyridoxine seen in patients with either hereditary or acquired disease.

Hereditary Sideroblastic Anemia
(Congenital Sideroachrestic Anemia, Hereditary Iron Loading Anemia)

The first description of the hereditary hypochromic type of anemia has been credited to Cooley[24a] and Rundles and Falls.[107] This disorder has been reported in siblings and in patients who have a family history of anemia. Nearly all of the reported cases have been males but females are not exempt. The anemia is usually noticed in childhood or in the early adult years and hemochromatosis often develops during the third and fourth decade. Early in the disorder patients often present with a history of weakness or easy fatigue; if hemochromatosis has developed, abdominal pain, heart failure, or thrombophlebitis are commonly seen. Physical examination usually discloses poor physical development associated with mild enlargement of the liver and spleen; sometimes increased pigmentation of the skin is apparent.

Laboratory examinations: classically the anemia is moderately severe, hypochromic and microcytic (MCV, 53 to 68 cu. microns; MCH, 18 to 20 micromicrograms; MCHC, 33 per cent) although in some cases included in this category it has been normocytic or macrocytic. The leukocyte count is normal; the differential count is usually normal but sometimes the lymphocytes are slightly increased. The platelet count is normal or diminished but in patients who have had splenectomy counts of a million or more are common. Reticulocyte counts are usually normal but counts as high as 15 per cent have been noted. The stained smear of the peripheral blood presents a striking appearance because of presence of marked anisochromia, anisocytosis, poikilocytosis, and leptocytosis. If the spleen has been removed many of the hypochromic erythrocytes contain iron-staining granules (siderocytes). Examination of the bone marrow reveals a very hyperplastic marrow with erythropoiesis of the normoblastic type; many young forms are present. If stains for iron are used, many of the nucleated cells are seen to be sideroblasts, normoblasts with granules of non-hemoglobin iron in the cytoplasm: they constitute from 80 to 95 per cent of the total (normal, 30 per cent). Ringed sideroblasts are considered by some to be almost pathognomonic of the disorder,[122] but they also occur in patients considered to have other disorders of iron metabolism.

The morphologic evidence of the disturbance in iron metabolism is confirmed by special studies. The serum iron is normal or increased, with values of 125 to 300 micrograms per 100 ml. reported. The degree of saturation of the transferrin may be normal but is usually greatly increased. Studies with radioactive iron have disclosed rapid clearance of the iron from the plasma associated with decreased utilization of the iron as measured by its appearance in the circulating erythrocytes; the picture is that of ineffective erythropoiesis. Iron absorption from the gastrointestinal tract must be increased early in the disorder but radioiron studies have given variable results; later in the disease absorption may diminish because of a build-up in tissue iron. Other evidence of abnormal hemoglobin metabolism in these patients is an increase in the coproporphyrin concentration and a decreased or normal protoporphyrin level in the erythrocytes.

Investigations have failed to disclose any evidence of significant hyperhemolysis. Fecal urobilinogen excretion is normal, serum bilirubin is normal or slightly increased, and red cell survival as measured by chromium tagged cells has been reported as normal or only slightly decreased. Electrophoresis has shown no increase in the A_2 hemoglobin and determinations of the fetal hemoglobin have been normal.

Treatment with iron, cobalt, vitamin B_{12}, and adrenocortical steroid is of no value; occasionally splenectomy is beneficial. The main therapeutic measures are pyridoxine, phlebotomies, and chelating agents. The administration of pyridoxine to some patients is followed by a partial hematologic response associated with symptomatic improvement. Such improvement warrants inclusion of the patient in the "pyridoxine-responsive anemia" group according to Horrigan and Harris.[62] Probably all patients thought to have the disorder should be given a trial on pyridoxine hydrochloride, 100 to 200 mg. a day. If phlebotomies can be tolerated they are advisable. Removal of iron in this way is the most effective means of preventing the development of severe hemochromatosis later in life and removal of some of the tissue iron sometimes leads to improvement in erythropoiesis. Some patients with this disorder do not tolerate phlebotomy; an effective chelating agent would be valuable in treatment.

Acquired Sideroblastic Anemia

Patients who have been reported as examples of "acquired sideroblastic anemia," "refractory anemia with sideroblastic bone marrow," "refractory normoblastic anemia," "refractory sideroblastic anemia," and as early examples of the Di Guglielmo syndrome appear to have the same or a very closely related syndrome that may be of diverse etiology.

The common features of the disorder, which usually appears in middle-aged or elderly males, are a moderately severe anemia associated with normoblastic hyperplasia of the bone marrow; the granulocyte and platelet counts may be normal or reduced and show no constant pattern. The anemia is the result of ineffective erythropoiesis; studies with radioactive iron have shown rapid clearance of the plasma iron but diminished utilization of the iron for the circulating erythrocytes. The serum iron level is usually increased, often over 200 micrograms per 100 ml., and saturation of the iron binding capacity is increased, sometimes reaching 100 per cent. Appropriate stains disclose greatly increased stores of iron in the marrow and a high percentage of sideroblasts; "ringed" sideroblasts are often present. The circulating erythrocytes are usually normocytic or slightly macrocytic, MCV 80 to 114 cu. microns, and normochromic; some patients have had a hypochromic microcytic anemia, and some have appeared to have a mixture of large and small cells. The reticulocyte count is normal or slightly increased and hemolysis of circulating red cells, as gauged by chromium survival studies, is only slightly increased.

The clinical course is often relatively benign but some patients develop hepatosplenomegaly and other features of hemochromatosis. Leukemia has developed in a number of the patients; an increase in myeloblasts and promyelocytes or other cells of the granulocytic series sometimes is evident months or years before the appearance of frank leukemia.

If the patients who respond partially to pyridoxine are separated from this group, the anemia is refractory to treatment other than transfusion. Because of the possible damaging effects of long-standing iron overload, an attempt to reduce the tissue iron by phlebotomy, which is rarely tolerated well, is advisable.

Secondary Sideroblastic Anemia Associated with Chemicals

A number of substances are known to inhibit heme synthesis.[54] Among the most important in clinical medicine are the antituberculous drugs and lead.

A relatively small number of patients with tuberculosis treated with isoniazid, cycloserine, or pyrazinamide, known to act as antagonists to pyridoxal-5-phosphate, have developed sideroblastic anemia.[54, 93] The disappearance of the anemia when the drugs were discontinued indicates that the drugs played an essential role. The stimulation of erythropoiesis and the improvement in the peripheral neuritis that follows the administration of pyridoxine while patients are being treated with INH point toward a deficiency or defective utilization of pyridoxine. Apparently incorporation of iron into protoporphyrin is defective.[54] Why only a small percentage of patients treated with these drugs develop the abnormality remains unclear.

The anemia of lead poisoning is usually mild, hemolytic and slightly hypochromic; basophilic stippling is present in the erythrocytes and reticulocytosis of varying degree is present. Sideroblasts are increased in the marrow. Other abnormalities are increased amounts of protoporphyrin and coproporphyrin in the erythrocytes accompanied by increased urinary excretion of delta-aminolevulinic acid, protoporphyrin III and uroporphyrin.[82] The swelling and disintegration of the mitochondria that have been revealed by electron microscopy are associated with some abnormality in the synthesis of hemoglobin involving several enzymatic reactions.[82] There is evidence that lead inhibits the synthesis of delta-aminolevulinic acid, the conversion of this substance to porphobilinogen, and the conversion of coproporphyrinogen III to protoporphyrin IX; in addition, movement of iron from the stroma of the cells into the mitochondria and its union with protoporphyrin to form heme are inhibited. Thus it appears that presence of lead inhibits, but does not block completely, nearly every step in the synthesis of heme.

Sideroblastic Anemia Associated with Other Diseases

Sideroblastic anemia has been observed in a number of diseases (see Table 5–3); often the clinical picture and the hematological abnormalities are not striking. The ringed sideroblasts usually disappear on successful treatment of the underlying disease or with the administration of pyridoxine and folic acid.[93] Ringed sideroblasts occur in hemolytic anemia when there is some associated defect in hemoglobin synthesis; they are seen in thalassemia and some acquired disorders, but not in hereditary spherocytosis.

Varying numbers of ringed sideroblasts, with or without anemia, have been observed in a number of diseases: few (1 to 4 per cent) in Di Guglielmo's syndrome, collagen disorders, megaloblastic anemia, malignant neoplasm, acute and chronic infections, uremia, liver disease, hemochromatosis, acquired hemolytic anemia, leukemia, and lymphoma; moderate numbers (5 to 21 per cent) in thalassemia major, myeloproliferative disorders, and lymphoma and leukemia after treatment; large numbers (37 to 77 per cent) in refractory normoblastic anemia and severe infection accompanied by leukopenia.[13] In two patients with lymphoma, the ringed sideroblasts appeared for the first time after treatment with alkylating agents and in one with chronic leukemia after treatment with 6-mercaptopurine. A reversible type of sideroblastic anemia has been reported in severe alcoholics with liver disease and folate deficiency.[57a, 57b]

The puzzling relationship of sideroblastic anemia to the Di Guglielmo syndrome and leukemia has been reviewed by Dameshek.[29] The frequent development of leukemia in patients who have acquired sideroblastic anemia, "refractory normoblastic anemia," or "aplastic anemia with a hypercellular marrow" has been noted many times.

Pyridoxine Responsive Anemia

The first report of a patient with pyridoxine responsive anemia was by Harris et al. in 1956 and since that time an increasing number of reports of similar patients have appeared although the disorder must still be considered a rare one.[30, 38, 49, 104, 123] One review included 72 patients.[62]

This disorder has been reported in patients from 8 to 87 years of age. About 80 per cent of the patients were males. Hepatomegaly, splenomegaly, and diffuse skin pigmentation have been noted in about half of the patients. Most patients have been well nourished; none has had other evidence of pyridoxine deficiency such as dermatitis, neuropathy, glossitis, or convulsions.

The reported hemoglobin levels have ranged from 3.8 to 11 gms. per 100 ml. Typically the erythrocytes are hypochromic and microcytic but in some patients they are hypochromic and normocytic or macrocytic; normochromic cells have been seen in a few patients. In the peripheral blood smear anisocytosis, poikilocytosis, and target cells are prominent; siderocytes are often increased. The reticulocytes are normal or low. The number of leukocytes and platelets shows no consistent variations but may be abnormal.

In about 80 per cent of the reported patients the bone marrow examination has disclosed normoblastic hyperplasia. Iron stains demonstrate a striking increase of iron in the reticuloendothelial cells and normoblasts. The number of sideroblasts is greatly increased and "ringed" sideroblasts have been observed. In a minority of the patients megaloblastic hyperplasia has been observed; in these patients macrocytosis is the rule and microcytosis the exception.

Characteristically the level of serum iron is increased, usually over 200 micrograms per 100 ml., and the iron binding capacity is 80 to 100 per cent saturated. Studies with radioactive iron have shown accelerated plasma clearance of injected iron and increased plasma iron turnover associated with subnormal or minimal incorporation of the radioiron into erythrocytes.

Other studies have shown a slight or moderate decrease in erythrocyte survival time as determined by the Cr^{51} method. Negative Coombs tests and a slight increase in the osmotic resistance to hypotonic saline have been reported. The free erythrocyte protoporphyrin is not increased as it is in iron deficiency.

The cause of the pyridoxine responsiveness in this group of patients has not been determined. The familial incidence of the disorder indicates that heredity may be an etiologic factor. There is no evidence of dietary deficiency in any of the patients reported, except one that was experimentally induced. Likewise, there is no evidence of malabsorption in most of the reported patients. Further evidence against the presence of a true deficiency of pyridoxine is the large amount of pyridoxine that is necessary to produce the remission, 10 to 100 mg. intramuscularly, or 200 mg. orally. Discontinuance of the pyridoxine has resulted in hematologic relapse in the reported patients who had previously responded, but the remission may be prolonged. The incompleteness of the remission in the majority of the reported patients suggests that a deficiency of pyridoxine is not the only defect. Response to treatment is often manifested by a reticulocytosis of from 2 to 50 per cent in from 4 to 10 days followed by a fall in the serum iron level.

Illustrative Case

A 19 year old white youth was first seen at the University of Virginia Hospital in 1954 because of anemia. He was known to have had anemia in infancy but was asymptomatic until 6 months before his visit, when he first experienced weakness, palpitation, and easy fatigue. At the initial examination the skin was hyperpigmented and the liver and spleen were both palpable 5 cm. below the costal margins. The hemoglobin was 4.4 grams per 100 ml., hematocrit 24 per cent, MCV 62 cu. microns, MCH 11 micromicrograms, MCHC 14 per cent. Marked hypochromia, anisocytosis, poikilocytosis, and microcytosis were apparent on the blood smear. Leukocyte and reticulocyte counts were normal. Hemoglobin electrophoresis and the alkali denaturation test were normal. Serum iron measured 325 micrograms per 100 ml. and iron binding capacity was completely saturated. Bone marrow aspiration disclosed the normoblastic type of erythropoiesis.

In August 1955 the patient underwent splenectomy without any improvement in his anemia. In October 1955 pyridoxine was started 50 mg. three times a day by mouth. On this regimen the hemoglobin rose from 4.7 grams to 10.3 grams per 100 ml. in about 2 months. He was given a maintenance dose of 50 mg. i.m. three times a week and did well on this treatment until 1960; then for some reason, he became lax, took his medication irregularly, and by June 1960 the hemoglobin was only 4.9 grams per 100 ml. Regular treatment was again started but in July 1960 he was admitted to his community hospital because of right upper quadrant pain and obstructive jaundice. Operation was performed and it was found that the biliary tract was obstructed with inspissated bile; no gall stones were found. Cholecystectomy was performed; postoperatively the patient developed biliary fistula, subdiaphragmatic abscess, and numerous other complications and after a rather lengthy illness died October 2, 1960.

Autopsy showed generalized peritonitis. There was advanced portal cirrhosis associated with heavy deposits of hemosiderin in the Kupffer's cells and in the parenchymal cells. Extensive fibrosis of the pancreas was present and associated with hemosiderin. Hemosiderin was also evident in the adrenal and pituitary glands. Erythroid and myeloid hyperplasia were apparent in the bone marrow.

Comment. This patient showed the characteristic features of hereditary sideroblastic anemia but the response to pyridoxine places it in a different category. Subsequent studies have shown a similar disease in one brother. The anemia was hypochromic and microcytic and was accompanied by elevation of the serum iron and saturation of the iron binding capacity. The liver and spleen were enlarged. The bone marrow was hyperplastic; erythropoiesis was normoblastic and numerous sideroblasts were present. The patient had a good but incomplete response to treatment with pyridoxine. Of particular interest in this disease is the fact that biopsy of the liver in 1955 revealed hemosiderin in the Kupffer's cells but was otherwise normal; at this time the patient had received less than 20 transfusions. At autopsy 5 years later the picture was typical of hemochromatosis.

Anemia Responsive to Crude Liver Extract

Two patients have been reported with hypochromic microcytic anemia, hyperferremia, anisocytosis, poikilocytosis anisochromasia, and leptocytosis accompanied by bone marrow hyperplasia of the normoblastic type who responded to crude liver extract administered orally but not to iron, vitamin B_{12}, or folic acid.[63] At the time of the report the effect of pyridoxine had not been determined in these patients although it was thought that pyridoxine was not a component of the liver extract which proved effective in their case. Crude liver extract was found to be ineffective in many of the pyridoxine responsive anemia patients who responded only partially and has also been found to be ineffective in at least some of the patients classified in the refractory group of sideroblastic anemias.

Iron Overload

Excessive iron is stored in the body in special circumstances. Ingestion of large amounts of iron, abnormally high intestinal absorption, and excess parenteral iron, usually administered in the form of transfusions, lead to excessive accumulation of iron. The most common clinical conditions associated with iron excess are idiopathic hemochromatosis, iron overload in the Bantu, hemosiderosis, and the group of anemias associated with abnormal utilization of iron.

Idiopathic Hemochromatosis

Idiopathic hemochromatosis is characterized by the slow increase of an excessive amount of iron in the body; the total of non-hemoglobin iron is greatly increased, being in the range of 20 to 40 grams compared to the normal of about 1.0 gram. Excessive iron deposits are found in the parenchymal cells of the liver, pancreas, heart, and adrenal glands; less striking increases are found in the skin, synovial membranes, kidneys, spleen, and other organs. Portal cirrhosis and pancreatic fibrosis usually occur. Pituitary failure as a result of iron deposition may be a serious development.[119] The clinical symptoms usually appear between the age of 40 and 60; over 90 per cent of the patients are men. The commonest symptoms are those associated with diabetes mellitus (weakness, weight loss, or hyperpigmentation of the skin) or those associated with heart failure or cirrhosis of the liver. Iron deposits in the myocardium are usually present in the patients with heart failure; the hyperpigmentation of the skin, which occurs in about 90 per cent of patients, is due mainly to increased melanin since excessive iron deposits are demonstrated only in about half of those with hyperpigmentation. Hepatomegaly is an almost constant finding on physical examination; splenomegaly and spider telangiectases occur in about half; ascites, signs of heart failure, and testicular atrophy occur in one third or less. Death is usually the result of heart failure (30 per cent), hepatic coma (15 per cent), hematemesis (15 per cent), hepatoma (14 per cent), or pneumonia (13 per cent).[39]

The disease is associated with an increased absorption of iron from the intestinal tract, but this apparently does not exceed 2 to 4 mg. a day. Neither the cause of the increased absorption nor the relationship of the iron deposits to the scarring of the organs is established with certainty. Although the portal cirrhosis is considered by some to be primary,[84] most authors have concluded that the disorder is the result of an inherited defect in the absorption of iron.[36, 39] It is probable that a defect in the function of the intestinal mucosa is responsible for the increased absorption because the intake of iron, the plasma transferrin, iron transport, and iron utilization apparently are normal. Evidence that supports the hereditary nature of the disease is the occurrence of the disorder in families and the demonstration of increased levels of serum iron in relatives who did not have the clinical disease.[32] In some patients, folate deficiency has seemed to produce an elevation of the serum iron and the deposition of iron in hepatic cells.[44a] The relationship of the tissue iron to the tissue damage has been the subject of some controversy. The failure to produce the disease by administering excessive amounts of iron orally has led to the concept that both the tissue damage and the increased iron absorption and deposition are the result of an unknown defect.[15] Nevertheless, a clinical picture of hemochromatosis has been reported in a 70 year old woman who took 1000 gm. of elemental iron over a 10 year period; autopsy confirmed the diagnosis.[69] At present the observations on patients with idiopathic hemochromatosis in the preclinical stage, which have disclosed that iron stores are excessive before cirrhosis develops,[10] similar observations on patients with hereditary iron loading anemia, and the clinical improvement that follows removal of iron all support the concept that iron deposition is responsible for the tissue damage.

Congenital iron overload in infants associated with hypotonia and minor anomalies without associated anemia or hyperhemolysis has been reported.[125] The hypothesis was advanced that the children were born with excessive iron which was the result of a genetically determined defect in the infants. The disorder ended fatally in both infants; no abnormalities of iron metabolism were demonstrated in either the father or the mother.

The best screening procedures for diagnosis are determinations of the serum iron and iron binding capacity. In over 80 per cent of the patients in one report the serum iron level was over 180 micrograms and the saturation of the transferrin was over 80 per cent.[36] Others state that usually the serum iron level is over 200 micrograms per 100 ml. and the transferrin is completely saturated or almost so, the main exceptions being when infection or neoplasm had occurred.[11] If the screening tests suggest hemochromatosis, a needle biopsy of the liver is usually done; study of the tissue allows a definitive diagnosis. Because of the familial incidence of the disease, any brothers and sons the patient may have should be studied for early detection of the disorder at a time when treatment will be easier and more beneficial.

Idiopathic hemochromatosis is treated by repeated phlebotomies, usually 500 ml. of whole blood each week. Some patients tolerate two or three phlebotomies a week. Each venesection removes 200 to 250 mg. of iron from the body. Two or three years of treatment is required to reduce the iron stores. Should anemia develop before the iron stores are depleted, a rest period is given. Maintenance bleeding of 1 to 2 liters of blood per year generally prevents excessive reaccumulation of iron.

Iron overload in the Bantu. Iron overload of a particular kind occurs almost exclusively among the Bantu in South Africa, Rhodesia, Bechuanaland, Nyasaland, Mozambique, and Ghana.[8, 11] The disease becomes manifest in late adolescence and is most severe between the ages of 40 and 60. The Bantu ingest excessive amounts of iron, sometimes as much as 100 mg. a day, not only because of the type of diet they consume but also because iron utensils are used in cooking and in the preparation of alcoholic drinks; although the positive daily balance is not often more than 2 or 3 mg., this increment is large enough to explain the heavy deposits found in middle age.[9] The disease is caused by excessive iron intake and not by an abnormality in intestinal function. In most patients iron deposits are confined to the liver and to the reticuloendothelial system and the distribution differs from that found in hemochromatosis; the total amount of tissue iron is probably about 15 grams, or less, and 10 grams or more of this may be in the liver. In the liver there is an association between severe hepatic siderosis and significant portal fibrosis or cirrhosis, particularly when the iron content of the liver is over 2 per cent by dry weight. In patients who develop cirrhosis other aggravating factors, such as alcoholism and malnutrition, may be important.

Hemosiderosis. Post-transfusional hemosiderosis is an important development in some patients with chronic bone marrow failure or hemolytic anemia who require frequent blood transfusions. Usually the iron is stored in the reticuloendothelial cells and is not found in the parenchymal cells; with this distribution hepatomegaly, splenomegaly, and hyperpigmentation of the skin often develop but are not accompanied by any serious disturbances in function. A second more serious form of this disorder has been recognized in which there is an accumulation of iron in parenchymal cells which is often associated with tissue damage and fibrosis; iron may be deposited in the parenchymal cells by transfer from the reticuloendothelial cells or by an increase in the intestinal absorption of iron.[17] Increased absorption is favored by hyperactive erythropoiesis and accumulation of iron in the liver is favored by a saturated state of the iron binding capacity; in the latter circumstance most of the iron absorbed in the gut is promptly deposited in the liver and does not gain access to the general circulation. Treatment with chelating agents may be helpful in some patients with this disorder who cannot be treated effectively with phlebotomies because of the anemia.

Idiopathic pulmonary hemosiderosis is a rare disorder characterized by widespread pulmonary capillary hemorrhages, hemoptysis, sudden falls in the hemoglobin level, hypochromic anemia, and reticulocytosis.[117] At times episodes of massive hemorrhage, dyspnea, cyanosis, and fever occur. It is seen most often in males, in childhood or early adult life. Later in the course of the disease, pulmonary hemosiderosis, fibrosis, dyspnea, and hepatosplenomegaly occur; cor pulmonale develops only occasionally. The cause of the disease is unknown; defects in the pulmonary epithelial cells and macrophages have been suggested;[76] iron is trapped in the macrophages which accumulate in the alveoli of the lungs. The disorder may be accompanied by gamma-A-immunoglobulin deficiency and possibly is a part of a generalized disorder of the lymphoreticular system.

Acute iron intoxication. Acute iron intoxication, rarely seen except in children who have ingested a large number of iron tablets, is potentially serious; mortality rates as high as 50 per cent have been reported in untreated patients.[66] Treatment with BAL, EDTA, and exchange transfusion have been occasionally successful. The most promising treatment utilizes deferoxamine, a chelating agent. A number of children have survived who were treated with gastric lavage followed by the instillation of 7000 mg. of deferoxamine methane sulfonate in 50 ml. of distilled water in the stomach; the same preparation was given intravenously, 15 mg. per kg. per hour over a 12 hour period.

A recent report recommends the following treatment for acute iron intoxication:[22]

1. General measures
   a. Induction of emesis
   b. Gastric lavage
   c. Suction and maintenance of clear airway
   d. Control of shock with I.V. fluids, blood, oxygen, vasopressor agents
   e. Correction of acidosis
2. Intramuscular deferoxamine mesylate (Desferal, Ciba) 1.0 gm. I.M., followed by 0.5 gm. I.M. q 4 h for 2 doses, or more if necessary (not more than 6.0 gm. in 24 hours).
3. Intravenous deferoxamine is recommended only if the patient is in cardiovascular shock. The rate of infusion should not be more than 15 mg. per kg. per hour I.V. slowly, followed by 0.5 gm. q 4 hr. for two doses or more, not to exceed 6.0 gm. in 24 hours.
4. Deferoxamine is contraindicated in patients with severe renal disease or anuria.

References

1. Adams, E. B., and Scragg, J. N.: Iron in the anemia of kwashiorkor. Brit. J. Haemat., *11*:676, 1965.
2. Bearn, A. G., and Parker, W. C.: Some observations on transferrin. In Gross, F., Ed.: Iron Metabolism. Springer-Verlag, Berlin, 1964, p. 60.
3. Bessis, M. D., and Breton-Gorius, J.: Iron metabolism in the bone marrow as seen by electron microscopy: a critical review. Blood, *19*:635, 1962.
4. Bessis, M. C., and Jensen, W. N.: Sideroblastic anaemia, mitochondria and erythroblastic iron. Brit. J. Haemat., *11*:49, 1965.
5. Beutler, E.: Iron enzymes in iron deficiency. I. Cytochrome C. Am. J. Med. Sc., *234*:517, 1957.
6. Beutler, E., and Blaisdell, R.: Iron enzymes in iron deficiency. II. Catalase in human erythrocyte. J. Clin. Invest., *37*:833, 1958.

7. Bjorkman, S. E.: Chronic refractory anemia with sideroblastic bone marrow. Blood, *11*:250, 1956.

8. Bothwell, T. H.: Iron overload in the Bantu. In Gross, F., Ed.: Iron Metabolism. Springer-Verlag, Berlin, 1964, p. 362.

9. Bothwell, T. H.: Pathophysiological and clinical aspects of iron overload. Series Haemat., *6*:56, 1966.

10. Bothwell, T. H., Cohen, I., Abrahams, O. L., and Perold, S. M.: A familial study in idiopathic hemochromatosis. Am. J. Med., *27*:730, 1959.

11. Bothwell, T. H., and Finch, C. A.: Iron Metabolism. Little, Brown & Co., Boston, 1962.

12. Bothwell, T. H., Pirzio-Biroli, G., and Finch, C. A.: Iron absorption: I. Factors influencing absorption. J. Lab. & Clin. Med., *51*:24, 1958.

13. Bowman, W. D., Jr.: Abnormal ("ringed") sideroblasts in various hematologic and non-hematologic disorders. Blood, *18*:662, 1961.

14. Brown, E. B., Jr., Dubach, R., and Moore, C. V.: Studies in iron transportation and metabolism. XI. Critical analysis of mucosal block by large doses of inorganic iron in human subjects. J. Lab. & Clin. Med., *52*:335, 1958.

15. Brown, E. B., Jr., Dubach, R., Smith, D. E., Reynafarje, C., and Moore, C. V.: Studies in iron transportation and metabolism. X. Long-term iron overload in dogs. J. Lab. & Clin. Med., *50*:862, 1957.

16. Brown, E. B., Jr., and Justus, B. W.: In vitro absorption of radioiron by everted pouches of rat intestine. Am. J. Physiol., *194*:319, 1958.

17. Byrd, R. B., and Cooper, T.: Hereditary iron-loading anemia with secondary hemochromatosis. Ann. Int. Med., *55*:103, 1961.

18. Callender, S. T.: Digestive absorption of iron. In Gross, F., Ed.: Iron Metabolism. Springer-Verlag, Berlin, 1964, p. 89.

19. Cartwright, G. E., Huguley, C. M., Jr., Ashenbrucker, H., Fay, J., and Wintrobe, M. M.: Studies on free erythrocyte protoporphyrin plasma iron and plasma copper in normal and anemic subjects. Blood, *3*:501, 1948.

20. Cartwright, G. E., et al.: Anemia of infection. II. The experimental production of hypoferremia and anemia in dogs. J. Clin. Invest., *25*:81, 1946.

21. Chodos, R. B., Ross, J. F., Apt, L., Pollycove, M., and Halkett, J. A. E.: Absorption of radioiron labelled foods and iron salts in normal and iron-deficient subjects and in idiopathic hemachromatosis. J. Clin. Invest., *36*:314, 1957.

22. Ciba Pharmaceutical Co.: Deferoxamine mesylate (Desferal Mesylate). Clin. Pharm. & Ther., *10*:595, 1969.

23. Committee on Iron Deficiency: Iron deficiency in the United States. J.A.M.A., *203*:407, 1968.

24. Conrad, M. E., Weintraub, L. R., and Crosby, W. H.: The role of the intestine in iron kinetics. J. Clin. Invest., *43*:963, 1964.

24a. Cooley, T. B.: A severe type of hereditary anemia with elliptocytosis: interesting sequence of splenectomy. Am. J. Med. Sc., *209*:561, 1945.

25. Cook, J. D., Layrisse, M., and Finch, C. A.: The measurement of iron absorption. Blood, *33*:421, 1969.

26. Crosby, W. H.: The control of iron balance by the intestinal mucosa. Blood, *22*:441, 1963.

27. Crosby, W. H.: Intestinal response to the body's requirement for iron. J.A.M.A., *208*:347, 1969.

28. Dameshek, W.: The Di Guglielmo syndrome. (Edit.) Blood, *13*:192, 1958.

29. Dameshek, W.: Sideroblastic anaemia: Is this a malignancy? Brit. J. Haemat., *11*:52, 1965.

30. Dawson, D. W., Leeming, J. T., Oelbaum, M. H., Pengelly, C. D. R., and Wilkinson, J. F.: Pyridoxine-responsive hypochromic anemia. Lancet, *2*:10, 1961.

31. Dawson, R. B., Rafal, S., and Weintraub, L. R.: Absorption of hemoglobin iron: The role of xanthine oxidase in the intestinal heme-splitting reaction. Blood, *35*:94, 1970.

32. Debre, R., Dreyfus, J. C., Frezal, J., Labie, D., Lamy, M., Maroteaux, P., Schapira, F., and Schapira, G.: Genetics in hemochromatosis. Ann. Human Genet., *23*:16, 1958.

33. Demulder, R.: Iron. Arch. Int. Med., *102*:254, 1958.

34. Dowdle, E. B., Schacter, D., and Schenker, H.: Active transport of Fe^{59} by everted segments of rat duodenum. Am. J. Physiol., *198*:609, 1960.

35. Drabkin, D. L.: Metabolism of the hemin chromoproteins. Physiol. Rev., *31*:345, 1951.

36. Dreyfus, J. C., and Schapira, G.: The metabolism of iron in haemochromatosis. In Gross, F., Ed.: Iron Metabolism. Springer-Verlag, Berlin, 1964, p. 296.

37. Ellis, L. D., Jensen, W. N., and Westerman, M. P.: An evaluation of depleted stores in a series of 1,332 needle biopsies. Ann. Int. Med., *61*:44, 1964.

38. Erslev, A. J., Lear, A. A., and Castle, W. B.: Pyridoxine-responsive anemia. New England J. Med., *262*:1209, 1960.

39. Finch, S. C., and Finch, C. A.: Idiopathic hemochromatosis, an iron storage disease. Medicine, *34*:381, 1955.
40. Finch, C. A., et al.: Iron metabolism: The pathophysiology of iron storage. Blood, *5*:983, 1950.
41. Fowler, W. M.: Chlorosis—an obituary. Ann. M. Hist., *8*:168, 1936.
42. Gitlin, D., Janeway, C. A., and Farr, L. E.: Studies on the metabolism of plasma proteins in the nephrotic syndrome. I. Albumin, gamma-globulin and iron-binding globulin. J. Clin. Invest., *35*:44, 1956.
43. Goodman, J. R., and Hall, S. G.: Accumulation of iron in mitochondria of erythroblasts. Brit. J. Haemat., *13*:335, 1967.
44. Granick, S.: Protein apoferritin and ferritin in iron feeding and absorption. Science, *103*:107, 1946.
44a. Greenberg, M. S., and Grace, N. D.: Folic acid deficiency and iron overload. Arch. Int. Med., *125*:140, 1970.
45. Gubler, C. J.: Absorption and metabolism of iron. Science, *123*:87, 1956.
46. Hahn, P. F., Balem, W. F., Ross, J. F., Balfour, W. M., and Whipple, G. H.: Radioactive iron absorption by the gastro-intestinal tract. J. Exper. Med., *78*:169, 1943.
47. Hallberg, L., and Solvell, L.: Absorption of a single dose of iron in man. Acta med. scandinav., *168*(Suppl. 358):19, 1960.
48. Hallen, L.: Part II. Gastric Secretion. Acta med. scandinav., Suppl. 90, 398, 1938.
49. Harris, J. W., Whittington, R. M., Weisman, R. J., and Horrigan, D. L.: Pyridoxine responsive anemia in human adult. Proc. Soc. Exper. Biol. & Med., *91*:427, 1956.
50. Haskins, D., Stevens, A. R., Jr., Finch, S., and Finch, C. A.: Iron metabolism: Iron stores in man as measured by phlebotomy. J. Clin. Invest., *31*:543, 1952.
51. Hayem, G.: Maladies du Sang. Masson et Cie., Paris, 1900.
52. Hegsted, D. M., Finch, C. A., and Kinney, T. D.: The influence of diet on iron absorption: II. The interrelation of iron and phosphorus. III. Comparative studies with rats, mice, guinea pigs and chickens. J. Exper. Med., *90*:147, 1949; *90*:137, 1949; *96*:115, 1952.
53. Heilmeyer, L.: In Wallerstein, R. O., and Mettier, S. R., Eds.: Iron in Clinical Medicine. University of California Press, Berkeley, Calif., 1958.
54. Heilmeyer, L.: Disturbances in Heme Synthesis. Charles C Thomas, Springfield, Ill., 1966.
55. Heilmeyer, L., Keller, W., Vivell, O., Keiderling, W., Betke, K., Wohler, F., and Schultze, H.: Kongenitale Atransferrinamie bei eine sieben jahre alten kind. Deutsche med. Wchnschr., *86*:1745, 1961.
56. Heilmeyer, L., and Ploetner, K.: Das Serumeisen und die Eisenmangelkrankheit, Pathogenese, Symptomatologic und Therapie. Jena, 1937.
57. Henderson, P. A., and Hillman, R. S.: Characteristics of iron dextran utilization in man. Blood, *34*:357, 1969.
57a. Hines, J. D.: Reversible megaloblastic and sideroblastic marrow abnormalities in alcoholic patients. Brit. J. Haemat., *16*:87, 1969.
57b. Hines, J. D., and Cowan, D. H.: Studies on the pathogenesis of alcohol-induced sideroblastic bone marrow abnormalities. New England J. Med., *283*:441, 1970.
58. Höglund, S.: Studies in iron absorption. VI. Transitory effect of oral administration of iron on iron absorption. Blood, *34*:505, 1969.
59. Höglund, S., and Reizenstein, P.: Studies in iron absorption. IV. Effect of humoral factors on iron absorption. Blood, *34*:488, 1969.
60. Höglund, S., and Reizenstein, P.: Studies in iron absorption. V. Effect of gastrointestinal factors on iron absorption. Blood, *34*:496, 1969.
61. Holmberg, C. G., and Laurell, C. B.: Studies on the capacity of serum to bind iron. A contribution to our knowledge of the regulation mechanism of serum iron. Acta physiol. scandinav., *10*:307, 1945.
62. Horrigan, D. L., and Harris, J. W.: Pyridoxin responsive anemias: An analysis of 62 cases. Advances Int. Med., *12*:103, 1964.
63. Horrigan, D. L., Whittington, R. M., Weisman, R., and Harris, J. W.: Hypochromic anemia with hyperferricemia responding to oral crude liver extract. Am. J. Med., *22*:99, 1957.
64. Huff, R. L., et al.: Plasma and red cell iron turnover in normal subjects and in patients having various hematopoietic disorders. J. Clin. Invest., *29*:1041, 1950.
65. Huff, R. L., and Judd, O. J.: Kinetics of Iron Metabolism. Advances in Biological and Medical Physics. Vol. IV. Academic Press, New York, 1956, p. 223.
66. Jacobs, J., Greene, H., and Gendel, B. R.: Acute iron intoxication. New England J. Med., *273*:1124, 1965.
67. Jandl, J. H., Inman, J. K., Simmons, R. L., and Allen, D. W.: Transfer of iron from the serum iron-binding protein to human reticulocytes. J. Clin. Invest., *38*:161, 1959.
68. Jandl, J. H., and Katz, J. H.: Plasma-to-cell cycle of transferrin. J. Clin. Invest., *42*:314, 1963.

69. Johnson, B. F.: Hemochromatosis resulting from prolonged oral iron therapy. New England J. Med., *278*:1100, 1968.

70. Johnston, F. A., Frenchman, R., and Boroughs, E. D.: The iron metabolism of young women on two levels of intake. J. Nutrition, *38*:479, 1949.

71. Katz, J. H.: Iron and protein kinetics studied by means of doubly labelled human crystalline transferrin. J. Clin. Invest., *40*:2143, 1961.

72. Katz, J. H.: The delivery of iron to the immature red cell—a critical review. Series Haemat., *6*:15, 1966.

73. Katz, J. H., and Jandl, J. H.: The role of transferrin in the transport of iron into the developing red cell. In Gross, F., Ed.: Iron Metabolism. Springer-Verlag, Berlin, 1964, p. 89.

74. Kimber, R. C., and Weintraub, L. R.: Malabsorption of iron secondary to iron deficiency. New England J. Med., *279*:453, 1968.

75. Krantz, S., Goldwasser, J., and Jacobson, L. O.: Studies on erythropoiesis. XIV. The relationship of humoral stimulation to iron absorption. Blood, *14*:654, 1959.

76. Krieger, I., and Brough, J. A.: Gamma-A Deficiency and Hypochromic Anemia Due to Defective Iron Mobilization. New England J. Med., *276*:886, 1967.

77. Lajtha, L. G.: In Stohlman, F. R., Jr., Ed.: Kinetics of Cellular Proliferation. Grune and Stratton, New York, 1959, p. 29.

78. Lajtha, L. G., and Suit, H. I.: Uptake of radioactive iron (Fe) by nucleated red cells in vitro. Brit. J. Haemat., *1*:55, 1955.

79. Lange, J.: De Morbo Virgineo. Medicinalium epistolarum miscellaneo. Wechelus, Basle, 1554, p. 74. (Quoted from Major, R. H.: Classic Descriptions of Disease. 3rd Ed. Charles C Thomas, Springfield, Ill., 1959, p. 487.)

80. Layrisse, M., Cook, J. D., Martinez, C., Roche, M., Kuhn, I., Walker, R. B., and Finch, C. A.: Food iron absorption: A comparison of vegetable and animal foods. Blood, *33*:430, 1969.

81. Lees, F., and Rosenthal, F. D.: Gastric mucosal lesions before and after treatment in iron deficiency anemia. Quart. J. Med., *27*:19, 1958.

82. London, I. M.: Biosynthesis of hemoglobin and its control in relation to some hypochromic anemias in man. Series Haematologica, *2*:1, 1965.

83. Loria, A., Sanchez-Medal, L., Lisker, R., de Rodriguez, E., and Labardini, J.: Red cell life span in iron deficiency anemia. Brit. J. Haemat., *13*:294, 1967.

84. MacDonald, R. A.: Idiopathic hemochromatosis. Arch. Int. Med., *107*:606, 1961.

85. MacDonald, R. A., and Mallory, G. K.: Hemochromatosis and hemosiderosis. A study of 211 autopsied cases. Arch. Int. Med., *105*:686, 1960.

86. MacGibbon, B. H., and Mollin, D. L.: Sideroblastic anemia in man: Observations on seventy cases. Brit. J. Haemat., *11*:59, 1965.

87. Magnus, E. M.: Folic acid activity in serum and red cells in patients with vitamin B-12 deficiency: Relation to treatment. Brit. J. Haemat., *11*:188, 1965.

88. Manis, J. G., and Schachter, D.: Active transport of iron by intestine: Effects of oral iron and pregnancy. Am. J. Physiol., *203*:81, 1962.

89. Manis, J. G., and Schachter, D.: Active transport of iron by intestine: Features of a two-step mechanism. Am. J. Physiol., *203*:73, 1962.

90. Mazur, A., Green, S., and Carleton, A.: Mechanism of plasma iron incorporation into hepatic ferritin. J. Biol. Chem., *235*:595, 1960.

91. Mendel, J. A., Weiler, R. J., and Mangalik, A.: Studies on iron absorption. II. The absorption of iron in experimental anemias of diverse etiology. Blood, *22*:450, 1963.

92. Middleton, E. J., Nagy, B., and Morrison, A. B.: Studies on the absorption of orally administered iron from sustained-release preparations. New England J. Med., *274*:136, 1966.

93. Mollin, D. L.: Introduction: Sideroblasts and sideroblastic anemia. Brit. J. Haemat., *11*:41, 1965.

94. Moore, C. V., and Dubach, R.: Metabolism and requirements of iron in the human. J.A.M.A., *162*:197, 1958.

95. Moore, C. V., and Dubach, R.: Observations on the absorption of iron from foods tagged with radioiron. Tr. A. Am. Physicians, *64*:245, 1951.

96. Murray, M. J., and Stein, N.: The effects on iron absorption of gastro-intestinal secretions from patients with iron-deficiency anemia and haemochromatosis. Brit. J. Haemat., *15*:87, 1968.

97. Murray, M. J., and Stein, N.: Effect of iron stores on gastric acid secretion by rats. Brit. J. Haemat., *15*:401, 1968.

98. Nixon, R. K., and Olson, J. P.: Diagnostic value of marrow hemosiderin patterns. Ann. Intern. Med., *69*:1249, 1968.

99. Noyes, W. D., Bothwell, T. H., and Finch, C. A.: The role of the reticuloendothelial cell in iron metabolism. Brit. J. Haemat., *6*:43, 1960.

100. Pirzio-Biroli, G., Bothwell, T. H., and Finch, C. A.: Iron absorption. II. The absorption of radioiron administered with a standard meal in man. J. Lab. & Clin. Med., *51*:37, 1958.

101. Pollycove, M.: Iron kinetics. In Wallerstein, R. O., and Mettier, S. R., Eds.: Iron in Clinical Medicine. University of California Press, Berkeley, Calif., 1958.

102. Ponka, P., and Neuwirt, J.: Regulation of iron entry into reticulocytes. I. Feedback inhibitory effect of heme on iron entry into reticulocytes and on heme synthesis. Blood, *33*:690, 1969.

103. Pribilla, W., Bothwell, T. H., and Finch, C. A.: Iron transport to the fetus in man. In Wallerstein, R. O., and Mettier, S. R., Eds.: University of California Press, Berkeley, Calif., 1958, p. 58.

104. Raab, S. O., Haut, A., Cartwright, G. E., and Wintrobe, M. M.: Pyridoxine-responsive anemia. Blood, *18*:285, 1961.

105. Rath, C. E., and Finch, C. A.: Chemical, clinical, and immunological studies on the products of human plasma fractionation. XXXVIII. Serum iron transport measurement of serum iron-binding capacity in man. J. Clin. Invest., *28*:79, 1949.

106. Rather, L. J.: Hemochromatosis and hemosiderosis. Am. J. Med., *21*:857, 1956.

106a. Roselle, H. A.: Association of laundry starch and clay ingestion with anemia in New York City. Arch. Int. Med., *125*:57, 1970.

107. Rundles, R. W., and Falls, H. F.: Hereditary (sex-linked) anemia. Am. J. M. Sc., *211*:641, 1946.

108. Rustung, E.: Studies of serum iron. Acta dermat.-venereol., Suppl. 21, *29*:1, 1949.

109. Sano, S., and Granick, S.: Mitochondrial coproporphyrinogen oxidase and protoporphyrin formation. J. Biol. Chem., *236*:1173, 1961.

110. Schade, A. L., and Caroline, L.: An iron-binding component in human blood plasma. Science, *104*:340, 1946.

111. Schade, S. G., Cohen, R. J., and Conrad, M. E.: Effect of hydrochloric acid on iron absorption. New England J. Med., *297*:672, 1968.

112. Schulz, J., and Smith, N. J.: A quantitative study of the absorption of iron salts in infants and children. A.M.A. J. Dis. Child., *95*:109, 1958.

113. Shahidi, N. T., Nathan, D. G., and Diamond, L. K.: Iron deficiency anemia associated with an error of iron metabolism in two siblings. J. Clin. Invest., *43*:510, 1964.

114. Sharney, L., Schwartz, L., Wasserman, L. R., Port, S., and Leavitt, D.: Pool systems in iron metabolism: with special reference to polycythemia vera. Proc. Soc. Exper. Biol. & Med., *87*:489, 1954.

115. Sheldon, J. H.: Haemochromatosis. Oxford University Press, London, 1935.

116. Smithies, O.: Variations in human serum beta globulins. Nature, *180*:1482, 1957.

117. Soergel, K. H., and Sommers, S. C.: Idiopathic pulmonary hemosiderosis and related syndromes. Am. J. Med., *32*:499, 1962.

118. Steinkamp, R., Dubach, R., and Moore, C. V.: Studies in iron transportation and metabolism. VIII. Absorption of radioiron from iron-enriched bread. Arch. Int. Med., *95*:181, 1955.

119. Stocks, A. E., and Martin, F. I. R.: Pituitary function in haemochromatosis. Am. J. Med., *45*:839, 1968.

120. Tompsett, S. L.: Factors influencing the absorption of iron and copper from the alimentary tract. Biochem. J., *34*:961, 1940.

121. Turnbull, A., and Giblett, E. R.: The binding and transport of iron by transferrin variants. J. Lab. & Clin. Med., *57*:450, 1961.

122. Verloop, M. C., Plodem, W., and Leunis, J.: Hereditary hypochromic hypersideraemic anaemia. In Gross, F., Ed.: Iron Metabolism. Springer-Verlag, Berlin, 1964, p. 376.

123. Verloop, M. C., and Rademaker, W.: Anaemia due to pyridoxine deficiency in man. Brit. J. Haemat., *6*:66, 1960.

124. Verwilghen, R., Reybrouck, G., Callens, L., and Cosemans, J.: Antituberculous drugs and sideroblastic anaemia. Brit. J. Haemat., *11*:65, 1965.

125. Vitale, L., Opitz, J. M., and Shahidi, N. T.: Congenital and familial iron overload. New England J. Med., *280*:642, 1969.

126. Vogler, W. R., and Mingioli, E. S.: Heme synthesis in pyridoxine-responsive anemia. New England J. Med., *273*:347, 1965.

127. Vogler, W. R., and Mingioli, E. S.: Porphyrin synthesis and heme synthetase activity in pyridoxine-responsive anemia. Blood, *32*:979, 1968.

128. Weintraub, L. R., Conrad, M. E., and Crosby, W. H.: Regulation of the intestinal absorption of iron by the rate of erythropoiesis. Brit. J. Haemat., *11*:432, 1965.

129. Weintraub, L. R., Dawson, R. B., and Rafal, S.: Absorption of hemoglobin iron: Release of iron from heme by intestinal xanthine oxidase. J. Clin. Invest., *47*:101a, 1968 (Abs. #299).

130. Weintraub, L. R., Weinstein, M. B., Huser, H., and Rafal, S.: Absorption of hemoglobin iron: Role of heme-splitting substance in intestinal mucosa. J. Clin. Invest., *47*:531, 1968.

131. Wheby, M. S.: Regulation of iron absorption. Gastroenterology, *50*:888, 1966.

132. Wheby, M. S., Conrad, M. E., Hedberg, S. E., and Crosby, W. H.: The role of bile in the control of iron absorption. Gastroenterology, *42*:319, 1962.

133. Wheby, M. S., and Jones, L. G.: Role of transferrin in iron absorption. J. Clin. Invest., *42*:1007, 1963.

134. Wheby, M. S., Jones, L. G., and Crosby, W. H.: Studies on iron absorption. Intestinal regulatory mechanism. J. Clin. Invest., *43*:1433, 1964.

134a. Whipple, G. H., and Robscheit-Robbins, F. S.: Iron and its utilization in experimental anemia. Am. J. M. Sc., *191*:11, 1936.

135. Widdowson, E. M., and McCance, R. A.: The absorption and excretion of iron before, during and after a period of very high intake. Biochem. J., *31*:2029, 1937.

136. Widdowson, E. M., and McCance, R. A., and Spray, C. M.: The chemical composition of the human body. Clin. Sc., *10*:113, 1951.

137. Yuile, C. L., Hayden, G. W., Bush, J. A., Tesluk, H., and Stewart, W. B.: Plasma iron and saturation of plasma iron. Binding protein in dogs as related to the gastrointestinal absorption of radioiron. J. Exper. Med., *92*:367, 1950.

Reviews and Monographs

Bothwell, T. H., and Finch, C. A.: Iron Metabolism. Little, Brown and Co., Boston, 1962.

Gross, F., Ed.: Iron Metabolism. Springer-Verlag, Berlin, 1964.

Moore, C. V.: Iron metabolism and nutrition. The Harvey Lectures, 1959–1960, p. 67. Academic Press, New York, 1961.

Wallerstein, R. O., and Mettier, S. R., Eds.: Iron in Clinical Medicine. University of California Press, Berkeley, Calif., 1958.

VI / Bone Marrow Failure

Classification

The disorder characterized by pancytopenia, which is usually diagnosed "aplastic anemia," "refractory anemia," or "chronic bone marrow failure," is probably a syndrome rather than a disease entity. The syndrome is sometimes present at birth but it may appear at any age. In some patients it develops after exposure to a drug or another chemical compound but in others it appears under no suspicious circumstances. The severity of the anemia, leukopenia, and thrombocytopenia varies in different patients and may vary at different times in the same patient. The cellularity of the bone marrow and the results obtained with the ferrokinetic studies may be different in patients who have similar abnormalities in the peripheral blood.[45] It is likely that different mechanisms are at fault in different patients; more precise information may establish that the syndrome includes several different diseases with different enzymatic or molecular defects.

Although an entirely satisfactory classification is not possible at present, a workable one is presented in Table 6–1. The relationship of this group to refractory sideroblastic anemia (Chapter V) and di Guglielmo's disease (Chapter XIII), which are not included in the classification, is uncertain. Whether the syndromes characterized by pancytopenia are related to erythrocytic hypoplasia is unknown. The difference in the hematologic features, the more frequent association with thymoma, the better prognosis with supportive measures, and the better response to therapeutic agents warrant placing the patients with erythrocytic hypoplasia in a separate group. In addition, some separation of the pancytopenia groups according to the microscopic appearance of the bone marrow and the ferrokinetic characteristics appear desirable in order to recognize the differences, even though the cause of these differences is poorly understood.

Table 6–1.   *Classification of Bone Marrow Failure (Aplastic Anemia)*

I. Hereditary (Congenital)
  A. Hypoplastic Anemia (Blackfan and Diamond[7])
  B. Pancytopenia
    1. With congenital deformities (Fanconi[11])
    2. Without congenital deformities (Estren and Dameshek[10])

II. Acquired (Chemicals or Idiopathic)
  A. Erythrocytic Hypoplasia
  B. Pancytopenia
    1. With hypocellular marrow
    2. With cellular marrow
      a. Inactive erythropoiesis
      b. Ineffective erythropoiesis

Aplastic Anemia

Ehrlich described the first case of aplastic anemia in 1888.[12] This patient was a 21 year old white woman who died about 1 month after the onset of an illness characterized by menorrhagia, retinal hemorrhages, and marked pallor. The peripheral blood, which showed marked anemia and leukopenia, was considered unusual in that no nucleated red cells were seen despite the severe anemia. This apparent lack of increase in blood production in response to the anemia was explained by the fatty, inactive appearance of the bone marrow at autopsy. Following Ehrlich's description similar cases of this acute fatal illness were reported. It was recognized also that a clinical picture identical with these "idiopathic" cases occurred as a result of exposure to toxic agents such as benzene, arsenicals, and roentgen rays. The concept of the disorder was broadened further by the inclusion of patients with the clinical picture and peripheral blood characteristic of "aplastic" anemia even though the bone marrow showed normal or increased cellularity.[61] In addition, cases have been considered to belong in this category if the anemia resulted from a failure of erythropoiesis when the anemia occurred alone or was associated with either neutropenia or thrombocytopenia.

Mechanism of the Anemia

The primary defect in patients with this type of anemia is the failure of the bone marrow to produce erythrocytes, and usually granulocytes and platelets, in normal numbers in spite of adequate amounts of all the known hematopoietic factors. The defect may be either an unresponsiveness of the erythropoietic tissues to adequate stimuli or the lack of some necessary stimulus. The presence of a defective response of the erythropoietic tissue is indicated by the reports of the presence of apparently adequate amounts of erythropoietin in the plasma of patients with hypoplastic anemia. The evidence available at present indicates that the defect in most patients is an inability of the erythropoietic tissue to respond to adequate stimuli.

Causative agents. The defective erythropoiesis may be the result of various forms of injury to the blood-forming tissue. In some patients the failure of erythropoiesis is clearly due to the effect on the bone marrow tissue of agents that are known to produce cellular damage if given in sufficient quantity. Included in this category are x-rays, chemicals, such as benzene, and drugs, such as nitrogen mustard, urethane, and the antimetabolites (antifolic compounds, 6-mercaptopurine). Prolonged nitrous oxide anesthesia (5 or 6 days) may also belong in this category.[21, 32] In other circumstances the damage to the bone marrow occurs as a result of some individual idiosyncrasy to drugs or chemicals that are ordinarily innocuous. Occasionally an infection appears to be the precipitating factor. Many times no adequate explanation for the aplasia is apparent and the case is classified as "idiopathic."

Total body radiation, administered therapeutically or received accidentally, may result in severe or even fatal aplastic anemia; less than 0.1 per cent of persons will survive an exposure of 700 rads, and 300 rads constitute the LD50. In addition, heavy partial body radiation, such as that currently used in the treatment of lymphomas and other malignancies, may induce marrow hypoplasia. Nevertheless, 3500 or 4000 rads may be given to much of the body, including the neck, mediastinum, paraaortic, and inguinal areas, with only temporary marrow depression. After a course of such treatment, from 4 to 6 months are usually necessary for the marrow to recover enough to tolerate chemotherapy in the usual dose.

Although the association has been known since 1955, two recent reports of over 20 patients have focused attention on the development of aplastic anemia during or after an attack of infectious hepatitis. [34, 52] Most of the reported patients were between 2 and 20 years of age, but some were middle-aged. At least three-fourths of the reported patients were male. Although aplastic anemia appeared during an attack of hepatitis, it usually developed after the hepatitis had subsided, sometimes after an interval as long as 26 weeks. The development of aplastic anemia is not related to the severity of the hepatitis; the aplastic anemia has been unusually severe and only 20 per cent of the reported patients have survived. How infectious hepatitis causes aplastic anemia is not apparent. Auto-immunity has not been a frequently recognized mechanism in aplastic anemia; failure of the liver to detoxify substances appears to be an unlikely explanation because many of the patients have normal liver function tests at the time the aplastic anemia first appears, sometimes months after the hepatitis. Another suggested explanation is that the hepatitis induces a genetic alteration in the hematopoietic cells, a theory consistent with the delayed appearance and severity of the aplasia.

Almost any drug or chemical may produce anemia or pancytopenia in a susceptible patient, but some are much more likely to do this than others. In a series of nearly 600 patients with aplastic anemia and pancytopenia compiled by the Registry on Blood Dyscrasias of the American Medical Association, the 10 most common offenders that were found are listed in Table 6–2.[56] Chloramphenicol was by far the commonest suspect, being the only drug administered in 113 cases. In another 150 patients the drug had been administered in association with other drugs with known or uncertain toxicity. The next most

Table 6–2. *Drugs or Chemical Most Often Associated with Pancytopenia*

1. Chloramphenicol
2. Phenylbutazone
3. Solvents (including benzene)
4. Sulfonamides
5. Insecticides (gamma benzene hexachloride, chlordane)
6. Methylphenylethylhydantoin
7. Gold
8. Mepazine
9. Chlorpromazine
10. Oral hypoglycemic agents

common drug, phenylbutazone, was reported in only 13 patients alone and in only 13 others in association with other drugs.

A recent report from California gives the following estimate of the incidence of aplastic anemia: (1) incidence in the U.S.A., two per one million population per year; (2) incidence in California, between one in 400,000 and one in 700,000; (3) incidence after chloramphenicol, between one in 24,000 and one in 132,000; (4) deaths after chloramphenicol, 4.5 grams, one in 36,000; 7.5 grams, one in 21,000; (5) incidence after phenylbutazone, one in 124,000; (6) incidence after atabrine in World War II, one in 50,000.[65] The best estimates place the incidence of aplastic anemia as one per 100,000 in patients receiving chloramphenicol.[2]

Observations on patients who developed anemia or pancytopenia after administration of chloramphenicol, and also studies on patients who were receiving this drug but had not developed abnormalities in the peripheral blood, indicate that the hematologic effects observed are the result of several factors. These are: (1) the qualitative action of the drug on cells of the hematopoietic system, (2) the quantity of the drug administered, and (3) an individual factor in the patient receiving the drug.[2, 40, 49, 53, 70] The ability of chloramphenicol to inhibit erythropoiesis was shown when it was demonstrated that a dose of 50 to 60 mg. per kg. for several days could inhibit the therapeutic response to specific treatment with vitamin B_{12} and iron.[53] Another investigation of the toxic effect of the drug indicates that bone marrow depression is a pharmacologic property of the drug. Bone marrow depression occurred regularly with blood levels of 25 micrograms per ml. which accompanied a daily dose of 50 mg. per kg. of body weight; a daily dose of 25 to 30 mg. per kg. produced adequate blood levels and was recommended. These studies indicate that chloramphenicol causes first depression of erythropoiesis and then depression of the other elements in the marrow. Depression of erythropoiesis is manifested by a rise in the serum iron level, a decrease in the iron utilization, and a fall in the circulating reticulocytes; vacuolization appears in the cytoplasm and nucleus of normoblasts in the bone marrow. Serial studies of the bone marrow of patients receiving chloramphenicol suggest that the marrow passes through a reversible phase of depression from which it recovers promptly, within 1 week if the drug is discontinued, and sometimes even if it is continued. This stage may be followed by a more severe depression which persists while the drug is being administered; recovery from the phase may be slow, or even absent, in some patients after the drug is discontinued. In the reported patients prolonged administration of the drug or high dosage levels are found much more often than "hypersensitivity" reactions to administration of the drug in very small doses or for very short periods, such as a day or two.[2, 6]

The mechanism by which chloramphenicol affects the bone marrow is uncertain. A direct effect is manifested by vacuolization of the red cell precursors, diminished iron uptake, and inhibition of the incorporation of heme in normoblasts and aminoacid in the leukocytes.[3] In addition, Weisberger and colleagues report that small amounts of chloramphenicol may block or reduce protein synthesis.[67] A series of experiments demonstrated that therapeutic concentrations of chloramphenicol inhibited the accelerated incorporation of C^{14} formate into reticulocyte ribosomes that was induced by added RNA or polyuridylic acid and suggested that chloramphenicol blocked the binding of messenger RNA to the ribosome and spared the ribosome bound RNA; the structural similarity between chloramphenicol and pyrimidine neucleotides raised the possibility that they might be competitive.

Another hypothesis concerning the action of the marrow cells has been advanced by Yunis and associates, who have reported that small amounts of chloramphenicol, 20 micrograms per ml., inhibit the incorporation of C^{14} leucine into the protein of mitochondria from human bone marrows;[39, 71] altered configuration of the mitochondria exposed to the drug was shown by electron microscopy. The mammalian mitochondria are much more sensitive to the drug than are the mammalian cytoplasmic ribosomes; the latter are much less sensitive than bacterial ribosomes. The observations support the hypothesis that the reversible bone marrow depression that is produced by chloramphenicol results from inhibition of the mitochrondria.

The observation that reticulocytopenia, inhibition of iron utilization, morphologic changes in the marrow, mild anemia, thrombocytopenia, and alteration in serum iron all reverted to normal when the drug was withdrawn has led to different opinions about the relation of these effects of the drug to the development of clinical aplastic anemia.

Yunis and coworkers have emphasized that two different types of marrow depression occur: the pharmacologic, which occurs in many patients and produces the commonly observed changes, and the pathologic, which occurs in a small percentage of patients and leads to persisting marrow aplasia, even after small doses. They have shown that when C^{14} formate uptake by marrow tissue was measured, there was a significantly lower uptake in formation of DNA and RNA in the marrow obtained from patients who had recovered from chloramphenicol-induced aplastic anemia as compared to the marrow of normal subjects.[69] The difference disappeared when the chloramphenicol concentration reached 250 micrograms per ml. The results suggested some abnormality in nucleic acid metabolism in the marrow of patients who had recovered from the dyscrasia.

The infrequent development of aplastic anemia in patients receiving chloramphenicol, the poor correlation between the dose of the drug and the development of aplastic anemia, the low incidence and good prognosis of the disease in blacks, and the occurrence of dyscrasias in some patients who received only small amounts of the drug for short periods all point toward some idiosyncrasy, possibly a hereditary defect, in the patients who develop aplastic anemia. The development of pancytopenia in the absence of demonstrable antibodies is best explained by some effect on the stem cell. Observations made on identical twins who developed aplastic anemia following the administration of chloramphenicol support the concept.[44] The similarities in the course of the disease in both patients suggested a genetic factor. During development of the disease in one patient, the authors observed that the youngest cells in the marrow disappeared first and were the first to reappear during recovery, a sequence which suggested that the failure of differentiated forms to develop from a damaged precursor cell was the primary event. The possibility that a drug causes aplastic anemia by an effect on an enzyme system in the stem cell is analogous to the effect produced by certain drugs in patients with varying degrees of G6PD deficiency; both the inherited defect and the drug are required to produce the clinical syndrome.

Weisberger has suggested that toxicity of chloramphenicol is the result of impaired metabolism of the drug.[67] Evidence advanced to support this concept is the observation that patients who have erythropoietic depression after the drug have a high serum level of free chloramphenicol; normally the free form is "detoxified," at least in part, by glycuronyl transferase in the liver. The increased incidence of toxicity in premature infants and other patients with liver disease supports the concept of a deficiency in this mechanism. The impaired clearance of chloramphenicol after an intravenous test dose was considered a reliable indicator of subsequent erythropoietic toxicity, and the only test currently available that can predict toxic effects;[60] an abnormal test or an abnormally high level of free chloramphenicol in the serum may be a contraindication to further use of the drug, or at least an indication for careful monitoring of the blood counts.

Whether or not the disastrous effects that chloramphenicol produces in a small percentage of patients are primarily the result of defective liver function, a subnormal enzyme system in the stem cell, or some other mechanism has not been established. Nevertheless, the delay of several months in the development of aplastic anemia in some patients after cessation of the drug, the sequential changes that have been observed in the blood and marrow, and the sequela of paroxysmal nocturnal hemoglobinuria that occurs occasionally all point to a major effect on the stem cell.

Idiopathic cases. In a large percentage of patients with this syndrome no acceptable cause for the marrow failure can be found. These cases are classified as "idiopathic." Although the mechanism of the anemia in this group is obscure, various possible explanations have been advanced. Bomford and Rhoads suggested that erythropoiesis might be damaged as a result of the failure of the liver to inactivate completely hormones and other chemicals in the body, with the result that a chemical compound toxic to the bone marrow might be produced by the abnormal metabolism of normal or innocuous compounds.[4] Another possibility, damage to the bone marrow by an auto-immune process, has been suggested as a result of the recognition of the role of antibodies in the production of hemolytic anemia, erythrocytic hypoplasia and thrombocytopenia purpura.[8, 17, 19, 29] Auto-antibodies against erythrocytes, leukocytes, and platelets have been reported in a patient with aplastic anemia who had never been transfused. An increase in the circulating blood of cells with the morphologic characteristics of the young lymphocyte which are undergoing DNA synthesis has been found in patients with idiopathic aplastic anemia but not in those who gave a history of exposure to toxic agents.[7] The similarity of the findings in this group to those in hemolytic anemia was interpreted as evidence to support the auto-immune hypothesis. A possible etiologic relationship between leukemia and aplastic anemia must also be considered, because leukemia sometimes develops in patients with aplastic anemia and both diseases have been reported to occur after exposure to benzol[5] or radiation. Still another possibility, which is suggested by the racial incidence and reports of a familial tendency, is the occurrence of a hereditary defect in the bone marrow that renders it more susceptible to either exogenous or endogenous toxins in later life.[40]

Some cases of "idiopathic" aplastic anemia may be the result of the gradual failure of an enzyme system in the stem cell. It is also possible, but not proved, that an enzyme system which is inherently weak or becomes so for some reason may, because of this deficiency, be badly or irreparably damaged not only by drugs but also by the ingestion of minute amounts of chemicals found in food from preservatives, herbicides, or pesticides. Inapparent viral infections, such as anicteric hepatitis, also may be responsible in some instances.

Hemolytic aspects.   Although the main feature of this syndrome is deficient erythropoiesis, hyperhemolysis as manifested by an increased fecal urobilinogen excretion is found in some patients. This occurs most often in patients who have cellular marrows. Studies that employ radioactive iron indicate that most such patients have ineffective erythropoiesis rather than an absence of erythropoiesis; iron is utilized in erythropoiesis but excessive hemolysis occurs in the marrow before the cells are released into the circulation. This increased intramedullary hemolysis is responsible for the evidences of hemolytic anemia in some patients with "aplastic" or "refractory" anemia. In other patients a decreased survival time of the circulating erythrocytes may be the only evidence of hemolysis.[66] When hyperhemolysis is present in patients who have not been transfused it is usually of such minor degree that anemia would not develop if the bone marrow were able to function normally. Increased hemolysis is seen most often in aplastic anemia in patients who have received numerous transfusions, when splenomegaly and hepatomegaly are often present.

Clinical Manifestations

Aplastic anemia may occur at any age. In one series about half of the patients developed the disorder after the age of 50 years;[49] men were affected more often than women, possibly as a result of a higher incidence of exposure to chemicals in occupations. In another series of 408 patients who had aplastic anemia following chloramphenicol therapy, 62 per cent were females; the peak incidence of the disease occurred between the ages of 3 and 7.[2] In this series, the amount of chloramphenicol ingested and the period during which it was taken varied considerably. Ten per cent developed the dyscrasia within 4 days of beginning therapy and 22 per cent developed it while taking the drug even though only 9 per cent had a previous exposure to the drug. The median time for development of symptoms was 38 days after the drug was stopped, but in 10 per cent aplasia did not develop until 130 days after the last dose of the drug. Aplastic anemia is rare in the black as compared to the white, and this is especially true of the "idiopathic" type.

The onset of the disorder is generally gradual and is characterized by increasing weakness and other evidences of anemia, such as exertional dyspnea, palpitation, and pallor. Weight loss is infrequent and night sweats are rare. In about one-third of the patients abnormal bleeding is the initial complaint. Although the onset is usually insidious, sometimes the disorder begins abruptly with marked weakness, fever, other evidence of infection, and hemorrhagic manifestations.

The most striking abnormality found on the physical examination is the pallor of the skin and mucous membranes. There is no yellowish tinge of the skin or sclerae. Grayish brown pigmentation of the skin and testicular atrophy occur in an appreciable percentage of patients with this disease; these abnormalities are found particularly in those who have been transfused, and it seems likely that they are due at least in part to transfusion hemosiderosis. In about one-half of the patients there is evidence of abnormal bleeding in the skin, mucous membranes, or retinae at the time of the initial examination. Although enlargement of the spleen, liver, and lymph nodes is unusual in the untreated patients, and indeed is strong evidence against the diagnosis in such circumstances, these organs have been found to be enlarged in about one-third of one group of patients who had been under observation and treatment for some time, probably because of the transfusions they had received.

Laboratory Examination

In a series of 50 patients studied at the University of Virginia Hospital the following peripheral blood conditions were noted: pancytopenia 37; anemia alone 7; anemia with leukopenia 4; anemia and thrombocytopenia 2.[40] The anemia was macrocytic (MCV > 94 cu. microns) in 60 per cent and normocytic in the remainder. A mild reticulocytosis of 2 to 5 per cent occurred at some time during the course of the disease in 21 patients, but an absolute increase in reticulocytes was rarely seen. Only 9 patients had reticulocyte counts that were persistently 0.1 per cent or less. In the same series of 50 patients, 41 had leukopenia. There was a relative lymphocytosis in 37 and an absolute lymphocytosis (over 3000 per cu.mm.) in 6. Only 5 had an absolute decrease in lymphocytes (less than 1500 per cu.mm.). The platelet counts varied from practically zero to normal levels but were markedly reduced in the majority of the patients.

The smear of the peripheral blood of patients with aplastic anemia manifests little poikilocytosis although the cells may be slightly macrocytic; significant poikilocytosis suggests some other diagnosis, such as hemolytic anemia, vitamin deficiency, iron deficiency, or myeloid metaplasia.

The marrow specimen obtained by aspiration or surgical biopsy usually shows decreased cellularity. In the authors' series the marrow was hypocellular in 74 per cent, normal in 16 per cent, and hypercellular in 10 per cent. Similar discrepancies between the cellularity and function of the bone marrow have been reported by others.[4, 48, 61] In Best's series of chloramphenicol-treated patients, the bone marrow was examined in 129 patients; 3 per cent were hypercellular and 7 per cent had normal cellularity; in 12 per cent one cell line was depressed, in 5 per cent it was two cell lines, and in 74 per cent all three cell lines were depressed (hypoplastic or aplastic).[2] In the bone marrow of many patients with this disease there is an increase in mononuclear cells that generally are classed as lymphocytes although their identity and origin are uncertain. The differential count of the cells in the bone marrow often reveals increased percentages of plasma cells and reticulum cells. (F.S.: I, 22–23.)

The results of other laboratory procedures are often interesting and sometimes are helpful in diagnosis. The level of the serum iron may be increased and the latent iron binding capacity may be saturated even before the patient has received any blood transfusions. The serum bilirubin level is usually normal but increased fecal urobilinogen excretion has been observed in some patients. Liver function tests are usually normal unless the patient has received a large number of transfusions which lead to increased iron deposition in the liver.

Differential Diagnosis

The disease which causes the most difficulty in differential diagnosis is leukemia. Even though careful studies of the blood and bone marrow do not reveal leukemia when the patient is first seen, the possibility that the patient may still develop evidence of leukemia at a later date continues to be a source of concern. The detection of significant enlargement of the spleen before the patient has been transfused should always raise the suspicion that the patient has leukemia, myelofibrosis, or some disease of the lymphoma group rather than aplastic anemia. The distinction between leukemia and aplastic anemia can usually be made as a result of the bone marrow examination and a careful study of the peripheral blood. Any significant increase in very young cells in the marrow or peripheral blood should raise the suspicion of leukemia even though a definite diagnosis cannot be made. Hypercellularity of the marrow and the presence of abnormal normoblasts with increased nuclear parachromatin suggest "preleukemia" and the need for careful follow-up studies. If what is considered a satisfactory marrow sample is not obtained after needle aspiration, a trephine or open surgical biopsy should be done to obtain a sample; some patients with leukemia have packed marrows or marrows that contain considerable reticulin tissue and yield only a very hypocellular or acellular specimen on aspiration. Although leukemia sometimes becomes manifest only months or years after the appearance of anemia, the distinction can be made in most patients after a relatively short period of observation. In the 14 autopsies in one series the diagnosis of aplastic anemia was confirmed in all but one patient.[40] In this patient, who had aplastic anemia while under observation for 5 years, the presence of acute myeloblastic leukemia became manifest 6 weeks before death. When leukemia appears some years after the onset of the anemia in a patient diagnosed as having aplastic anemia, a question of the relationship of the two diagnoses arises. The question is whether or not the patient has both aplastic anemia and leukemia, possibly from the same or related causative factors, or only leukemia that has masqueraded as aplastic anemia.

Aplastic anemia must be distinguished from pernicious anemia, but this is usually not difficult because of the differences in appearance of the skin and the tongue, and the absence of central nervous system involvement in aplastic anemia. Most patients with aplastic anemia retain the ability to secrete hydrochloric acid and this finding is sufficient to practically exclude pernicious anemia from consideration. Examination of the bone marrow, even though hypocellular, generally permits the identification of erythropoiesis as the normoblastic type rather than the megaloblastic type seen in untreated pernicious anemia. Examination of the smear of peripheral blood also helps to distinguish between the two diseases; even when the anemia is severe and macrocytic in aplastic anemia, a smear of the peripheral blood usually shows but little poikilocytosis and anisocytosis.

At times the problem of the differential diagnosis between the idiopathic aplastic anemia and anemia associated with generalized carcinomatosis may arise. The finding of young leukocytes and nucleated red cells in the peripheral blood suggests the possibility of carcinomatosis of the bone marrow. The presence of metastases can be established sometimes by a bone marrow aspiration which reveals the malignant cells and at other times by radiographic study of the skeleton which discloses evidence of osseous involvement.

Treatment

The most desirable form of treatment of aplastic anemia caused by drugs and chemicals is prevention. Regular blood counts should be made on patients taking drugs that are known to produce blood dyscrasias. McCurdy has recommended that patients receiving chloramphenicol receive serial reticulocyte counts. If the reticulocyte count drops abruptly or falls below 0.5 per cent, bone marrow examination should be made;[37] if erythropoietic activity is diminished or vacuoles are present in the young normoblasts, the drug should be discontinued. Unfortunately, careful and repeated assessment of the blood and marrow while the drug is being administered may not indicate the patients who will develop aplastic anemia later. A drug, such as chloramphenicol, which is known to be potentially dangerous should not be used if a safer one will be effective. Some unfortunate instances of aplastic anemia have occurred in patients who were treated with potentially dangerous drugs for minor illnesses, illnesses which probably would have ended in recovery if treated with safer preparations or simple supportive measures.

The treatment of this disorder is unsatisfactory in general, but nevertheless the patient is treated as effectively as possible in the hope that recovery or remission will occur. The most effective form of treatment is the removal of the cause. For this reason patients should be questioned carefully about exposure to drugs or chemicals and should be removed from contact with any suspicious offenders.

In most patients, particularly with disease of the idiopathic type, the most important treatment is blood transfusion. Although the decision regarding the number and frequency of transfusions must be an individual one for each patient, the hematocrit seldom need be raised to levels higher than 33 or 34 per cent. If the blood is returned to the normal level, whatever active erythro-poiesis that is present may be depressed. The vast majority of patients accom-modate to a lower than normal level of hemoglobin without disagreeable symptoms. Dangers of transfusion that restrict their usefulness are hemolytic transfusion reactions, febrile reactions to the leukocytes in the transfusion, the danger of infectious hepatitis, and the long-term danger of exogenous hemo-chromatosis.

Platelet concentrates prepared from fresh blood collected in plastic con-tainers are often helpful in controlling hemorrhage due to thrombocytopenia; usually platelets from four units of blood are administered at one time. Platelets given in this way are effective for a few days initially but the time becomes shortened as the recipient develops platelet antibodies. Nevertheless, with such treatment it may be possible to tide an adult over the dangers of hemor-rhage for several weeks or even a few months while waiting for the marrow to recover. A longer term of treatment is not practical in adults; although the volume of blood and platelets required is more easily managed in children, the long-term use is usually defeated by the development of platelet antibodies even when splenectomy has been performed. A satisfactory method of platelet typing might avoid this complication.

The results of treatment with large doses of oxymetholone have been encouraging. Sanchez-Medal et al. reported their experience with 14 children and 55 adults treated with oxymetholone and related compounds.[54] The remis-sion rate was 48 per cent in the whole group and 70 per cent in those treated for more than 2 months. Twenty-two patients remained in remission from 1 to 5 years without maintenance therapy, eight relapsed after therapy was dis-continued but responded to further treatment, and four required continued treatment. A response was noted in from several weeks to 6 months of treat-ment; clinical remission was accompanied by increased cellularity of the bone marrow, reticulocytosis, and stabilization of hemoglobin levels so that further transfusions were not required; improvement in the leukocytes and thrombo-cytes was slower. Oxymetholone and related compounds appeared to be equally effective. Some patients developed hirsutism and hoarseness and gained weight, but the most serious side effect was a hepatotoxic reaction. Although nine patients became jaundiced and five died, it was difficult or impossible to assess the importance of the oxymetholone in this development. The authors recom-mended dose of 2 mg. per kg. per day, even though some patients had remis-sions on 1 mg. per day. Other authors have reported similarly favorable results with the same agents in smaller series.[1, 58]

How androgens exert their effect and why some patients with aplastic anemia respond and others do not remain unclear. In experimental animals, androgens produce an increase in the incorporation of radioactive iron into red cells followed by an increase in the red cell mass; in vitro studies of the marrow cultures of children disclosed that in about half testosterone caused a great increase in the uptake of labeled thymidine within a few hours (evidence of DNA synthesis).[25] Androgens also increased production of the renal ery-thropoietin factor or erythropoietin.[18, 43] That this is not the explanation of the mechanism of the action of androgen in aplastic anemia is apparent because patients with the disorder have high circulating levels of erythropoietin, even when untreated; in addition, when patients respond to androgens the leuko-cytes and platelets as well as the red cells increase. It has been suggested that androgen may in some way condition the stem cell so that it can respond to erythropoietin; the demonstration that estrogens inhibit or restrict the effect of erythropoietin on the stem cell is suggestive supporting evidence. One little understood aspect of the response to androgen is the long lag phase between beginning treatment and response, which may be as much as 2 or 3 months.

Antibiotic drugs should be used when infection is present, but their use as prophylactic agents appears inadvisable because of the emergence of resistant strains of bacteria and the development of fungus infections. Gray, necrotic "agranulocytic" ulcers sometimes occur in the vagina, pharynx, intestine, or rectum, and may be a source of septicemia. Any unnecessary trauma to the skin and mucous membranes is to be avoided.

Clinical Course and Prognosis

Aplastic anemia is a serious disorder but the outlook for survival with the treatment available has improved considerably. In one series of 62 patients reported in 1919, only three patients survived more than a year.[59] In 1941, Bomford and Rhodes reported that in their series of 66 patients, 15 recovered completely; many of these cases developed as the result of toxic exposure to chemicals.[4] In a series of 62 patients seen at the University of Virginia Hospital, 40 have died and 22 are living. Of the 40 patients who died, 50 per cent survived for one year, 35 per cent for 3 years, 20 per cent for 5 years, and 10 per cent for 10 years. Of the patients who are still alive, over 50 per cent have survived 5 years or more (Fig. 6–1). Similar results have been reported by others.[35, 55] In recovery from aplastic anemia the increase in platelets lags behind that of the other blood elements; thrombocytopenia of varying degree may remain after the other values have returned to normal, as shown in Figure 6–2. which illustrates the course of a patient (Case 1) who recovered from aplastic anemia which developed after administration of chloramphenicol and sulfonamide.

The prognosis is best when the offending agent can be recognized and eliminated, giving the marrow a chance to recover before it has been damaged too severely. The outlook is better in patients who have erythrocytic hypoplasia than in those who have pancytopenia. Patients who have a severe pancytopenia associated with what appears to be a totally aplastic marrow have a very poor prognosis. Most such patients do not respond to any form of treatment and supportive measures such as transfusions, platelet packs, and antibiotics rarely prolong survival more than a few months. Contrary to the experience of some,[35, 64] in our patients a hypocellular or acellular marrow, severe reticulo-cytopenia (0.1 per cent or less), thrombocytopenia (less than 10,000 per cu.mm.), and severe leukopenia (leukocytes less than 1000 per cu.mm.) have indicated a worse than average prognosis.

The clinical course of the disease is extremely variable. Some patients have an acute illness with septicemia, fever, prostration, and bleeding; the outlook for such patients is poor and death usually occurs within a matter of a few days,

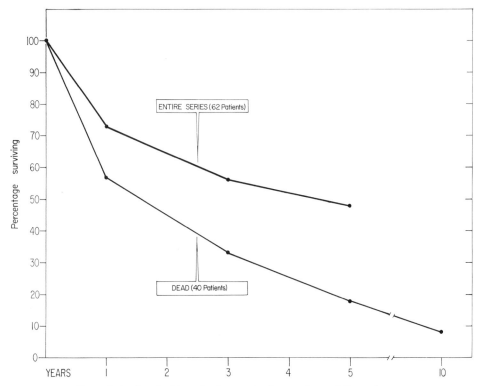

Figure 6–1. Survival in aplastic anemia, from estimated time of onset.

weeks, or months. Fortunately, many patients have a longer and more benign course extending over a period of years. Death in these patients is most often the result of hemorrhage, either gastrointestinal or intracranial; infections such as septicemia or pneumonia also are often terminal complications. Serious infections are more likely to occur in patients who have an absolute neutrophil count of less than 500 cu.mm.; in addition infection almost invariably causes a further fall in the neutrophil count, often accompanied by a reduction in the platelet and reticulocyte counts.[64] Some patients die from coexisting disorders, such as vascular disease, or from complications of therapy, and a few develop leukemia as a terminal event. More recently, the development of paroxysmal nocturnal hemoglobinuria has been recognized as a sequela to aplastic anemia in some patients.[15b, 36]

The place of prednisone and related compounds in treatment is uncertain. When bleeding is a problem, prednisone in doses of from 10 to 60 mg. a day may be beneficial because of its effect on the capillaries. Although the use of prednisone has been followed by remission in aplastic anemia and chronic erythrocytic hypoplasia, the remission rate is smaller and the incidence of complications is greater than when oxymethelone is used in aplastic anemia.

Splenectomy has been effective in some patients with chronic erythrocytic hypoplasia and in some with pancytopenia.[20] Although there are exceptions,[8] the experience of most clinics is that few patients respond well to splenectomy and for this reason the operation cannot be considered a standard method of

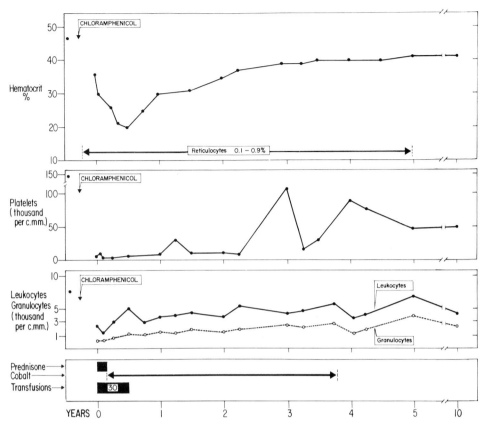

Figure 6–2. Course of aplastic anemia following treatment with chloramphenicol in a woman aged 62 at onset.

treatment. Splenectomy is most likely to be helpful if there is an associated hemolytic component and evidence of splenic sequestration of red cells can be demonstrated. Neither the presence of hyperhemolysis nor the presence of a cellular marrow gives any assurance that splenectomy will be effective in a particular patient. Hyperhemolysis may be a feature of the disease initially but it is more likely to become prominent after the patient has received numerous transfusions. If the patient requires a 500 ml. blood transfusion oftener than every 10 days, and is not bleeding, excessive hemolysis is probably present.

The transplantation of bone marrow, a subject of considerable study at present, offers hope for a more definite form of therapy in the future but has been successful in only a few special situations thus far.

Paroxysmal noctural hemoglobinuria, a rare disorder, developed in 15 per cent of 46 patients with aplastic anemia seen by Lewis and Dacie;[36] the same authors found that of 60 patients with PNH, 15 had earlier been diagnosed as having aplastic anemia. PNH may develop as long as 6 years after the diagnosis of aplastic anemia is made.[15b] The disorder is characterized by intravascular hemolysis associated with ahaptoglobinemia, reduced red cell acetylcholinesterase, hemosiderinuria, leukopenia, variable degrees of thrombocytopenia, episodes of abdominal pain, and venous thrombosis. Presumably there is an

acquired defect in the red cell membrane which permits hemolysis to be produced by complement in vivo without the action of antibody. Maximum lysis
occurs at pH 6.8 when complement sensitive sites in the cell are most exposed.
The most acceptable explanation for the development of this disorder in
patients with aplastic anemia is that the stem cell has undergone a somatic
mutation which has resulted in the development of two red cell populations,
one with a membrane defect that makes it extremely sensitive to complement
and susceptible to hyperhemolysis and the other with a normal life span. A
further interesting but unfortunate association has been the development of
acute myeloblastic leukemia in several patients with paroxysmal nocturnal
hemoglobinuria.[24, 26, 27]

Erythrocytic Hypoplasia (Pure Red Cell Anemia)

Erythrocytic hypoplasia, which may be congenital or may develop at any
time from childhood to old age, is characterized by normocytic (or slightly
macrocytic) anemia, usually severe, associated with normal leukocyte and platelet
counts. The reticulocytes, although sometimes slightly increased, usually are
greatly reduced and often number less than 0.1 per cent. Normoblasts may not
be found in an examination of the bone marrow and at best are scarce. In these
patients the danger is that of severe anemia; hemorrhage and infections are
usually not problems. Nevertheless, some patients who appear to have simple
erythrocytic hypoplasia at onset later develop thrombocytopenia or pancytopenia and become vulnerable to the complications seen in aplastic anemia.
Most patients with erythrocytic hypoplasia require periodic transfusions to
maintain a satisfactory red cell volume (Fig. 6–3). In some, however, treatment
with corticosteroids produces a gratifying response manifested by reticulocytosis, increased normoblasts in the bone marrow, and a return of the peripheral blood count to normal; at times relapse occurs when the drug is discontinued and readministration of the steroid may or may not produce another
remission. In acquired erythrocytic hypoplasia, some instances are classified as
"idiopathic" and others are associated with thymoma or follow exposure to
drugs.

The association of erythrocytic hypoplasia and thymoma was first reported
by Matras and Priesel in 1928.[8a] Since that time, more than 50 patients, all but
one over 40 years of age, have been reported.[23] Thymomas have been found
in 50 per cent of adults with pure red cell anemia and erythrocytic hypoplasia
occurs in less than 10 per cent of patients with thymoma; the meaning of the
association is uncertain. There is no convincing evidence that the thymus is
concerned in erythropoiesis; in accord with the concept that nearly any abnormality of the thymus can lead to an abnormality in the immune mechanism,
it has been suggested that the thymoma may be responsible for an auto-immune
mechanism directed against either the red cell precursors or erythropoietin.
When a patient with pure red cell anemia is seen, thymoma should be searched
for. If one is found, thymectomy probably is indicated, although of 25 patients

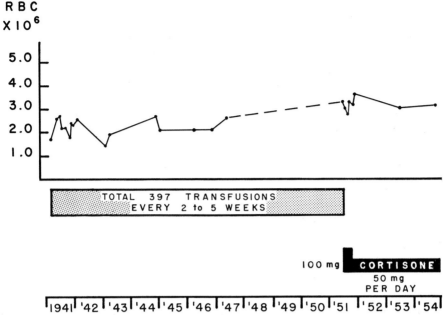

Figure 6-3. Chart showing response of a patient with chronic erythrocytic hypoplasia to treatment with cortisone. Although this patient required an average of 400 ml. of blood per week for 10½ years, no further transfusions were necessary after the institution of treatment with cortisone. (From Mohler and Leavell: Ann. Int. Med., vol. 49, 1958.)

treated with thymectomy, only three had a good and lasting remission; three more responded well to corticosteroid treatment after thymectomy. Splenectomy was largely ineffective, but again, subsequent treatment with corticosteroid produced some benefit. The outlook is not good for patients with this syndrome. Seventeen of a group of 50 died within 6 months; the mean survival in those who obtained remission was 47 months, for those who did not have a remission, 18 months.

Pure red cell aplasia associated with drug therapy has been reported in 40 patients.[46] Twenty-one cases followed treatment with chloramphenicol. Other drugs that have been connected with aplasia of the red cells are sulfathiazole, arsphenamine, penicillin, phenobarbital, chenopodium, isoniazid, tolbutamide, diphenylhydantoin sodium, phenylbutazone and chlorpropamide. Ten of 12 patients reported in detail recovered when the drug was stopped and one recovered when riboflavin was given with the drug.[68]

The mechanism of the anemia in patients with red cell aplasia is uncertain and may not be the same in every patient. Recent reports of the demonstration in the plasma of gamma-G antibody to erythroblast nuclei and a gamma-G fraction that inhibited heme synthesis, with disappearance of these antibodies as well as the anemia after treatment with 6-mercaptopurine and cyclophosphamide, point strongly toward an important role of antibodies in the development of the syndrome.[29, 30] A different interpretation was advanced for a patient who repeatedly developed red cell aplasia while taking Dilantin.[68] Investigation disclosed that Dilantin inhibited the uptake of C^{14} formate into DNA but not into RNA. Antibodies could not be demonstrated by the methods used; nevertheless it is interesting that the patient, a 17 year old boy, took the drug for 2 years before developing anemia, went through a period when a 2 week exposure to the drug would produce anemia, then finally became resistant to toxic effects of the drug.

Aplastic Anemia in Children

The syndrome of aplastic anemia, both congenital and acquired, occurs in children as well as adults. In 1927 Fanconi described three siblings with bone marrow hypoplasia, pancytopenia and congenital anomalies.[15] In 1967 he reviewed the abnormalities seen in 129 patients with this syndrome.[15a] Listed as the chief criteria for Fanconi's anemia were the following: (1) pancytopenia, (2) hyperpigmentation, (3) malformation, especially of the skeleton, (4) small stature since birth, (5) hypogonadism, and (6) familial occurrence (the familial occurrence need not be evident). Of the skeletal manifestations, abnormalities in development of the thumb and the radius are most common; manifestations of anemia and thrombocytopenia usually do not appear until 7 or 8 years after birth. Early in the disease, hyperactive megaloblastic or "megaloblastoid" marrow may be present. Other common symptoms and signs found in 129 cases include microsomy in 60 per cent, microcephaly in 40 per cent, malformation of the kidneys in 28 per cent, strabismus in 22 per cent, and mental retardation in 17 per cent. Both hypoplastic and normally cellular marrows have been found in patients thought to have this syndrome.[10] Other syndromes that have been described in infants are the familial hypoplastic anemia characterized by pancytopenia without associated congenital anomalies[14] and a type of hypoplastic anemia which affects the red cell series solely or predominantly.[11]

Aplastic anemia in children, defined as physiologic and anatomic failure of the bone marrow with marked decrease of blood-forming elements in the marrow, peripheral pancytopenia, and no splenomegaly, hepatomegaly, or lymphadenopathy, differs in some respects from the disorder in adults.[57] The prospect for remission when treated only by supportive measures is very poor, even worse than for adults. The history of exposure to a possible toxic chemical is obtained in a high percentage of cases; in one group of 17 children from 5 months to 13 years of age with aplastic anemia, a history of exposure to naphthalene, chloramphenicol, or DDT was obtained in 12. Withdrawal of the suspected agent and administration of testosterone and corticosteroids produced a remission in a high percentage of patients; 9 of 17 patients treated with these preparations (testosterone or methyl testosterone, 1 to 2 mg. per kg. of body weight per day, and triamcinolone, 8 to 20 mg. per day) obtained complete remissions after being treated for 2½ to 15 months. When the drugs were discontinued, a partial hematologic relapse occurred for about 2 months; this was followed by spontaneous recovery by the third month. Similarly gratifying responses to this regime occurred in 6 of 7 patients from 2 to 10 years of age who had congenital aplastic anemia. The response in this group differed from that of the acquired group in that the platelet response was incomplete; furthermore, persistent pancytopenia recurred in several patients when the drugs were discontinued and maintenance dosage of the drug was found to be necessary. Despite these encouraging early results, it has been reported that in children treated in this way the overall mortality rate remained more than 50 per cent.[1] More promising results have been reported recently; treatment with oxymetholone, 2 to 6.5 mgm. per kg. per day, has been followed by good results in five patients[1] and at present appears to be the treatment of choice. Repeated platelet transfusions may be valuable in children; such treatment may prevent fatal hemorrhage and enable the patient to survive until remission occurs.[33]

The clinical course of acquired aplastic anemia in children treated with supportive care has been reported.[22] The study included 33 children, from 10 months to 14 years old, seen between the years 1951 and 1968. They were treated with supportive measures but without androgens; 16 patients (48.4 per cent) died, 15 have recovered, and two are still being transfused. The report emphasizes that the approximately 50 per cent survival is the same as that seen after treatment with corticosteroids and testosterone. This group of patients also provided some interesting figures about the time of recovery and those who survived; the mean time of recovery from anemia was 10 months; from leukopenia, 12 months; and from thrombocytopenia, 18.9 months.

Illustrative Cases

CASE 1

Aplastic Anemia

A 61 year old white housewife had numerous urinary tract infections which were treated with sulfonamides over a period of years. On two occasions in the spring of 1959 she took 1.0 gm. of chloramphenicol and in September 4.0 gm.; she had a small but undetermined quantity of sulfonamide in the spring and in October. In June her hematocrit was 43 per cent, white blood count 4200 per cu.mm., platelets and differential count normal. On December 7, 1959 she noticed ecchymoses of the skin; at that time the hematocrit was 36 per cent, white blood count 2600 cu.mm., and platelets 5000 per cu.mm. A bone marrow aspiration was hypocellular.

Prednisone was prescribed with some symptomatic improvement in her purpura, but on January 19, 1960 she was admitted to the hospital acutely ill with chills, temperature (103° F.), and hypotension; septicemia was suspected but not proved. Her hematocrit was 26 per cent, white blood count 1500 (20 per cent granulocytes), platelets 2500 per cu.mm. The bone marrow was very hypocellular. She responded to antibiotics and transfusions, but similar febrile episodes, gastrointestinal bleeding, and periarticular ecchymoses occurred during the next two months. During this time she received 15 transfusions. She then began to improve, less frequent transfusions were necessary, and none was needed after July, 1960. The course of her blood counts is shown in Figure 6–2.

Comment. This patient developed aplastic anemia following repeated treatments with sulfonamide and chloramphenicol. Frequent transfusions were necessary for the first six months of the illness but none has been necessary since that time. She was treated with prednisone, androgen, and cobalt; her improvement began while on the last drug but it is doubtful if any of the agents were responsible. The blood counts improved gradually; the hematocrit and leukocyte count returned to normal but thrombocytopenia has persisted for 10 years.

Chronic Erythrocytic Hypoplasia

CASE 2

A white government official, who had been admitted to the hospital several times between 1920 and 1950 because of hemorrhages from a duodenal ulcer, was admitted in January 1956 at the age of 82 because of mild congestive heart failure and was found to have a normochromic, normocytic type of anemia. Admission blood studies showed the following: Hb. 6.5 gm. per 100 ml., R.B.C. 2.5 mil. per cu.mm., Hct. 20 per cent, W.B.C. 5500 per cu.mm., retics. 0.6 per cent, differential count (per cent), segs. 50, lymphs. 37, monocytes 10, basophils 2. The platelets were normal in number. The serum iron was 127 μg. per 100 ml. and the unsaturated iron binding protein was 185 μg. per 100 ml. Blood urea was normal. The bone marrow obtained by aspiration appeared active and normoblastic. No cause for the anemia was found and he was treated with blood transfusions.

Treatment and course. The anemia recurred and failed to respond to oral iron, folic acid, vitamin B$_{12}$, or cobaltous chloride. In July 1956 examination of the bone marrow disclosed almost complete absence of erythropoiesis and slightly depressed myelopoiesis. During the period from January to July he received transfusions amounting to an average of 1500 ml. of whole blood every month. In August 1956, when the R.B.C. was 1.4 mil. per cu.mm., Hb. 3.9 gm. per 100 ml., Hct. 11 per cent, retics. 0 per cent, prednisone was started in a dose of 20 mg. daily. Striking improvement followed and the bone marrow reverted toward normal. On a maintenance dose of 10 to 15 mg. of prednisone a day the hematocrit remained in the range of 38 to 41 per cent for 6½ months without transfusions.

Unfortunately an exacerbation of a previously mild diabetes occurred and the symptoms of peripheral neuritis became so severe that prednisone was discontinued in February 1957. The neurologic symptoms subsided but on April 9, 1957, the hematocrit had fallen to 16 per cent. Subsequently the anemia failed to respond to prednisone, testosterone, or cobalt, and transfusions were required regularly until his death at home in March 1961. The leukocyte and platelet counts remained normal and the reticulocyte count was usually zero. Extensive studies failed to reveal any apparent cause for this anemia. An autopsy was not performed.

Comment. This elderly clerical worker had aplastic anemia of the chronic erythrocytic hypoplasia type. This syndrome is characterized by anemia with almost complete absence of reticulocytes and erythrocytic hypoplasia in the bone marrow; the levels of the leukocytes and platelets in the circulating blood are normal. Anemia of this type generally pursues a chronic course refractory to all therapy except transfusions but in some patients it responds to treatment with prednisone, thymectomy, or other measures. The symptoms generally are due to anemia; bleeding and infections are rarely serious problems.

References

1. Allen, D. M., Fine, M. H., Necheles, T. F., and Dameshek, W.: Oxymetholone therapy in aplastic anemia. Blood, *32*:83, 1968.
2. Best, W. R.: Chloramphenicol-associated blood dyscrasias (a review of cases submitted to the A.M.A. Registry). J.A.M.A., *201*:181, 1967.
3. Bithell, T. C., and Wintrobe, M. M.: Drug-induced aplastic anemia. Seminars in Hematology, *4*:194, 1967.
4. Bomford, R. R., and Rhoads, C. P.: Refractory anemia. I. Clinical and pathological aspects. Quart. J. Med., *10*:175, 1941.
5. Bowditch, M., and Elkins, H. B.: Chronic exposure to benzene (benzol). J. Indust. Hyg. & Toxicol., *21*:321, 1939.
6. Cone, T. E., Jr., and Abelson, S. M.: Aplastic anemia following two days of chloramphenicol therapy. Case report of a fatality in a 6-year-old girl. J. Pediat., *41*:340, 1952.
7. Cooper, I. A., and Firkin, B. G.: The presence of deoxyribonucleic and (DNA) synthesizing cells in patients with refractory anemia. Blood, *24*:415, 1964.
8. Crosby, W. H., et al.: Panels in therapy. XII. Hypoplastic-aplastic anemia. Blood, *12*:193, 1957.
8a. Dameshek, W., Brown, S. M., and Rubin, A. D.: "Pure" red cell anemia (erythroblastic hypoplasia) and thymoma. Seminars in Hematology, *4*:222, 1967.
9. Daniel, T. M., Suhrland, L. G., Weisberger, A. S.: Supression of the anamestic response to tetanus toxoid in man by chloramphenicol. New England J. Med., *123*:367, 1965.
10. Dawson, J. P.: Congenital pancytopenia associated with multiple congenital anomalies (Fanconi type). Pediatrics, *15*:325, 1955.
11. Diamond, L. K., and Blackfan, K. D.: Hypoplastic anemia. Am. J. Dis. Child., *56*:464, 1938.
12. Ehrlich, P.: Ueber einen Fall von Anämie mit Bermerkungen über regenerative Veränderungen des Knochenmarks. Charité-Ann., *13*:300, 1888.
13. Ellis, L. D., Jensen, W. N., and Westerman, M. P.: Needle biopsy of bone and marrow. Arch. Int. Med., *114*:213, 1964.
14. Estren, S., and Dameshek, W.: Familial hypoplastic anemia of childhood. Am. J. Dis. Child., *73*:671, 1947.
15. Fanconi, G.: Familiäre infantile perniziösaartige Anämie perniözioses Blutbild und Konstitution. Jahrb. f. Kinderh., *117*:257, 1927.
15a. Fanconi, G.: Familial constitutional panmyelocytopathy, Fanconi's anemia (F.A.). Seminars in Hematology, *4*:233, 1967.
15b. Gardner, F. H., and Blum, S. F.: Aplastic anemia in paroxysmal nocturnal hemoglobinuria, mechanisms and therapy. Seminars in Hematology, *4*:250, 1967.
16. Gardner, F. H., and Pringle, J. C., Jr.: Androgens and erythropoiesis. Arch. Int. Med., *107*:846, 1961.
17. Gasser, C.: Pure red cell anemia due to auto-antibodies; immune type of aplastic anemia (erythroblastopenia). Le sang, *26*:6, 1955.
18. Gordon, A. S., Mirand, E. A., Wenig, J., Katz, R., and Zanjani, E. D.: Androgen actions on erythropoiesis. Ann. N.Y. Acad. Sci., *149*:318, 1968.
19. Havard, C. W. H.: An investigation of refractory anaemias. Quart. J. Med., *31*:21, 1962.
20. Heaton, L. D., Crosby, W., and Cohen, A.: Splenectomy in the treatment of hypoplasia of the bone marrow with a report of twelve cases. Ann. Surg., *146*:637, 1957.
21. Henriksen, E.: Tetanus og N_2O—narkose Svaer knoglemarvsintoxication some følge af protraheret kvaelstrofforiltenarkose. Nord. med., *56*:1418, 1956.
22. Heyn, R. M., Ertel, I. J., and Tubergen, D. G.: Course of acquired aplastic anemia in children treated with supportive care. J.A.M.A., *208*:1372, 1969.
23. Hirst, E., and Robertson, T. I.: The syndrome of thymoma and erythroblastopenic anemia. Medicine, *46*:225, 1967.
24. Holden, D., and Lichtman, H.: Paroxysmal noctural hemoglobinuria with acute leukemia. Blood, *33*:283, 1969.

25. Jacobson, W., Sidman, R. L., and Diamond, L. K.: The effect of testosterone on the uptake of triatiated thymidine by the bone marrow of children. Ann. N.Y. Acad. Sci., *149*:389, 1968.

26. Jenkins, D. E., and Hartmann, R. C.: Paroxysmal nocturnal hemoglobinuria terminating in acute myeloblastic leukemia. Blood, *33*:274, 1969.

27. Kaufmann, R. W., Schechter, G. P., and McFarland, W.: Paroxysmal nocturnal hemoglobinuria terminating in acute granulocytic leukemia. Blood, *33*:287, 1969.

28. Kennedy, B. J.: Stimulation of erythropoiesis by androgenic hormones. Ann. Int. Med., *57*:917, 1962.

29. Krantz, S. B., and Kao, V.: Studies on red cell aplasia. I. Demonstration of a plasma inhibitor to heme synthesis and an antibody to erythroblast nuclei. Acad. Sci. U.S.A., *58*:493, 1967.

30. Krantz, S. B., and Kao, V.: Studies on red cell aplasia. II. Report of a second patient with an antibody to erythroblast nuclei and a remission after immuno-suppressive therapy. Blood, *34*:1, 1969.

31. Lange, R. D., et al.: Refractory anemia occurring in survivors of the atomic bombing in Nagasaki, Japan. Blood, *10*:312, 1955.

32. Lassen, H. C. A., Henriksen, E., Neukirch, F., and Kristensen, H. S.: Treatment of tetanus. Severe bone-marrow depression after prolonged nitrous-oxide anaesthesia. Lancet, *270*:527, 1956.

33. Levin, R. H., Barrett, P. V. D., Cline, M. J., Berlin, N. I., and Freireich, E. J.: Platelet therapy and red cell defect in aplastic anemia. Arch. Int. Med., *11*:278, 1964.

34. Levy, R. N., Sawitsky, A., Florman, A. L., and Rubin, E.: Fatal aplastic anemia after hepatitis. New England J. Med., *273*:1118, 1965.

35. Lewis, S. M.: Course and prognosis in aplastic anemia. Brit. Med. J., *1*:1027, 1965.

36. Lewis, S. M., and Dacie, J. V.: The aplastic anaemia-paroxysmal nocturnal haemoglobinuria syndrome. Brit. J. Haemat., *13*:236, 1967.

37. McCurdy, P. R.: Chloramphenicol bone marrow toxicity. J.A.M.A., *176*:106, 1961.

38. McGuire, L. B.: Aplastic anemia in an adult with two remissions on androgen. Va. Med. Monthly, *91*:207, 1964.

38a. Manyan, D. R., and Yunis, A. A.: Effect of chloramphenicol treatment in ferrochelatase in dogs. Biochem. Biophys. Res. Comm., *41*:926, 1970.

39. Martelo, O. J., Manyan, D. R., Smith, U. S., and Yunis, A. A.: Chloramphenicol and bone marrow mitochondria. J. Lab. & Clin. Med., *74*:927, 1969.

40. Mohler, D., and Leavell, B. S.: Aplastic anemia. An analysis of 50 cases. Ann. Int. Med., *49*:326, 1958.

41. Movitt, E. R., Mangum, J. F., and Porter, W. R.: Idiopathic true bone marrow failure. Am. J. Med., *34*:500, 1963.

42. Murray, W. D., and Webb, J. N.: Thymoma associated with hypogammaglobulinaemia and pure red cell aplasia. Am. J. Med., *41*:974, 1966.

43. Naets, J. P., and Wittek, M.: The mechanism of action of androgens on erythropoiesis. Ann. N.Y. Acad. Sci., *149*:366, 1968.

44. Nagoa, T., and Mauer, A. M.: Concordance for drug-induced aplastic anemia in identical twins. New England J. Med., *281*:7, 1969.

45. Pollycove, M., and Lawrence, J. H.: Ferrokinetics of refractory anemia. Proceedings of the Eighth International Congress of Hematology, 1960, p. 42.

46. Recker, R. R., and Hynes, H. E.: Pure red blood cell aplasia associated with chlorpropamide therapy. Arch. Intern. Med., *123*:445, 1969.

47. Reynafarje, C., and Faura, J.: Erythrokinetics in the treatment of aplastic anemia with methandrostenolone. Arch. Int. Med., *120*:654, 1967.

48. Rhoads, C. P., and Miller, D. K.: Histology of the bone marrow in aplastic anemia. Arch. Path., *26*:648, 1938.

49. Rich, M. L., Ritterhoff, R. J., and Hoffman, R. J.: A fatal case of aplastic anemia following chloramphenicol (Chloromycetin) therapy. Ann. Int. Med., *33*:1459, 1950.

50. Rosenthal, L., and Blackman, A.: Bone-marrow hypoplasia following use of chloramphenicol eye drops. J.A.M.A., *191*:136, 1965.

51. Rubin, D., Weisberger, A. S., Botti, R. E., and Storaasli, J. P.: Changes in iron metabolism in early chloramphenicol toxicity. J. Clin. Invest., *37*:1286, 1958.

52. Rubin, E., Gottlieb, C., and Vogel, P.: Syndrome of hepatitis and aplastic anemia. Am. J. Med., *45*:88, 1968.

53. Saidi, P., Wallerstein, R. O., and Aggeler, P. M.: Effect of chloramphenicol on erythropoiesis. J. Lab. & Clin. Med., *57*:247, 1961.

54. Sanchez-Medal, L., Gomez-Leal, A., Duarte, L., and Rio, M. G.: Anabolic androgenic steroids in the treatment of acquired aplastic anemia. Blood, *34*:283, 1969.

55. Scott, J. L., Cartwright, G. E., and Wintrobe, M. M.: Acquired aplastic anemia: An analysis of thirty-nine cases and review of the pertinent literature. Medicine, *38*:119, 1959.

56. Semi-annual Tabulation of Reports Compiled by the Registry on Blood Dyscrasias (March 20, 1963). American Medical Association, Chicago, 1963.

57. Shahidi, N. T., and Diamond, L. K.: Testosterone-induced remission in aplastic anemia on both acquired and congenital types. New England J. Med., *264*:953, 1961.

58. Silinik, S. J., and Firkin, B. G.: An analysis of hypoplastic anemia with special reference to the use of oxymetholone (Adroyd) in its therapy. Aust. Ann. Med., *17*:224, 1968.

59. Smith, L. W.: Report on an unusual case of aplastic anemia. Am. J. Dis. Child., *17*:174, 1919.

60. Suhrland, L. G., and Weisberger, A. S.: Delayed clearance of chloramphenicol from serum in patients with hematologic toxicity. Blood, *34*:466, 1969.

61. Thompson, W. P., Richter, M. N., and Edsall, K. S.: An analysis of so-called aplastic anemia. Am. J. M. Sc., *187*:77, 1934.

62. Tsai, S. Y., and Levin, W. C.: Chronic erythrocytic hypoplasia in adults. Am. J. Med., *22*:322, 1957.

63. Vilter, R. W., Jarrold, T., Will, J. J., Mueller, J. F., Friedman, B. I., and Hawkins, V. R.: Refractory anemia with hyperplastic bone marrow. Blood, *15*:1, 1960.

64. Vincent, P. C., and Gruchy, G. C.: Complications and treatment of acquired aplastic anemia. Brit. J. Haemat., *13*:977, 1967.

65. Wallerstein, R. O., Condit, P. K., Kasper, C. K., Brown, J. W., and Morrison, F. R.: Statewide study of chloramphenicol therapy and fatal aplastic anemia. J.A.M.A., *208*:2045, 1969.

66. Wasserman, L. R., Stats, D., Schwartz, L., and Fudenberg, H.: Symptomatic and hemopathic hemolytic anemia. Am. J. Med., *18*:1961, 1955.

67. Weisberger, A. S.: Mechanisms of action of chloramphenicol. J.A.M.A., *209*:97, 1969.

68. Yunis, A. A., Arimura, G. K., Lutcher, C. L., Blasquez, J., and Halloran, M.: Biochemical lesion in Dilantin-induced erythroid aplasia. Blood, *30*:587, 1967.

69. Yunis, A. A., and Bloomberg, G. R.: Chloramphenicol toxicity: Clinical features and pathogenesis. Prog. in Hematolog., *4*:138, 1964.

70. Yunis, A. A., and Harrington, W. J.: Patterns of inhibition by chloramphenicol of nucleic acid synthesis in human bone marrow and leukemic cells. J. Lab. & Clin. Med., *56*:831, 1960.

71. Yunis, A. A., Smith, U. S., and Restrepo, A.: Reversible bone marrow suppression from chloramphenicol. Arch. Int. Med., *126*:272, 1970.

VII / Hemolytic Anemia

The erythrocytes normally have a life span of about 120 days. When the erythrocyte is destroyed or disintegrates, the iron of the hemoglobin is stored in the cells of the reticuloendothelial system. In these same cells heme is converted into the unconjugated form of bilirubin, which is then transported in the plasma to the liver where the bilirubin is conjugated and excreted through the biliary system; in the bowel, bilirubin is converted into fecal urobilinogen.

Whether the senescent red cells are phagocytized by the reticuloendothelial cells or are fragmented in the circulation before the particles are engulfed by these cells has not been established. Whatever the actual mechanism, reticuloendothelial cells in any part of the body, particularly the bone marrow, the liver, the spleen, and the lymph nodes, participate in the process. Splenectomy in an otherwise normal individual produces no significant increase in the life span of the erythrocytes; this indicates that the spleen is not essential for the physiologic destruction of the cells. The concept has evolved that the erythrocyte is destroyed because its metabolic activity fails, its reserves are exhausted, and it is no longer able to maintain itself. The abnormalities which have been detected in older cells, such as increases in density, osmotic fragility, and mechanical fragility, are probably manifestations of underlying changes in the metabolic status of the cells. The aging process in the red cells appears to be primary; when this has reached a certain point, the cells, or their disintegrating fragments, are taken up by reticuloendothelial cells in any part of the body.

Hemolytic anemias are characterized by a shortened life span of the red cells. An increase in the number of cells destroyed is usually accompanied by enlargement of the spleen, a rise in the level of unconjugated bilirubin in the plasma, and elevation of the fecal urobilinogen excretion. Compensatory erythroid hyperplasia occurs in the marrow and increased numbers of reticulocytes appear in the peripheral blood. In stained smears of the peripheral blood there is usually visible evidence of hereditary or acquired abnormality in

178

the structure of the erythrocytes in the form of spherocytosis, poikilocytosis, anisocytosis, or basophilic stippling.

In most patients with hemolytic anemia, red cell destruction is extravascular in the reticuloendothelial system. In a limited number of hemolytic disorders, red cells are destroyed intravascularly with resulting hemoglobinuria. Hemoglobin released in the plasma is bound by an α_2-globulin, haptoglobin, which is capable of binding two molecules of hemoglobin. When the threshold of haptoglobin binding is exceeded, in the range of 90 to 130 mg. of hemoglobin per 100 ml. of plasma, hemoglobin appears in the urine. Other indications of intravascular hemolysis are increases in plasma hemoglobin, methemalbumin, and lactic dehydrogenase, decreased or absent haptoglobin, and hemosiderinuria. Staining for hemosiderin in the urine sediment is a sensitive indicator of intravascular hemolysis and may remain positive long after gross hemoglobinuria has cleared.

Erythrocyte Metabolism and Methemoglobinemia

The red blood cell is the site of numerous metabolic activities designed to maintain cellular integrity and to transport oxygen and carbon dioxide. Four main areas of red cell metabolism which are crucial to normal red cell survival and function may be identified. These are the red cell membrane, the pentose phosphate shunt–glutathione system, glycolysis by the Embden-Meyerhof pathway, and hemoglobin. Abnormalities in any of these areas of metabolism will result in impaired red cell survival and function.

The Red Cell Membrane

The details of the structure and organization of the erythrocyte membrane are still a subject of controversy. Basically it is composed of a bimolecular lipid leaflet consisting of phospholipid and cholesterol sandwiched between an inner protein lining rich in sulfhydryl groups and a lesser amount of surface protein rich in sialic acid, which gives the red cell its negative charge. [9, 12, 17, 24, 48, 48a] In addition, the membrane contains the blood group antigens and a number of enzymes such as ATPase and cholinesterase.[12, 34, 35]

Two essential attributes of the red cell membrane are its deformability and permeability characteristics. The red cell, which averages about 7 microns in diameter, must traverse passages less than 3 microns in diameter in the microcirculation of the bone marrow and spleen.[47, 49] In order to accomplish this feat the membrane must remain pliable because any decrease in deformability will lead to sequestration and destruction by the reticuloendothelial system.[45a]

The permeability properties of the erythrocyte membrane are important in controlling the volume of the red cell and in preventing colloid osmotic hemolysis. Because the red cell contains a relatively high concentration of molecules, such as hemoglobin, phosphorylated intermediates, and glutathione, which do not cross the red cell membrane, there is a slightly positive osmotic gradient towards the inside of the erythrocyte.[23] If this osmotic force were unopposed, water would enter the cell in excess of its capacity and hemolysis would ensue. The erythrocyte protects itself from osmotic lysis by active cation transport and a relative impermeability to cations. The red cell membrane is freely permeable to water and the anions, chloride and bicarbonate, which traverse the membrane in less than a second.[50]

In contrast, the exchange of sodium ion and potassium ion proceeds much more slowly with a halftime of over 30 hours.[38] This allows the red cell "time" to adjust its volume by the active transport of sodium ion along with water out of the cell. The intracellular:extracellular ratio for K^+ is 25:1 and for Na^+ is 1:12.[45] The passive movements of these cations is in the direction of their electrochemical gradients, with Na^+ leaking into the cell and K^+ leading out. These electrochemical gradients are maintained by active transport with Na^+ being pumped out while K^+ is pumped in. The energy for active transport is provided by ATP, which is derived from glycolysis. The energy is released by action of ATPase residing in the red cell membrane.[16, 31, 40] The volume control of the red cell depends on a combination of the permeability of the membrane and the rate of the cation pump. Any disturbance which increases permeability or curtails the production of ATP for active transport may lead to colloid osmotic hemolysis.

Pentose Phosphate Shunt–Glutathione System

Approximately 90 per cent of the glucose utilized by the mature red cell is converted to lactate by the anaerobic enzymatic steps of the Embden-Meyerhof pathway and the remaining 10 per cent is metabolized by the oxidative pentose phosphate pathway.[27] The pentose phosphate shunt is important to the red cell as the pathway for the generation of NADPH (Fig. 7–1). NADPH along with reduced glutathione (GSH) is the main line of defense of the red cell against oxidative injury.[22] When the red cell is exposed to a variety of oxidant drugs, which function as electron transport agents in oxidation-reduction reactions, or after a number of infections, hydrogen peroxide is formed. This is reduced by the following series of interrelated reactions:[7, 26]

1. Red cell + oxidant $\longrightarrow H_2O_2$

2. $H_2O_2 + 2\,GSH \xrightarrow{\text{glutathione peroxidase}} 2H_2O + GSSG$

3. $GSSG + NADPH + H^+ \xrightarrow{\text{glutathione reductase}} 2\,GSH + NADP^+$

4. $G\text{–}6\text{–}P + NADP^+ \xrightarrow{\text{glucose–6–phosphate dehydrogenase}} 6\text{–}PG + NADPH + H^+$

$\qquad$ (G–6–P = glucose–6–phosphate; 6–PG = 6–phosphogluconate)

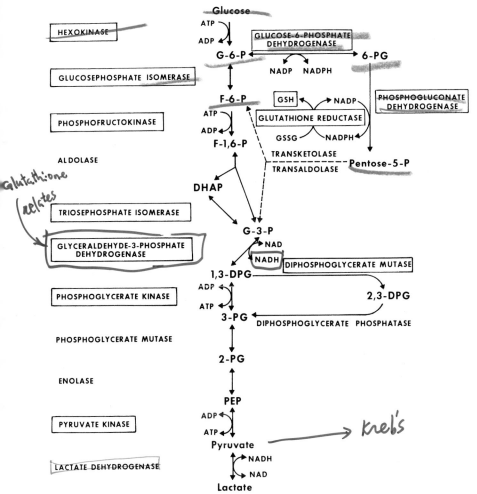

Figure 7–1. Glycolytic and pentose phosphate shunt pathways. Deficiencies of the enclosed enzymes have been associated with hereditary hemolytic anemia.

In order for glutathione peroxidase to remain effective in reducing H_2O_2 to H_2O, a continuous supply of GSH must be available. This is accomplished by the reduction of GSSG to GSH by glutathione reductase, which in turn requires NADPH as a cofactor. A deficiency of glutathione peroxidase, glutathione reductase, or glucose–6–phosphate dehydrogenase or an inability to synthesize glutathione leads to defective reduction of H_2O_2. When H_2O_2 accumulates, hemoglobin is irreversibly oxidized and precipitated as Heinz bodies.[22] Rifkin has shown that the precipitated Heinz bodies are attached to the red cell membrane; being rigid bodies they interfere with the deformability of the membrane which leads to the cell's sequestration and lysis by the spleen and reticuloendothelial system.[32, 33] The formation of Heinz bodies appears to be the common pathway of hemolysis in anemias secondary to defects in the pentose phosphate shunt–glutathione systems, unstable hemoglobins, and thalassemia.

Although the red cell is rich in catalase, which also decomposes H_2O_2, it does not appear to be as physiologically important to the red cell as glutathione peroxidase,[26] since a hereditary deficiency of catalase[1] is not associated with hemolytic anemia, whereas a deficiency of glutathione peroxidase is.[29, 41]

Glycolysis

Figure 7–1 shows the anaerobic metabolism of glucose by the Embden-Meyerhof pathway and the aerobic metabolism of glucose by the pentose phosphate shunt. In contrast to nucleated cells which contain mitochondria and metabolize glucose via the Krebs cycle, yielding 38 moles of ATP per mole of glucose utilized, the mature red cell contains no mitochondria and the yield of ATP is only 2 moles per mole of glucose metabolized.[27]

The energy of ATP is used by the red cell primarily for the active transport of Na^+ and K^+ and is important in controlling the volume of the cell.[28] ATP also has a role in maintaining the permeability, shape characteristics, and deformability of the red cell membrane.[23a, 45a, 47] Any deficiency in the supply of ATP resulting from a lack of the substrate glucose or from a deficiency of some enzyme in the Embden-Meyerhof pathway will lead to failure of the cation pump and, ultimately, to colloid osmotic hemolysis. In addition, decreased erythrocyte ATP levels lead to less bound Ca^{++} with a concomitant increase in membrane Ca^{++}, resulting in increased membrane rigidity and permeability.[23a]

The erythrocyte is unique among cells utilizing anaerobic glycolysis in that it contains an unusually large amount of 2,3-diphosphoglycerate (2,3 DPG) and no glycogen.[2] It has recently been shown by Chanutin and Curnish[6] and by Benesch and Benesch[3] that 2,3-DPG plays a key role in controlling oxygen-hemoglobin dissociation. This compound has a strong affinity for hemoglobin and in the presence of high levels of 2,3-DPG oxygen is released more readily to the tissues. It has been demonstrated that patients with anemia or living at high altitudes respond with an increase in 2,3-DPG which renders their hemoglobin more efficient in delivering oxygen to the tissues.[30] On the other hand, patients with hexokinase deficiency have lower than normal levels of 2,3-DPG with an increased affinity of their hemoglobin for oxygen.[10]

Another important function of the glycolytic pathway is the generation of

NADH which is the physiological cofactor for the reduction of methemoglobin to oxyhemoglobin.[19, 20]

Hemoglobin

Although more than 100 abnormal hemoglobins have been described in man, only a few of these have been of pathologic importance in the genesis of hemolytic anemia. These have usually involved amino acid substitutions which render the hemoglobin susceptible to structural change under certain conditions, such as the molecular stacking with tactoid formation, which occurs with sickle hemoglobin when oxygen tension is reduced, and the precipitation of unstable hemoglobins with Heinz body formation upon exposure to oxidant drugs. These changes impair membrane deformability and lead to red cell destruction.

The function of the erythrocyte is to carry oxygen from the lungs to the cells of the body and to transport carbon dioxide to the lungs. Under normal circumstances the hemoglobin molecule in the mature erythrocyte is in a stable state and there is no degradation or resynthesis during the life span of the cell. However, hemoglobin does change constantly, from the reduced to the oxidized state. When the iron is in the reduced form, hemoglobin can bind and transport oxygen. Ferric or oxidized hemoglobin, which is known as methemoglobin, is not able to function as an oxygen transport system.

Two methemoglobin reductase systems are of importance in maintaining hemoglobin in the reduced state. Both pathways are dependent on carbohydrate metabolism for the regeneration of reduced pyridine nucleotides and are referred to as NADH methemoglobin reductase[37] and NADPH methemoglobin reductase.[18] The NADH dependent system appears to be the major pathway under physiologic conditions.[19, 20] These reactions function so efficiently that not more than 1 per cent of the hemoglobin in the erythrocyte is in the oxidized state.[14, 18]

Methemoglobinemia. Methemoglobinemia of greater than 1.5 to 2.0 gm. per 100 gm. hemoglobin will produce cyanosis and concentrations in the order of 70 gm. per 100 gm. hemoglobin are probably lethal.[4, 20] Significant amounts of methemoglobin may occur in a variety of disorders.

1. A genetically determined abnormality in the NADH methemoglobin reductase system is not uncommon.[5, 15, 36] The condition appears benign though patients may complain of mild dyspnea on exertion and have slight compensatory erythrocytosis. The blood may contain 20 to 45 per cent methemoglobin. Family studies indicate a recessive autosomal mode of inheritance. The condition requires no therapy, but the cyanosis will respond to methylene blue, which activates the NADPH methemoglobin reductase system.

A severe degree of NADH reductase deficiency has been found in association with mental retardation.[21]

A form of methemoglobinemia transmitted by an autosomal dominant gene has been described in which erythrocyte NADH and NADPH methemoglobin reductase concentrations and hemoglobin structure appear normal but erythrocyte glutathione synthesis appears to be depressed.[43] The reduction in glutathione concentration is believed to affect the function of the sulfhydryl dependent enzyme glyceraldehyde-3-phosphate dehydrogenase, reducing the availability of NADH to the NADH dependent methemoglobin reductase system.[44]

2. A genetically determined altered structure of the hemoglobin molecule may result in methemoglobinemia and the abnormal hemoglobin has been designated hemoglobin M.[39] A number of variants of hemoglobin M have been described.[20] The mechanism by which methemoglobin accumulates in these patients has not been completely elucidated. It has been suggested that the ferric iron in methemoglobin M forms a complex with a ligand provided by the abnormal amino acid substitution in the hemoglobin molecule and that this complex resists enzymatic reduction.[13, 25] The abnormality appears to be transmitted as an autosomal characteristic and the homozygous state is probably incompatible with life. In the heterozygous state only 25 to 35 per cent of the hemoglobin is methemoglobin, suggesting a lowered rate of synthesis.

3. Toxic methemoglobinemia.

An elevated level of methemoglobin is also found following the introduction into the body of compounds that preferentially oxidize hemoglobin and exceed the capacity of the normal blood cell reducing systems. Among the most important offenders are nitrites, sulfonamides, and aniline derivatives.[11, 42] Methemoglobinemia with cyanosis has also been observed in individuals taking the antimalarial drugs, primaquine and chloroquine. Such individuals have been found to be heterozygous for NADH methemoglobin reductase deficiency.[8]

Sulfhemoglobin is another compound that is not capable of carrying oxygen. Its formation represents an irreversible change in hemoglobin and it persists until the destruction of the red blood cell. It is unaffected by methylene blue or ascorbic acid. Some source of sulfur, such as a sulfur-containing drug or chronic constipation, plus the ingestion of a drug which will oxidize hemoglobin, is thought necessary for its production. The syndrome of enterogenous cyanosis is probably related to the formation of either methemoglobin or sulfhemoglobin secondary to disturbed bowel function.[11]

Classification

Any process that shortens the life span of the erythrocyte results in hyperhemolysis; if erythropoiesis is unable to compensate for the increased hemolysis, anemia appears. A diminished life span of the erythrocytes has been demonstrated in almost every type of anemia found in association with disease. In many instances the shortening of the life span is slight, not more than the normal marrow can compensate for if it functions normally. If the degree of hyperhemolysis is minor, the anemia is more properly considered a reflection of inadequate marrow function. The term "hemolytic anemia" is usually reserved for those patients who have a severe degree of hyperhemolysis associated with anemia. The term "hemolytic disease" is a broader one that includes patients without anemia who have appreciable hyperhemolysis which is compensated by augmented erythropoiesis.

A number of different abnormalities affect the red cell and cause hemolytic anemia. As knowledge about the nature of these disorders increases, more precise names will come into use and a more satisfactory classification will become possible.

For the present it is convenient to classify hemolytic disorders according to whether they are hereditary or acquired, as shown in Table 7–1.

Table 7–1. *Classification of Hemolytic Disease*

I. Hereditary hemolytic disorders
 A. Erythrocyte membrane defects
  1. Hereditary spherocytosis
  2. Hereditary elliptocytosis
  3. Stomatocytosis
  4. Selective increase in membrane lecithin
 B. Pentose phosphate shunt–glutathione system enzyme deficiencies
  1. Glucose–6–phosphate dehydrogenase
  2. Others: 6–phosphogluconate dehydrogenase, glutathione reductase, glutathione synthetase, glutathione peroxidase
 C. Glycolytic enzyme deficiencies
  1. Pyruvate kinase
  2. Others: diphosphoglyceromutase, triosephosphate isomerase, glucosephosphate isomerase, phosphoglycerate kinase, phosphofructokinase, hexokinase, glyceraldehyde–3–phosphate dehydrogenase, ATPase
 D. Hemoglobinopathies
  1. Sickle cell anemia
  2. Hemoglobin C disease
  3. Thalassemia
  4. Combinations: sickle cell–hemoglobin C disease, sickle cell–thalassemia disease, sickle cell–hemoglobin D disease, and others
  5. Unstable hemoglobins: Zurich, Köln, Genova, Sydney, Hammersmith, Gun Hill, and others
II. Acquired hemolytic disorders
 A. Antibody-mediated
  1. Isoantibodies
   a. Transfusion reactions
   b. Erythroblastosis fetalis
  2. Drug-induced antibodies
   a. Quinidine
   b. Penicillin
   c. Methyldopa
  3. Autoantibodies _CLL_
   a. Idiopathic
   b. Secondary – malignancies, connective tissue disease, mycoplasma pneumonia, paroxysmal cold hemoglobinuria
 B. Paroxysmal nocturnal hemoglobinuria
 C. Mechanical hemolysis
  1. March hemoglobinuria
  2. Cardiac hemolytic anemia
  3. Microangiopathic hemolytic anemia
 D. Infections
  1. Malaria
  2. Bacterial infections
  3. Viral infections
 E. Chemical
 F. Physical agents
 G. Hypersplenism

Hereditary Hemolytic Disorders

ERYTHROCYTE MEMBRANE DEFECTS

Hereditary Spherocytosis

History

The history of this disorder has been reviewed by Dreyfus.[67] Formerly credit for the first detailed clinical description of "congenital hemolytic icterus" was usually given to Minkowski's report in 1900.[83] Because of Chauffard's discovery of two of the characteristic features of the disease, namely, reticulocytosis and the increased hypotonic saline fragility of the red cells,[55, 56, 83] the disorder was sometimes referred to as the "hemolytic anemia of the Chauffard and Minkowski type." Vanlair and Masius' report in 1871, in which spherocytes were described, has been rediscovered only recently[94] and, as a result, credit for the first clear description of this disease has been given to these authors.[67, 100]

Mechanism of Disease

Hereditary spherocytosis is believed to be inherited as an autosomal dominant.[99, 100] According to this concept at least one parent and one-half the offspring of the patient should be affected. However, apparent exceptions have been observed in families that were studied carefully.[90, 100] Consideration of these apparent exceptions has led to the suggestion that they may be explained in one of the following ways: (1) the testing method may be inadequate to detect the anomaly in the parents and siblings, possibly because of factors of gene penetrance or expressivity; (2) some patients may develop spherocytosis as a result of gene mutation; (3) the disease in the exceptional cases that appears to be hereditary spherocytosis is in reality similar to it but is not identical with it; (4) the legal parents are not the biological parents.[99, 100] The first and third possibilities are considered most likely.

Patients with hereditary spherocytosis manifest the evidences of a hemolytic process, such as increased fecal urobilinogen excretion, elevation of the indirect reacting serum bilirubin in the plasma, splenomegaly, reticulocytosis, and normoblastic hyperplasia in the bone marrow. Although the anemia is cured by splenectomy, an intracorpuscular defect has been shown by Dacie and Mollison[61] to be the primary factor in the increased hemolysis. They demonstrated that erythrocytes from normal donors survived from 100 to 130 days when transfused into patients with hereditary spherocytosis; in contrast, erythrocytes that were obtained from a patient with hereditary spherocytosis 4 days prior to splenectomy and 1 year after splenectomy disappeared from the circulation in 14 days and 19 days respectively when transfused into normal recipients. The importance of both the intracorpuscular defect and the spleen in the hyperhemolysis in this disease was further demonstrated by Emerson.[68] He observed that erythrocytes from a patient with hereditary spherocytosis, both before and after splenectomy, had shortened survival times when transfused into a normal recipient; erythrocytes from the same patient had a normal survival time when transfused into an otherwise normal recipient whose spleen had been removed because of trauma.

Ever since the increased osmotic fragility of the erythrocytes in hereditary spherocytosis was first described, efforts have been made to find some link between this peculiarity and the increased destruction of the erythrocytes in vivo. Haden demonstrated that the increased susceptibility of the erythrocytes in the disease to hypotonic saline is related to their increased thickness and "microspherocytic" shape.[70] The observation that microspherocytosis and increased osmotic fragility persisted after splenectomy suggested that the defects in the red cell were the result of an inherited abnormality of the erythrocyte.[70] Ham and Castle found that sterile incubation caused an increase in the spheroidicity and osmotic fragility of human erythrocytes and postulated that abnormally susceptible erythrocytes would be hemolyzed more easily than normal cells by erythrostasis in the spleen, which might be compared to incubation in vitro.[71] This concept implies selective sequestration of the abnormal "spherocytes" in the spleen because normal erythrocytes survive normally in patients with hereditary spherocytosis.[61, 69, 86] Such selective sequestration has been demonstrated in experiments that utilized mixtures of different types of cells that could be identified by differential agglutination. Identifiable normal erythrocytes were transfused into patients with hereditary spherocytosis prior to splenectomy; when the spleen was studied after its removal it was found that the patient's cells had been selectively retained by the spleen.

Although selective sequestration by the spleen of the abnormal red cells in hereditary spherocytosis has been clearly demonstrated, the mechanism by which this is accomplished is not entirely clear. In experiments that utilized millipore filters with 5 micron pores, Jandl and his associates observed that only the most spheroidal cells were retained by the filter.[78] A spherical erythrocyte is considerably less deformable than a biconcave one and it is not surprising that many of these cells are trapped by the microcirculation of the spleen where they may be required to pass through apertures less than 3 microns in diameter.[47, 49] However, the spherical shape of the cell does not appear to be the entire answer. Crosby and Conrad showed that flattening of the spherocyte by producing iron deficiency did not prevent sequestration of the cells by the spleen and did not improve red cell survival.[58] A possible explanation for this observation may come from the work of LaCelle and Weed,[79] who have used a micropipette technique to measure the deformability of the red cell membrane. They have found an increased rigidity of the membrane of red cells from patients with hereditary spherocytosis even before the cell becomes spherical.

Although the basic red cell lesion has not yet been determined in hereditary spherocytosis, a number of metabolic abnormalities have been demonstrated which help to explain the cells' particular vulnerability to erythrostasis both in vitro and in vivo. Jacob and Jandl,[73, 74] amplifying the observations of earlier workers,[53, 72] have shown an increased permeability to the passive influx of sodium. The red cell compensates for this leak by increasing the rate of active transport of sodium out of the cell with a concomitant increase in glucose and ATP utilization.[73, 74, 84, 89, 92] This mechanism is effective as long as sufficient glucose is available to the cell. In the spleen where erythrostasis occurs, glucose may fall to inadequate levels,[76, 77] ATP generation declines, sodium leaks into the cell faster than it can be pumped out and eventually osmotic swelling and lysis occurs.

When red cells from patients with hereditary spherocytosis are incubated in the absence of glucose for prolonged periods they first begin to swell, a change which can be explained by the permeability lesion described above; later the cells lose volume, become smaller, and assume the microspheroidal shape characteristic of the disease. This change requires another explanation. A spherocyte is formed when there is an alteration in the ratio of surface area to volume. Since the spherocyte in hereditary spherocytosis is a small one, it must follow that the cell has lost surface area. This has been shown to be the case by Reed and Swisher,[91] who have demonstrated excessive membrane lipid loss upon incubation. The composition of lipid in the membrane of red cells in hereditary spherocytosis is normal[64] and when lipid is lost from the membrane the proportions of the various lipids in the membrane remain the same, indicating that whole fragments of the membrane are lost.[91, 96] This has been shown directly by electron microscopy of incubated red cells[95] and accounts for the loss of surface area with subsequent microspherocytosis.[96] Cooper and Jandl have proposed that fragmentation is a late irreversible event signaling the imminent demise of the cell, whereas an earlier selective loss of membrane cholesterol may lead to reversible sphering.[51, 76] They infused ^{51}Cr-labeled red cells from a patient with hereditary spherocytosis into patients with obstructive jaundice and observed improvement in osmotic fragility and red cell survival. Since bile acids in the plasma of patients with obstructive jaundice block the transfer of cholesterol from red cells to plasma, they postulated that an increase in membrane cholesterol was responsible for the improvement in red cell survival they observed.

Recently Weed and his associates have emphasized the role of calcium in membrane rigidity.[23a, 46, 79] As intracellular calcium increases an actinomycin-like protein on the inner surface of the membrane undergoes a sol to gel transformation which is reversed by ATP. They have postulated that the red cell membrane in hereditary spherocytosis may have an increased affinity for calcium since the spherocytic red cell is more sensitive to falling levels of ATP and increase in calcium than the normal red cell.

From these observations it can be seen how the spleen is ideally suited to bring out the red cell defects in hereditary spherocytosis. When erythrostasis occurs, ATP depletion follows, leading to intracellular accumulation of sodium, loss of membrane lipid, sphering, enhancement of calcium effect on membrane protein, rigidity of the membrane, and ultimately sequestration by the microcirculation of the spleen.

Clinical Manifestations

Hereditary spherocytosis occurs in both sexes, but it is rare in blacks.[54] Clinical evidence of the disease may appear soon after birth or not until after middle age.

The severity of the disease varies greatly in different patients. In some the clinical manifestations are so mild that the disease is asymptomatic and the patients lead an active normal life. In such individuals the diagnosis can be established only after a careful study of the blood because the anemia may be mild, or even absent, if the bone marrow is able to compensate for the hyperhemolysis. More often the patient has the symptoms of a mild chronic illness. Some patients do not realize that they have been feeling subnormal until after splenectomy produces an increased sense of well-being.

In many patients the course of the disease is associated with episodes of severe illness, the so-called "crisis." These attacks are characterized by the sudden onset of fever, abdominal discomfort, nausea, vomiting, and rapidly increasing weakness and pallor. Tachycardia and low blood pressure are usually present and shock may develop. Some patients appear severely ill and lethargic and lapse into unconsciousness. It was formerly thought that the episode of crisis was caused by a marked increase in the severity of hemolysis, but the recent studies of such episodes indicate that the majority are the result of a combination of decreased erythropoiesis and a continuation of the usual degree of hemolysis. Owren described the occurrence of an "aplastic crisis" characterized by rapidly increasing anemia, leukopenia, and thrombocytopenia that accompanied a fall in the reticulocyte count, and a decrease in the plasma bilirubin and the development of an aplastic picture in the bone marrow.[86] The occurrence of episodes of this type in several members of a family at the same time suggests that some intercurrent infection is the causative factor. Other attacks labeled as crisis that are associated with increasing jaundice may be in reality attacks of biliary colic and infection. In these circumstances the features of obstructive jaundice and infection are superimposed on those of hyperhemolysis. Cholelithiasis occurs in over half the patients over the age of 10, and in only about 5 per cent of those under 10 years of age.[52] In one group of 14 patients over 11 years of age, cholelithiasis occurred in 12.[100]

The most constant abnormality found on physical examination is splenomegaly of mild or moderate degree. In most patients the spleen is firm and does not extend below the level of the umbilicus but in some patients it fills the entire left half of the abdominal cavity. The liver is often palpable but is rarely significantly enlarged. The patient with hereditary spherocytosis has been described as "more jaundiced than sick," but the degree of clinical jaundice is usually mild unless there is associated dysfunction of the biliary tract. Both the pallor and the jaundice may be so mild as to be overlooked on the physical examination. In patients with hereditary spherocytosis, growth and development are usually normal. Abnormalities such as tower skull, polydactyly, skeletal defects, and infantilism have been reported in this disease but appear to be uncommon.[99]

Laboratory Examination

The anemia is usually moderate and erythrocyte counts of 3.0 to 3.5 mil. per cu.mm. are common. The erythrocyte count may be normal if the hemolytic process is fully compensated, or markedly reduced if there is an episode of crisis.

The MCV is usually normal or slightly reduced, the result of the presence of both small spherocytes and large young red cells. The MCHC is character-

istically increased because the hemoglobin is densely packed in the microspherocytes that have lost more surface area than cellular contents by fragmentation. Figure 7–2 shows a stained blood smear showing many characteristic
microspherocytes. A reticulocytosis of from 5 to 20 per cent or more is found
regularly unless erythropoiesis is depressed because of an aplastic crisis or for
some other reason. During an aplastic crisis reticulocytes may disappear from
the peripheral blood.[62, 86] In the usual patient the bone marrow undergoes
hyperplasia of the normoblastic type. During an aplastic crisis the marrow may
be either aplastic or unusually cellular; the appearance depends on whether the
specimen is obtained near the onset of crisis or during the recovery phase.

Study of the patient discloses other features common to hemolytic anemias
of all types, such as an elevation of the level of serum bilirubin, an increase in
the excretion of fecal urobilinogen and urinary urobilinogen, and normal or elevated levels of the serum iron. In one series, the serum bilirubin level ranged
from 0.4 to 5.7 mg. per 100 ml., but in 80 per cent it was below 3.0 mg.[100] Levels
higher than 4.0 mg. per 100 ml. are unusual unless complications are present.

Increased fragility of erythrocytes in hypotonic saline solutions has been
recognized as a characteristic feature of hereditary spherocytosis. When normal
erythrocytes are tested in saline solutions hemolysis begins in concentrations of
about 0.45 per cent and is complete at 0.30 per cent. In most patients with hereditary spherocytosis hemolysis begins at concentrations of from 0.50 per cent to
0.75 per cent and is complete at 0.40 per cent. The test has been modified so that
results may be expressed quantitatively.[60, 100] When incubated for 24 hours at
37° C. erythrocytes from patients with hereditary spherocytosis show a greater
increase in osmotic fragility than do normal cells.[100] In mildly affected cases the

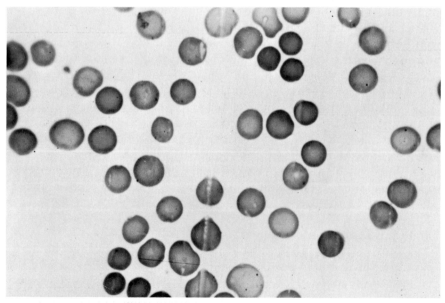

Figure 7–2. Peripheral blood smear of a patient with hereditary spherocytosis showing
many microspherocytes.

abnormal osmotic fragility may not be evident until after incubation, and for this reason an incubated osmotic fragility is prefered. Microspherocytes have not only an increased hypotonic saline fragility but also an increased mechanical fragility.[69, 93] The autohemolysis test performed by incubating whole blood under sterile conditions for 48 hours is abnormal and is corrected to nearly normal by the addition of glucose.[60] Normally less than 2 per cent hemolysis occurs in the autohemolysis test, whereas in hereditary spherocytosis usually 20 to 30 per cent of the red cells hemolyze.

Differential Diagnosis

The diagnosis may be difficult if the patient is seen for the first time during an episode of aplastic crisis or during an attack of biliary colic when the hemolytic nature of the underlying disorder may not be suspected. As a rule the presence of mild anemia, splenomegaly, and slight icterus suggests the diagnosis. The presence of hyperhemolysis is confirmed by finding reticulocytosis, increased urobilinogen excretion, and elevation of the indirect reacting bilirubin in the blood.

Hereditary spherocytosis is generally distinguished from other types of hemolytic anemia by the family history and the hypotonic fragility test. However, the presence of microspherocytes and increased osmotic fragility does not establish the disorder as hereditary spherocytosis, for these sometimes occur in other types of hemolytic anemia. Increased osmotic fragility has been found in auto-immune hemolytic anemia, myelosclerosis, leukemia, erythroblastosis fetalis, lymphadenoma, ovarian dermoid cyst, uremia, lymphosarcoma, pneumonia, and after the administration of hemolytic poisons such as acetylphenylhydrazine, sulfanilamide, and arsenic. Non-specific spherocytosis can usually be distinguished from hereditary spherocytosis by the autohemolysis test. Spherocytosis which occurs secondary to antibody injury, uremia, and other disorders will be accompanied by an increase in auto-hemolysis but, unlike hereditary spherocytosis, this will not be improved by the addition of glucose. At times study of the blood of siblings and parents is necessary to establish the diagnosis of hereditary spherocytosis in an individual patient. The Coombs antiglobulin test, hemoglobin electrophoresis, and the alkali denaturation test are often helpful in distinguishing hereditary spherocytosis from other hemolytic anemias, such as the hemoglobinopathies and auto-immune hemolytic disease.

Treatment

Splenectomy was first performed on a patient with this disease by Wells in 1887, some years before the nature of the disease was recognized.[63] It has been established since then that the procedure almost invariably relieves the anemia and jaundice.[60, 98, 100] The serum bilirubin level returns to normal promptly and the erythrocyte count generally becomes normal in from 2 to 4 weeks (Fig. 7–3). Although spherocytosis is less marked after splenectomy, both the spherocytosis

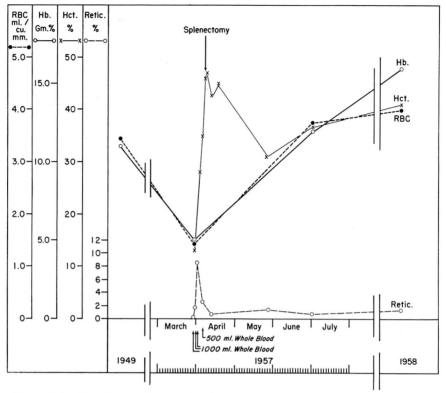

Figure 7–3. Hereditary spherocytosis, showing results of splenectomy. The patient was admitted during an "aplastic crisis" when the reticulocytes were nearly zero; despite transfusions the reticulocytes rose within a few days.

and increased osmotic fragility persist after operation.[60, 100] Operation appears to be indicated in virtually all patients with this disease except those with the mildest form of the disorder, unless there are other contraindications to surgery. Splenectomy may be done in infancy if the anemia is severe, but postponement to late childhood if possible is recommended by Dacie.[60] If the patient has cholelithiasis, cholecystectomy may be performed at the time of splenectomy, but at times it may be more prudent to perform the operations separately.

Folic acid, iron, and vitamin B_{12} are without value in the uncomplicated case of hereditary spherocytosis. Transfusions may be necessary during episodes of "crisis," particularly if splenectomy must be done at such a time, but do not constitute a regular form of treatment.

Illustrative Case

This white woman was first admitted to the University of Virginia Hospital in March of 1957, at the age of 38, for fever, weakness, and anemia. She had been told at another hospital in 1940 that she was anemic and should have a splenectomy but she declined to have the operation. She had noted intermittent episodes of jaundice all of her life. Her brother and daughter had a similar anemia for which splenectomy had been performed. On admission she was acutely ill and febrile. Physical examination was normal except for an enlarged spleen palpable 4 cm. below the left costal margin.

Laboratory examination. Admission blood studies: Hct. 13 per cent, Hb. 5.2 gm. per 100 ml., MCV 89, MCH 35, MCHC 40, W.B.C. 5400 per cu.mm., serum bilirubin 1.0 mg. per 100 ml., no reticulocytes were seen. Spherocytes were seen on peripheral blood smear. Erythroid hyperplasia was evident in the bone marrow. Osmotic fragility was increased, as was the autohemolysis test which was improved by glucose.

Course. Splenectomy was performed and results are shown in Figure 7–3. Her gall bladder was also removed and showed chronic cholecystitis but no stones were found. She is no longer anemic.

Comment. The diagnosis of hereditary spherocytosis was readily established in this patient by the presence of spherocytes on the blood smear, increased osmotic fragility, abnormal auto-hemolysis test improved by glucose, splenomegaly, and family history of hemolytic anemia which responded to splenectomy.

She also represents the problem these patients may have with aplastic crises accompanied by a marked fall in hematocrit which may be life threatening. This is one of the main reasons for recommending splenectomy when this diagnosis is made.

Hereditary Elliptocytosis

Elliptocytosis in man was reported first by Dresbach in 1904; the cells were seen in a healthy 22 year old mulatto male.[66] The disorder is inherited as an autosomal dominant.[59, 80] It is usually manifested as an asymptomatic trait, but about 12 per cent of the persons with elliptocytosis have evidence of increased hemolysis and some have frank hemolytic anemia.[51, 87, 97] The disorder is usually recognized by the elliptical appearance of the erythrocytes. Poikilocytes, microcytes, and other abnormal forms occur only when there is increased hemolysis. The MCV, MCH, and MCHC are usually normal. No abnormality of the hemoglobin has been demonstrated by electrophoresis or by other means. Patients with hemolytic anemia have a moderately severe anemia, hemoglobin in the range of 7.5 to 9.2 grams per 100 ml., accompanied by normal leukocyte and platelet counts. The osmotic fragility test and the auto-hemolysis test have been abnormal in some patients and normal in others. An increased membrane permeability to the passive influx of sodium, similar to that seen in hereditary spherocytosis, has been described.[102] Splenomegaly occurs in patients with anemia and studies with tagged erythrocytes have indicated a shortened survival time associated with an increased uptake of radioactivity over the spleen. Splenectomy usually relieves the anemia although the abnormal appearance of the erythrocytes persists. (F.S.: I, 10.)

Other Erythrocyte Membrane Defects

Stomatocytosis in association with hemolytic anemia and abnormal red cell osmotic fragility has been reported in a number of different families.[80-82, 85, 101] The characteristic feature that all patients with this disorder have in common is a morphological alteration of their red blood cells consisting of a slit or mouth-like opening in the central part of the red cell. Such red cells have been called stomatocytes. Patients with stomatocytosis and hemolytic anemia probably represent a heterogeneous group of red cell disorders rather than a specific biochemical entity, as there has been decreased glucose-6-phosphate dehydrogenase in one family,[80] low erythrocyte glutathione in another patient,[82] and marked increase in permeability to univalent cations in two other families.[85, 101] The increase in cation permeability and osmotic fragility is similar to that seen in hereditary spherocytosis but differs in that the red cells of patients with stomatocytosis do not display membrane lipid loss and do not become spherocytes. In one of the families reported by Oski and his associates,[85] the hemolytic process was quite mild in the face of a much more severe cation leak than is seen in hereditary spherocytosis, emphasizing the importance of additional membrane lesions in hereditary spherocytosis. Acquired reversible stomatocytosis with hemolytic anemia has been observed in some patients as a complication of alcohol ingestion.[65]

Jaffé and Gottfried have reported an hereditary hemolytic anemia in a large family from the Dominican Republic.[75] The disorder is inherited as an autosomal dominant and is characterized by an increased content of the phospholipid, lecithin, in the red cell membrane. Both unincubated and incubated osmotic fragility of the erythrocytes were less than normal.

PENTOSE PHOSPHATE SHUNT–GLUTATHIONE SYSTEM ENZYME DEFICIENCIES

Glucose-6-Phosphate Dehydrogenase Deficiency

History

In 1926, Cordes noted that the antimalarial drug pamaquine caused hemolytic anemia in some patients.[120] Earle, in 1948, made the observation that only the erythrocytes of blacks hemolyzed after taking pamaquine.[126] The Korean War in the early 1950's first focused major attention on this problem when large numbers of American blacks stationed in Korea developed acute hemolytic anemia after taking primaquine for treatment or prophylaxis of malaria. A study group was formed under the direction of Alving that was responsible for contributing much of the early information to the understanding of this type of anemia.[124, 125] This also stimulated an upsurge of interest in red cell metabolism in general. They quickly learned that patients who had had hemolysis while taking pamaquine also had hemolysis after taking primaquine.[129] They demonstrated that Heinz body formation was a prominent part of the hemolytic process[107] and in 1956 a deficiency of red cell glucose-6-phosphate dehydrogenase

(G-6-PD) was shown to be the basic red cell defect.[117] A number of detailed reviews are available.[104, 105, 118, 137a, 154]

Clinical Manifestations

Glucose-6-phosphate dehydrogenase deficiency is transmitted on the X chromosome with full expression in the hemizygous male and partial expression in the heterozygous female.[119] In the United States the disorder is found most frequently in blacks. Approximately 10 to 13 per cent of male American blacks have G-6-PD deficiency, 20 per cent of female blacks are carriers, and 3 per cent of black women react to oxidant drugs. Less than 1 per cent of whites of Northern European origin have the deficiency but the disorder is prevalent among whites in the Mediterranean area, being as high as 48 per cent in Sardinian males.[154] The disorder is world-wide and it has been estimated that over 100 million people have this deficiency.[118] Since the areas of highest incidence correspond to areas where there is a high incidence of malaria, it has been postulated that G-6-PD deficiency confers some resistance against the malarial parasite.[104]

When a patient with G-6-PD deficiency is exposed to an oxidant drug or some other type of oxidant stress, the following sequence of events occurs: acute hemolysis is evident between the second and fourth day and is accompanied by hemoglobinuria. The hematocrit continues to fall for 7 to 12 days and approximately 30 to 50 per cent of the red cell mass is destroyed. During this time Heinz bodies are seen and the bilirubin may be elevated. As the reticulocyte response reaches its peak (around 10 to 12 days) the hematocrit begins to rise again and gradually returns to normal levels in 4 to 5 weeks, even though the offending drug is continued. It has been shown with radioiron labeling that in black patients the older population of red cells are hemolyzed and the younger red cells are relatively resistant to this type of drug-induced hemolysis.[106] This correlates well with G-6-PD activity, which decreases as red cells age.

Table 7–2 lists some of the drugs which have been reported to produce hemolysis in G-6-PD deficient patients. All of these drugs are oxidants in that they have the ability to transport electrons and serve as catalysts in oxidation-reduction reactions. Most of the offending drugs are aromatic amines.[104, 105]

Hemolytic anemia may be precipitated in G-6-PD deficient patients not only by oxidant drugs but also by infection. In a series of hemolytic episodes in G-6-PD deficient patients reviewed by Burka and his colleagues,[114, 115] infection

Table 7–2. Some Drugs Which Produce Hemolysis of G-6-PD-Deficient Red Cells

1. Antimalarials—primaquine, pamaquine
2. Sulfonamides—sulfanilamide, sulfapyridine, sulfisoxazole, sulfamethoxy-pyridazine, sulfacetamide, sulfoxone, salicylazosulfapyridine
3. Nitrofurans—nitrofurantoin, furaltadone (altafur), nitrofurazone
4. Analgesics—acetanilid, acetophenetidin (phenacetin), and aspirin in large doses
5. Diuretics—thiazides, acetazolamide
6. Hypoglycemic agents—tolbutamide, chlorpropamide
7. Miscellaneous—chloramphenicol, para-aminosalicylic acid (PAS), vitamin K, naphthalene (moth balls), fava beans

alone was a more frequent cause of hemolysis than drugs alone. The episodes were associated with both bacterial and viral infections and were particularly common with infectious hepatitis.[145] In addition, diabetic acidosis may induce a hemolytic episode.[127]

Whites from the Mediterranean area and blacks who have G-6-PD deficiency are not anemic and have no difficulty unless they are exposed to oxidative stress. On the other hand, whites of Northern European origin usually have a mild hemolytic anemia at all times which is made worse by oxidants.[138] These patients would have been classified as congenital non-spherocytic hemolytic anemia before the specific red cell enzyme deficit was established.

Laboratory Examination

In the black and the Mediterranean white, routine hematologic tests are normal except during a hemolytic episode brought on by exposure to some oxidant. During that time, signs of hemolysis are present, including hemoglobinuria and bilirubinemia. The red cells usually show Heinz bodies early in the course of the hemolytic episode. In patients with congenital non-spherocytic hemolytic anemia secondary to G-6-PD deficiency, the usual findings of chronic hemolysis are present.

Much of the laboratory evaluation in G-6-PD deficiency has been directed towards detecting individuals with the deficiency in order to avoid exposure to offending agents and to diagnose the cause of acute hemolysis in a likely candidate, such as a black male.

Although a number of screening tests have been proposed, the most useful in the authors' hands have been the methemoglobin reduction test[113] and the cyanide-ascorbate test.[131] The methemoglobin reduction test has the advantage of employing simple reagents, sodium nitrite and methylene blue, and may be read visually. However, it is not sensitive enough to pick up heterozygous females and is often equivocal after an acute hemolytic episode when most of the older red cells with the lowest G-6-PD levels have been lysed. In this situation the test must be repeated several months later. The cyanide-ascorbate test has the advantage of screening not only for G-6-PD deficiency but also for other enzymes in the pentose phosphate shunt–glutathione system; glutathione reductase, glutathione synthetase, and glutathione peroxidase. All of these enzymes are necessary for the effective reduction of the hydrogen peroxide generated by ascorbic acid. The test can also be read visually and has the advantage of detecting most of the heterozygous females. It is also usually positive during an acute hemolytic episode. For these reasons we feel that this is the screening test of choice.

Variants of Glucose-6-Phosphate Dehydrogenase

More than 23 mutants of G-6-PD have been described.[135] Different types of G-6-PD have been distinguished electrophoretically and by enzyme kinetics. The two major electrophoretic types are A^+ and B^+. Whites have only type B^+; 82 per cent of blacks have type B^+ and 18 per cent have A^+. Black females may have both types. Yoshida and his colleagues have shown that the faster moving A^+ differs from B^+ only by the substitution of aspartic acid for asparagine.[163] Whites with G-6-PD deficiency have deficiency of the B^- type. In blacks, although type B^+ is the most common, the common deficiency is of A^- type and rarely of the B^- type. No biochemical difference has been found between A^+ and A^- types except that the A^- type enzyme in deficient blacks is degraded more rapidly than normal. This may account for the older red cells showing the more marked deficiency.

OTHER DEFICIENCIES OF THE PENTOSE PHOSPHATE SHUNT–GLUTATHIONE SYSTEM

Although a number of patients have been described with erythrocyte 6-phosphogluconate dehydrogenase deficiency, sufficient clinical information has not been reported to determine whether they had mild hemolysis or were susceptible to oxidative stress.[111, 112] On the other hand, patients with deficiencies of glutathione reductase[116, 160] glutathione synthetase,[108, 139, 146] and glutathione peroxidase[29, 41] who have chronic hemolytic anemia and susceptibility to oxidants have been reported. These are very rare and probably transmitted as an autosomal recessive, except for glutathione reductase deficiency, which has been reported to be relatively common in Germany, but not in the United States, and is thought to be transmitted as an autosomal dominant.[160] However, Beutler has pointed out that flavin compounds stimulate glutathione reductase activity, and that some patients who were thought to have hereditary glutathione reductase deficiency were in reality suffering from riboflavin deficiency.[105a]

GLYCOLYTIC ENZYME DEFICIENCIES

In 1953 Dacie and his colleagues popularized the concept of the congenital non-spherocytic hemolytic anemias characterized by the absence of spherocytes or abnormal hemoglobin accompanied by normal osmotic fragility of fresh red cells.[122] The next year Selwyn and Dacie divided this group of patients into type I and II based on the autohemolysis test; type I patients had normal or slightly increased autohemolysis which was improved by glucose and type II had increased autohemolysis which was not improved by the addition of glucose.[150] It is apparent now that G-6-PD deficiency corresponds to type I and pyruvate kinase deficiency to type II. As more specific enzyme deficiencies become delineated in patients with hereditary hemolytic anemia, the descriptive term "congenital non-spherocytic hemolytic anemia" should drop from usage.[123]

Pyruvate Kinase Deficiency

In 1961, Valentine and his associates[156] demonstrated a deficiency in red cell pyruvate kinase to be the cause of hereditary hemolytic anemia corresponding generally to the type II congenital non-spherocytic hemolytic anemia described by Dacie. This was the first time a specific enzyme defect had been discovered in the main pathway of glycolysis, the Embden-Meyerhof pathway. It is the most common of the glycolytic enzyme deficiencies associated with hemolytic anemia. Over 95 documented cases have been reported.[110, 133, 144, 151, 152, 158]

The patients have ranged in age from birth to 65 and have been predominantly of Northern European ancestry. The deficiency is transmitted as an autosomal recessive, with heterozygous family members having about half the normal amount of enzyme activity but showing no signs of disease. The great variation in the severity of the anemia in homozygous patients suggests genetic polymorphism, but this has not been clearly established.[130] Splenectomy often ameliorates the anemia, particularly in severe cases, although the hemolytic anemia persists at a lesser degree of severity.

Osmotic fragility of fresh erythrocytes is normal but increases greatly after incubation. Auto-hemolysis is markedly abnormal and is not improved by the addition of glucose, but it is lessened by adding ATP. The reticulocyte count is often between 20 and 50 per cent, and may be even higher after splenectomy. In the more severe cases the erythrocyte membrane appears to be damaged, with crenated red cells that resemble acanthocytes appearing on the peripheral blood smear.[141]

Although most patients with pyruvate kinase deficiency hemolytic anemia have low red cell ATP levels as a result of their metabolic block, the severity of the anemia does not correlate well with ATP levels and the specific sequence of biochemical events leading to red cell destruction remains to be clarified.[130, 155]

OTHER GLYCOLYTIC ENZYME DEFICIENCIES

Since pyruvate kinase deficiency hemolytic anemia was described in 1961, patients with hereditary hemolytic anemia secondary to seven additional enzyme deficiencies involving the anaerobic glycolytic pathway have been described: 2,3-diphosphoglyceromutase,[109, 137, 149] triosephosphate isomerase,[147, 148] hexokinase,[134, 140, 157] glucosephosphate isomerase,[103, 143] phosphoglycerate kinase,[136, 156] phosphofructokinase,[153, 162] and glyceraldehyde-3-phosphate dehydrogenase.[142] The position of these enzymes in the Embden-Meyerhof pathway is shown in Figure 7–3. In addition to these glycolytic enzymes, a deficiency in red cell ATPase, a membrane enzyme, has also been reported as a cause of hemolytic anemia.[121, 128]

Most of these enzyme deficiencies have been shown to be transmitted as an autosomal recessive and are consequently rare, there being only a few families reported with each type of deficiency. The hereditary erythrocyte enzyme deficiencies have recently been reviewed by Jaffé.[132]

HEMOGLOBINOPATHIES

More than 100 abnormal hemoglobins have been described in man, but relatively few have been associated with clinical disease. Heller has proposed a classification of the hemoglobinopathies based on their functional characteristics.[279]

Group 1. Abnormal hemoglobins without physiologic aberrations. This constitutes the largest group and although these hemoglobin mutants are of genetic and biochemical interest they are without clinical significance.

Group 2. "Aggregating" hemoglobins. Hemoglobins S and C fall into this group, as structural changes occur in the red cell because of tactoid formation of hemoglobin S and crystal formation of hemoglobin C.

Group 3. "Unbalanced" synthesis of hemoglobins. This group consists of the thalassemia syndromes in which one type of hemoglobin chain is synthesized in excess of other hemoglobin chains, with the excess chains precipitating as Heinz bodies.

Group 4. Unstable hemoglobins. These hemoglobins, which usually involve an amino acid substitution in the region of heme attachment, are susceptible to oxidative denaturation with precipitation as Heinz bodies. Hemoglobins Zurich, Köln, Seattle, and many others belong to this group.

Group 5. Hemoglobins with abnormal heme function. This group includes the M hemoglobins that are associated with methemoglobinemia; hemoglobins Chesapeake, Rainier, and others which have an increased affinity for oxygen with compensatory polycythemia; and hemoglobin Kansas and others which have a decreased affinity for oxygen.

Sickle Cell Anemia

History

The first case of sickle cell anemia was described by Herrick in 1910.[190] This patient, a 20 year old male black from the West Indies, had most of the classic clinical and hematologic features of the disease. In addition to the usual morphology of many of his erythrocytes, which had the shape of a sickle, this patient had cardiac enlargement, icterus, anemia, normoblasts in the peripheral blood, and leukocytosis. Huck established the fact that the sickling property resides in the cell and not in the plasma.[194] Ponder showed that red cells washed free of hemoglobin do not sickle[220] and Harris showed that stroma-free solutions of deoxygenated sickle hemoglobin form sickle tactoids.[186] Hahn and Gillespie demonstrated that sickling is a reversible reaction related to the degree of oxygenation of the hemoglobin in the erythrocyte.[185] A most important contribution was made by Pauling, Itano, Singer, and Wells in 1949 when they established that sickle cell anemia is a molecular disease.[215, 216] They demonstrated that hemoglobin obtained from patients with sickle cell anemia differed electrophoretically from that present in erythrocytes of normal individuals and concluded that the abnormality resided in the protein portion of the molecule. The nature of the defect was further characterized by Ingram, who showed that the molecule of sickle cell hemoglobin differs from a molecule of normal hemoglobin only by having glutamic acid replaced by valine in the beta chain.[196] The studies of Neel and others have shown that the molecular abnormality of hemoglobin is genetically controlled.[169, 212, 213] The complete amino acid sequence of the alpha and beta chains of sickle and normal hemoglobin have been described.[192]

Mechanism of the Anemia

The sickling property is a gene-transmitted abnormality that is heterozygous in persons with sickle cell trait and homozygous in individuals with sickle cell anemia.[169, 212, 213] The consequence of this defect is found in the globin portion of the hemoglobin molecule and not in the heme portion.[215, 216] Sickle cell hemoglobin and normal hemoglobin differ in that the beta peptide chain in each half of the sickle cell hemoglobin molecule contains valine in the sixth position, where glutamic acid is found in normal hemoglobin.[196] Thus it appears that of almost 300 amino acids present in each half of the hemoglobin molecule, hemoglobin S and hemoglobin A differ in only one amino acid. The substitution of valine for glutamic acid with the resultant loss of the carboxyl group explains the electrophoretic differences in these two hemoglobins. In addition, efforts have been made to explain the unusual chemical and clinical manifestations of the disease by this molecular peculiarity.

The sickle cell hemoglobin tends to polymerize and form tactoids under conditions of lowered oxygen tension[219] and lowered pH.[186] Sickling of erythrocytes is reversible and thought to be the result of realignment of the hemoglobin molecules in the cell envelope rather than the actual crystallization of the hemoglobin molecules.[186] Murayama, using scale models of the hemoglobin molecule, has proposed the following explanation for the molecular stacking of deoxgenated S hemoglobin. The substitution of valine for glutamic acid in the sixth position of the beta chain allows an intramolecular hydrophobic bond to form betweed the valines in the first and sixth positions at the amino terminal end of the beta chain. This cyclization of the two ends of the beta chain forms a "key" arrangement which fits into a complementary site in the alpha chains of an adjacent molecule so that molecular stacking occurs. When S hemoglobin is oxygenated, the two beta chains move closer together by approximately 7 Å leading to disruption of the "lock" and "key" arrangement and unsickling of the S hemoglobin. Based on electron microscopy, Murayama has also proposed that when hemoglobin S sickles, microtubules are formed, consisting of six monofilaments of hemoglobin twisted around a hollow center.[210, 211]

Erythrocytes from patients with sickle cell anemia will sickle in the physiologic ranges of oxygen concentration, but a marked lowering of the oxygen tension is necessary to produce sickling in individuals with the sickle cell trait. It has been assumed that this difference between erythrocytes that contain only sickle hemoglobin and those that contain both normal and sickle hemoglobin forms the basis for the different clinical manifestations of sickle cell anemia and sickle cell trait. Individuals who have the sickle cell trait are essentially asymptomatic and remain so unless the oxygen saturation of the blood is reduced to an abnormal degree or acidosis develops. Patients who are homozygous for hemoglobin S have sickle cell anemia, a chronic illness characterized by anemia and the occurrence of infarctions in various organs of the body.

The anemia, which is hemolytic in type, is the result of the intracorpuscular defect. Erythrocytes from normal individuals survive for about 120 days when transfused into patients with sickle cell anemia, but erythrocytes from patients with sickle cell anemia have a much shorter survival time when transfused into normal recipients. Studies that utilized the analysis of N^{15}-hemin disappearance and fecal stercobilin N[15] appearance indicate complete random destruction of the red cells, a shortened survival time of the erythrocytes (16 days in one patient), and no evidence of more than one population of cells.[197] It has been suggested that the excessive destruction of the erythrocytes is the result of the increase in mechanical fragility that has been demonstrated when the erythrocytes assume the sickle cell form.[186] According to this explanation, the erythrocytes become sickled under the oxygen tensions that occur in the body normally and in this form both the mechanical fragility of the cells and the amount of trauma that they encounter in the circulation are increased.

A serious complication of sickle cell anemia is the "hypoplastic or aregenerative crisis."[227] Systemic infections may depress erythropoiesis and although they are of little note in persons with a normal red cell life span, they may be life-threatening in patients with a shortened red cell life span. The transient marrow aplasia may be responsible for a sudden increase in the severity of the anemia.

The development of the lesions that occur in the various organs of the body is usually attributed to thrombosis and infarction or to ischemic necrosis and hemorrhage;[178, 203] either ischemia or thrombosis would be favored by the packing and stasis of the sickle shaped erythrocytes in the capillaries under conditions of lowered oxygen tension. It has been suggested that the assumption of the sickle form is associated with an increase in viscosity which leads to a "vicious cycle" of increased deoxygenation, increased sickling, and increased stasis.[184]

Clinical Manifestations

Sickle cell trait and sickle cell anemia have been found almost entirely in the black race. The incidence of the sickling trait varies in different parts of the world and is about 9 per cent in American blacks. Sickle cell anemia has a frequency of about one-fortieth that of the trait.[209]

Sickle cell anemia is characterized by the occurrence of symptoms in virtually any part of the body. These symptoms are sometimes bizarre and vary greatly from patient to patient and from time to time in the same patient. Most patients with sickle cell anemia, both children and adults, continue in a mild state of chronic illness with stable levels of erythrocytes and serum bilirubin, but nearly all patients at one time or another experience episodes of more severe symptoms, the attacks of so-called "crisis." Different types of attacks have been described as "crisis."

The aregenerative type of hypoplastic crisis, manifested by erythrocytic hypoplasia or aplasia in the marrow, marked decrease in the number of reticulocytes in the circulating blood, and a rapidly increasing anemia, usually follows bacterial or viral infection and need not be associated with any pain. The factors which are responsible for the bone marrow failure, which often is associated with a precipitous fall in the hemoglobin level, are not understood. The authors have observed the same patient with sickle cell anemia during several attacks of pneumonoccal pneumonia; on some occasions a hypoplastic crisis developed and at other times pneumococcal pneumonia was not associated with significant change in the values of the circulating blood.

Another type of attack called "crisis" is that associated with localizing signs of disease. These are thought to be the result of erythrostasis and anoxia or infarction. Infarction of the spleen, kidney, bone, and lungs and localized neurologic lesions are examples of this type. Patients with sickle cell anemia also have other illnesses, such as acute appendicitis, renal colic, and gall bladder disease, that must be distinguished from the episodes of "crisis."

A third type of painful "crisis" is the most puzzling of all. The onset is quite sudden and may occur when a patient awakes in the morning or after an afternoon nap. The attack usually begins with aching pain in one or both knees or legs. It increases steadily in severity and in extent and often progresses to the back, the abdomen, both arms, the neck, and the head. The pain may involve almost the entire body within 10 minutes or after several hours; at times it does not progress beyond one or several extremities, or one side of the body. Sometimes the attacks are mild and last but a day or two. More often the pain is severe and may not be completely relieved by aspirin or narcotics. The frequency of these attacks varies greatly; attacks occur in some patients every few weeks, in some several times a year, and in others only at intervals of years. Nearly all patients emphasize the suddenness of the onset of the attack. Respiratory infections, insect bites, fever, a feeling of nervousness, and various indications precede some attacks, but in others the patient feels perfectly well and is engaged in nothing more strenuous than talking with members of the family when the attack begins abruptly. Fever is not invariably present, peripheral blood counts remain unchanged and the patient manifests no cyanosis, shock, or localized vascular insufficiency.

The most common cutaneous manifestations of the disease are indolent ulcers or scars on the lower legs, which can be found on about 75 per cent of the older children or adults with the disease. Ulceration is rare in very young children.[85] The ulcers, which have sharply defined edges, are usually single but may be multiple and bilateral (Fig. 7–4).

Various types of cardiac abnormalities have been reported in from 50 to 91 per cent of the patients.[165, 229] The commonest of these is an apical systolic murmur which occurs in the majority. Although they are rare, mitral, aortic, and pulmonic diastolic murmurs have been reported. Cardiac enlargement, which often involves both ventricles, is a common finding and has been attributed to the chronic anemia.[230] Cor pulmonale occurs in some patients, possibly as a result of repeated pulmonary infarctions and pulmonary hypertension.[201, 230] Electrocardiographic abnormalities, such as a prolonged PR interval and minor changes in the ST segment and T wave, occur but are non-specific.

Symptoms referable to the genitourinary tract are not common but may be dramatic and serious. Episodes of hematuria may occur as a complication of both sickle cell trait and sickle cell disease.[204, 164] The bleeding is usually unilateral and recurrent and may be marked. Some patients have been operated upon for suspected tumor because of unilateral hematuria associated with an abnormal intravenous pyelogram. A defect in the capacity of the kidney to concentrate the urine has been noted in most patients with sickle cell anemia and in many with sickle cell trait.[202, 218, 227a] The defect may be temporarily corrected by transfusion with normal red blood cells in young patients, but this is not often true in adults who have had time to develop irreversible structural damage to the renal

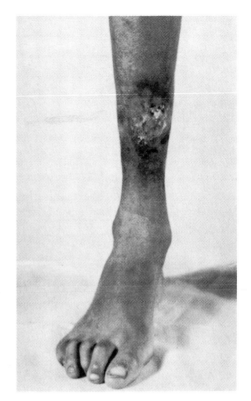

Figure 7-4. Typical leg ulcer in sickle cell anemia.

medulla. The pathogenesis of hematuria and hyposthenuria is incompletely understood. Sickling of the erythrocytes of patients with sickle cell disease and sickle cell trait is thought to occur in the medullary capillaries as the result of a combination of reduced oxygen tension and hyperosmolality (and perhaps reduced pH). The resulting engorgement and vascular obstruction is particularly evident in the peritubular areas and local ischemia is believed to lead to degeneration of the tubular epithelium, extravasation of blood around the collecting tubules, and in some instances to papillary necrosis.[164, 186, 218] Chronic renal insufficiency may occasionally be seen in older patients. Glomerular congestion and enlargement early in the course of the disease, followed by progressive ischemia, fibrosis and obliteration of the glomeruli, is believed responsible for the progressive decline in glomerular filtration rate late in the course of the disorder.[171]

Priapism has been reported in a number of patients; it sometimes persists from 10 to 36 days and is often followed by complete impotence.

Nearly all patients with sickle cell anemia at one time or another complain of gastrointestinal symptoms such as anorexia, nausea, vomiting, or jaundice. Severe pain may occur in any part of the abdomen and at times it is difficult to decide whether surgical intervention is indicated. Such pains may be due to infarction of the spleen or some other organ, or may be related to cholelithiasis, which has been reported to have an incidence of 25 per cent. In a group of 47 patients ranging in age from 12 to 58 years old with sickle cell anemia, study suggested that one-third of the patients over 10 years of age had gall stones and chronic cholecystitis although less than 10 per cent had signs or symptoms attributable to this complication.[168] Elective cholecystectomy has been recommended in patients who have gall stones because the risk of operation does not seem great and it is difficult to distinguish jaundice with cholangitis and gall stones from that caused by sickling and hepatic stasis.[168] Some patients with sickle cell anemia develop right upper quadrant pain, tenderness, rapid and marked enlargement of the liver, and greatly elevated direct-acting serum bilirubin. In such patients it may be difficult to decide whether it is an attack of severe fulminating hepatitis, possibly from transfusions, hepatic vein thrombosis, or generalized hepatic congestion with sickle cells that has developed.

A wide variety of central nervous system manifestations has been reported in patients of all ages.[195] These include hemiplegia, aphasia, dysphagia, nystagmus, drowsiness, coma, headache, convulsions, and stiff neck. Electroencephalographic abnormalities are common in children.[191] Evidence of the neurologic involvement may subside completely, but some patients die during these episodes and others develop a spastic paralysis that persists. The lesions in the central nervous system are presumed to be the result of vascular accidents or circulatory disturbances of a transient nature.

Characteristic conjunctival vascular abnormalities consisting of comma-shaped capillary segments seemingly isolated from the rest of the vascular network are often seen with a hand lens or slit lamp in patients with sickle cell anemia.[182, 214] Funduscopic examination of the retina of patients with sickle cell anemia or sickle cell trait may reveal marked tortuosity and dilatation of the retinal vessels (Fig. 7–5). In addition, one may find neovascularization and microaneurysms, stasis, or thrombosis of retinal vessels and retinal hemorrhages.[206]

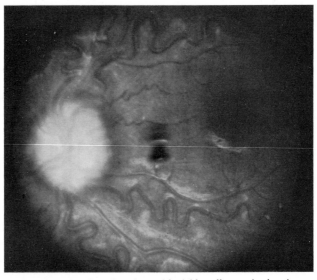

Figure 7–5. Ophthalmic fundus of patient with sickle cell anemia showing marked tortuosity and dilatation of retinal vessels.

Sickle cell anemia is often accompanied by symptoms or signs referable to the joints and skeleton. Pain in the joints is common, but actual swelling of the joints is rare. Skeletal abnormalities are usually demonstrable only by roentgenograms; the commonest manifestations are "fish tailing" of the vertebral bodies and radiolucent areas of necrosis in these or other bones.[179, 207] The "hair on end" appearance of the skull sometimes occurs but is not common. Other abnormalities that can be demonstrated radiologically in some patients are gallstones, pulmonary infarcts, and cardiac enlargement. In young children attacks of dactylitis, particularly in the hands, are common.

Bone marrow infarction, recognized by the necrotic appearance of the marrow aspirate, has long been considered a possible source of pulmonary and cerebral emboli; more recently it has been suspected to be a cause of painful crisis.[174a]

Sickle cell anemia in infants is an especially serious disease. In one report, 10 of 64 patients died during the first year of life; the causes of death were pneumonia, crisis, sepsis with meningococcus, pseudomonas, and salmonella organisms, and diarrhea.[221] The disease was first manifested by dactylitis, particularly in the hands but also in the feet, with or without any x-ray abnormalities, infection, crisis, and with non-specific symptoms termed a "failure to thrive." Fulminant pneumococcemia may terminate fatally within a few hours after onset.[200] Predisposing factors may be a deficiency of pneumococcal serum opsonizing activity[228] and functional asplenia,[217] which have been reported in sickle cell anemia. Intravascular coagulation has been present in some of the children with septicemia. Sudden death in children also occurs during crisis.[198] Extreme pallor, weakness, lethargy, tachycardia, and cold clammy skin are the most common manifestations of shock. The principal finding at autopsy has been severe congestion of internal organs, especially the liver and spleen, with sickled erythrocytes.

Although the presence of sickle cell trait usually is associated with no manifestation of disease, important exceptions occur. Hematuria, which may be persistent and very troublesome, occurs in patients with sickle cell trait. Patients with sickle cell trait flying at high altitudes have developed splenic infarction; others have died suddenly while involved in very strenuous physical exercise.[199] In the last two conditions, anoxia, dehydration, and acidosis are probably responsible for the attacks.

Salmonella osteomyelitis has been reported in a number of patients with sickle cell anemia and it has been established that there is an increased incidence of this infection in the disease.[193a] Bacteremia and multiple foci of involvement, particularly in the long bones, occur. Pus may collect beneath the skin or in the joints after spontaneous rupture of a subperiosteal abscess through the periosteum. The reason for the increased susceptibility of patients with sickle cell anemia is not clear; a possible factor may be that the macrophages have a diminished capacity to phagocytize and kill salmonella organisms as a result of erythrophagocytosis by the reticuloendothelial cells.[182a, 201a] Local ischemia or infarction and splenic atrophy with functional asplenia may also be important.

Functional asplenia, possibly the result of a diversion of splenic blood flow through intravascular shunts, has been reported in children with splenomegaly; splenic function was restored when transfusions raised the level of normal cells to 50 per cent, probably by reducing the blood viscosity.[216a]

Laboratory Examination

In the usual patient with sickle cell anemia the hemoglobin and erythrocyte count are reduced to about half the normal values. The anemia is normocytic and normochromic unless complicating factors are present. On the stained smear of peripheral blood a few sickled forms may be seen but the most prominent features are marked anisocytosis, poikilocytosis, and the presence of target cells; nucleated red cells are often present (Fig. 7–6). Fragmented cells and other abnormalities usually seen in impact hemolysis have been observed in patients with sickle cell anemia and pulmonary emboli.[167] The leukocyte count is usually between 12,000 and 16,000 per cu.mm.; the reported counts have ranged from 4000 to 69,000 per cu.mm.[189, 225] The platelet count is usually normal but counts over 1,000,000 per cu.mm. sometimes occur.

The laboratory evidences of a hemolytic process are found unless a hypoplastic phase is present. The reticulocyte count is often over 20 per cent and although the level of the indirect reacting bilirubin in the serum is increased, it usually does not exceed 3.0 mg. per 100 ml. unless there is some associated hepatic or biliary complication. Fecal urobilinogen excretion is increased, and average daily excretions between 200 and 750 mg. have been reported.[222, 223] The daily fecal urobilinogen excretion varies spontaneously and decreases after transfusions of whole blood. The plasma iron level is normal or elevated and the latent iron binding capacity is normal.

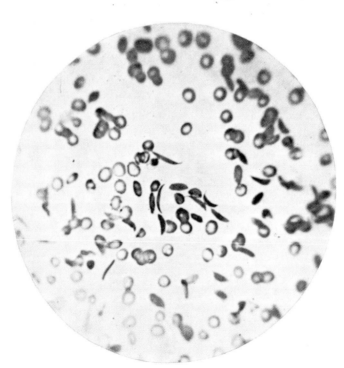

Figure 7–6. Erythrocytes in sickle cell anemia; Wright's stain. (Courtesy of Dr. B. E. Washburn and the Virginia Medical Monthly, vol. 15, 1911.)

Examination of the bone marrow usually reveals erythrocytic hyperplasia of the normoblastic type associated with hyperplasia of the myeloid cells. Occasionally, a long-continued marrow hyperplasia leads to folate deficiency which may be manifested by the megaloblastic type of erythropoiesis. During a hypoplastic crisis, acute transient marrow aplasia has been reported. Sickling of the adult erythrocytes and of the nucleated red cells may be observed in material obtained from the marrow. Long filamentous erythrocytes are observed more often in the marrow preparations than in preparations made from the peripheral blood.

The sedimentation rate in patients whose red cells sickle is not increased as much as is usually the case in patients with a comparable degree of anemia. Prolonged stasis of venous blood causes an increased retardation of the sedimentation rate.

The erythrocytes of sickle cell anemia are abnormally resistant to hypotonic saline; in one series the average figure for beginning hemolysis was 0.35 per cent and for completion was 0.22 per cent.[177a] Some of the cells are not hemolyzed in distilled water. The mechanical fragility of the cells is normal when they are in the discoid form but becomes increased if sickling is produced by exposure to carbon dioxide.[177]

The characteristic sickling phenomenon can be demonstrated in moist sealed cover slip preparations that were first introduced by Emmel.[181] The undesirable features of the cover slip method are the time required for the sickling to take place, even in patients with sickle cell anemia, and the occurrence of false negative results. At least 14 other tests that produce sickling have been described.[205] The sodium metabisulfite method has proved to be satisfactory in our experience (Fig. 7–7).[384] The use of hemoglobin electrophoresis has proved to be essential in distinguishing patients with sickle cell anemia from those who have the sickle cell trait combined with some unrelated anemia, and from those patients who are heterozygous for two abnormal hemoglobins.[291]

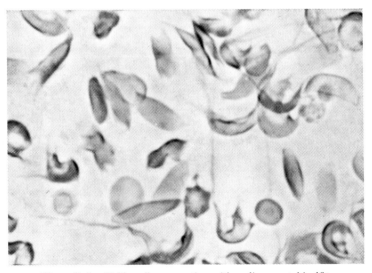

Figure 7–7. Sickle cell preparation with sodium metabisulfite.

Differential Diagnosis

There is usually no difficulty in establishing the diagnosis of sickle cell anemia if the possibility is considered. A positive test for sickling indicates that the individual has either the heterozygous sickling trait or sickle cell anemia. The demonstration of the sickling phenomenon in a patient who has anemia does not establish the diagnosis of sickle cell anemia because the sickle cell trait is common in blacks who may have anemia from some other cause. An incorrect diagnosis of sickle cell anemia may be made in patients with sickle cell trait who have chronic blood loss or pernicious anemia, unless proper studies are carried out. Unless the patient has been transfused recently, the diagnosis of sickle cell anemia can nearly always be established or excluded by hemoglobin electrophoresis. The discovery of a relatively mild degree of anemia associated with a positive sickling test in a patient who has significant splenomegaly should arouse the suspicion that the patient has a combination of sickle cell trait plus some other hemoglobin abnormality, such as hemoglobin C, rather than sickle cell anemia. Hemoglobin electrophoresis is the most valuable method of distinguishing sickle cell anemia from sickle cell–hemoglobin C disease and other disorders that are due to the occurrence of sickle cell hemoglobin with some other abnormal hemoglobin. When the second amino acid substitution of hemoglobin Memphis occurs in conjunction with homozygous hemoglobin S, there is an ameliorating effect on the blood viscosity of sickle cell disease so that painful crises are rare.[284] Amino acid analysis is necessary to establish the diagnosis, since the electrophoretic pattern is that of homozygous hemoglobin S.[283, 284]

If the diagnosis of sickle cell anemia is not considered the disease may be mistaken for acute rheumatic fever when the patient presents with anemia, joint complaints, fever, cardiac enlargement, and cardiac murmurs. The absence of the severe pains, swelling, and tenderness of the joints that are usually seen in rheumatic fever may help to distinguish between these two diseases. In other patients with signs of acute intra-abdominal disease, it may be difficult to make the correct diagnosis because patients with sickle cell anemia sometimes develop acute surgical emergencies just as any other patients do, but also they develop signs of acute intra-abdominal disease as the result of sickle cell anemia alone. Both possibilities must be considered when the patient is seen and the decision must be made on the basis of the evidence available at that time. Sickle cell anemia must be differentiated from other diseases that cause ulcers of the extremities and from those that produce symptoms or signs of involvement of the central nervous system. Sickle cell anemia has been confused at times with rheumatoid arthritis, osteomyelitis, poliomyelitis, meningitis, cerebrovascular accident, infectious hepatitis, and other diseases.[205]

Course and Prognosis

Sickle cell anemia is a serious disorder and few patients survive the third decade. Many patients die during childhood. Rarely will a patient live to a ripe old age.[175] Death comes most often from infections such as pneumonia and chronic pyelonephritis with renal failure. Other causes of death are heart failure, bone marrow and fat emboli,[225] shock with abdominal crisis, complications in the central nervous system, tuberculosis, and sarcoidosis.[183, 193]

The occurrence of pregnancy has been considered a serious matter in the patients with sickle cell anemia who reach the childbearing age. The incidence of spontaneous abortion, stillbirth, and death soon after birth is probably increased. Hazards to the mother are heart failure, pulmonary embolism, shock, cerebrovascular accidents, and uremia.[205] Pyelonephritis occurs frequently. Pregnancy appears to be a greater problem in sickle cell–hemoglobin C disease than in sickle cell anemia.[227b]

In some patients with sickle cell anemia physical development is greatly retarded and hypogonadism occurs. In other patients the growth and development seem to follow a normal pattern. The reason for these differences in patients with sickle cell anemia is not apparent, but the differences in development are not due solely to differences in the severity of the anemia.

Treatment

The treatment of sickle cell anemia is generally unsatisfactory. Transfusions are the only means of returning the blood to normal levels that are available at present. Transfusions are not used to maintain the blood in the normal range because patients with this disease adjust very well to their lowered hemoglobin levels. Transfusions are valuable during periods of aplastic crisis, abdominal crisis, and at any other time when the patient is severely ill. They are also advantageous in carrying patients through pregnancy or operations, because multiple transfusions depress erythropoiesis and reduce the number and percentage of sickle cells in the peripheral circulation (Fig. 7–8).[180] Partial exchange transfusions which combine the removal of the patient's blood with replacement of normal packed cells raise the hemoglobin level and lower the concentration of sickle cells more quickly than transfusion alone. Exchange is particularly desirable in patients who have frank or incipient heart failure and can be accomplished without an increase in blood volume. Whether or not such a treatment will, when carried out at regular intervals, reduce the frequency of attacks of crisis remains uncertain. The value of these measures in crisis and in pregnancy has been confirmed by several reports.[172, 224]

Splenectomy is sometimes beneficial in children. The beneficial effect seems to be related to the size of the spleen.[226] In most adults with the disease the spleen is markedly reduced in size, probably because of repeated infarctions, and splenectomy has little place in the treatment.

Various measures have been used in an effort to reduce the sickling and thereby relieve or reduce the severity of the clinical symptoms in these patients. In this category are cortisone, ACTH, tolazoline, sodium bicarbonate, acetazolamide and urea. None of these agents can be considered to be of proven value at the present time. Double blind trials have failed to show any value of phenothiazine[208] or low molecular weight dextran.[166]

Patients are often critically ill during episodes of "crisis." At such times blood transfusions, antibiotics, and measures to relieve pain are necessary. The short-term use of antibiotics appears justified even though the presence of an

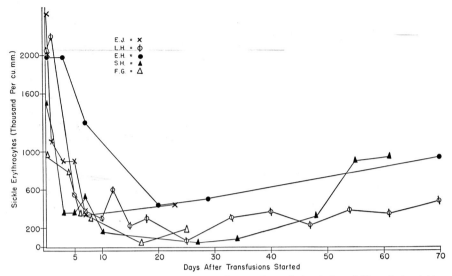

Figure 7–8. The effect of transfusion on the number of circulating sickle cells in sickle cell anemia. (From Donegan, MacIlwaine, and Leavell: Am. J. Med., vol. 17, 1954.)

infection cannot be established, because these episodes are so often preceded by an infection. Oxygen is of no value in the treatment of sickle cell crisis unless pulmonary disease is present, because the hemoglobin is fully oxygenated in the lungs.

It has been pointed out recently that the hyposthenuria associated with sickle cell disease and sickle cell trait requires careful attention to fluid balance. Clinical hydration is maintained as long as free access to fluids is allowed and no stressful situation occurs. Negative water balance may occur early in the course of sickle cell crisis and will respond to fluid therapy. The possible role of negative fluid balance in sickle cell crisis remains to be determined.[188]

Hematuria should be treated conservatively with blood replacements as needed. Surgery should be avoided.

Priapism, a painfully serious complication that often leads to impotence, has been treated successfully in at least two patients with a derivative of venom of the pit viper (Arvin), which leads to defibrination.[170]

In view of the fact that treatment has not been very effective in sickle cell anemia, more emphasis should be placed on its possible prevention. Scott has pointed out that although this disease occurs once in 500 births in blacks and has a median survival of only 20 years, relatively little attention has been given to public education of the populations affected.[225a] Because of the availability of simple tests to detect those with sickle cell trait, it should be possible to greatly reduce the incidence of the disease by education and genetic counseling.

Illustrative Case

This patient, a male black, was first admitted to the hospital at the age of 12 because of fever, cough, and pleuritic pain of 1 week's duration. For some years he had been troubled with recurring chronic ulcers in the lower tibial region. A brother 10 years of age had a similar illness characterized by recurring attacks of fever and chronic ulceration of the legs. One sister had died 10 days previously of unknown cause. The patient's father, mother, and four siblings were alive and well.

Physical examination. Temperature 105, pulse 120, respirations 26, and blood pressure 105/55. The patient was alert, thin, and appeared acutely ill. The veins in both fundi were extremely tortuous. A systolic murmur was present. Above the left internal malleolus there was an ulcer 4 cm. in diameter.

Laboratory examination. Admission blood studies: Hb. 4.0 gm. per 100 ml., R.B.C. 1.4 mil. per cu.mm., W.B.C. 22,000 per cu.mm., reticulocytes 0.1 per cent. The leukocyte differential count was normal but a few sickled erythrocytes and many target cells were present on the fixed stained smear. A moist coverslip preparation was positive for sickling. A chest roentgenogram showed increased bronchial markings and an infiltrate in the left lower lobe.

Treatment and course. A diagnosis of sickle cell anemia with pneumonia was made. The patient was given blood transfusions and penicillin and made an uneventful recovery. Before discharge from the hospital on the sixteenth day, the leukocyte count had fallen to 11,000 per cu.mm. and the reticulocyte count had risen to 5.4 per cent despite numerous transfusions.

This patient was observed for 8 years, during which time his course was characterized by chronic ill health and exacerbations of acute illnesses. The erythrocyte count was usually in the range of 1.5 to 2.0 mil. per cu.mm. and the reticulocyte count was usually 25 or 30 per cent. The growth and development were subnormal. The extremities were long and thin, the trunk was short, and no secondary sex characteristics developed. At the age of 20 he weighed but 80 pounds and appeared to be about 10 years of age. He was hospitalized on four occasions because of pneumonia. In some of these attacks the reticulocyte count was 0.1 per cent and the serum bilirubin was less than 1.0 mg. per 100 ml.; in others the reticulocyte count was 18 per cent and the serum bilirubin was 3.0 mg. per 100 ml. Repeated roentgenograms revealed progressive enlargement of the heart. In December 1954 when he was 21 years old this patient was hospitalized with congestive heart failure and severe anemia. He failed to respond to the usual measures and died in acute heart failure.

Postmortem. The testes appeared to be prepubertal, and a section through the prostate gland disclosed only a few glands that appeared immature. The heart was moderately hypertrophied. The right atrium and ventricle were markedly dilated. The pulmonary artery was greatly dilated from its point of origin, but no thrombi were demonstrated in the larger branches. Microscopic examination of the lungs disclosed emphysema, thickening of the walls of the smaller pulmonary arteries that produced complete obliteration of the lumen in some areas, and multiple small granulomatous lesions. The lymph nodes from various parts of the body were enlarged and contained innumerable discrete epithelioid cell granulomas. These granulomatous lesions were diagnosed as Boeck's sarcoid. The spleen was scarred and contracted and weighed only 28 grams. The bone marrow was hyperplastic.

Comment.   Many of the commonest features of sickle cell anemia
were evident in this young black who had a severe hemolytic anemia,
chronic ill health, and retarded physical development. He had ulcerations of the lower legs, a systolic murmur over the precordium, and a
tortuous "corkscrew" appearance of the retinal veins. During his first
admission he apparently had an episode of "aplastic crisis." Other
attacks of pneumonia of equal severity did not produce such depression of the bone marrow. He died at the age of 21 of heart failure
associated with cor pulmonale. As is often the case, the spleen was
scarred and smaller than normal. The presence of Boeck's sarcoid that
was demonstrated at the postmortem examination was not suspected
ante mortem.

Homozygous Hemoglobin C Disease

Hemoglobin C was first described by Itano and Neel.[281] Instances of homozygous hemoglobin C disease have been reported by a number of observers.[276,]
[289, 292, 294, 296] The disease occurs almost exclusively in blacks, in whom the
incidence of hemoglobin C trait has been found to be about 2 or 3 per cent.[291]
The patients that have been reported have presented a fairly uniform clinical
picture characterized by splenomegaly, mild or moderately severe hemolytic
anemia, and recurrent jaundice. A report of the disease in one patient who was
74 years of age indicates that the disorder is consistent with a normal life span.[296]

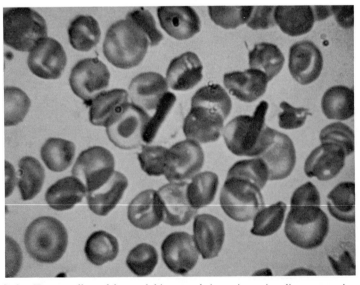

Figure 7-9.   Target cells and hemoglobin crystals in an isotonic saline suspension of erythrocytes from the peripheral blood of a patient with homozygous hemoglobin C disease after splenectomy. Note persistence of the cellular membrane about the hemoglobin crystal in the center of
the picture. (F.S.: I, 21.)

The hemoglobin values in the reported cases have varied from 8.7 to 12.5 gm. per 100 ml.[295] The most prominent feature of the stained smear is the presence of numerous target cells that often constitute from 50 to 100 per cent of the erythrocytes. The osmotic fragility of the red cells is decreased. Hemoglobin electrophoresis discloses the presence of only hemoglobin C. Mild reticulocytosis is often present. The erythrocytes have a decreased life span and the fecal urobilinogen excretion is increased.[295] Intraerythrocytic hemoglobin crystals have been observed in patients, particularly after splenectomy (Fig. 7–9).[276, 296] The mechanism of the anemia is the crystalization of hemoglobin which decreases red cell deformability and increases blood viscosity.[270, 285] The amino acid substitution is lysine for glutamic acid at the sixth position of the amino terminal end of the beta chain.[274]

Thalassemia

Synonyms: Mediterranean Anemia, Cooley's Anemia

History

Archeologic data, based on characteristic skeletal changes, indicate that thalassemia may have originated over 50,000 years ago in a valley south of Italy and Greece now covered by the Mediterranean.[266]

Thalassemia, or "Cooley's anemia", was first recognized as a clinical entity by Cooley and Lee, who described five cases of this disorder in 1925.[237] A similar but much less severe disease found in adolescents and adults was reported in 1940 by Wintrobe, Matthews, Pollack, and Dobyns.[262] As a result of studies on the genetics of the disease, Valentine and Neel concluded that these disorders were related and suggested that the term "thalassemia major" be used to denote the severe form of the disease, which appeared to be the homozygous condition, and the name "thalassemia minor" be given to the milder form, which appeared to be the heterozygous state.[259]

Mechanism of Disease

The thalassemia syndromes may be currently viewed as a result of a biochemical defect in the synthesis of hemoglobin. No amino acid substitution has been demonstrated and the hemoglobin once formed is normal in structure.[244] The explanation for decreased hemoglobin synthesis in thalassemia is unclear, but most likely involves some alteration in the messenger RNA that directs the synthesis of a specific hemoglobin chain.[234, 247, 249, 260, 261] Recent work by Schwartz showing decreased beta chain synthesis in the reticulocytes but not in the nucleated red cells of patients with beta thalassemia suggests an unstable messenger RNA.[255]

Four pairs of genes are responsible for the synthesis of the various subunits of hemoglobin: alpha (α) chains, beta (β) chains, gamma (γ) chains, and delta

(δ) chains. Dimers of these different type chains combine with another type of dimer to form the particular four-chain hemoglobin molecule. In the adult, hemoglobin A ($\alpha_2\beta_2$) accounts for about 95 per cent of the hemoglobin, hemoglobin A$_2$ ($\alpha_2\delta_2$) for 1 to 3 per cent, and hemoglobin F ($\alpha_2\gamma_2$) for less than 2 per cent.[247] A deficiency in the synthesis of any one of these chains may lead to one of the thalassemia syndromes. It is convenient to classify thalassemia by the deficient subunit.

Beta thalassemia. A defect in the synthesis of beta chains is by far the most common type of thalassemia.[260] When the patient inherits the abnormal gene from both parents and is homozygous for the defect, severe anemia, thalassemia major, results. When the patient is heterozygous for the defect, the anemia is mild and is termed thalassemia minor. For reasons which are not entirely clear, some homozygous patients have a milder than usual course and some heterozygous patients have a more severe course than usual. Such patients are said to have thalassemia intermedia.

In thalassemia major there is a marked diminution in beta chain synthesis, and there appears to be a compensatory increase in hemoglobin F, which ranges from 20 to 90 per cent.[247, 260] Most patients with thalassemia minor have normal or only slightly increased hemoglobin F but have a significant increase in hemoglobin A$_2$ in the range of 3 to 7 per cent.[247, 260] A few patients with thalassemia minor have increased hemoglobin F rather than A$_2$ and probably represent a variant.[247, 260]

It is heterozygous beta thalassemia that interacts with other types of beta chain hemoglobinopathies. Such double heterozygotes may synthesize very little hemoglobin A, which results in the clinical picture of the homozygote for the other abnormal hemoglobin. This is the case in sickle cell–thalassemia disease, in which nearly all of the hemoglobin may be hemoglobins S and F.

Another variant of beta thalassemia is hemoglobin Lepore, which is manifested by a mild hypochromic anemia and red cell morphology characteristic of thalassemia.[252] In this circumstance there is not only decreased synthesis of beta chains but also a structural alteration in the beta chain which is an amalgam of the N–terminal end of a delta chain and the C–terminal end of a beta chain.[232] Hemoglobin Lepore is associated with a decrease in hemoglobin A, slight increase in hemoglobin F, and a normal or decreased amount of hemoglobin A$_2$. Hemoglobin Lepore appears to be very similar to hemoglobin Pylos.[241]

Alpha thalassemia. Patients heterozygous for alpha thalassemia have a clinical picture similar to that in heterozygous beta thalassemia, displaying a mild microcytic hypochromic anemia with erythrocytosis and poikilocytosis.[247, 249, 260] They differ from beta thalassemia in that there is no enhanced production of hemoglobin A$_2$ or F because there is diminished production of alpha chains, which those hemoglobins contain.[245] Alpha thalassemia does not interact with beta chain hemoglobinopathies such as hemoglobin S or C but does with hemoglobinopathies involving the alpha chain, hemoglobins I[231] and Q.[238]

Homozygous alpha thalassemia is usually not compatible with life; the infant is stillborn or dies shortly after birth. Studies of the blood of such infants have shown a hemoglobin composed of four gamma chains (γ_4) which is referred to as Bart's hemoglobin. This hemoglobin has virtually no Bohr effect and binds oxygen nearly irreversibly at the oxygen tension of tissues.[243] Infants with alpha thalassemia trait may also have small amounts of Bart's hemoglobin at birth but it disappears as gamma chain synthesis ceases.[239, 243]

Hemoglobin H disease is another form of alpha thalassemia occuring in families with heterozygous alpha thalassemia. The clinical picture most nearly resembles, that of thalassemia intermedia.[242] Hemoglobin H is composed of a tetramer of four beta chains (β_4) and is probably a result of the increased synthesis of beta chains over alpha chains with polymerization of the excess beta chains to form hemoglobin H.[242] This hemoglobin migrates more rapidly than hemoglobin A on starch block electrophoresis and may account for from 10 to 34 per cent of the total hemoglobin.[254] Like Bart's hemoglobin, it has a high affinity for oxygen that inhibits its capacity to deliver oxygen to the tissues.[236, 242] Hemoglobin H is also unstable and susceptible to oxidation with precipitation of hemoglobin into large Heinz bodies which may be seen with supravital stains on blood smears, particularly after splenectomy.

Delta and gamma thalassemia. Although the clinical syndromes of thalassemia consist of the alpha and beta types, a decrease in the synthesis of gamma and delta chains has been described but has no clinical sequelae.[240, 249]

Mechanism of the Anemia

Nathan and his associates[249, 250] have stressed the role of unbalanced hemoglobin synthesis in the pathogenesis of the hemolytic anemia seen in thalassemia. They view the relative overproduction of normal chains as more important as a cause of pathology in thalassemia than the underproduction of other hemoglobin chains. In beta thalassemia the alpha chains, which are produced in excess, polymerize to form an unstable hemoglobin that readily precipitates to form Heinz bodies — the inclusion bodies that have been observed in thalassemic cells.[233, 249] The precipitation of rigid Heinz bodies renders the red cell vulnerable to fragmentation and sequestration in any area of restricted passage in the microcirculation, particularly the spleen.[257] It has also been shown that the precipitation of Heinz bodies in thalassemic red cells causes increased membrane permeability to cations, which aggravates their susceptibility to lysis.[250] In alpha thalassemia, a similar situation exists when excess beta chains polymerize to form hemoglobin H, with subsequent Heinz body formation.

In addition to the increased destruction of thalassemic red cells in the circulation, there is also evidence for ineffective erythropoiesis with destruction of red cell precursors within the bone marrow and defective iron utilization.[260]

Clinical Manifestations

Thalassemia occurs mainly in families of Mediterranean origin, particularly those from Italy, Greece, Sicily, and Syria, but it also is seen in blacks and in Southeast Asia.[248] In a large Italian population in Rochester, N. Y., the incidence of thalassemia minor has been estimated at one in 25 persons, and of thalassemia major as one of 2368 births.[251]

Thalassemia minor, the heterozygous form of the disease, is largely asymptomatic. It is the type seen most often in adults. In its mildest form, which may be found by chance or in the study of the family of a patient with the major form of the disease, the only apparent abnormality in the routine laboratory tests may be the presence of leptocytosis. Other patients with this mild form of the disease have more pronounced hypochromic microcytosis and mild reductions in hemoglobin and hematocrit associated with an elevated red cell count. In patients with thalassemia minor appropriate studies often demonstrate an increased osmotic resistance of the red cells associated with an increase in hemoglobin A_2. Splenomegaly, slight reticulocytosis, and mild icterus are sometimes present. The occurrence of "intermediate" forms of thalassemia with moderately severe anemia is not well understood. It appears likely that many instances of the intermediate form are in reality patients in whom the heterozygous thalassemia gene is associated with some other unrecognized hemoglobin abnormality.

Thalassemia major, the homozygous form of the disease, is a severe disorder that generally becomes manifest early in childhood, nearly always in the first decade. Pallor and easy fatigue often appear in the first few years of life. As the disease progresses the diagnosis may be suggested by the patient's appearance. The head often appears unduly large. The prominence of the malar eminences associated with depression of the bridge of the nose and the muddy yellowish color of the skin was termed "Mongolian" by Cooley and Lee.[237] Marked splenomegaly and hepatomegaly are usually present. The abdomen often protrudes because the spleen may fill the left half of the abdominal cavity. Chronic leg ulcers sometimes occur, but are not common.[256] Evidence of abnormalities of the cardiovascular system in the form of cardiac enlargement, edema, pleural effusions, and ascites is not unusual. Skeletal defects may be prominent but they are not pathognomonic of thalassemia. The changes in the skull consist of a thinning of the inner and outer table associated with a widening of the diploë, which may contain prominent vertical striations that produce the "hair on end" appearance of the skull. Alterations in the long bones, which are less striking, consist of widening of the medullary canals, thinning of the cortices, osteoporosis, and heavy trabeculations near the ends of the shaft. Because of defective iron utilization coupled with increased iron absorption and blood transfusion therapy, iron overload with the clinical picture of hemochromatosis is a common complication.

Thalassemia major must be considered a fatal disease at present because the majority of patients do not survive to adult life. The prognosis appears worse if the disease becomes manifest early in life. Death is usually caused by an intercurrent infection or complications of iron overload.

Laboratory Examination

Thalassemia major is characterized by a microcytic hypochromic type of anemia.[260] The anemia is usually severe but the erythrocyte count may range from 1.0 mil. per cu.mm. to 4.0 mil. per cu.mm. The MCV is often less than 60 to 70 cu. microns. The reduction in the MCHC is not as pronounced as the decrease in the MCH.[256] Stained films of the peripheral blood show a severe degree of poikilocytosis, anisocytosis, and polychromatophilia. The erythrocytes appear small and hypochromic. Many stippled cells and "target" cells are present.

Nucleated red cells, which are almost invariably present, are often numerous and sometimes outnumber the leukocytes. Reticulocytosis is usually present and is accompanied by normoblastic hyperplasia in the bone marrow. Leukocyte counts in the range of 10,000 to 25,000 per cu.mm. are common and immature forms sometimes appear in the peripheral blood. The platelet count is generally normal. (F.S.: I, 16–19.)

In thalassemia minor the erythrocyte count is often normal or increased even though the hemoglobin and hematocrit are reduced. In some such cases there may be a mild reticulocytosis and slight hyperbilirubinemia. Target cells, anisocytosis, poikilocytosis, polychromatophilia, and stippling are evident in the blood smear and are much more prominent than one would expect from the degree of anemia that is present.

Other features common to most hemolytic anemias are usually present in thalassemia major. These are elevation of the indirect reacting bilirubin in the serum, increased excretion of urobilinogen in the feces and urine, elevation of the serum, iron, and decrease in the latent iron binding capacity. In addition, the erythrocytes are abnormally resistant to hemolysis in hypotonic saline; hemolysis may not be complete at 0.2 per cent saline or even in distilled water.

One of the characteristic hematologic features of thalassemia is the presence of large amounts of hemoglobin F.[256] Hemoglobin of this type constitutes from 50 to more than 90 per cent of the hemoglobin in some patients with thalassemia major.[246] The presence of hemoglobin A_2, usually in increased amounts, is found in nearly all patients with thalassemia minor when hemoglobin electrophoresis is performed on starch slabs.[246]

Diagnosis

The appearance of the typical patient with thalassemia major may suggest the diagnosis. In thalassemia major the diagnosis usually is not difficult because of the evident hepatosplenomegaly, the presence of aniso-poikilocytosis, target cells, and normoblasts on the blood smear, evidence of hemolysis, and the presence of increased amounts of hemoglobin F.

Although the diagnosis of thalassemia major is rarely difficult the distinction between the milder forms of thalassemia and other types of hemolytic anemia and hemoglobinopathies is not always easy. The occurrence of hypochromic microcytosis—with or without anemia—target cells, nucleated red cells, and stippled cells in the peripheral blood of a young person with hepatosplenomegaly suggests the diagnosis. At other times, the presenting problem may be a hypochromic microcytic anemia that must be distinguished from iron deficiency. In doubtful cases either the determination of the plasma iron level, which is low in iron deffciency and normal or high in thalassemia, or an evaluation of iron stores in the bone marrow is helpful. The finding of microcytic erythrocytosis in a patient is sometimes the first indication that the patient has thalassemia minor. The demonstration of increased resistance of the erythrocytes in the hypotonic saline test supports the diagnosis. The demonstration of an increase of hemoglobin A_2 by electrophoresis is helpful in establishing the diagnosis. The recognition of the presence of a thalassemia gene in patients who have some other inherited hemoglobinopathy may be very difficult. For example, a person who is heterozygous for hemoglobin S and the thalassemia gene may appear to have sickle cell anemia clinically and show only hemoglobins S and F on electrophoresis because of the suppression of hemoglobin A. Studies of other members of the family may be necessary to establish the true nature of the disorder.

Therapy

Patients with thalassemia minor rarely need treatment. In thalassemia major, blood transfusions are the only effective means of correcting the anemia. The question of how vigorous transfusion therapy should be has not been determined. Some hematologists feel that the hemoglobin should be maintained in the range of 7 gm. per cent to avoid symptoms of anemia and give as few transfusions as possible to avoid adding to the problem of iron overload. Others feel that thalassemic children do better if their hemoglobin level is maintained in the range of 10 gm. per cent. Wolman and others have presented evidence that children whose blood levels are maintained at a level nearer normal have an improved rate of growth, less bone malformation, and decrease in hepatosplenomegaly and cardiomegaly, and in general they are more active and feel better.[235, 253, 263, 265] Although this is accomplished at the expense of increasing the iron burden, this is balanced to some degree by diminished iron absorption and better tissue oxygenation, which may be a factor in the toxicity of iron to tissues.

The removal of excess storage iron by iron chelating agents such as desferrioxamine has been tried by a number of investigators in thalassemic patients. Although initially a significant excretion of chelated iron in the urine occurs, this soon diminishes to the point that the relatively small loss of iron over an extended period does not merit the time, expense, and toxicity of administering chelating agents.[260]

Splenectomy may be helpful in patients in whom significant red cell sequestration by the spleen is demonstrated and in patients in whom marked splenomegaly causes discomfort. Although splenectomy may often decrease the blood transfusion requirement, other clinical problems are not benefited and the patient's life is not prolonged. Also, Smith and his co-workers have emphasized the increased incidence of severe infections after splenectomy, particularly in children under 2 years of age.[258]

Other important features in the management of thalassemia include prompt treatment of infection, which is a frequent complication in this disorder, and folic acid therapy when folic acid deficiency occurs as a result of increased utilization of folate by a hyperactive bone marrow.[260]

Illustrative Case

A 5½ year old white male was admitted to the hospital for transfusion therapy. Anemia, first noted at 4 months of age, was treated with iron. It was not until he was 21 months old that the diagnosis of thalassemia major was established. At that time the hemoglobin was 5.6 gm. per 100 ml., hct. 20 per cent, and reticulocytes 11.5 per cent. There was an increase in both fetal and A₂ hemoglobins. The liver was felt 7 cm. below the right costal margin and the spleen at the level of the iliac crest. A program of blood transfusions every four weeks was instituted in an effort to keep the patient's hemoglobin near normal levels. On this regime the patient did well, with nearly normal growth and development.

Laboratory Examination. At the time of admission to the University of Virginia Hospital, the hemoglobin was 9.0 gm. per cent and hematocrit 25 per cent. Leukocyte and platelet counts were normal. Microcytosis, hypochromia, target cells, anisocytosis, and poikilocytosis were seen on the peripheral blood smear. The serum iron was 147 micrograms per cent and total iron binding capacity 196 micrograms per cent, with 75 per cent saturation. Serum folate was 1.6 nanograms per ml. The bone marrow examination disclosed erythroid hyperplasia with increased iron stores and slight megaloblastic changes.

Family Studies. Both parents, a brother, and a sister of the patient have mild anemia with target cells and hypochromia on the blood smear. All have increased levels of hemoglobin A₂ but normal hemoglobin F, consistent with the diagnosis of thalassemia minor.

Comment. Although the patient was undoubtedly anemic at birth, the correct diagnosis of thalassemia was not made until he was nearly 2 years of age. Iron therapy for a year and a half aggravated the iron overload problem.

Once thought of, the diagnosis of thalassemia major was readily made on the basis of a microcytic hypochromic hemolytic anemia, target cells, high serum iron, elevated fetal hemoglobin, hepatosplenomegaly, and findings of thalassemia minor in the parents and siblings. The patient developed folic acid deficiency with a megaloblastic marrow, a not uncommon complication of a chronically hyperactive bone marrow. The patient has done well with a vigorous transfusion program, but the long-term effects of the increased iron burden remain to be seen.

Combinations and Other Hemoglobinopathies

SICKLE CELL–HEMOGLOBIN C DISEASE

Hemoglobin C was first recognized as a new hemoglobin in a study of patients who were diagnosed as atypical sickle cell anemia but instead proved to have sickle cell-hemoglobin C disease.[281] The presence of both hemoglobin C and hemoglobin S was demonstrated by electrophoresis. In the reported patients, the major portion of the hemoglobin has been of the C type.[298]

The clinical features of this disease have been described by several authors.[282, 292] The disease is generally much milder than sickle cell anemia, but severe episodes of crisis may occur in some patients; pregnancy may be associated with serious complications. In adults the spleen is usually considerably enlarged, in contrast to sickle cell anemia, in which a small spleen is an almost constant feature. The anemia is usually mild or moderate in degree and the hematocrit and hemoglobin values range from 70 to 100 per cent of normal, except during episodes of crisis. The reticulocyte count is normal or slightly increased.[292] On fixed stained smears of the peripheral blood, from 50 to 100 per cent of the erythrocytes appear as target cells and intra-erythrocytic hemoglobin crystals have been described in patients who have had splenectomy.[275] Sickling can be demonstrated in moist preparations. The osmotic fragility of the erythrocytes is decreased. The diagnosis is established by electrophoresis, which reveals the presence of both hemoglobin S and hemoglobin C. Exchange transfusion during the last trimester of pregnancy has been reported to be effective in lessening the complications of pregnancy.[224]

SICKLE CELL–THALASSEMIA DISEASE

Sickle cell–thalassemia disease probably was first described by Silvestroni and Bianco in 1946, before electrophoretic studies of hemoglobin were made.[288a] The majority of the patients with this disease are whites of Greek or Italian stock and blacks.[298] It has been possible to demonstrate that the patient with this disease is a double heterozygote for the two abnormal genes present in the parents.[287]

The disease resembles sickle cell anemia, but the severity of the anemia, the frequency of painful crisis and leg ulcers, and the degree of splenomegaly vary greatly from one patient to another. The hematologic characteristics are microcytic hypochromic anemia, erythrocytic sickling in moist preparations, and the presence of numerous target cells on the fixed smear. Reticulocytosis is usually present. It is the beta type of thalassemia that interacts with S hemoglobin since both genes affect the beta chain. In some patients virtually all the hemoglobin is S and F so that family studies are necessary to establish the diagnosis of sickle cell–thalassemia disease.

SICKLE CELL–HEMOGLOBIN D DISEASE

Hemoglobin D was described first by Itano.[280] It has been found to be more common among non-blacks in some parts of the world, but is more common in blacks than in whites in the United States. The incidence in blacks in the United States has been reported to be 1:1000[293] and 4:1000.[272]

Sickle cell–hemoglobin D disease has been the subject of several reports.[269, 293] The patients who have this disorder are normally developed, often remain asymptomatic for long periods, and may have little or no anemia. The concentration of hemoglobin S may vary from 25 to 75 per cent in these patients.[269] Attacks that resemble mild episodes of sickle cell crisis occur. Differentiation of this disorder from sickle cell anemia may be difficult because in both diseases sickling occurs in preparations of fresh blood, and filter paper electrophoresis at pH 8.6 shows only a single concentration peak that has the mobility of S hemoglobin. In some instances the differentiation can be made by comparing the solubilities of the reduced forms of the hemoglobin, because the solubility of reduced hemoglobin D is normal but that of reduced hemoglobin S is decreased.[280] Differential solubility studies may not be conclusive, and in such circumstances electrophoresis on agar at pH 6.2 may be utilized to differentiate the two hemoglobins.[293] Homozygous hemoglobin D disease has also been reported.[273]

Less Common Syndromes

Thalassemia–hemoglobin C disease and thalassemia–hemoglobin E disease are similar clinically and hematologically. Splenomegaly, mild hypochromic anemia, target cells, and increased resistance to hypotonic saline occur in both diseases.[271, 290, 297, 298]

Hemoglobin Memphis has a glutamine for glutamic acid substitution at the twenty-third position in the alpha chain.[283, 284] Patients doubly heterozygous for this hemoglobin and hemoglobin S are indistinguishable from the usual patient with sickle cell trait. However, when hemoglobin Memphis occurs in combination with homozygous hemoglobin S, the clinical picture is considerably milder than what is usually seen in sickle cell disease.[283] The anemia is not much different, but painful crises are rare. This has been attributed to a decrease in viscosity conferred by the alpha chain substitution. The electrophoretic pattern is that of hemoglobin SS, and amino acid analysis is necessary to establish the diagnosis.

Two abnormal hemoglobins which sickle and migrate electrophoretically as hemoglobin C have been described. They have the usual valine for glutamic acid substitution of hemoglobin S, but in addition they have a second amino acid substitution in the beta chain. In hemoglobin Harlem, the second substitution is asparagine for aspartic acid at the seventy-third position;[267] in hemoglobin Georgetown the second substitution has not been established.[278, 286] Only heterozygous patients with these hemoglobinopathies have been observed. They have no clinically apparent disease except for the individuals who are heterozygous for hemoglobin Harlem and have a renal concentrating defect.[267]

UNSTABLE HEMOGLOBINS

Carrell and Lehman[268] have used the term "unstable hemoglobin hemolytic anemia" to refer to a group of similar disease syndromes. The clinical picture is characterized by a congenital hemolytic anemia, red cell inclusions which are typical Heinz bodies, excretion of a dipyrrole of the bilifuscin-mesobilifuscin type in the urine, and splenomegaly. The hemoglobin is heat-labile and precipitates when a hemolysate is incubated at 50° C. for several hours. In the past, most of these disorders have probably been called congenital Heinz body hemolytic anemia.

More than 20 abnormal hemoglobins of this type have been described (hemoglobins Zurich, Köln, Genova, Sydney, Hammersmith, Gun Hill, Seattle, Olmsted, Santa Ana, and others).[268, 277, 279a, 281a] These abnormal hemoglobins have in common an amino acid substitution in the region where heme is attached to globin, which has been referred to as the "heme pocket." The comparatively high stability of normal hemoglobin is dependent on the interaction of the globin molecule with the heme groups, and amino acid substitutions in that area render the molecule unstable.[268, 274, 279, 288]

The anemia in these patients is usually mild except upon exposure to oxidant drugs. Such exposure causes an acute hemolytic episode similar to that seen in glucose-6-phosphate dehydrogenase deficiency. The main treatment is avoidance of oxidant drugs, but splenectomy has also been of benefit in some of these patients.[268] The amino acid substitution is usually "silent" in that electrophoretic mobility is normal and amino acid analysis must be carried out to establish the diagnosis. However, a presumptive diagnosis may be made by demonstrating heat-labile hemoglobin plus Heinz bodies in the red cells. Several reviews of the unstable hemoglobins and other hemoglobinopathies are available.[268, 274, 279, 279a, 288]

Acquired Hemolytic Disorders

ANTIBODY MEDIATED

Transfusion reactions are discussed in Chapter XVI.

Erythroblastosis Fetalis

History

The term "erythroblastosis" was first used by Rautman in 1912.[322] In 1932 Diamond, Blackfan, and Baty reviewed two cases with universal edema, 12 with icterus gravis neonatorum, and six with anemia of the newborn and concluded that these three disorders were closely related and dependent on the same underlying process.[306] In 1939 Levine and Stetson reported the case of a group "O" 25 year old secundipara who delivered a macerated stillborn fetus and suffered a severe hemolytic reaction when transfused with her husband's group O blood; the mother was shown to have an isoagglutinin independent of M, N, and P blood factors that reacted with the blood of 45 of 50 group O donors.[313] In 1941 Landsteiner and Wiener reported their studies of the Rh agglutinogen in human blood; these indicated that the factor is inherited as a mendelian dominant independent of other blood groups.[311] In the same year Levine and co-workers studied the incidence of the Rh factor in mothers and fathers of patients with erythroblastosis. They concluded that iso-immunization with Rh explained 91 per cent of the cases and thought that other factors were responsible for 9 per cent. They also concluded that the Rh factor was limited to the red cells and was not present in the saliva and other tissues.[312, 314] In 1943 Mollison demonstrated that Rh-positive red cells were eliminated rapidly after transfusion into infants with erythroblastosis during the first 14 days of life but Rh-negative cells were eliminated at the normal rate.[317] The value of exchange transfusion with Rh-negative blood was demonstrated by Wallerstein in 1946.[324] The value of this form of treatment in preventing the most serious aspect of the disease, kernicterus, was shown in 1950 by Allen, Diamond, and Vaughan.[301]

Mechanism of Disease

The anemia in erythroblastosis fetalis is hemolytic in type.[300, 314, 317] The destruction of the fetal red cells is caused by the presence in the fetal circulation of iso-antibodies that are formed in the mother in response to a blood group antigen that the mother lacks. Agglutinogens A, B, and D are strongly antigenic and the others are less so. Allen and Diamond state that A and B incompatibilities are responsible for about two-thirds of the cases of erythroblastosis fetalis, D (Rh) for about one-third, and other blood factors for 2 or 3 per cent.[300] The occurrence of ABO hemolytic disease is virtually limited to group A or B offspring of group O mothers.[325] A possible explanation for difference in response of the group O mothers has been afforded by studies of the size of the antibodies.[323] Group O mothers tend to form IgG isohemagglutinins which traverse the placental barrier but group A and B mothers tend to form IgM isohemagglutinins, a size that is unlikely to enter the fetal circulation. Immunization with Rh antigen results first in the apperance of IgM antibodies, but on continued immunization the IgG antibodies appear. There is considerable individual difference in the ability to form antibodies and less than 10 per cent of the Rh-negative mothers who have Rh-positive husbands become sensitized; even if the husband is homozygous Rh-positive (DD), the wife may have many children without becoming sensitized.[308]

The method of sensitization of the mother to the fetal red cells in the cases of Rh (D) incompatibilities is an intriguing problem. Although the administration of incompatible blood by transfusion or by intramuscular injection may be responsible for sensitization in women prior to pregnancy, the iso-antibody formation in mothers is usually the result of pregnancy. Allen and Diamond report that quantities of blood as small as 0.1 to 1.0 ml. may be sufficient to produce sensitization. Using an acid elution technique to demonstrate fetal hemoglobin in erythrocytes, it has been demonstrated that small quantities of fetal red cells gain access to the maternal circulation throughout pregnancy. This occurs most frequently during the last trimester.[305] Postpartum, approximately 50 per cent of the mothers can be shown to have fetal red cells in their circulation. In a small percentage transplacental bleeding is sufficient to lead to anemia in the newborn infant or in stillbirth.[305]

Kernicterus, circumscribed areas of yellow coloring in the brain that involve the nuclear areas particularly, is one of the most serious manifestations of erythroblastosis fetalis. It causes death within 7 days in 70 per cent of the babies who have this complication.[309] The brain damage, which is not present at birth, has been shown to be related to the level of the serum bilirubin, since kernicterus occurs in 50 per cent of babies whose level of the serum bilirubin is over 30 mg. per 100 ml. In newborn babies, the ability of the liver to convert indirect reacting bilirubin (unconjugated bilirubin) to the direct reacting form (bilirubin-glucuronide) for excretion is poorly developed; the deficiency is even more marked in premature infants.[303] Defects in the glucuronyl transferase and uridyldiphosphoglucose dehydrogenase activity that is necessary for the synthesis of bilirubin-glucuronide have been demonstrated in the livers of fetal and newborn guinea pigs and support the hypothesis that the glucuronide-conjugating mechanism is inadequately developed in human newborns and prematures. When this mechanism is defective, even though the level of serum bilirubin may not be greatly elevated at birth, the level of the serum bilirubin rises rapidly after birth if hemolytic anemia is present. Unconjugated bilirubin has been identified as the pigment present in the brain in infants dying with kernicterus.

It is also possible that other pigments may be important in kernicterus. Fatalities from kernicterus have occurred in patients with serum bilirubin levels as low as from 1 to 6 mg. per 100 ml.; in such patients the plasma has been shown to have increased levels of heme pigments with an absorption maximum in the range of 405 to 415 mμ., which is different from the absorption maximum for bilirubin, 460 mμ.[299] It has been suggested that in patients with early kernicterus and relatively low serum bilirubin levels methemalbumin may interfere with the ability of the bilirubin to bind to the serum proteins.[320] Brown, Zuelzer, and Robinson have demonstrated that the serum bilirubin concentration is not always a gauge of the diffusible or total body bilirubin.[303a] If the bilirubin cannot bind with the protein in the vascular spaces, the plasma level may be low even though bilirubin has diffused into the cells in appreciable quantities. This shift may be of special importance in premature infants who have lower serum albumin levels than full term infants.[303a]

Clinical Manifestations

Erythroblastosis is reported to occur in about 1 per cent of pregnancies.[300] About one-fifth of the affected infants die in utero or are born critically ill with anemia at the time of birth.

Many erythroblastotic infants appear normal at birth. Jaundice is said to be invariably absent at birth,[300] but it may appear within 2 or 3 hours and may increase rapidly thereafter unless treatment is instituted. Petechial hemorrhages sometimes develop soon after birth. Hepatomegaly and splenomegaly occur almost invariably in Rh disease. When erythroblastosis is due to A or B incompatibility the spleen is often enlarged but to a lesser degree than in Rh disease. Pulmonary edema, pleural effusions, ascites, and edema may be manifestations of heart failure. Kernicterus, which usually becomes manifest late in the second day of life, is rare in the absence of considerable jaundice.[299, 309] Any infant with erythroblastosis should have frequent and careful neurologic examinations. In the early stages kernicterus may be accompanied by no more than minimal neurologic signs that are easily missed. When the kernicterus is more pronounced, the affected infant has a high-pitched cry, irritability, tremor, and an overactive but incomplete Moro reflex; opisthotonos, twitching, convulsions, and respiratory distress may also occur. If the child has kernicterus and survives, sequelae, such as deafness, mental retardation, athetoid movements, and spastic ataxia, develop.

Laboratory Examination

Anemia is considered to be present if the hemoglobin level of the cord blood is less than 13.0 gm. per 100 ml.,[318] if the hemoglobin level of the venous blood is less than 15 gm. per 100 ml.,[300] or if the hemoglobin level of capillary blood is less than 16.0 gm. per 100 ml. on the first day.[318] A hemoglobin level of less than 9.0 gm. per 100 ml. at birth indicates anemia of severe degree. Reticulocytosis is usually present. A high percentage of reticulocytes indicates a severe hemolytic process even if associated with a normal level of hemoglobin. Nucleated red cells are commonly present in the peripheral blood, but may be absent in one-third of the cases on the first day.[318] Elevated leukocyte counts are the rule and have little prognostic value. Thrombocytopenia often occurs in severe cases.

The normal level of serum bilirubin on cord blood is considered to be from 0.8 to 2.6 mg. per 100 ml.[318] The level of indirect reacting serum bilirubin in newborn babies at 48 hours rarely exceeds 13 mg. per 100 ml. In erythroblastosis the level of the serum bilirubin may be normal at birth and rise rapidly thereafter. For this reason frequent determinations are most important in the management of these patients.

Diagnosis

Erythroblastosis fetalis must be distinguished from other causes of anemia, such as hereditary spherocytosis and hemorrhage, and from other causes of jaundice, such as infectious hepatitis, bacterial infections, syphilis, cytomegalic inclusion disease, and fungus infection, that occur during the first days of life.[300] Nucleated red cells occur in the peripheral blood in a number of disorders but the occurrence of large numbers of normoblasts or reticulocytes usually indicates that the presence of hemolytic disease of some type is probable.

The possibility of erythroblastosis, particularly Rh disease, should be suspected in pregnant women who give a history of a normal pregnancy followed by pregnancies that ended with jaundiced infants, abortion, or stillbirth. In about 40 to 50 per cent of the cases of ABO hemolytic disease the firstborn child is affected.[325] The presence of marked edema or pallor at birth or the appearance of jaundice during the first 24 hours may be the first indication of the disease in the infant. However, all the abnormal clinical findings characteristic of the disease are sometimes absent at birth and for this reason the laboratory examinations are often of greater importance than the clinical features.

Every effort is made to make an antenatal diagnosis of erythroblastosis by the use of appropriate laboratory procedures whenever possible. All pregnant women should be typed to determine the ABO group and tested for the Rh factor routinely; if the prospective mother is Rh-negative, the father should be tested for Rh factor and the mother should be tested for possible Rh sensitization at seven months and within two or three weeks of delivery.[300] If anti-Rh antibodies are not detected at that time erythroblastosis is unlikely; if antibodies are present, regardless of the titer, the physician is alerted for the possibility of the disease. A positive Coombs (antiglobulin) test on the fetal red cells (cord blood or infant's blood) definitely establishes the diagnosis. If the husband is Rh-positive the wife should be checked carefully for sensitization in each pregnancy, because a normal course in preceding pregnancies is no guarantee that iso-immune disease will not develop in subsequent pregnancies.

Agglutinogens A and B were formerly considered to be responsible for from 5 to 9 per cent of the cases of erythroblastosis,[307, 314] but more recent studies place the incidence at about 66 per cent.[300] Erythroblastosis due to ABO incompatibility is usually much milder than that due to Rh incompatibility; ABO incompatibility between mother and fetus exists in 20 per cent of pregnancies but erythroblastosis fetalis occurs in only 5 per cent of these (1 per cent of the total). A possible explanation for the lower incidence and milder nature of ABO disease as compared to anti-Rh disease is that the agglutinogens A and B occur on other tissue cells of the fetus as well as on the erythrocytes. In such a circumstance the other tissue cells may take up the antibodies and spare the erythrocytes. Rh agglutinogen apparently is largely or exclusively confined to the erythrocytes, and consequently in this situation the red cells alone suffer from the reaction with antibodies.[300, 310] Erythroblastosis due to ABO incompatibility is rarely associated with severe anemia. Marked hepatomegaly or splenomegaly is unusual. The most significant clinical feature is the occurrence of jaundice during the first 24 hours. When erythroblastosis is suspected, an antiglobulin (Coombs) test should be done on the baby's blood and tests for ABO and Rh factors should be done on the blood of the mother and the baby. The occurrence of A, B, or Rh incompatibility between mother and child, accompanied by reticulocytosis and elevated serum bilirubin in the child, is strong presumptive evidence of erythroblastosis.[300] The indirect antiglobulin (Coombs) test performed on the infant's serum is nearly always positive in disease of this type.

Prevention

A major advance in the management of Rh hemolytic disease has been the observation that the administration of an adequate dose of anti-Rh gamma globulin to an Rh-negative mother within 72 hours of delivery of an Rh-positive infant will prevent sensitization to the Rh antigen in nearly all patients so treated. The failure rate is in the order of 1 per cent or less.[304, 321]

The background for this form of treatment rests on observations by Nevanlinna and Vaino[319] that the risk of Rh hemolytic disease is much less in those instances in which the mother and fetus are ABO incompatible. This naturally occurring protection is thought to be due to antibody destruction of fetal red cells before the mother has sufficient exposure to the Rh antigen to become immunized. In a similar fashion the passive administration of anti-Rh gamma globulin prevents sensitization of the Rh-negative mother by Rh-positive fetal red cells.

This type of prophylaxis is of no benefit to the mother who has already been sensitized by previous pregnancies or by blood transfusions.[321] Mothers who have a significant anti-Rh titer and give birth to a Coombs-positive infant, therefore, should not be treated with anti-Rh gamma globulin, as this will not prevent an anamnestic response to antigenic challenge. All other Rh-negative mothers who are in danger of becoming sensitized should receive adequate amounts of anti-Rh gamma globulin soon after delivery.[304, 321] As more and more Rh-negative mothers receive proper prophylaxis the incidence of erythroblastosis fetalis should be greatly reduced.

Treatment

Infants with erythroblastosis should be treated in a hospital that is properly equipped and staffed to follow the course of the disease and carry out exchange transfusion at any time of day or night. Once the diagnosis of hemolytic disease of the newborn has been established the treatment will depend on the severity of the disease. Mild forms of the disease may need no treatment other than careful observation. Therapy is directed toward preventing kernicterus that is due to the toxic action of the unconjugated bilirubin on cells in the brain. The indications for exchange transfusions in erythroblastosis fetalis listed by Allen and Diamond are:[300]

1. Anemia: hemoglobin of less than 13 gm. per 100 ml. on venous blood or less than 15 gm. per 100 ml. in capillary blood.

2. Increased serum bilirubin (indirect reacting type): over 7 mg. per 100 ml. on cord blood; a rapidly rising serum level; exchange transfusion is performed as often as necessary to keep the serum level less than 20 mg. per 100 ml.

3. Prematurity, except in the mildest cases.

4. History of a previous baby with kernicterus.

5. Reticulocyte count above 15 per cent.

6. Maternal anti-Rh titer of 1:64 or higher.

Zuelzer and Cohen state that, as a general rule, exchange transfusion is performed if the serum bilirubin level in full term infants exceeds the following: 10 mg. per 100 ml. in the first 24 hours; 14 mg. per 100 ml. in the second 24 hours; 17 mg. in the third or fourth day.[325]

The exchange transfusion performs several important functions. In addition to lowering the level of serum bilirubin in the infant's blood, it removes cells that are susceptible to hemolysis, lowers the antibody content of the blood, and supplies albumin that enables the infant's blood to bind a larger amount of bilirubin. Repeated exchange transfusions may be required to keep the serum bilirubin level below 20 mg. per 100 ml. Following an exchange transfusion the infant is observed carefully and the serum bilirubin level is measured as often as is considered necessary. The risk (mortality rate) of exchange transfusion is said to be between 1 and 2 per cent for term infants and about 4 per cent for premature infants.[325] This factor must be considered when deciding whether to do exchange transfusion; it is particularly pertinent when the procedure is considered for nonerythroblastotic infants who are jaundiced.

Fresh blood is used for transfusion whenever possible. It is preferable to obtain the blood for transfusion prior to the birth of the infant. In cross-matching for transfusion the prospective donor cells should be tested against the mother's serum.[300, 317] Prospective donors should be of the same Rh and ABO groups as the mother; Rh-negative blood of the mother's group is used if it is fairly certain that the disease is due to anti-Rh agglutinins. Group O blood is used when the destruction is thought to be due to anti-A or anti-B agglutinins.[317] ABO agglutinins in the donor blood incompatible with the baby's cells should be of low titer and should be neutralized with A and/or B specific substances. If no compatible donor can be found, the mother's red cells, separated from her plasma that contains the antibodies, may be used.[300] When the mother's blood is not available for cross-matching, it is best to select a group O Rh-negative donor to cross-match with the baby's blood.

If edema of congestive heart failure secondary to anemia is present, phlebotomy is often necessary in order to lower the venous pressure. The oxygen-carrying capacity of the blood can be increased by means of transfusion with packed red cells, which only partially replaces the blood volume.

Induction of labor at about the 37th week has been recommended in an effort to prevent stillbirth.[300] Before advising this course the dangers of prematurity must be considered.

Amniocentesis and intrauterine transfusion have a useful place in the management of severe erythroblastosis.[302, 316] Amniotic fluid should be examined only when anti-Rh antibody is already known to be present, since there is a risk of sensitizing an unsensitized mother with this procedure. If antibody is present, or if there is a history of an erythroblastotic infant, amniocentesis should be performed beginning at the twenty-third to the twenty-fifth week of gestation.[316]

The purpose of examining the amniotic fluid is to detect those severely affected infants who may be saved by intrauterine transfusion. Since early delivery and exchange transfusion carry less risk, intrauterine transfusion should be reserved for the more severely affected infant.[302] The timing of the procedure is important because once the infant becomes hydropic, transfusion is usually of no benefit.

Several examinations of the amniotic fluid are necessary to gauge whether the bilirubin-like pigment in the fluid is increasing. Based on criteria established by Liley[315] and modified by others,[302] a decision can be made by measuring the pigment in the amniotic fluid as to which fetuses should have intrauterine transfusion. In one large series consisting of 218 transfusions carried out on 100 fetuses, two-thirds of those who were transfused before the twenty-sixth week of gestation survived.[302]

Other approaches to the treatment of hyperbilirubinemia of the newborn are the use of phototherapy[301a] and phenobarbital.[306a, 324a] Phototherapy is based on the observation that the plasma level of indirect bilirubin decreases when an infant is exposed to light of the wavelengths between 300 and 600 mμ, which causes the oxidative breakdown of bilirubin. Since there is no good evidence at present that phototherapy significantly reduces the incidence of subsequent neurologic damage, retarded motor development, or kernicterus in the human, and since the long-term possible toxic effects are as yet unknown, this type of therapy should be used with the same kind of caution reserved for any new drug that becomes available for the treatment of newborn infants. Although it may have a role in the treatment of the jaundice of prematurity and in infants with mild hemolytic disease secondary to ABO incompatibility, it should not be used in the infant with Rh erythroblastosis, since this might delay indicated exchange transfusion.[301a]

Phenobarbital lowers the serum bilirubin by accelerating the conjugation and transport of bilirubin by the liver. It has been used in an effort to ameliorate neonatal jaundice by administering the drug to both the mother during the last few weeks of pregnancy and the newborn infant.[306a, 324a] There are conflicting reports concerning the efficacy of this form of therapy, and more information is needed before its proper role as a therapeutic agent in jaundice of the newborn can be determined.

Illustrative Case

The patient was the product of the seventh pregnancy of a 38 year old white female. The mother was type A, Rh-negative and father was type A, Rh-positive. There had been two previous neonatal deaths due to erythroblastosis. Saline antibodies were positive in 1:4 dilution and indirect Coombs test was positive in dilution of 1:64. Pregnancy was uneventful; labor lasted 6 hours and 21 minutes and terminated in a normal spontaneous delivery.

The baby appeared to be in fair condition in the delivery room. He was well developed and weighed 2700 gm. The skin was grayish in color, and was covered with multiple small ecchymoses. The umbilical cord was icteric. The baby was active when stimulated and cried vigorously. The spleen edge extended 5 cm. over the left costal margin and the liver 7 cm. below the right costal margin.

Laboratory Examination and Treatment. Initial blood examination: total bilirubin 4 mg.; Hct. 25 per cent; Hb. 7.0 gm. per 100 ml.; W.B.C. 13,000 per cu.mm.; nucleated red cells 150 per 100 leukocytes. Coombs test was positive.

A diagnosis of erythroblastosis was made and an exchange transfusion was performed. After exchange transfusion the serum bilirubin level was 2.4 mg. per 100 ml. and the hematocrit 29 per cent. The leukocyte count was 4800 per cu.mm. Five hours later another exchange transfusion was performed at a time when the serum bilirubin had risen to 6 mg. per 100 ml. and the nucleated red cell count had reached 337 per 100 leukocytes. After the second exchange transfusion serum bilirubin level was 2.7 mg. per 100 ml. and the hematocrit was 36 per cent. No further exchange transfusions were necessary and the patient was discharged on the thirteenth day, at which time he was eating well and appeared healthy. At this time the hematocrit was 46 per cent, the white count was 12,000 per cu.mm. and the blood smear contained 5 nucleated red cells per 100 white cells.

Comment. This patient illustrates many of the common features of erythroblastosis. The father was Rh-positive, the mother was Rh-negative. Two siblings had died previously in the neonatal period because of erythroblastosis. The disease was anticipated in this patient. At birth, pallor, ecchymoses, splenomegaly, and hepatomegaly were present; the antiglobulin test was positive. Because of the previous history in the family and the severe anemia, exchange transfusion was performed even though the serum bilirubin level was only slightly elevated at the time of birth. The necessity of the second exchange is debatable. Although the level of the serum bilirubin level was not greatly elevated, exchange transfusion was considered to be the safest course, mainly because of the rate of increase in the bilirubin level. The patient made an uneventful recovery.

Immune Drug-Induced Hemolytic Anemia

The Coombs positive hemolytic anemias induced by drugs are relatively rare but are important as they afford insight into the various mechanisms by which exogenous agents may induce red cell antibodies. Three types of antibody induction are exemplified by the drugs: quinidine, penicillin, and methyldopa[333, 380] (Table 7–3).

QUINIDINE TYPE

This type of drug-induced anemia was first described following the use of stibophen (Fuadin) for the treatment of schistosomiasis.[341, 348] The immune mechanism involved has been clarified by Shulman in his studies on patients with (quinidine-related hemolysis.[372] He has presented evidence in favor of the concept that the positive Coombs test is caused by the attachment of antigen-antibody complexes to the red cell. The drug acts as a hapten which serves as an antigen when it is bound to some plasma protein. The antibody is directed against the protein-bound circulating drug, and then as a secondary effect the antigen-antibody complex combines with the red cell surface, usually with the fixation of complement. The antigen-antibody complex dissociates from the red cell, leaving only complement behind, so that a non-gamma (anticomplement) Coombs serum may be necessary to detect this type of drug reaction.

Quinidine is much more likely to produce immune thrombocytopenia than immune hemolytic anemia.[329] Shulman has proposed that the type of antibody that a patient has against quinidine determines whether he will develop thrombocytopenia or anemia.[372] People more commonly respond with IgG antibody, and the target for this drug-antibody complex is the platelet. The rare patient who develops IgM quinidine antibodies has a hemolytic anemia because the IgM-drug complex is attracted to the red cell. As further substantiation of this concept, patients have been reported who have had both IgG and IgM antibodies against quinidine and have had both thrombocytopenia and hemolytic anemia.[345, 372]

Other drugs which are thought to produce immune hemolytic anemia by a similar mechanism are: quinine,[362] para-aminosalicylic acid,[358] phenacetin,[358, 362] mephenytoin,[373] isoniazid,[365] chlorpropamide,[357a] and sulfonamides.[337, 371] They are rarely the cause of immune hemolytic anemia; only a few cases have been reported with each drug. The clinical picture is usually one of an acute hemolytic anemia with intravascular hemolysis and hemoglobinuria.[380] The anemia subsides promptly when the offending drug is discontinued, although the anticomplement Coombs test may remain positive for several weeks.

Table 7–3. *Immune Drug-Induced Hemolytic Anemia*

PROTOTYPE DRUG	MECHANISM	TYPE OF ANTIBODY
Quinidine	Antigen-antibody complex	IgM
Penicillin	Hapten binding to red cell	IgG
Methyldopa	Induction of anti-Rh IgG antibodies	IgG

PENICILLIN TYPE

Although circulating antibodies to penicillin occur frequently in patients receiving this antibiotic, Coombs-positive hemolytic anemia secondary to penicillin is rare and occurs only under special circumstances.[333, 380]

The breakdown derivatives of penicillin, benzylpenicilloyl acid, and benzylpenaldic acid are firmly bound to the red cell by covalent bonds.[355] In this situation the red cell is an "innocent bystander" and antibodies reacting with penicillin injure the carrier red cell leading to hemolysis. In order for this to become clinically significant, large amounts of penicillin must be given before sufficient penicillin is bound to red cells to cause a positive Coombs test. In most of the recorded cases, penicillin was administered intravenously at dosages greater than 10 million units a day.[364, 374] Also, the type of antibody response against penicillin is important. In most patients, circulating antibodies to penicillin are of the IgM class, and it is only the rare patient who responds to penicillin with a high titer of IgG antibody who develops a Coombs-positive hemolytic anemia.[333, 380] However, it should be kept in mind, particularly in patients who are taking large doses of penicillin for subacute bacterial endocarditis whose anemia begins to get worse rather than better.

This complication has been reported mainly with penicillin, but in vitro cross reactions with ampicillin and methicillin have been observed.[363] Coombs-positive hemolytic anemia has also been reported after large dose treatment with cephalothin, but in most patients the positive Coombs test after cephalothin therapy is due to non-specific binding of IgG and is not associated with hemolysis.[346, 354, 361] Unlike the quinidine type of immune hemolytic anemia, that associated with penicillin is not accompanied by intravascular hemolysis.[380] The Coombs test becomes negative and hemolysis ceases once the penicillin is discontinued.

METHYLDOPA TYPE

The association of Coombs-positive hemolytic anemia with methyldopa (Aldomet) therapy was first recognized by Carstairs, Worlledge, Dacie, and associates in 1966.[330] They noted that several patients who had what appeared to be typical idiopathic auto-immune hemolytic anemia were taking methyldopa. They then surveyed a group of hypertensive patients taking methyldopa and found that 20 per cent of them had a positive Coombs test but most of them did not have hemolytic anemia, the incidence of clinical hemolysis being about 1 per cent.[380] These observations have been amply confirmed by others,[357, 381] and over 60 patients with methyldopa-induced hemolytic anemia have been reported, making this type of immune drug-induced hemolytic anemia more common than the quinidine and penicillin types combined.[380]

It usually takes from 3 to 6 months of methyldopa therapy for the Coombs test to become positive, and this delay is not shortened when a previously Coombs-positive patient is restarted on the drug. The Coombs test gradually becomes negative when the methyldopa is stopped, but this may take anywhere from 1 month to 2 years, depending on the initial strength of the Coombs test. However, there does not appear to be any correlation between the rate of recovery and the total dose of methyldopa or the length of therapy. The clinical and hematological findings are identical to those of a patient with idiopathic auto-immune hemolytic anemia.[380]

In contrast to the quinidine and penicillin types of immune hemolytic anemia, which require the presence of the drug for a positive Coombs test, methyldopa induces a positive Coombs test that remains positive long after the drug is discontinued. Furthermore, antibodies eluted from the patient's red cells will react with normal red cells without the presence of methyldopa and the reaction is not blocked by methyldopa or its derivatives.[357]

The antibody on the red cell after methyldopa therapy is identical to the type usually seen in idiopathic auto-immune hemolytic anemia. It is of the IgG class, is most active at 37° C, and has Rh specificity.[357] The mechanism whereby methyldopa induces antibodies against the red cell is unclear. It is possible that antibodies against methyldopa or one of its derivatives cross react with the Rh locus on the red cell, or that the drug alters the Rh locus during red cell development, rendering the locus antigenic. Another proposed explanation is that methyldopa releases from inhibition clones of lymphocytes, which then form antibodies against normal red cell antigens. As yet there is no firm evidence to support any of these hypotheses. Methyldopa is not unique in producing this type of immune hemolysis, as mefanamic acid (Ponstan) has been reported to produce a similar picture in three patients receiving the drug for rheumatoid arthritis.[370]

The fact that methyldopa and mefanamic acid can induce a Coombs-positive hemolytic anemia identical to that seen in idiopathic auto-immune hemolytic has important implications for our understanding of the idiopathic type. It is likely that other drugs and exogenous agents such as bacteria and viruses may also induce red cell antibody formation.

Auto-Immune Hemolytic Anemia

History

The history of "acquired" hemolytic anemia has been reviewed by Dameshek and Schwartz.[339] The first recognizable description of this type of anemia has been credited to Hayem.[336] The "non-congenital" type of hemolytic icterus, which appeared either during the course of other illnesses or without known cause, was also described by Widal, Abrami, and Brulé in 1908.[378, 379] The name "acquired" hemolytic icterus was given to these cases. The occurrence of reticulocytosis and auto-agglutination, the absence of apparent hereditary influences, and the absence of significant abnormalities in the hypotonic saline test were noted.

The discovery of the antiglobulin or Coombs test in 1945 by Coombs, Mourant, and Race[331] was followed by a marked increase in interest in this syndrome. This has led to numerous studies on the demonstration, production, action, and nature of "auto-antibodies." Most of these studies have been reviewed by Dacie.[336, 337a, 338] At the present time this type of anemia is often spoken of as "auto-immune hemolytic anemia."

Patients with auto-immune hemolytic anemia have the usual manifestations of a hemolytic process, such as shortened erythrocyte survival time, increased fecal urobilinogen excretion, elevated serum bilirubin, anemia, reticulocytosis, and splenomegaly. The distinguishing feature is the positive Coombs antiglobulin test which identifies antibodies on the red cell surface. The disorder occurs during the course of some diseases, particularly those of the lymphoma group, but also appears in patients in whom no primary disease can be demonstrated. In the former circumstance the disorder is classified as secondary or symptomatic; in the latter circumstance patients are classified as "primary" or "idiopathic."

Pathogenesis

The type of antibody attached to the red cell determines the mechanism of hemolysis. IgM antibodies have been referred to as saline antibodies, complete antibodies, agglutinins, and hemolysins. Because they are large, they can combine with antigen sites on adjacent red cells, causing agglutination in saline or in the circulation. IgM antibodies fix complement which, if present in sufficient amounts, causes lysis of red cells in saline and intravascular hemolysis in vivo. Such antibodies are called hemolysins; those causing just agglutination are referred to as agglutinins. Red cells agglutinated by IgM antibodies in the circulation are removed primarly by the liver and to a lesser extent by the spleen.[353] Examples of IgM antibodies are the major blood group antibodies, anti-A and anti-B and cold agglutinins.

IgG antibodies have been referred to as incomplete or sensitizing antibodies. Although they have two combining sites like IgM antibodies, because of their smaller size and the normal distance between negatively charged red cells, they coat the red cell surface but do not cause agglutination in saline or in the general circulation. The major importance of the development of the Coombs antiglobulin test is in the detection of this type of red cell antibody.[331] IgG antibodies usually do not fix complement nor lead to intravascular hemolysis or agglutination, and red cells coated with IgG antibodies are removed from the circulation primarily by the spleen.[353] Red cells coated with IgG antibodies do not agglutinate in saline but do when suspended in a high protein media such as albumin. In the spleen, where the plasma protein concentration is higher than in the general circulation, IgG-coated red cells begin to agglutinate and are sequestered.[353]

Another important factor in the destruction of IgG-coated erythrocytes by the spleen is that mononuclear cells in the spleen as well as circulating monocytes have a receptor site for IgG.[356] This appears to be specific for IgG, and these cells do not react with other immunoglobulins or plasma proteins.[356] When IgG-coated red cells become attached to splenic phagocytes, the erythrocyte may be lysed or, more commonly, a portion of the red cell membrane may be removed, leading to erythrocyte fragmentation, spherocytosis, and ultimately sequestration and lysis by the spleen. In most cases of idiopathic auto-immune hemolytic anemia, the antibody involved is IgG.[336, 338, 343] IgA antibodies are rarely involved in Coombs-positive hemolytic anemia.

The antibodies involved in Coombs-positive hemolytic anemia may also be classified according to whether they react optimally at 37° C (warm antibodies) or at lower temperatures (cold antibodies).[336, 338] The IgG antibodies seen in idiopathic auto-immune hemolytic anemia, Rh isoantibodies, and those induced by methyldopa are of the warm variety, whereas the IgM red cell antibodies found after mycoplasma pneumonia and chronic cold hemagglutinin disease are examples of cold antibodies.[338] These cold antibodies fix complement, and at 37° C, or room temperature, the IgM antibody which fixed complement at a lower temperature dissociates from the red cell, leaving only complement on the red cell surface. It is therefore important to use a non-gamma (anticomplement) Coombs serum when checking for red cell antibodies at room temperature in order not to miss cold antibodies.

For a number of years there was controversy as to whether the globulins on the red cell surface were really antibodies to red cells, because these globulins reacted with nearly all red cells they were tested against with no apparent specificity. Then it was learned that the antigens involved were very common ones ("public antigens") which occur on the red cells of all but a few individuals.[375] In idiopathic auto-immune hemolytic anemia and in methyldopa hemolytic anemia, the IgG antibodies have been found, with only rare exceptions, to be directed against antigens of the Rh system.[336, 338, 357] When Weiner and Vos used Rh null red cells (cells containing no Rh locus) to test for antibody specificity in idiopathic auto-immune hemolytic anemia, they found specificity to the Rh locus in about 70 per cent of the sera.[376] In high titer cold agglutinin hemolytic anemia following mycoplasma pneumonia, the antibodies have anti-I specificity, in infectious mononucleosis they have anti-i specificity, and in paroxysmal cold hemoglobinuria the Donath-Landsteiner antibody is directed against the P antigen.[336, 338]

Although a number of hypotheses have been proposed, there is no completely satisfactory one to explain why a patient develops autoantibodies against his own red cells. The main theories expounded are: (1) alteration of red cell antigen, (2) cross reaction with a red cell antigen, and (3) induction of lymphoid cells to produce antibodies against normal red cells.

It is possible that viruses, bacteria, or drugs such as methyldopa might alter red cell antigens, particularly the Rh locus, so that the red cells become antigenic for normal lymphoid cells. There is no experimental evidence to support this theory, and the fact that eluted antibodies react as strongly with normal cells from other donors as with the patient's red cells makes this explanation unlikely.

The observation that mycoplasma infection produces a Coombs-positive hemolytic anemia, and that syphilis is associated with most cases of the Donath-Landsteiner antibody in paroxysmal cold hemoglobinuria, has raised the possibility that antibodies against mycoplasma and the spirochete may cross react with I and P antigens of the red cell, and in a similar fashion other exogenous agents may produce cross reactions.[337a] Again, there is little experimental evidence to substantiate this hypothesis, and the fact that autoantibodies persist long after the exogenous agent is presumably gone casts doubt on this theory.

Small amounts of autoantibodies are present normally, and it is possible that some exogenous agent interferes with the normal immune regulatory system in such a way that autoantibody titers increase sufficiently to cause clinically apparent disease. The observation that most secondary immune hemolytic anemias are associated with lymphoproliferative disorders has led to the theory of a mutation of a clone of lymphocytes which make antibodies against normal red cell antigens. The fact that this type of antibody as well as that studied in chronic cold hemagglutinin disease is usually homogeneous, in terms of immunoglobin light chains and subclasses of heavy chains, supports the concept that the antibodies are monoclonal in origin and may have arisen from a mutant strain of lymphocytes.[338] In contrast, the antibodies observed in idiopathic autoimmune hemolytic anemia[327, 344] and methyldopa-induced anemia[328] are heterogenous with respect to light chains and subclasses of heavy chains. This suggests that normal lymphoid tissue is responding to chronic exogenous antigenic stimulation.

Clinical Manifestations

Auto-immune hemolytic anemia may arise in association with some other disease, when it is termed "secondary" or "symptomatic." It may also occur when no other disease is demonstrable, in which circumstance it is classified as "primary" or "idiopathic." In several large series, about 50 per cent of patients have been classified as idiopathic, with a range of 25 to 60 per cent.[334, 336, 338, 340, 343] The secondary cases have occurred most often in association with mycoplasma pneumonia, chronic lymphocytic leukemia, lymphosarcoma, Hodgkin's disease, disseminated lupus, and infectious mononucleosis. Less common associated diseases are sarcoidosis, tuberculosis, Felty's syndrome, carcinoma, and ovarian teratoma.[338]

The idiopathic disorder occurs at any age in either sex, but females are affected more often than males. The severity and duration of the disease may vary greatly. At times the onset of the disease is sudden and the course is rapid and fulminating. In such patients the course is characterized by high temperature, rapidly progressing weakness, and dyspnea. Anemia becomes more severe, icterus is usually apparent, and hemoglobinuria sometimes occurs. It is in this type of patient that hemolysins are more likely to be demonstrated. More often the course of the disorder is a chronic one that persists with varying degrees of severity over a period of months or years. Spontaneous remissions sometimes occur. Exacerbations of the disease are said to occur more often in the winter months.[334] When the disorder is associated with the cold type of auto-antibodies, Raynaud's phenomena and hemoglobinuria may appear on exposure to cold. A subacute form that is intermediate in severity between the acute and chronic form also occurs.

In secondary auto-immune hemolytic disease, the clinical features are those of the underlying disorder plus those associated with the hemolytic anemia. At times the hemolytic element may be so severe that it dominates the clinical picture and at other times it may be merely an incidental finding. When hemolytic anemia follows mycoplasma pneumonia, the anemia, which may be severe, usually appears suddenly at the end of the second or third week of illness and disappears spontaneously in 1 or 2 weeks.[334, 336] In diseases such as lymphosarcoma the hemolytic anemia may precede other evidence of the primary disease by months, or it may not appear until after the underlying disease has been under observation and treatment for several years.[366] The development of auto-immune hemolytic disease may be the first manifestation of a recurrence of carcinoma of the bowel.

The main abnormalities on physical examination in the idiopathic cases are pallor and splenomegaly. In addition, patients with the secondary type may manifest evidence of the underlying disease, such as lymphadenopathy, hepato-megaly, or evidence of disease in the skin, lungs, and gastrointestinal tract.

Laboratory Examination

Any degree of anemia may occur in either the idiopathic or symptomatic forms of disease. In one series of 57 cases the hemoglobin varied from 2.5 gm. to 12.5 gm. per 100 ml.[334] The anemia is usually macrocytic (MCV > 94 cu. microns) because of reticulocytosis, but a stained smear of the peripheral blood often reveals many microcytes, polychromatophilia, poikilocytosis, and the presence of normoblasts. Spherocytosis is often present during periods of crisis and is usually absent during quiescence. Reticulocytosis is usually present, but reticulocytopenia occurs in some patients. Leukocytosis is common during periods of active hemolysis and the count may exceed 30,000 per cu.mm.; the increase is mainly in the granulocytic series and myelocytes may be found in the peripheral blood. Neutropenia sometimes occurs in chronic cases but is unusual during episodes of crisis. Erythrophagocytosis by monocytes is sometimes evident on plain smears or on smears made from the buffy coat and may suggest the diagnosis. The platelet count is usually normal or moderately reduced but severe thrombocytopenia is found in some patients.

The osmotic fragility is increased during the acute phase when spherocytes are prominent but is usually normal during periods of quiescence.[382] The auto-hemolysis test shows increased hemolysis after incubation which is not decreased by glucose and may be increased further by the addition of glucose.[336] Hemo-globin electrophoresis reveals the normal A type of hemoglobin.

Of fundamental importance in the diagnosis of auto-immune hemolytic anemia is the demonstration of a positive direct Coombs test. The direct Coombs test is the demonstration of gamma globulin or complement attached to washed red cells, and the indirect Coombs test is the demonstration of antibodies in the patient's serum which react with other individuals' red cells and may be either autoantibodies or isoantibodies. In auto-immune hemolytic anemia, the direct Coombs test is regularly positive, and in some patients, usually those with more severe anemia, the indirect Coombs test is also positive.

Coombs sera may be prepared by immunizing rabbits against whole human serum, in which case it is referred to as broad spectrum and detects all the immunoglobulins and complement to some extent. More specific and sensitive Coombs sera may be prepared by immunizing a rabbit against one of the purified immunoglobulins or complement. Since IgA is rarely if ever involved in immune hemolytic anemia and IgM is usually detected only when the test is performed at low temperatures, common practice is to use anti-IgG Coombs sera (often referred to as gamma) and anti-complement Coombs sera (often referred to as non-gamma).

When these two types of Coombs sera are used, most cases of auto-immune hemolytic anemia fall into one of three patterns: IgG, IgG plus complement, or complement alone.[338, 343] In idiopathic auto-immune hemolytic anemia due to warm antibodies, most of the cases show a pattern of IgG, a lesser number IgG plus complement, and only a few cases complement alone.[338, 343, 359a] When the hemolytic anemia is caused by a cold antibody either spontaneously (chronic cold hemagglutinin disease) or secondary to a lymphoma or a connective tissue disorder, usually only complement can be detected on the red cell.[338, 343, 359a] It should be pointed out that when the Coombs test is performed on large numbers of hospitalized patients or normal blood donors, a significant number will show only complement reactions and have no evidence of excessive hemolysis.[338]

Treatment and Prognosis

Treatment of the patient with auto-immune hemolytic disease is directed toward both the hemolytic anemia and the underlying disease. Blood transfusion, adrenocorticosteroid preparations, and splenectomy are the most important measures for the treatment of the anemia. Blood transfusion may be lifesaving during episodes of crisis and may be necessary periodically in patients with the chronic type of disorder who have failed to respond satisfactorily to splenectomy or steroids. The use of packed red cells for transfusions after the plasma and leukocytes have been removed from the blood often reduces the incidence of febrile transfusion reactions. Cross-matching is sometimes difficult because of the presence of the abnormal antibody in the patient's blood. In patients for whom no compatible donor blood can be found and whose need for transfusion is urgent, the least incompatible blood available should be used.

Splenectomy induces a complete remission in about 40 to 50 per cent of patients.[334, 377] It is more likely to be helpful in cases of the idiopathic variety than in the symptomatic group. Although the response to splenectomy is unpredictable and relapse may occur at any time after an apparently good postoperative response,[335, 382] the use of Cr^{51} to measure splenic sequestration is valuable in selecting patients that are most likely to respond to splenectomy.[352] In a series of 45 patients reported by Allgood and Chaplin, 68 per cent obtained a complete remission after splenectomy, and 44 per cent remained cured without supplementary corticosteroid therapy.[326] They noted that a negative indirect Coombs test and IgG type antibody predisposed to a favorable response to splenectomy, and others have noted[343] that a good response to previous corticosteroid therapy makes a satisfactory response to splenectomy more likely. They also pointed out that although significant splenic sequestration of Cr^{51}-labeled red cells presaged a good result from splenectomy, the lack of significant red cell sequestration did not preclude a good response.[326]

Treatment with the adrenocortical steroid drugs produces improvement in many patients with this type of anemia, although the mechanism of the action of these preparations is not clear. In the group of patients reported by Allgood and Chaplin, 84 per cent obtained an initial partial or complete remission following a single course of steroid therapy, but only 16 per cent were able to maintain the remission when steroids were discontinued.[326] Because of the high frequency of relapse when steroids are discontinued and the many deleterious side effects of prolonged steroid therapy, splenectomy should not be delayed in those patients in whom large doses of corticosteroids are necessary to control the hemolytic process.

Immunosuppressive therapy with such drugs as azothioprine, 6-mercaptopurine, chlorambucil, and cyclophosphamide has met with variable success in the treatment of auto-immune hemolytic anemia.[332, 338, 351, 369] This type of therapy is usually reserved for the more refractory patient who has not responded to splenectomy or to corticosteroid therapy. Although such therapy has been effective in some patients, it carries the risk of bone marrow depression associated with these drugs.

In patients with chronic cold hemagglutinin disease with high titers of cold agglutinins, corticosteroid therapy and splenectomy have rarely been of any benefit.[338, 343, 368] Immunosuppressive therapy has been successful in lowering the antibody titer and improving the anemia in some of these patients.[350] Dacie reported a good response to chlorambucil therapy in three of nine patients with chronic cold hemagglutinin disease.[338]

In the very acute type of illness, a more aggressive plan of treatment is often necessary. In this circumstance numerous blood transfusions, intravenous steroids, and splenectomy all may be utilized in the space of a few days.

If the hemolytic anemia is of the secondary variety, appropriate therapy should be directed at the primary disease as soon as feasible. If this is one of the collagen diseases, corticosteroid therapy of the hemolytic process may be all that is necessary. If the underlying disorder is a carcinoma or an ovarian cyst, definitive surgical treatment is usually indicated. If lymphosarcoma is present the anemia may improve following treatment with chemotherapy, but simultaneous therapy with prednisone or some related compound is usually necessary, at least in the beginning of the course of therapy.[334, 366] Therapy of the lymphoma with x-ray or chemotherapeutic agents may also cause an exacerbation of the hemolytic process.[366]

The prognosis of patients with the secondary type of anemia is mainly that of the underlying disease. The prognosis is generally favorable when the disorder follows a virus infection and is poor when it is associated with malignancy or one of the collagen diseases. Patients with a negative indirect Coombs test and IgG antibodies on their red cells generally respond better to therapy and have a more favorable prognosis than those patients whose red cells are also coated with complement.[326] The presence of complement is more likely to be associated with underlying disease than is the presence of IgG alone.[343] The commonest causes of death are cardiac failure caused by anemia, acute renal failure, septicemia, and pulmonary emboli.[326, 334] The occurrence of severe anemia, reticulocytopenia, thrombocytopenia, and leukopenia appears to be associated with a poor prognosis.

Illustrative Case

This 53 year old white housewife had been under observation for 5 years as a tuberculosis suspect but the diagnosis was never established. On a periodic chest roentgenogram it was noted that hilar adenopathy had developed and the patient was admitted to the hospital for investigation. The patient admitted vague chest pains and irregular cough on occasions. She denied weight loss, pruritus, or other symptoms.

Physical Examination. The posterior cervical and axillary lymph nodes were enlarged and measured 0.5 to 1 cm. in diameter. The spleen was felt two fingerbreadths below the left costal margin. Physical examination was otherwise within normal limits.

Laboratory Examination. Admission blood studies: Hb. 7.1 gm. per cent; hematocrit 27 per cent; R.B.C. 1.9 mil. per cu.mm.; retics. 22.3 per cent; W.B.C. 18,000 per cu.mm. Differential count (per cent): bands 4, segmented 50, lymphocytes 40, monocytes 1, eosinophils 4, basophils 1. The serum protein was 8.9 gm. per 100 ml., albumin 3.5 gm. per 100 ml., globulin 5.4 gm. per 100 ml. The direct antiglobulin (Coombs) test was positive and the Wassermann test was anticomplementary. Blood cultures, tuberculin skin test, platelet counts, and examination for L.E. cells were normal. Plasma electrophoresis indicated increased total protein, increased gamma globulin, decreased albumin, and beta globulin with two peaks; the pattern was considered suggestive of Boeck's sarcoid. Bone marrow aspiration revealed marked normoblastic hyperplasia; plasma cells and eosinophils appeared to be slightly increased.

Regular roentgenograms and laminograms of the chest suggested a slight enlargement in the right hilus area. On bronchoscopy no mass was visualized. Biopsies of the right prescalene node and right axillary node were interpreted as "hyperplastic lymphadenitis."

Treatment and Course. The patient was thought to have a hemolytic anemia of the auto-immune type. Although sarcoid, lymphosarcoma, and disseminated lupus were suspected as underlying primary diseases, no diagnosis could be established. Accordingly the patient was given prednisone 20 mg. every 8 hours beginning on June 24. On June 26 this was reduced to 10 mg. four times a day and at discharge on July 3 the dose was reduced to 5 mg. three times a day. There was a striking improvement in her blood count, and on September 16 her hematocrit was 42 per cent, and the reticulocyte count had fallen to 1.5 per cent. On November 4, 1 month after her prednisone dosage had been reduced to 2.5 mg. three times a week, the patient was asymptomatic and the hematocrit was 39 per cent.

Comment. This patient had evidence of a hemolytic anemia and the positive direct Coombs test indicated that the anemia was of the extracorpuscular or auto-immune type. No primary diagnosis was established and the case might be considered to be "idiopathic." However, various features strongly suggest the presence of some underlying disease, and in this circumstance the patient must be examined periodically for additional evidence of some primary disorder. The anemia has responded well to treatment with prednisone for 2 years, although the Coombs test remains positive.

Paroxysmal Cold Hemoglobinuria

Paroxysmal cold hemoglobinuria is a rare disorder. The sudden attacks of intravascular hemolysis and hemoglobinuria that occur on exposure to cold are due to the presence of an auto-hemolysin in the serum. The attacks are precipitated by chilling of the body and hemolysis occurs during the subsequent warming. Donath and Landsteiner demonstrated that hemolysis occurs in paroxysmal cold hemoglobinuria because of the presence of an auto-hemolysin in the patient's blood.[342] The hemolysin in the patient's plasma unites with the patient's erythrocytes in the presence of complement at temperature of 15° or less. In the presence of the complement, hemolysis occurs on warming. The hemolysin is not active at body temperature or at room temperature.[347] The Wassermann reaction is reported to be positive in over 90 per cent of patients with the disorder and unquestionable clinical evidence of syphilis is found in about 30 per cent.[336, 359] The Donath-Landsteiner hemolysin is an IgG antibody;[338, 349] it bears no constant relationship to the Wassermann antibody but has anti-P specificity.[338]

The attacks are precipitated by exposure to cold but there is a wide range of variability in the amount of chilling that is necessary; no more than the opening of a door from an unheated room may be required.[359] The interval between the chilling and the onset of symptoms may vary from a few minutes to 7 or 8 hours. The prodromal period is apt to be associated with malaise, headache, abdominal cramps, and pains in the back and legs. The actual paroxysm is usually manifested by a shaking chill followed by a temperature rise to 102° or 104° F that lasts for several hours. After the chill the voided urine usually appears dark red or brown; urine of this character may be passed in only the first or first few specimens after the chill, or over a period of 2 or 3 days. Severe, reversible acute renal failure may develop during an attack.[360] During the episode mild jaundice, splenomegaly, and hepatomegaly are often demonstrable. Severe leukopenia that is the result of the virtual disappearance of the granulocytes from the peripheral blood also occurs.[367]

Treatment during an attack consists of keeping the patient in a warm environment and administering transfusions when necessary. Between episodes exposure to cold is avoided and any underlying disease is treated. Many patients remain asymptomatic during these intervals.

The diagnosis is made by the history and by abnormalities that can be demonstrated in the laboratory tests. The degree of the anemia and the evidence of blood regeneration depend on the severity of the hemolysis. Hemoglobinemia, hemoglobinuria, and a positive antiglobulin (Coombs) test can be demonstrated during an attack. More specific tests establish the diagnosis. In various modifications of the Donath-Landsteiner test hemolysis is demonstrated after the blood has been chilled in vitro.[336, 384] Paroxysmal cold hemoglobinuria must be distinguished from the hemoglobinuria that follows exposure to cold in patients with cold agglutinins; the latter disorder occurs in association with mycoplasma pneumonia and hemolysis occurs only when the agglutinin is present in high titer.

PAROXYSMAL NOCTURNAL HEMOGLOBINURIA

Paroxysmal nocturnal hemoglobinuria (PNH), or the Marchiafava-Micheli syndrome, is a rare disorder of unknown cause that occurs in both sexes.[337, 347,]

[367, 383, 386, 388, 393, 395] Although the disease has been reported in patients $5\frac{1}{2}$ and 52 years of age, it usually appears during the third or fourth decade.[367] The disease is characterized by intravascular hemolysis and hemoglobinuria that is usually more marked during or immediately after sleep, chronicity, spontaneous remissions and exacerbations, and refractoriness to therapy. It has been demonstrated that the increased hemolysis is due to an intracorpuscular defect, since erythrocytes from patients with paroxysmal nocturnal hemoglobinuria have a diminished survival time when transfused into normal subjects, but erythrocytes from normal individuals survive normally when transfused into patients with paroxysmal nocturnal hemoglobinuria.[387, 390] Autosurvival studies on three patients, utilizing Cr^{51}-tagged cells, have shown half-survival times of 2, 7, and 17 days; however, in each instance a portion of the cell population survived for prolonged periods and suggested the presence of a double population.[397] The reticulocytes and young red cells appear to be most sensitive to hemolysis.[401]

The exact nature of the red cell defect in PNH is yet to be defined. The most characteristic abnormality and the abnormality leading directly to hemolysis is an increased sensitivity to complement. Rosse and Dacie have shown that PNH red cells are approximately 25 times more sensitive to the hemolytic effects of complement than are normal red cells, and they have also demonstrated two populations of red cells in PNH patients based on sensitivity to complement.[407, 408] Yachnin has shown that complement may become attached to PNH red cells and the complement sequence be completed without the presence of antibody.[410–412]

Acetylcholinesterase activity of PNH red cells is very low or absent.[294, 295] This is probably a secondary rather than a primary defect, since in vivo experiments with acetylcholinesterase inhibitors have shown no detrimental effect[405] and familial deficiency of erythrocyte acetylcholinesterase is not associated with hemolysis or positive serologic tests for PNH.[400]

Normal red cells can be made to take on many of the characteristics of PNH red cells by in vitro treatment with large amounts of sulfhydryl-containing compounds, such as glutathione and cysteine.[404, 409] This suggests that some alteration in erythrocyte membrane sulfhydryl groups may be responsible for enhanced sensitivity to complement, but as yet this remains speculative.

The diagnosis of PNH is usually based on a positive acidified serum or Ham's test.[337, 384] This test is very specific, and when done properly rarely gives either false positive or false negative results.[337, 338, 395] An interesting exception is a hereditary anemia referred to as congenital normoblastic binuclearity.[385] These patients' red cells are particularly sensitive to an isoagglutinin present in most normal sera, and consequently give a positive Ham test with most, but not all, sera. The sugar water test is negative.

The sugar water test of Hartman and Jenkins[396] is also a sensitive test in the diagnosis of PNH and is based on the enhancement of complement by low ionic strength solutions. This test also has high specificity for PNH when properly performed.[396a]

Many cases of PNH are preceded by a period of pancytopenia before the anemia becomes frankly hemolytic.[337, 383, 388, 391, 393, 403] In at least 25 per cent of PNH patients aplastic anemia has been diagnosed previously, and the diagnosis of PNH should always be considered and tested for in such patients.[403] It is tempting to speculate that the abnormal population of PNH red cells arises as a mutation following bone marrow injury. Since PNH has been recorded to follow familial aplastic anemia,[389] drug-induced aplastic anemia,[406] and idiopathic aplastic anemia,[403] it is likely that the mutation is related to disordered hematopoiesis which follows bone marrow hypoplasia rather than due to any specific etiological agent.

The treatment of PNH has been unsatisfactory. The administration of alkali and splenectomy have been of no benefit. A combination of iron and androgen therapy has been reported to improve the anemia,[395] but not infrequently iron therapy may lead to an acute worsening of the anemia because of an increase in reticulocytes, which are more sensitive to the hemolytic action of complement.[401, 408a] Corticosteroids have been shown to be helpful in some patients, but large doses may be necessary and severe relapses may occur when the dosage is lowered or they are discontinued.[392]

The course of the disease is a chronic one which may continue for many years in some patients. Infections, antisera, and menstruation may precipitate hemolytic crises.[395] In fatal cases, death is caused not only by anemia and infections during acute episodes, but also by thromboses of cerebral, coronary, portal, hepatic, and pulmonary vessels.[337] The disorder may terminate in acute myeloblastic leukemia.[398, 399, 402]

MECHANICAL HEMOLYSIS

Mechanical damage to the red cell as a cause of hemolytic anemia can be divided into three categories: (1) erythrocyte injury secondary to impact of red cells in the microcirculation against a flat surface, as in march hemoglobinuria, (2) erythrocyte damage secondary to valvular heart disease, and (3) red cell damage secondary to obstructive disease of small blood vessels.

March Hemoglobinuria

Although hemoglobinuria occurring in a soldier after a long and strenuous march was reported as long ago as 1881 by Fleicher,[420] it was not until 1964 that Davidson[421] focused attention on trauma to red cells in the superficial capillaries of the feet against a hard flat surface as the cause of hemolysis. He noted that the common denominator in such cases was walking or running on a hard surface and that equally strenuous exercise such as swimming, cycling, or running on a soft surface did not cause hemoglobinuria. He and others also demonstrated that this type of hemoglobinuria could be prevented by putting rubber insoles into the runners' shoes.[421, 422]

This type of impact hemolysis has also been reported in a young man indulging in vigorous karate exercises involving considerable trauma to the ulnar surfaces of his hands.[430]

Since most individuals do not have hemoglobinuria after walking or running on a hard surface, an intrinsic red cell defect which is brought out by this kind of stress has been looked for, but none has been found.[429] Chaplin and his associates reported the case of a young man who had hemoglobinuria and a congenital heart lesion with chronically depressed haptoglobin levels. They postulated that the relatively low haptoglobin levels made the patient more prone to exceed the capacity of haptoglobin after traumatic intravascular hemolysis, with hemoglobinuria occurring as a consequence.[419]

Cardiac Hemolytic Anemia

Many patients with valvular heart disease, both those with prosthetic valve replacements and those who have had no operation, have a decreased red cell survival because of trauma to erythrocytes as they pass through the heart.[425] In many patients the degree of hemolysis is slight and easily compensated for by increased red cell production, so that anemia is mild or absent. Hemolysis in such patients usually goes unrecognized unless special studies are done. On the other hand, hemolysis is marked in some patients, resulting in severe anemia with hemoglobinuria and the expected adverse effects on cardiac function.

Table 7–4 lists the types of cardiac abnormalities that have been associated with mechanical hemolysis. Although many types of operative procedures and prosthetic devices have been associated with hemolysis, replacement of the aortic valve by a prosthesis has been the most common offender. In one series of 317 operative cases involving the aortic valve, approximately 10 per cent developed clinically significant hemolytic anemia.[427]

Although the mechanism whereby turbulence of blood across a diseased or artificial heart valve leads to red cell fragmentation and intravascular hemolysis is not entirely clear, in most instances there is a significant regurgitant jet stream resulting from separation, tearing, or malposition of the artificial valve. This usually occurs in the high flow aortic area, but has also been observed with faulty mitral prosthetic valves[432] and with severe mitral insufficiency without surgery.[433] The damage to the red cells is apparently caused by turbulent flow and shearing forces as erythrocytes become adherent to fibrin deposits on the prosthetic or diseased valve. Nevaril and his associates have shown in vitro that a shearing force of 3000 dynes per cm² causes erythrocyte fragmentation and hemolysis, a shear stress similar to that which has been estimated to occur across an insufficient aortic valve.[426]

The diagnosis of traumatic hemolysis in cardiac patients is not difficult to make if one is aware of the possibility of its occurrence and looks for laboratory

Table 7–4. *Types of Cardiac Abnormalities Associated with Mechanical Hemolysis*

Operated Patients	Unoperated Patients
Aortic valve replacement	Aortic disease
Mitral valve replacement	Stenosis
Repair of atrial septal defect	Insufficiency
Repair of tetralogy of Fallot	Coarctation
Repair of atrioventricular canal defect	Mitral disease
	Insufficiency

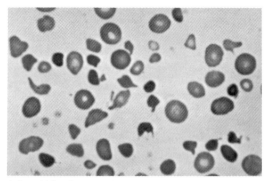

Figure 7–10.   Peripheral blood smear showing schistocytes and red cell fragmentation. (From Davidson and Henry: Todd-Sanford Clinical Diagnosis by Laboratory Methods. Philadelphia, W. B. Saunders, 1969.) (F.S.: I, 7–8.)

abnormalities that accompany intravascular hemolysis. There is increased plasma hemoglobin, decreased plasma haptoglobin, increased serum lactic dehydrogenase, and hemosiderinuria. The appearance of schistocytes (distorted and fragmented red cells) on the peripheral blood smear denotes traumatic damage to erythrocytes in the circulation (Fig. 7–10).

Prolonged hemosiderinuria and hemoglobinuria may lead to iron deficiency which aggravates the anemia.[423] As the anemia becomes more severe, cardiac output is increased, which heightens the degree of turbulence across the valve and makes the traumatic hemolysis worse. For this reason any iron deficiency should be treated promptly. At times correcting the iron deficiency is enough to lead to a compensated hemolytic state, but usually it is necessary to repair the defective valve in order to correct both the anemia and cardiac dysfunction.

Microangiopathic Hemolytic Anemia

The term "microangiopathic hemolytic anemia" was introduced in 1962 by Brain, Dacie, and Hourihane to describe hemolytic anemia occurring in a variety of disorders which have in common disease of the small blood vessels.[413, 415] They were struck by the similarity between the blood smears in these patients and those previously described in patients with traumatic hemolysis secondary to valvular heart disease. In both instances burr cells, helmet cells, fragmented cells, and spherocytes were noted.

They postulated that the mechanism of hemolysis was trauma to red cells by turbulent flow across abnormal valves in one and squeezing through partially obstructed and abnormal small vessels in the other.

Table 7–5 lists the types of disorders which have been associated with microangiopathic hemolytic anemia. They all have in common disease of the microcirculation with partial obstruction to the flow of erythrocytes. In nearly all instances the renal vasculature is involved,[414] but obstruction of other vessels may also cause fragmentation and traumatic lysis of erythrocytes. This has been observed in patients with disseminated carcinoma with small vessel involve-

Table 7-5. *Causes of Microangiopathic Hemolytic Anemia*

Thrombotic thrombocytopenic purpura
Purpura fulminans
Hemolytic-uremic syndrome of childhood
Acute glomerulonephritis
Renal cortical necrosis
Polyarteritis
Malignant hypertension
Eclampsia
Lupus erythematosus
Carcinomatosis involving small blood vessels
Rejection of renal homografts

ment[415] and in purpura fulminans when only the blood vessels of the skin are involved.[424]

Microangiopathic hemolytic anemia has been produced experimentally in animals by inducing the generalized Shwartzman reaction,[417] by the injection of thrombin,[416] by rapid defibrination from injecting a purified coagulant fraction of Malayan pit-viper venom (Arvin),[428] and by producing malignant hypertension with a combination of salt overload and the administration of desoxycorticosterone.[431] In these models, red cells have been observed to become enmeshed in fibrin clots, to be adherent to fibrin deposited on vessel walls, and at times to become adherent to damaged endothelium. This red cell adherence plus the force of blood flow through partially occluded small vessels leads to shear stresses which cause erythrocyte fragmentation and traumatic hemolysis.[418]

The importance of a careful examination of the peripheral blood smear in any patient with anemia needs repeated emphasis. This simple procedure is particularly valuable in patients with impact hemolysis in whom the characteristic finding of fragmented and distorted red cells may provide the first clue to the nature of the pathologic mechanism of the anemia and the type of underlying disease. It is important to make the diagnosis of microangiopathic hemolytic anemia not only as a clue to the underlying disease, which may be treated, but also as an indication for heparin therapy, which in some instances may prevent progressive and irreversible impairment of renal function.[413, 414]

References

ERYTHROCYTE METABOLISM AND METHEMOGLOBINEMIA

1. Aebi, H., Heiniger, J. P., and Suter, H.: Some properties of red cells and other tissues from normal and acatalatic humans. Biochem. J., *89*:63, 1963.
2. Bartlett, G. R.: Human red cell glycolytic intermediates. J. Biol. Chem., *234*:445, 1959.
3. Benesch, R., and Benesch, R. E.: The effect of organic phosphates from the human erythrocyte on the allosteric properties of hemoglobin. Biochem. Biophys. Res. Commun., *26*:162, 1967.
4. Bucklin, R., and Myint, M. K.: Fatal methemoglobinemia due to well water nitrates. Ann. Int. Med., *52*:703, 1960.
5. Cawein, M., Behlen, C. H. II, Lappat, E. J., and Cohen, J. E.: Hereditary diaphorase deficiency and methemoglobinemia. Arch. Int. Med., *113*:578, 1964.
6. Chanutin, A., and Curnish, R. R.: Effect of organic and inorganic phosphates on the oxygen equilibrium of human erythrocytes. Arch. Biochem. Biophys., *121*:96, 1967.

7. Cohen, G., and Hochstein, P.: Glucose-6-phosphate dehydrogenase and detoxification of hydrogen peroxide in human erythrocytes. Science, 134:1756, 1961.

8. Cohen, R. J., Sachs, J. R., Wicker, O. J., and Conrad, M. E.: Methemoglobinemia provoked by malarial chemoprophylaxis in Vietnam. New England J. Med., 270:1127, 1968.

9. Davson, H.: Growth of the concept of the paucimolecular membrane. Circulation, 26:1022, 1962.

10. Delivoria-Papadopoulos, M., Oski, F. A., and Gottlieb, A. J.: Oxygen-hemoglobin dissociation curves: effect of inherited enzyme defects of the red cell. Science, 165:601, 1969.

11. Finch, C. A.: Methemoglobinemia and sulfhemoglobinemia. New England J. Med., 239:470, 1948.

12. Firkin, B. G., and Wiley, J. S.: The red cell membrane and its disorders. Prog. Hemat., 5:26, 1966.

13. Gerald, P. S., and George, P.: Second spectroscopically abnormal methemoglobin associated with hereditary cyanosis. Science, 129:393, 1959.

14. Gibson, Q. H.: The reduction of methaemoglobin in red blood cells and studies on the cause of idiopathic methaemoglobinaemia. Biochem. J., 42:13, 1948.

15. Gibson, Q. H., and Harrison, D. C.: Familial idiopathic methaemoglobinemia. Five cases in one family. Lancet, 253:941, 1947.

16. Hoffman, J. F.: Cation transport and structure of the red-cell plasma membrane. Circulation, 26:1201, 1962.

17. Hoffman, J. F.: The red cell membrane and the transport of sodium and potassium. Am J. Med., 41:666, 1966.

18. Huennekens, F. M., Liu, L., Myers, H. A. P., and Gabrio, B. W.: Erythrocyte metabolism. III. Oxidation of glucose. J. Biol. Chem., 227:253, 1957.

19. Jaffé, E. R.: Hereditary methemoglobinemias associated with abnormalities in the metabolism of erythrocytes. Am. J. Med., 41:786, 1966.

20. Jaffé, E. R., and Heller, P.: Methemoglobinemia in man. Progr. Hemat., 4:48, 1964.

21. Jaffé, E. R., Neumann, G., Rothberg, H., Wilson, F. T., Webster, R. M., and Wolff, J. A.: Hereditary methemoglobinemia with and without mental retardation. A study of three families. Am. J. Med., 41:42, 1966.

22. Jandl, J. H.: The Heinz body hemolytic anemias. Ann. Int. Med., 58:702, 1963.

23. Jandl, J. H.: Analytical review: leaky red cells. Blood, 26:367, 1965.

23a. LaCelle, P. L.: Alteration of membrane deformability in hemolytic anemia. Seminars in Hemat., 7:355, 1970.

24. Lewis, S. M., Osborn, J. S., and Stuart, P. R.: Demonstration of an internal structure within the red blood cell by ion etching and scanning electron microscopy. Nature, 20:614, 1968.

25. Liddell, J., and Lehmann, H.: Defects of hemoglobin and of methemoglobin reductase. Ann. N.Y. Acad. Sci., 123:207, 1965.

26. Mills, G. L., and Randall, H. T.: Hemoglobin catabolism. II. The protection of hemoglobin from oxidative breakdown in the intact erythrocyte. J. Biol. Chem., 232:589, 1958.

27. Murphy, J. R.: Erythrocyte metabolism. II. Glucose metabolism and pathways. J. Lab. & Clin. Med., 55:286, 1960.

28. Murphy, J. R.: Erythrocyte metabolism. V. Active cation transport and glycolysis. J. Lab. & Clin. Med., 61:567, 1963.

29. Necheles, T. F., Maldonado, N., Barquet-Chediak, A., and Allen, D. M.: Homozygous erythrocyte glutathione-peroxidase deficiency: clinical and biochemical studies. Blood, 33:164, 1969.

30. Oski, F. A., Gottlieb, A. J., Delivioria-Papadopoulous, M., and Miller, W. W.: Red-cell 2,3-diphosphoglycerate levels in subjects with chronic hypoxemia. New England J. Med., 280:1165, 1969.

31. Post, R. L., Merritt, L. R., Kinsolving, C. R., and Albright, C. D.: Membrane adenosine triphosphatase as a participant in the active transport of sodium and potassium in the human erythrocyte. J. Biol. Chem., 235:1796, 1960.

32. Rifkind, R. A.: Destruction of injured red cells in vivo. Am. J. Med., 41:711, 1966.

33. Rifkind, R. A., and Davon, D.: Heinz body anemia—an ultrastructural study. I. Heinz body formation. Blood, 25:885, 1965.

34. Schrier, S. L.: Studies of the metabolism of human erythrocyte membranes. J. Clin. Invest., 42:756, 1963.

35. Schrier, S. L.: Organization of enzymes in human erythrocyte membranes. Am. J. Physiol., 210:139, 1966.

36. Scott, E. M.: The relation of diaphorase of human erythrocytes to inheritance of methemoglobinemia. J. Clin. Invest., 39:1176, 1960.

37. Scott, E. M., and McGraw, J. C.: Purification and properties of diphosphopyridine nucleotide diaphorase of human erythrocytes. J. Biol. Chem., 237:249, 1962.

38. Sheppard, C. W., and Martin, W. R.: Cation exchange between cells and plasma of mammalian blood. I. Methods and application to potassium exchange in human blood. J. Gen. Physiol., *33*:703, 1950.

39. Singer, K.: Hereditary hemolytic disorders associated with abnormal hemoglobins. Am. J. Med., *18*:633, 1955.

40. Solomon, A. K.: Red cell membrane structure and ion transport. J. Gen. Physiol., *43*:1, 1960.

41. Steinberg, M., Brauer, M. J., and Necheles, T. F.: Acute hemolytic anemia associated with erythrocyte glutathione-peroxidase deficiency. Arch. Int. Med., *25*:302, 1970.

42. Ternberg, J. L., and Luce, E.: Methemoglobinemia: a complication of silver nitrate treatment of burns. Surgery, *63*:328, 1968.

43. Townes, P. L., and Lovell, G. R.: Hereditary methemoglobinemia: a new variant exhibiting dominant inheritance of methemoglobin A. Blood, *18*:18, 1961.

44. Townes, P. L., and Morrison, M.: Investigation of the defect in a variant of hereditary methemoglobinemia. Blood, *19*:60, 1962.

45. Valberg, L. S., Holt, J. M., Paulson, E., and Szivek, J.: Spectrochemical analysis of sodium, potassium, calcium, magnesium, copper, and zinc in normal human erythrocytes. J. Clin. Invest., *44*:379, 1965.

45a. Weed, R. I.: The importance of erythrocyte deformability. Am. J. Med., *49*:147, 1970.

46. Weed, R. I., LaCelle, P. L., and Merrill, E. W.: Metabolic dependence of red cell deformability. J. Clin. Invest., *48*:795, 1969.

47. Weed, R. I., and Weiss, L.: The relationship of red cell fragmentation occurring within the spleen to cell destruction. Trans. Assoc. Am. Phys., *79*:426, 1966.

48. Weinstein, R. S.: The structure of cell membranes. New England J. Med., *281*:86, 1969.

48a. Weinstein, R. S., and McNutt, N. S.: Ultrastructure of red cell membranes. Seminars in Hemat., 7:259, 1970.

49. Weiss, L., and Tavassoli, M.: Anatomical hazards to the passage of erythrocytes through the spleen. Seminars in Hemat., 7:372, 1970.

50. Whittam, R.: Transport and Diffusion in Red Blood Cells. Edward Arnold Ltd., London, 1964.

HEREDITARY SPHEROCYTOSIS AND OTHER ERYTHROCYTE MEMBRANE DEFECTS

51. Baker, S. J., Jacob, E., Rajan, K. T., and Gault, E. W.: Hereditary haemolytic anaemia associated with elliptocytosis: a study of three families. Brit. J. Haem., 7:210, 1961.

52. Bates, G. C., and Brown, C. H.: Incidence of gallbladder disease in chronic hemolytic anemia (spherocytosis). Gastroenterology, *21*:104, 1952.

53. Bertles, J. F.: Sodium transport across the surface membrane of red blood cells in hereditary spherocytosis. J. Clin. Invest., *36*:816, 1957.

54. Butterworth, C. E., Kracke, R. R., and Riser, W. H., Jr.: Hereditary spherocytic anemia in the Negro. Blood, *5*:793, 1950.

55. Chauffard, A.: Pathogenie de l'ictère congénital des adults. Semaine Med., *27*:25, 1907.

56. Chauffard, A., and Fiessinger, N.: Ictère congénital hémolytique avec lesions globulaires. Bull. et Mem. Soc. Med. Hop. Paris, *24*:1169, 1907.

57. Cooper, R. A., and Jandl, J. H.: The role of membrane lipids in the survival of red cells in hereditary spherocytosis. J. Clin. Invest., *48*:736, 1969.

58. Crosby, W. H., and Conrad, M. E.: Hereditary spherocytosis: observations on hemolytic mechanisms and iron metabolism. Blood, *15*:662, 1960.

59. Cutting, H. O., McHugh, W. J., Conrad, F. G., and Marlow, A. A.: Autosomal dominant hemolytic anemia characterized by ovalocytosis. Am. J. Med., *39*:21, 1965.

60. Dacie, J. V.: The congenital anaemias. Part I in The Haemolytic Anaemias: Congenital and Acquired. 2nd Ed. Grune & Stratton, New York, 1960.

61. Dacie, J. V., and Mollison, P. L.: Survival of normal erythrocytes after transfusion to patients with familial hemolytic anaemia. Lancet, *1*:550, 1943.

62. Dameshek, W., and Bloom, M. L.: The events in the hemolytic crisis of hereditary spherocytosis, with particular reference to the reticulocytopenia, pancytopenia, and an abnormal splenic mechanism. Blood, *3*:1381, 1948.

63. Dawson of Penn, Lord.: Haemolytic icterus. Brit. Med. J., *1*:921, 1931.

64. DeGier, J., Ban Deenen, L. L. M., Verloop, M. L., and Van Gastel, Z.: Phospholidid and fatty acid characteristics of erythrocytes in some cases of anemia. Brit. J. Haemat., *10*:246, 1964.

65. Douglass, L. L., and Twomey, J. J.: Transient stomatocytosis with hemolysis: a previously unrecognized complication of alcoholism. Ann. Int. Med., *72*:159, 1970.

66. Dresbach, M.: Elliptical human red corpuscles. Science, *19*:469, 1904.

67. Dreyfus, C.: Chronic hemolytic jaundice. Bull. New England Med. Center, *4*:122, 1942.
68. Emerson, C. P.: Influence of the spleen on the osmotic behavior and the longevity of red cells in hereditary spherocytosis: a case study. Boston Med. Quart., *5*:65, 1954.
69. Emerson, C. P., Jr., Shenn, S. C., Ham, T. H., and Castle, W. B.: The mechanism of blood destruction in congenital hemolytic jaundice. J. Clin. Invest., *26*:1180, 1947.
70. Haden, R. L.: The mechanism of the increased fragility of the erythrocytes in congenital hemolytic jaundice. Am. J. Med. Sci., *188*:441, 1934.
71. Ham, T. H., and Castle, W. B.: Relation of increased hypotonic fragility and erythrostasis to the mechanism of hemolysis in certain anemias. Trans. Assoc. Am. Physicians, *55*:127, 1940.
72. Harris, E. J., and Prankerd, T. A.: The rate of sodium extrusion from human erythrocytes. J. Physiol., *121*:470, 1953.
73. Jacob, H. S.: Abnormalities in the physiology of the erythrocyte membrane in hereditary spherocytosis. Am. J. Med., *41*:734, 1966.
74. Jacob, J. S., and Jandl, J. H.: Increased cell membrane permeability in the pathogenesis of hereditary spherocytosis. J. Clin. Invest., *43*:1704, 1964.
75. Jaffé, E. R., and Gottfried, E. L.: Hereditary nonspherocytic hemolytic disease associated with altered phospholipid composition of erythrocytes. J. Clin. Invest., *47*:1375, 1968.
76. Jandl, J. H.: Hereditary spherocytosis. In Beutler, E. (Ed.): Hereditary Disorders of Erythrocyte Metabolism. Grune & Stratton, New York, 1968, p. 209.
77. Jandl, J. H., and Aster, R. H.: Increased splenic pooling and the pathogenesis of hypersplenism. Am. J. Med. Sci., *253*:383, 1967.
78. Jandl, J. H., Simmons, R. L., and Castle, W. B.: Red cell filtration and the pathogenesis of certain hemolytic anemias. Blood, *18*:133, 1961.
79. LaCelle, P. L., and Weed, R. I.: Abnormal membrane deformability. A model for the hereditary spherocyte. J. Clin. Invest., *48*:48a, 1969.
80. Lock, S. P., Smith, R. S., and Hardisty, R. M.: Stomatocytosis: a hereditary red cell anomaly associated with haemolytic anaemia. Brit. J. Hemat., *7*:303, 1961.
81. Meadow, S. R.: Stomatocytosis. Proc. Roy. Soc. Med., *60*:13, 1967.
82. Miller, G., Townes, P. L., MacWhinney, J. B.: A new congenital hemolytic anemia with deformed erythrocytes ("stomatocytes") and remarkable susceptibility of erythrocytes to cold hemolysis in vitro. I. Clinical and hematologic studies. Ped., *35*:906, 1965.
83. Minkowski, O.: Über eine hereditäre, unter dem Bilde eines chronischen ikterus mit Urobilinurie, Splenomegalie and Nierensiderosis verlaufende Affektion. Verhandl. Dtsch. Cong. f. Inn. Med., *18*:316, 1900 (Quoted from Dacie, J. V.[60])
84. Mohler, D. N.: Adenosine triphosphate metabolism in hereditary spherocytosis. J. Clin. Invest., *44*:1417, 1965.
85. Oski, F. A., Naiman, J. L., Blum, S. F., Zarkowsky, H. S., Whaun, J., Shohet, S. B., Green, A., and Nathan, D. G.: Congenital hemolytic anemia with high-sodium, low-potassium red cells. New England J. Med., *280*:909, 1969.
86. Owren, P. A.: Congenital hemolytic jaundice. The pathogenesis of the "hemolytic crisis." Blood, *3*:231, 1948.
87. Ozer, F. L., and Mills, G. L.: Elliptocytosis with haemolytic anemia. Brit. J. Haemat., *10*:468, 1964.
88. Pearson, H. A.: The genetic basis of hereditary elliptocytosis with hemolysis. Blood, *32*:972, 1968.
89. Prankerd, T. A. J.: Studies on the pathogenesis of haemolysis in hereditary spherocytosis. Quart. J. Med., *29*:199, 1960.
90. Race, R. R.: On the inheritance and linkage relations of acholuric jaundice. Ann. Eugenics, *11*:365, 1942.
91. Reed, C. F., and Swisher, S. N.: Erythrocyte lipid loss in hereditary spherocytosis. J. Clin. Invest., *45*:777, 1966.
92. Robinson, M. A., Loder, P. B., de Gruchy, G. C.: Red-cell metabolism in non-spherocytic congenital haemolytic anemia. Brit. J. Haemat., *7*:327, 1961.
93. Shen, S. C., Castle, W. B., and Fleming, E. M.: Experimental and clinical observations on increased mechanical fragility of erythrocytes. Science, *100*:387, 1944.
94. Vanlair and Masius: Bull. Acad. roy. Med. de Belgique, *5*:515, 1871. (Quoted from Dreyfus, C.[67])
95. Weed, R. I., and Bowdler, A. J.: Metabolic dependence of the critical hemolytic volume of human erythrocytes: relationship to osmotic fragility and autohemolysis in hereditary spherocytosis and normal red cells. J. Clin. Invest., *45*:1137, 1966.
96. Weed, R. I., and Reed, C. F.: Membrane alterations leading to red cell destruction. Am. J. Med., *41*:681, 1966.
97. Weiss, H. J.: Hereditary elliptocytosis with hemolytic anemia. Am. J. Med., *35*:455, 1963.

98. Welch, C. S., and Dameshek, W.: Splenectomy in blood dyscrasias. New England J. Med., 242:601, 1950.

99. Young, L. E.: Hereditary spherocytosis. Am. J. Med., 18:486, 1955.

100. Young, L. E., Izzo, M. J., and Platzer, R. F.: Hereditary spherocytosis. I. Clinical hematologic and genetic features in 28 cases with particular reference to the osmotic and mechanical fragility of incubated erythrocytes. Blood, 6:1073, 1951.

101. Zarkowski, H. S., Oski, F. A., Shaafi, R., Shohet, S. B., and Nathan, D. G.: Congenital hemolytic anemia with high sodium, low potassium red cells. I. Studies of membrane permeability. New England J. Med., 278:573, 1968.

102. Zipursky, A., Peters, J. C., Rowland, M. R., and Israels, L. G.: An abnormality in erythrocyte sodium transport in hereditary elliptocytosis. J. Pediat., 67:939, 1965.

ENZYME DEFICIENCY HEMOLYTIC ANEMIA

103. Baughan, M. A., Valentine, W. N., Paglia, D. E., Ways, P. O., Simons, E. R., and DeMarsh, Q. B.: Hereditary hemolytic anemia associated with glucose phosphate isomerase (GPI) deficiency — a new enzyme defect of human erythrocytes. Blood, 32:236, 1968.

104. Beutler, E.: Glucose-6-phosphate dehydrogenase deficiency. In Stanbury, J. B. Wyngaarden, J. B., and Frederikson, D. S. (Eds.): The Metabolic Basis of Inherited Disease. 2nd Ed. McGraw-Hill, New York, 1966, p. 1060.

105. Beutler, E.: Drug-induced hemolytic anemia. Pharmacol. Rev., 21:73, 1969.

105a. Beutler, E.: Effect of flavin compounds on glutathione reductase activity: in vivo and in vitro studies. J. Clin. Invest., 48:1957, 1969.

106. Beutler, E., Dern, R. J., and Alving, A. S.: The hemolytic effect of primaquine. IV. The relationship of cell age to hemolysis. J. Lab. & Clin. Med., 44:439, 1954.

107. Beutler, E., Dern, R. J., and Alving, A. S.: The hemolytic effect of primaquine. VI. An in vitro test for sensitivity of erythrocytes to primaquine. J. Lab. & Clin. Med., 45:40, 1955.

108. Boivin, P., Galand, C., André, R., and Debray, J.: Anémies hémolytiques congénitales avec déficit isolé en glutathion réduit par déficit en glutathione synthétase. Nouv. Rev. Franc. Hemat., 6:859, 1966.

109. Bowdler, A. J., and Prankerd, T. A. J.: Studies in congenital nonspherocytic haemolytic anaemias with specific enzyme defects. Acta Haemat., 31:65, 1964.

110. Bowman, H. S., and Procopio, F.: Hereditary non-spherocytic hemolytic anemia of the pyruvate-kinase deficient type. Ann. Int. Med., 58:567, 1963.

111. Brewer, G. J.: 6-Phosphogluconate dehydrogenase and glutathione reductase. In Yunis, J. J. (Ed.): Biochemical Methods in Red Cell Genetics. Academic Press, New York, 1969, p. 139.

112. Brewer, G. J., and Dern, P. J.: A new inherited enzymatic deficiency of human erythrocytes: 6-phosphogluconate dehydrogenase deficiency. Amer. J. Human Genet., 16:472, 1964.

113. Brewer, G. J., Tarlov, A. R., and Alving, A. S.: Methemoglobin reduction test: a new simple in vitro test for identifying primaquine sensitivity. Bull. World Health Organ., 22:633, 1960.

114. Burka, E. R.: Infectious disease: a cause of hemolytic anemia in glucose-6-phosphate dehydrogenase deficiency. Ann. Int. Med., 70:222, 1969.

115. Burka, E. R., Weaver, Z. III., Marks, P. A.: Clinical spectrum of hemolytic anemia associated with glucose-6-phosphate dehydrogenase deficiency. Ann. Int. Med., 64:817, 1966.

116. Carson, P. E., Brewer, G. J., and Ickes, C. E.: Decreased glutathione reductase with susceptibility to hemolysis. J. Lab. & Clin. Med., 58:804, 1961.

117. Carson, P. E., Flanagan, C. L., Ickes, C. E., and Alving, A. S.: Enzymatic deficiency in primaquine-sensitive erythrocytes. Science, 24:484, 1956.

118. Carson, P. E., and Frischer, H.: Glucose-6-phosphate dehydrogenase deficiency and related disorders of the pentose phosphate pathway. Am. J. Med., 41:744, 1966.

119. Childs, B., Zinkham, W., Browne, E. A., Kimbro, E. L., and Torbert, J. V.: A genetic study of a defect in glutathione metabolism of the erythrocyte. Bull. Johns Hopkins Hosp., 102:21, 1958.

120. Cordes, W.: Experiences with plasmochin in malaria: preliminary reports. 15th Annual Report, United Fruit Co., 1926, p. 26.

121. Cotte, J., Kissin, C., Mathieu, M., Poncet, J., Monnet, P., Salle, B., and Germain, D.: Observation d'un cas de déficit partial en ATPase intraérythrocytaire. Rev. Franc. Etudes Clin. Biol., 13:284, 1968.

122. Dacie, J. V., Mollison, P. L., Richardson, N., Selwyn, J. G., and Shapiro, L.: Atypical congenital hemolytic anemia. Quart. J. Med., 22:79, 1953.

123. de Gruchy, G. C., Santamaria, J. N., Parson, I. C., and Crawford, H.: Nonspherocytic congenital hemolytic anemia. Blood, 16:1371, 1960.

124. Dern, R. J., Beutler, E., and Alving, A. S.: The hemolytic effect of primaquine. II. The natural course of the hemolytic anemia and the mechanism of its self-limited character. J. Lab. & Clin. Med., *44*:171, 1954.

125. Dern, R. J., Weinstein, I. M., LeRoy, G. V., Talmage, D. W., and Alving, A. S.: The hemolytic effect of primaquine. I. The localization of the drug-induced hemolytic defect in primaquine-sensitive individuals. J. Lab. & Clin. Med., *43*:303, 1954.

126. Earle, D. P., Jr., Bigelow, F. S., Zubrod, C. G., and Kane, C. A.: Studies on the chemotherapy of the human malarias. IX. Effect of primaquine on the blood cells of man. J. Clin. Invest., *27*:121, suppl., 1948.

127. Gant, F. L., and Winks, G. F., Jr.: Primaquine sensitive hemolytic anemia complicating diabetic acidosis. Clin. Res., *9*:27, 1961. (Abstract)

128. Harvald, B., Hanel, K. H., Squires, R., and Trap-Jensen, J.: Adenosine-triphosphatase deficiency in patients with nonspherocytic haemolytic anaemia. Lancet, *2*:18, 1964.

129. Hockwald, R. S., Arnold, J., Clayman, C. B., and Alving, A. S.: Status of primaquine. IV. Toxicity of primaquine in Negroes. J.A.M.A., *149*:1568, 1952.

130. Hsu, T. H. J., Robinson, A. R., and Zuelzer, W. W.: Genetic polymorphism of hemolytic anemia associated with erythrocyte pyruvic kinase deficiency. Blood, *28*:977, 1966 (Abstract).

131. Jacob, H. S., and Jandl, J. H.: Screening test for glucose-6-phosphate dehydrogenase deficiency. New England J. Med., *274*:1162, 1966.

132. Jaffé, E. R.: Clinical profile: hereditary hemolytic disorders and enzymatic deficiencies of human erythrocytes. Blood, *35*:116, 1970.

133. Keitt, A. S.: Pyruvate kinase deficiency and related disorders of red cell glycolysis. Am. J. Med., *41*:762, 1966.

134. Keitt, A. S.: Hemolytic anemia with impaired hexokinase activity. J. Clin. Invest., *48*:1997, 1969.

135. Kirkman, H. N., Kidson, C., and Kennedy, M.: Variants of human glucose-6-phosphate dehydrogenase. Studies of samples from New Guinea. In Beutler, E. (Ed.): Hereditary Disorders of Erythrocyte Metabolism. Grune & Stratton, New York, 1968, p. 126.

136. Kraus, A. P., Langston, M. F., Jr., and Lynch, B. L.: Red cell phosphoglycerate kinase deficiency. A new cause of non-spherocytic hemolytic anemia. Biochem. Biophys. Res. Commun., *30*:173, 1968.

137. Löhr, G. W., and Waller, H. D.: Zur Biochemie einiger angeborener hämolytischer Anämien. Folia Haemat. (Frankfurt) *8*:377, 1963.

137a. Mohler, D. N.: Glucose-6-phosphate dehydrogenase deficiency. M.C.V. Quarterly, *6*:42, 1970.

138. Mohler, D. N., and Crockett, C. L., Jr.: Hereditary hemolytic disease secondary to glucose-6-phosphate dehydrogenase deficiency: report of three cases with special emphasis on ATP metabolism. Blood, *23*:427, 1964.

139. Mohler, D. N., Majerus, P. W., Minnich, V., Hess, C. E., and Garrick, M. D.: Glutathione synthetase deficiency as a cause of hereditary hemolytic disease. New England J. Med., *283*:1253, 1970.

140. Necheles, T. F., Rai, U. S., and Cameron, D.: Congenital non-spherocytic hemolytic anemia associated with unusual erythrocyte hexokinase abnormality. J. Lab. Clin. Med., *76*:593, 1970.

141. Oski, F. A., Nathan, D. G., Sidel, V. W., and Diamond, L. K.: Extreme hemolysis and red-cell distortion in erythrocyte pyruvate kinase deficiency. New England J. Med., *270*:1023, 1964.

142. Oski, F. A., and Whaun, J. M.: Hemolytic anemia and red cell glyceraldehyde-3-phosphate dehydrogenase deficiency. Clin. Res., *17*:601, 1969. (Abstract)

143. Paglia, D. E., Holland, P., Baughan, M. A., and Valentine, W. N.: Occurrence of defective hexosephosphate isomerization in human erythrocytes and leukocytes. New England J. Med., *280*:66, 1969.

144. Paglia, D. E., Valentine, W. N., Baughan, M. A., Miller, D. R., Reed, C. F., and McIntyre, O. R.: An inherited molecular lesion of erythrocyte pyruvate kinase. Identification of a kinetically aberrant isozyme associated with premature hemolysis. J. Clin. Invest., *47*:1929, 1968.

145. Phillips, S. M., and Silvers, N. P.: Glucose-6-phosphate dehydrogenase deficiency, infectious hepatitis, acute hemolysis, and renal failure. Ann. Int. Med., *70*:99, 1969.

146. Prins, H. K., Oort, M., Looms, J. A., Zürcher, C., and Beckers, T.: Congenital nonspherocytic hemolytic anemia associated with glutathione deficiency of the erythrocytes. Hematologic, biochemical and genetic studies. Blood, *27*:145, 1966.

147. Schnieder, A. S., Valentine, W. N., Baughan, M. A., Paglia, D. E., Shore, N. A., and Heins, H. L., Jr.: Triosephosphate isomerase deficiency. A multisystem inherited enzyme disorder. Clinical and genetic aspects. In Beutler, E. (Ed.): Hereditary Disorders of Erythrocyte Metabolism. Grune & Stratton, New York, 1968, p. 265.

148. Schneider, A. S., Valentine, W. N., Hattori, M., and Heins, H. L., Jr.: Hereditary hemolytic anemia with triosphosphate isomerase deficiency. New England J. Med., *272*:229, 1965.

149. Schröter, W.: Kongenitale nichtsphärocytäre hämolytische Anämie bei 2,3-Diphosphogly-ceratmutase-Mangel der Erythrocyten im frühen Säughlingsalter. Klin. Wschr., *43*:1147, 1965.

150. Selwyn, J. G., and Dacie, J. V.: Autohemolysis and other changes resulting from the incubation in vitro of red cells from patients with congenital hemolytic anemia. Blood, *9*:414, 1954.

151. Tanaka, K. R., and Valentine, W. N.: Pyruvate kinase deficiency. In Beutler, E. (Ed.): Hereditary Disorders of Erythrocyte Metabolism. Grune & Stratton, New York, 1968, p. 229.

152. Tanaka, K. R., Valentine, W. N., and Miwa, S.: Pyruvate kinase (PK) deficiency hereditary nonspherocytic hemolytic anemia. Blood, *19*:267, 1962.

153. Tarin, S., Kono, N., Nasu, T., and Nishikawa, M.: Enzymatic basis for the coexistence of myopathy and hemolytic disease in inherited muscle phosphofructose kinase deficiency. Biochem. Biophys. Res. Commun., *34*:77, 1969.

154. Tarlov, A. R., Brewer, G. J., Carson, P. E., and Alving, A. S.: Primaquine sensitivity. Arch. Int. Med., *109*:209, 1962.

155. Twomey, J. J., Moser, R., Hudson, W., O'Neal, F., and Alfrey, C.: ATP metabolism in pyruvate kinase (PK) deficient erythrocytes. Clin. Res., *14*:437, 1966 (Abstract).

156. Valentine, W. N., Hsieh, H. S., Paglia, D. E., Anderson, H. M., Baughan, M. A., Jaffé, E. R., and Garson, O. M.: Hereditary hemolytic anemia associated with phosophoglycerate kinase deficiency in erythrocytes and leukocytes. A probable x-chromosome-linked syndrome, New England J. Med., *280*:528, 1969.

157. Valentine, W. N., Oski, F. A., Paglia, D. E., Baughan, M. A., Schneider, A. S., and Nauman, J. L.: Hereditary hemolytic anemia with hexokinase deficiency. Role of hexokinase in erythrocyte aging. New England J. Med., *276*:1, 1967.

158. Valentine, W. N., and Tanaka, K. R.: Pyruvate kinase deficiency hereditary hemolytic anemia. In Stanbury, J. B. et al. (Eds.): The Metabolic Basis of Inherited Disease. 2nd Ed. McGraw-Hill, Inc., New York, 1965, p. 1051.

159. Valentine, W. N., Tanaka, K. R., and Miwa, S.: A specific erythrocyte glycolytic enzyme defect (pyruvate kinase) in three subjects with congenital non-spherocytic hemolytic anemia. Trans. Assoc. Amer. Physicians, *74*:100, 1961.

160. Waller, H. D.: Glutathione reductase deficiency. In Beutler, E. (Ed.): Hereditary Disorders of Erythrocyte Metabolism. Grune & Stratton, New York, 1968, p. 185.

161. Waller, H. D., and Gerok, W.: Schwere strahleninduzierte Hämolyse bei hereditärem Mangel an reduziertem Gluthion in Blutzellen. Klin. Wschr., *42*:948, 1964.

162. Waterburg, L., and Frenkel, E. P.: Phosphofructokinase deficiency in congenital nonsphero-cytic hemolytic anemia. Clin. Res., *17*:347, 1969. (Abstract.)

163. Yoshida, A.: The structure of normal and variant human glucose-6-phosphate dehydrogenase. In Beutler, E. (Ed.): Hereditary Disorders of Erythrocyte Metabolism. Grune & Stratton, New York, 1968, p. 146.

SICKLE CELL ANEMIA

164. Allen, T. D.: Sickle cell disease and hematuria: a report of cases. J. Urol., *91*:177, 1964.

165. Anderson, W. W., and Ware, R. L.: Sickle cell anemia. Am. J. Dis. Child., *44*:1055, 1932.

166. Barnes, P. M., Hendrickse, R. G., and Watson-Williams, E. J.: Low molecular weight dextran in treatment of bone pain crises in sickle cell disease—a double-blind trial. Lancet, *2*:1271, 1965.

167. Barreras, L., Diggs, L. W., and Bell, A.: Erythrocyte morphology in patients with sickle cell anemia and pulmonary emboli. J.A.M.A., *203*:569, 1968.

168. Barrett-Connor, E.: Cholelithiasis in sickle cell anemia. Am. J. Med., *45*:889, 1968.

169. Beet, E. A.: The genetics of the sickle cell trait in a Bantu tribe. Ann. Eugenics, *14*:19, 1949.

170. Bell, W. R., and Pitney, W. R.: Management of priapism by therapeutic defibrination. New England J. Med., *280*:649, 1969.

171. Bernstein, J., and Whitten, C. F.: A histologic appraisal of the kidney in sickle cell anemia. Arch. Path., *70*:407, 1960.

172. Brody, J. I., Goldsmith, M. H., Parks, S. K., and Soltys, H. D.: Symptomatic crises of sickle cell anemia treated by limited exchange transfusion. Ann. Int. Med., *72*:327, 1970.

173. Callender, S. T. E., and Nickel, J. F.: Survival of transfused sickle cells in normal subjects and of normal red blood cells in patients with sickle cell anemia. J. Lab. & Clin. Med., *32*:1397, 1947.

174. Callender, S. T. E., Nickel, J. F., Moore, C. V., and Powell, E. O.: Sickle cell disease: studied by measuring the survival of transfused red blood cells. J. Lab. & Clin. Med., *34*:90, 1949.

174a. Charache, S., and Page, D. L.: Infarction of bone marrow in the sickle-cell disorders. Ann. Int. Med., *67*:1195, 1967.

175. Charache, S., and Richardson, S. N.: Prolonged survival of a patient with sickle cell anemia. Arch. Int. Med., *113*:844, 1964.

176. Clinicopathologic conference, a patient with sickle cell anemia surviving forty-eight years. Am. J. Med., *48*:226, 1970.

177. Diggs, L. W.: The sickle cell phenomenon. The rate of sickling in moist preparations. J. Lab. & Clin. Med., *17*:913, 1932.

177a. Diggs, L. W., and Bibb, J.: The erythrocyte in sickle cell anemia; morphology, size, hemoglobin content, fragility and sedimentation rate. J.A.M.A., *112*:695, 1939.

178. Diggs, L. W., and Ching, R. E.: The pathology of sickle cell anemia. South. Med. J., *27*:839, 1934.

179. Diggs, L. W., Pulliam, H. N., and King, J. C.: The bone changes in sickle cell anemia. South. Med. J., *30*:249, 1937.

189. Donegan, C. C., MacIlwaine, W. P., and Leavell, B. S.: Hematologic studies in patients with sickle cell anemia following multiple transfusions. Am. J. Med., *17*:29, 1954.

181. Emmel, V. E.: A study of the erythrocytes in a case of severe anemia with elongated and sickle-shaped red blood corpuscles. Arch. Int. Med., *20*:586, 1917.

182. Fink, A. I., Funahansi, T., Robinson, M., and Watson, R. J.: Conjunctival blood flow in sickle cell disease. Arch. Ophthal., *66*:82, 1961.

182a. Gill, F. A., Kaye, D., and Hook, E. W.: The influence of erythrophagocytosis on the interaction of macrophages and *Salmonella* in vitro. J. Exper. Med., *124*:173, 1966.

183. Greenberg, S. R., Atwater, J., and Israel, H. L.: Frequency of hemoglobinopathies in sarcoidosis. Ann. Int. Med., *62*:125, 1965.

184. Greenberg, N. S., Kass, E. H., and Castle, W. B.: Studies on the destruction of red blood cells. XII. Factors influencing the role of S hemoglobin in the pathologic physiology of sickle cell anemia and related disorders. J. Clin. Invest., *36*:833, 1957.

185. Hahn, E. V., and Gillespie, E. B.: Sickle cell anemia: report of a case greatly improved by splenectomy. Experimental study of sickle cell formation. Arch. Int. Med., *39*:233, 1927.

186. Harris, J. W., Brewster, H. H., Ham, T. H., and Castle, W. B.: Studies on destruction of the red blood cells. X. The biophysics and biology of sickle cell disease. Arch. Int. Med., *97*:145, 1956.

187. Harrow, B. R., Sloane, J. A., and Liebman, N. C.: Roentgenologic demonstration of renal papillary necrosis in sickle cell trait. New England J. Med., *268*:969, 1963.

188. Hatch, F. E., and Diggs, L. W.: Fluid balance in sickle cell disease. Arch. Int. Med., *116*:10, 1965.

189. Henderson, A. B.: Sickle cell anemia. Clinical study of fifty-four cases with autopsy. Am. J. Med., *9*:757, 1950.

190. Herrick, J. B.: Peculiar elongated and sickle-shaped red blood corpuscles in a case of severe anemia. Arch. Int. Med., *6*:517, 1910.

191. Hill, F. S., Hughes, J. G., and Davis, B. C.: Electroencephalographic findings in sickle cell anemia. Pediatrics, *6*:277, 1950.

192. Hill, R. J., Konigsberg, W., Guidotti, G., and Craig, L. C.: Structure of human hemoglobin: I. The separation of the $\alpha-$ and $\beta-$ chains and their amino acid composition. J. Biol. Chem., *237*:1549, 1962.

193. Hirschman, R. J., and Johns, C. J.: Hemoglobin studies in sarcoidosis. Ann. Int. Med., *62*:129, 1965.

193a. Hook, E. W., Campbell, C. G., Weens, H. S., and Cooper, G. R.: *Salmonella* osteomyelitis in patients with sickle-cell anemia. New England J. Med., *257*:403, 1957.

194. Huck, J. G.: Sickle cell anemia. Bull. Johns Hopkins Hosp., *34*:335, 1923.

195. Hughes, J. G., Diggs, L. W., and Gillespie, C. E.: The involvement of the nervous system in sickle cell anemia. J. Pediat., *17*:66, 1940.

196. Ingram, V. M.: A specific chemical difference between the globins of normal human and sickle cell anaemia haemoglobin. Nature, *178*:792, 1956. Conference on Hemoglobin, National Academy of Sciences, 1958, Pub. 557, p. 233.

197. James, G. W. III, and Abbott, L. D., Jr.: Erythrocyte destruction in sickle-cell anemia: Simultaneous N[15]-hemin and N[15] stercobilin studies. Proc. Soc. Exper. Biol. & Med., *88*:398, 1955.

198. Jenkins, M. E., Scott, R. B., and Baird, R. C.: Studies in sickle cell anemia. XVI. Sudden death during sickle cell crisis. J. Ped., *56*:30, 1960.

199. Jones, S. R., Binder, R. A., and Donowho, E. M., Jr.: Sudden death in sickle cell trait. New England J. Med., *282*:323, 1970.

200. Kabins, S. A., and Lerner, C.: Fulminant pneumococcemia in sickle cell anemia. J.A.M.A., *211*:467, 1970.

201. Kampmeier, R. H.: Sickle cell anemia as a cause of cerebrovascular disease. Arch. Neurol. & Psychiat., *36*:1323, 1936.

201a. Kaye, D., Gill, F. A., and Hook, E. W.: Factors influencing host resistance to *Salmonella* infections: The effects of hemolysis and erythrophagocytosis. Am. J. Med. Sci. *254*:101, 1967.

202. Keitel, H. G., Thompson, D., and Itano, H. A.: Hyposthenuria in sickle cell anemia: a reversible renal aspect. J. Clin. Invest., *35*:998, 1956.

203. Kimmelstiel, P.: Vascular occlusion and ischemic infarction in sickle cell disease. Am. J. Med. Sci., *216*:11, 1948.

204. Knochel, J. P.: Hematuria in sickle cell trait. Arch. Int. Med., *123*:160, 1969.

205. Leavell, B. S., and MacIlwaine, W. A.: Sickle cell anemia. In Bean, W. B.: Monographs in Medicine. Series 1. William & Wilkins Co., Baltimore, 1952.

206. Lieb, W. A., Geeracts, W. J., and Guerry, E. III: Sickle-cell retinopathy. Ocular and systemic manifestations of sickle cell disease. Acta Ophthal. (Kobenhavn) Suppl., *58*:1, 1959.

207. Macht, S. H., and Roman, P. W.: The radiologic changes in sickle cell anemia. Radiology, *51*:697, 1948.

208. Mahmood, A.: A double-blind trial of a phenothiazine compound in the treatment of clinical crisis of sickle cell anaemia. Brit. J. Haemat., *16*:181, 1969.

209. Margolis, M. P.: Sickle cell anemia. A composite study and survey. Medicine, *30*:357, 1951.

210. Murayama, M.: Molecular mechanism of red cell sickling. Science, *153*:145, 1966.

211. Murayama, M.: Tertiary structure of sickle cell hemoglobin and its functional significance. J. Cell Physiol., *67*:211, 1966.

212. Neel, J. V.: The inheritance of the sickling phenomenon with particular reference to sickle cell disease. Blood, *6*:389, 1951.

213. Neel, J. V.: Genetic aspects of abnormal hemoglobins. Conference on hemoglobin, National Academy of Sciences, Pub. 557, 1958, p. 253.

214. Paton, D.: The conjunctival sign of sickle-cell disease. Arch. Ophthal., *68*:627, 1962.

215. Pauling, L., Itano, H. A., Singer, S. J., and Wells, I. C.: Sickle cell anemia, a molecular disease. Science, *110*:543, 1949.

216. Pauling, L. et al.: Sickle cell anemia hemoglobin. Science, *111*:459, 1950.

216a. Pearson, H. A., Cornelius, E. A., Schwartz, A. D., Zelson, J. H., Wolfson, S. L., and Spencer, R. P.: Transfusion-reversible functional asplenia in young children with sickle-cell anemia. New England J. Med., *283*:334, 1970.

217. Pearson, H. A., Spencer, R. P., and Cornelius, E. A.: Functional asplenia in sickle cell anemia. New England J. Med., *281*:923, 1969.

218. Perillie, P. E., and Epstein, F. H.: Sickling phenomena produced by hypertonic solutions; a possible explanation for the hyposthenuria of sickle cell anemia. J. Clin. Invest., *42*:570, 1963.

219. Perutz, M. F., and Mitchison, J. M.: State of haemoglobin in sickle cell anaemia. Nature, *166*:677, 1950.

220. Ponder, E.: Red cell cytochemistry and architecture. Ann. N.Y. Acad. Sci., *48*:579, 1947.

221. Porter, F. S., and Thurman, W. G.: Studies in sickle cell disease. Am. J. Dis. Child., *106*:35, 1963.

222. Reinhard, E. H., Moore, C. V., Dubach, R., and Wade, L. J.: Effect of breathing 80 to 100 percent oxygen on the erythrocyte equilibrium in patients with sickle cell anemia. J.A.M.A., *121*:1245, 1943.

223. Reinhard, E. H., Moore, C. V., Dubach, R., and Wade, L. J.: Depressant effects of high concentrations of inspired oxygen on erythrocytogenesis. Observations on patients with sickle cell anemia with a description of the observed toxic manifestations of oxygen. J. Clin. Invest., *23*:682, 1944.

224. Ricks, P.: Further experiences with exchange transfusion in sickle cell anemia and pregnancy. Am. J. Obstet. & Gyn., *100*:1087, 1968.

225. Ryerson, C. S., and Terplan, K. L.: Sickle cell anemia. Two unusual cases with autopsy. Folia Haemat., *53*:353, 1935.

225a. Scott, R. B.: Health care priority and sickle cell anemia. J.A.M.A., *214*:731, 1970.

226. Shotton, D., Crockett, C. L., Jr., and Leavell, B. S.: Splenectomy in sickle cell anemia: report of a case and review of the literature. Blood, *6*:365, 1951.

227. Singer, K., Motulsky, A. G., and Wile, S. A.: Aplastic crisis in sickle cell anemia. A study of its mechanism and its relationship to other types of hemolytic crises. J. Lab. & Clin. Med., *35*:721, 1950.

227a. Statius van Eps, L. W., Pinedo-Veels, C., DeVries, G. H., and DeKonig, J.: Nature of concentrating defect in sickle-cell nephropathy. Lancet, *1*:450, 1970.

227b. Symposium on hemoglobinopathies in pregnancy. Clin. Obstet. & Gyn., *12*:13, 1969.

228. Winkelstein, J. A., and Drachman, R. H.: Deficiency of pneumococcal serum opsonizing activity in sickle cell disease. New England J. Med., *279*:459, 1968.

229. Winsor, T., and Burch, G. E.: The electrocardiogram and cardiac state in active sickle cell anemia. Am. Heart J., *29*:685, 1945.

230. Wintrobe, M. M.: The cardiovascular system in anemia: with a note on the particular abnormalities in sickle cell anemia. Blood, *1*:121, 1946.

THALASSEMIA

231. Atwater, J., Schwartz, I. R., Erslev, A. J., Montgomery, T. L., and Tocantins, L. M.: Sickling of erythrocytes in patients with thalassemia–hemoglobin-I disease. New England J. Med., *263*:1215, 1960.

232. Baglioni, C.: Fusion of two polypeptide chains in hemoglobin lepore and its interpretation as genetic deletion. Proc. Nat. Acad. Sci., *48*:1880, 1962.

233. Bank, A., and Marks, P. A.: Excess α chain synthesis relative to β chain synthesis in thalassemia major and minor. Nature, *212*:1198, 1966.

234. Bank, A., and Marks, P. A.: Protein synthesis in cell-free human reticulocyte system: ribosome function in thalassemia. J. Clin. Invest., *45*:330, 1966.

235. Beard, M. E., Necheles, T. F., and Allen, D. M.: Clinical experience with intensive transfusion therapy in Cooley's anemia. Ann. N.Y. Acad. Sci., *165*:415, 1969.

236. Benesch, R., and Benesch, R. E.: Properties of haemoglobin H and their significance in relation to function of haemoglobin. Nature, *202*:773, 1964.

237. Cooley, T. B., and Lee, P.: Series of cases of splenomegaly in children with anemia and peculiar bone changes. Trans. Am. Pediat. Soc., *47*:29, 1925.

238. Dormandy, K. M., Lock, S. P., and Lehmann, H.: Haemoglobin Q-alpha-thalassemia. Brit. Med. J., *1*:1582, 1961.

239. Fessas, P., and Mastrohalos, N.: Demonstration of small components in red cell haemolysates by starch-gel electrophoresis. Nature, *183*:30, 1959.

240. Fessas, P., and Stamatoyannopoulos, G.: Absence of haemoglobin A_2 in an adult. Nature, *195*:1215, 1962.

241. Fessas, P., Stamatoyannopoulas, G., and Karaklis, A.: Hemoglobin "Pylos": study of a hemoglobinopathy resembling thalassemia in the heterozygous homozygous and double heterozygous state. Blood, *19*:1, 1962.

242. Gabuzda, T. G.: Analytic review, Hemoglobin H and the red cell. Blood, *27*:568, 1966.

243. Harton, B. F., Thompson, R. B., Dozy, A. M., Nechtman, C. M., Nichols, E., and Henswain, T. H. J.: Inhomogeneity of hemoglobin VI. The minor hemoglobin components of cord blood. Blood, *20*:302, 1962.

244. Ingram, V. M.: The Hemoglobins in Genetics and Evolution. Columbia University Press, New York, 1963.

245. Kan, Y. W., Schwartz, E. and Nathan, D. G.: Globin chain synthesis in the alpha thalassemia syndromes. J. Clin. Invest., *45*:2515, 1968.

246. Lehmann, H.: Inheritance of human haemoglobin. Brit. Med. Bull., *15*:40, 1959.

247. Marks, P. A.: Thalassemia syndromes: biochemical, genetic and clinical aspects. New England J. Med., *275*:1363, 1966.

248. Minnich, V., Na-Nakorn, S., Chongchareonsuk, S., and Kochaseni, S.: Mediterranean anemia. A study of 32 cases in Thailand. Blood, *9*:1, 1954.

249. Nathan, D. G., and Gunn, R. B.: Thalassemia: the consequence of unbalanced hemoglobin synthesis. Am. J. Med., *41*:819, 1966.

250. Nathan, D. G., Stossel, T. B., Gunn, R. B., Zarkowsky, H. S., and Laforet, M. T.: Influence of hemoglobin precipitation on erythrocyte metabolism in alpha and beta thallassemia. J. Clin. Invest., *48*:33, 1969.

251. Neel, J. V., and Valentine, W. N.: The frequency of thalassemia. Am. J. Med. Sci., *209*:568, 1945.

252. Pearson, H. A., Gerald, P. S., and Diamond, L. K.: Thalassemia intermedia due to interaction of Lepore trait with thalassemia trait: report of three cases. J. Dis. Child., *97*:464, 1959.

253. Piomelli, S., Danoff, S. J., Becker, M. H., Lipera, M. J., and Travis, S. F.: Prevention of bone malformation and cardiomegaly in Cooley's anemia by early hypertransfusion regimen. Ann. N.Y. Acad. Sci., *165*:427, 1969.

254. Rigas, D. A., Koler, R. D., and Osgood, E. E.: New hemoglobin possessing a higher electrophoretic mobility than normal adult hemoglobin. Science, *121*:372, 1955.

255. Schwartz, E.: Heterozygous beta thalassemia: balanced globin synthesis in bone marrow cells. Science, *167*:1513, 1970.

256. Singer, K.: Hereditary hemolytic disorders associated with abnormal hemoglobins. Am. J. Med., *18*:633, 1955.

257. Slater, L. M., Muir, W. A., and Weed, R. I.: Influence of splenectomy on insoluble hemoglobin inclusion bodies in β thalassemic erythrocytes. Blood, *31*:766, 1968.

258. Smith, C. H., Erlandson, M. E., Stern, G., and Schulman, I.: The role of splenectomy in the management of thalassemia. Blood, *15*:197, 1960.

259. Valentine, W. N., and Neel, J. V.: Hematologic and genetic study of the transmission of thalassemia. Arch. Int. Med., *74*:185, 1944.

260. Weatherall, D. J.: The Thalassemia Syndromes. F. A. Davis Co., Philadelphia, 1965.

261. Weatherall, D. J., Clegg, J. B., and Naughton, M. A.: Globin synthesis in thalassemia: in vitro study. Nature, *208*:1061, 1965.
262. Wintrobe, M. M., Matthews, E., Pollack, R., and Dobyns, B. M.: A familial hemopoietic disorder in Italian adolescents and adults. J.A.M.A., *114*:1530, 1940.
263. Wolff, J. A., and Lukem, K. H.: Management of thalassemia: a comparative program. Ann. N.Y. Acad. Sci., *165*:423, 1969.
264. Wolman, I. J.: Transfusion therapy in Cooley's anemia: growth and health as related to long-range hemoglobin levels, a progress report. Ann. N.Y. Acad. Sci., *119*:736, 1964.
265. Wolman, I. J., and Ortolani, M.: Some clinical features of Cooley's anemia patients as related to transfusion schedules. Ann. N.Y. Acad. Sci., *165*:407, 1969.
266. Zaino, E. C.: Paleontologic thalassemia. Ann. N.Y. Acad. Sci., *119*:402, 1964.

OTHER HEMOGLOBINOPATHIES

267. Bookchin, R. M., Davis, R. P., and Ranney, H. M.: Clinical features of hemoglobin C Harlem, a new sickling hemoglobin variant. Ann. Int. Med., *68*:8, 1968.
268. Carrell, R. W., and Lehmann, H.: The unstable haemoglobin haemolytic anaemias. Semin. Hemat., *6*:116, 1969.
269. Cawein, M. J., Lappat, E. J., Brangle, R. W., and Farley, Z. H.: Hemoglobin S-D disease. Ann. Int. Med., *64*:62, 1966.
270. Charache, S., Conley, L. L., Waugh, D. F., Ugoretz, R. J., and Spurrell, R.: Pathogenesis of hemolytic anemia in homozygous hemoglobin C disease. J. Clin. Invest., *40*:1795, 1967.
271. Chernoff, A. I.: Studies on hemoglobin E. J. Lab. & Clin. Med., *44*:780, 1954.
272. Chernoff, A. I.: On the prevalence of hemoglobin D in the American Negro. Blood, *11*:907, 1956.
273. Chernoff, A. I., Smith, G., and Steinkamp, R.: Homozygous hemoglobin D disease. J. Lab. & Clin. Med., *48*:795, 1956.
274. Conley, J. C. L., and Charache, S.: Inherited hemoglobinopathies. Hosp. Pract., *4*:35, 1969.
275. Diggs, L. W., and Bell, A.: Intraerythrocytic hemoglobin crystals in sickle cell–hemoglobin C disease. Blood, *25*:218, 1965.
276. Diggs, L. W., Kraus, A. P., Morrison, D. B., and Rudnicki, R. P. T.: Intraerythrocytic crystals in a white patient with hemoglobin C in the absence of other types of hemoglobin. Blood, *9*:1172, 1954.
277. Fairbanks, V. F., Opfell, R. W., and Burgert, E. O., Jr.: Three families with unstable hemoglobinopathies (Köln, Olmsted and Santa Ana) causing hemolytic anemia with inclusion bodies and pigmenturia. Am. J. Med., *46*:344, 1969.
278. Gerald, P. S., and Path, C. E.: Hemoglobin C Georgetown; first abnormal hemoglobin due to two different mutations in the same gene. J. Clin. Invest., *45*:1012, 1966.
279. Heller, P.: Hemoglobinopathic dysfunction of the red cell. Am. J. Med., *41*:799, 1968.
279a. Huehns, E. R.: Diseases due to abnormalities of hemoglobin structure. Ann. Rev. Med., *21*:157, 1970.
280. Itano, H. A.: A third abnormal hemoglobin associated with hereditary hemolytic anemia. Proc. Nat. Acad. Sci., *37*:775, 1951.
281. Itano, H. A., and Neel, J. V.: A new inherited abnormality of human hemoglobin. Proc. Nat. Acad. Sci., *36*:613, 1950.
281a. Jacob, H. S.: Mechanisms of Heinz body formation and attachment to red cell membrane. Seminars in Hemat., *7*:341, 1970.
282. Kaplan, E., Zuelzer, W., and Neel, J. V.: A new inherited abnormality of hemoglobin and its interaction with sickle cell hemoglobin. Blood, *6*:1240, 1951.
283. Kraus, A. P., Miyaji, T., Iuchi, I., and Kraus, L. M.: A new variety of sickle cell anemia with clinically mild symptoms due to an α chain variant of hemoglobin ($\alpha^{23\ Glu\ NH_2}$). J. Lab. & Clin. Med., *66*:886, 1965.
284. Kraus, L. M., Miyaji, T., Iuchi, I., and Kraus, A. P.: Characterization of $\alpha^{23\ Glu\ NH_2}$ in hemoglobin Memphis. Hemoglobin Memphis S, a new variant of molecular disease. Biochemistry, *5*:3701, 1966.
285. Lessin, L. S., Jensen, W. N., and Porter, E.: Molecular mechanism of hemolytic anemia in homozygous hemoglobin C disease. J. Exper. Med., *130*:443, 1969.
286. Pierce, L. E., Path, L. E., and McCoy, K.: A new hemoglobin variant with sickling properties. New England J. Med., *268*:862, 1963.
287. Powell, W. N., Rodarte, J. G., and Neel, J. V.: The occurrence in a family of Sicilian ancestry of the traits for both sickling and thalassemia. Blood, *5*:887, 1950.
288. Ranney, H. M.: Clinically important variants of human hemoglobin. New England J. Med., *282*:144, 1970.

288a. Silvestroni, E., and Bianco, I.: Singulare associazone di "anemia microcitica" constituzionale con "depranocitiro-anemia" in sogetto di razza bianca. Policlinico (sez. Prat.) *53*:265, 1946.
289. Singer, K., Chapman, A. Z., Goldberg, S. R., Rubinstein, H. M., and Rosenblum, S. A.: Studies on abnormal hemoglobins. IX. Pure (homozygous) hemoglobin C disease. Blood, *9*:1023, 1954.
290. Singer, K., Kraus, A. P., Singer, L., Rubinstein, H. M., and Goldberg, S. R.: Studies on abnormal hemoglobins X. A new syndrome: hemoglobin C–thalassemia disease. Blood, *9*:1032, 1954.
291. Smith, E. W., and Conley, C. L.: Filter paper electrophoresis of human hemoglobins with special reference to the incidence and clinical significance of hemoglobin C. Bull. Johns Hopkins Hosp., *93*:94, 1953.
292. Smith, E. W., and Conley, C. L.: Clinical features of the genetic variants of sickle cell disease. Bull. Johns Hopkins Hosp., *94*:289, 1954.
293. Smith, E. W., and Conley, C. L.: Sickle cell–hemoglobin D disease. Ann. Int. Med., *50*:94, 1959.
294. Spaet, T. H., Alway, R. H., and Ward, G.: Homozygous type C hemoglobin. Pediatrics, *12*:483, 1954.
295. Tanaka, K. R., and Clifford, G. O.: Homozygous hemoglobin C disease: report of three cases. Ann. Int. Med., *49*:30, 1958.
296. Wheby, M. S., Thorup, O. A., and Leavell, B. S.: Homozygous hemoglobin C disease in siblings; further comment on intraerythrocytic crystals. Blood, *11*:266, 1956.
297. Zuelzer, W., and Kaplan, E.: Thalassemia–hemoglobin C disease. A new syndrome presumably due to the combination of the genes for thalassemia and hemoglobin C. Blood, *9*:1047, 1954.
298. Zuelzer, W. W., Neel, J. V., and Robinson, A. R.: Abnormal hemoglobins. Progr. Hemat., *1*:91, 1956.

ERYTHROBLASTOSIS FETALIS

299. Abelson, N. M., and Boggs, T. R., Jr.: Plasma pigments in erythroblastosis fetalis. Pediatrics, *17*:452, 1956.
300. Allen, F. H., Jr., and Diamond, L. K.: Erythroblastosis fetalis. New England J. Med., *257*:659, 1957; *257*:705, 1957; *257*:761, 1957.
301. Allen, F. H., Jr., Diamond, L. K., and Vaughan, V. C.: Erythroblastosis fetalis. Prevention of kernicterus. Am. J. Dis. Child., *80*:779, 1950.
301a. Behrman, R. E., and Hsia, D. Y. Y.: Summary of a symposium on phototherapy for hyperbilirubinemia. J. Pediat., *75*:718, 1969.
302. Bowman, J. M., Friesen, R. F., Bowman, W. D., McInnis, A. L., Barnes, P. H., and Grewar, D.: Fetal transfusion in severe Rh isoimmunization. J.A.M.A., *207*:1101, 1969.
303. Brown, A. K., and Zuelzer, W. W.: Studies on the neonatal development of the glucuronide conjugating system. J. Clin. Invest., *37*:332, 1958.
303a. Brown, A. K., Zeulzer, W. W., and Robinson, A. R.: Studies in hyperbilirubinemia. II. Clearance of bilirubin from plasma and extravascular space in newborn infants during exchange transfusion. Am. J. Dis. Child., *93*:274, 1957.
304. Clarke, C. A.: Prevention of rhesus iso-immunization. Semin. Hemat., *6*:201, 1969.
305. Cohen, F., Zuelzer, W. W., Gustafsan, D. C., and Evans, M. M.: Mechanisms of isoimmunization. I. The transplacental passage of fetal erythrocytes in homospecific pregnancies. Blood, *23*:621, 1964.
306. Diamond, L. K., Blackfan, K. D., and Baty, J. M.: Erythroblastosis fetalis and its association with universal edema of the fetus, icterus gravis neonatorum and anemia of the newborn. J. Pediat., *1*:269, 1932.
306a. Doxiadis, S.: Phenobarbital prophylaxis for neonatal jaundice. Hosp. Pract., *5*:115, 1970.
307. Dunn, H. G.: Hemolytic disease of the newborn due to ABO incompatibility. Am. J. Dis. Child., *85*:655, 1953.
308. Ernster, L., Herlin, L., and Zetterstrom, R.: Experimental studies on the pathogenesis of kernicterus. Pediatrics, *20*:647, 1957.
309. Hsia, D. Y., Allen, F. H., Jr., Gellis, S. S., and Diamond, L. K.: Erythroblastosis fetalis. VIII. Studies of serum bilirubin in relation to kernicterus. New England J. Med., *247*:668, 1952.
310. Kelsall, G. A., Vos, G. H., Kirk, R. L., and Shield, J. W.: The evaluation of cord blood hemoglobin, reticulocyte percentage and maternal antiglobulin titer in the prognosis of hemolytic disease of the newborn. Pediatrics, *20*:221, 1957.
311. Landsteiner, K., and Wiener, A. S.: Studies on an agglutinogen (Rh) in human blood reacting with antirhesus sera and with human isoantibodies. J. Exper. Med., *74*:309, 1941.
312. Levine, P., Katzin, E. M., and Burnham, L.: Isoimmunization in pregnancy. J.A.M.A., *116*:825, 1941.

313. Levine, P., and Stetson, R. E.: Unusual cases of intragroup agglutination. J.A.M.A., *113*:126, 1939.
314. Levine, P., Vogel, P., Katzin, E. M., and Burnham, L.: Pathogenesis of erythroblastosis fetalis: statistical evidence. Science, *94*:371, 1941.
315. Liley, A. W.: Intrauterine transfusion of fetus in hemolytic disease. Brit. Med. J., *2*:1107, 1963.
316. Little, B., McCutcheon, E., and Desforges, J. F.: Amniocentesis and intrauterine transfusion in Rh-sensitized pregnancy. New England J. Med., *27*:332, 1966.
317. Mollison, P. L.: Survival of transfused erythrocytes in hemolytic disease of the newborn. Arch. Dis. Child., *18*:161, 1943.
318. Mollison, P. L., and Cutbush, M.: Haemolytic disease of the newborn: criteria of severity. Brit. Med. J., *1*:123, 1949.
319. Nevanlinna, H. R., and Vaino, T.: The influence of mother-child ABO incompatibility on Rh immunization. Vox Sang., *1*:26, 1956.
320. Odell, G. B.: Studies in kernicterus. I. The protein binding of bilirubin. J. Clin. Invest., *38*:823, 1959.
321. Pollack, W., Gorman, J. G., and Freda, V. J.: Prevention of Rh hemolytic disease. Progr. Hemat., *6*:121, 1969.
322. Rautmann, H.: Über Blutbildung bei fötaler allgemeiner Wassersucht. Beitr. Path. Anat., *54*:332, 1912.
323. Rosen, F. S.: The macroglobulins. New England J. Med., *267*:546, 1962.
324. Wallerstein, H.: Treatment of severe erythroblastosis by simultaneous removal and replacement of blood of the newborn infant. Science, *103*:583, 1946.
324a. Wilson, J. T.: Phenobarbital in the neonatal period. Pediatrics, *43*:324, 1969.
325. Zuelzer, W. W., and Cohen, F.: ABO hemolytic disease and heterospecific pregnancy. Pediat. Clin. North America, *4*:405, 1957.

DRUG-INDUCED AND AUTO-IMMUNE HEMOLYTIC ANEMIA

326. Allgood, J. W., and Chaplin, H., Jr.: Idiopathic acquired auto-immune hemolytic anemia. A review of forty-seven cases treated from 1955 through 1965. Am. J. Med., *43*:254, 1967.
327. Bakemeier, R. F., and Leddy, J. P.: Heavy chain:light chain relationships among erythrocyte autoantibodies. J. Clin. Invest., *46*:1033, 1967.
328. Bakemeier, R. F., and Leddy, J. P.: Erythrocyte autoantibody associated with alpha-methyldopa: heterogeneity of structure and specificity. Blood, *32*:1, 1968.
329. Bolton, F. G., and Dameshek, W.: Thrombocytopenic purpura due to quinidine. I. Clinical studies. Blood, *11*:527, 1956.
330. Carstairs, K. L., Breckenridge, A., Dollery, C. T., and Worlledge, S. M.: Incidence of a positive direct Coombs test in patients on methyldopa. Lancet, *2*:133, 1966.
331. Coombs, R. R. A., Mourant, A. E., and Race, R. R.: A new test for the detection of weak and "incomplete" Rh agglutinins. Brit. J. Exper. Path., *26*:255, 1945.
332. Corley, L. E., Lessner, H. E., and Larsen, W. E.: Azathioprine therapy of "autoimmune" diseases. Am. J. Med., *41*:404, 1966.
333. Croft, J. D., Jr., Swisher, S. N., Jr., Gilliland, B. L., Bakemeier, R. F., Leddy, J. P., and Weed, R. I.: Coombs-test positively induced by drugs: mechanisms of immunologic reactions and red cell destruction. Ann. Int. Med., *68*:176, 1968.
334. Crosby, W. H., and Rappaport, H.: Autoimmune hemolytic anemia. I. Analysis of hematologic observations with particular reference to their prognostic value. A survey of 57 cases. Blood, *12*:42, 1957.
335. Dacie, J. V.: The auto-immune hemolytic anemias. Am. J. Med., *18*:810, 1955.
336. Dacie, J. V.: The Auto-immune haemolytic anemias. Part II in The Haemolytic Anaemias, Congenital and Acquired. 2nd Ed. Grune & Stratton, New York, 1962.
337. Dacie, J. V.: Drug-induced hemolytic anaemias, paroxysmal nocturnal haemoglobinuria, haemolytic disease of the newborn. Part IV in The Haemolytic Anaemias, Congenital and Acquired. 2nd Ed. Grune & Stratton, New York, 1967.
337a. Dacie, J. V.: Autoimmune haemolytic anaemias. Brit. Med. J., *2*:381, 1970.
338. Dacie, J. V., and Worlledge, S. M.: Auto-immune hemolytic anemias. Progr. Hemat., *6*:82, 1969.
339. Dameshek, W., and Schwartz, S. O.: Acute hemolytic anemia (acquired hemolytic icterus, acute type). Medicine, *19*:231, 1940.
340. Dausset, J., and Colombani, J.: The serology and the prognosis of 128 cases of autoimmune hemolytic anemia. Blood, *14*:1280, 1959.
341. DeTorregrosa, M. V. V., Rosada, A. L. R., and Montella, E.: Hemolytic anemia secondary to stibophen therapy. J.A.M.A., *186*:598, 1963.

342. Donath, J., and Landsteiner, R.: Ueber paroxysmalen Hämoglobinurie. München med. Wchnschr., *51*:1590, 1904.
343. Eyster, M. E., and Jenkins, D. E., Jr.: Erythrocyte coating substances in patients with positive direct antiglobulin reactions. Correlation of γ G globulin and complement coating with underlying diseases, overt hemolysis and response to therapy. Am. J. Med., *46*:360, 1969.
344. Eyster, M. E., Nachman, R. L., Christenson, W. N., and Engel, R. L., Jr.: Structural characteristics of red cell auto-antibodies. J. Immun., *96*:107, 1966.
345. Freedman, A. L., Barr, R. S., Brody, E. A.: Hemolytic anemia due to quinidine: observations on its mechanism. Am. J. Med., *20*:806, 1956.
346. Gralnick, H. R., Wright, L. D., Jr., and McGinniss, M. D.: Coombs positive reactions associated with sodium cephalothin therapy. J.A.M.A., *199*:725, 1967.
347. Ham, T. H.: Hemoglobinuria. Am. J. Med., *18*:990, 1955.
348. Harris, J. W.: Studies on the mechanism of a drug-induced hemolytic anemia. J. Lab. Clin. Med., *44*:809, 1954.
349. Hinz, C. F.: Serologic and physiochemical characterization of Donath-Landsteiner antibodies from six patients. Blood, *22*:600, 1963.
350. Hippe, E., Jensen, K. B., Olesen, H., Lind, K., and Thomsen, P. E. B.: Chlorambucil treatment of patients with cold agglutinin syndrome. Blood, *35*:68, 1970.
351. Hitzig, W. H., and Massemo, L.: Treatment of autoimmune hemolytic anemia in children with azathioprine (Imuran). Blood, *28*:840, 1966.
352. Jandl, J. H., Greenberg, M. S., Yonemoto, R. H., and Castle, W. B.: Clinical determination of the sites of red cell sequestration in hemolytic anemia. J. Clin. Invest., *35*:842, 1956.
353. Jandl, J. H., Richardson-Jones, A., and Castle, W. B.: Destruction of red cells by antibodies in man. I. Observations of the sequestration and lysis of red cells altered by immune mechanisms. J. Clin. Invest., *36*:1428, 1957.
354. Kaplan, K., Reisberg, B., and Weinstein, L.: Cephaloridine: studies of therapeutic activity and untoward effects. Arch. Int. Med., *121*:168, 1968.
355. Levine, B. B., and Redmond, A. P.: Immune mechanisms of penicillin-induced Coombs' positivity in man. J. Clin. Invest., *46*:1085, 1967 (Abstract).
356. LoBuglio, A. F., Cotran, R. J., and Jandl, J. H.: Red cells coated with immunoglobin G: binding and sphering by mononuclear cells in man. Science, *158*:1582, 1967.
357. LoBuglio, A. F., and Jandl, J. H.: The nature of the alpha-methyldopa red-cell antibody. New England J. Med., *276*:658, 1967.
357a. Logue, G. L., Boyd, A. E., III, and Rosse, W. F.: Chlorpropamide-induced immune hemolytic anemia. New England J. Med., *283*:900, 1970.
358. Mac Gibbon, B. H., Loughridge, C., Hourihane, W., O'B. D., and Boyd, D. W.: Autoimmune haemolytic anemia with acute renal failure due to phenacetin and p-amino-salicylic acid. Lancet, *1*:7, 1960.
359. MacKenzie, G. M.: Paroxysmal hemoglobinuria. Medicine, *8*:159, 1929.
359a. MacKenzie, M. R., and Creevy, N. C.: Hemolytic anemia with cold-detectable IgG antibodies. Blood, *36*:549, 1970.
360. Mohler, D. N., Farris, B. L., and Pearre, A. A.: Paroxysmal cold hemoglobinuria with acute renal failure. Arch. Int. Med., *112*:36, 1963.
361. Moltlan, L., Reidenberg, M. M., and Eichman, M. F.: Positive direct Coombs' test due to cephalothin. New England J. Med., *277*:123, 1967.
362. Muirhead, E. E., Halden, E. R., and Groves, M.: Drug-dependent Coombs (antiglobulin test) and anemia: observations on quinine and acetophenetidin (Phenacetin). Arch. Int. Med., *101*:87, 1958.
363. Nesmith, L. W., and Davis, J. W.: Hemolytic anemia caused by penicillin. J.A.M.A., *203*:27, 1968.
364. Petz, L. D., and Fudenberg, H. H.: Coombs-positive hemolytic anemia caused by penicillin administration. New England J. Med., *274*:171, 1966.
365. Robinson, M. G., and Foadi, M.: Hemolytic anemia with positive Coombs test. Association with isoniazid therapy. J.A.M.A., *208*:656, 1969.
366. Rosenthal, M. C., Pisciotta, A. V., Kominos, Z. D., Goldberg, H., and Dameshek, W.: The auto-immune hemolytic anemia of malignant lymphocytic disease. Blood, *10*:197, 1955.
367. Ross, J. F.: Hemoglobinemia and the hemoglobinurias. New England J. Med., *233*:691, 732, 1945.
368. Schubothe, H.: The cold hemagglutinin disease. Semin. Hemat., *33*:27, 1966.
369. Schwartz, R., and Dameshek, W.: The treatment of autoimmune hemolytic anemia with 6-mercaptopurine and thioguanine. Blood, *19*:483, 1962.
370. Scott, G. L., Myles, A. B., and Bacon, P. A.: Autoimmune haemolytic anaemia and mefanamic acid therapy. Brit. Med. J., *3*:534, 1968.
371. Shinton, N. K., and Wilson, L.: Autoimmune haemolytic anaemia due to phenacetin and p-aminosalicylic acid. Lancet, *1*:226, 1960.

372. Shulman, N. R.: A mechanism of cell destruction in individuals sensitized to foreign antigens and its implications in autoimmunity. Ann. Int. Med., 60:506, 1964.
373. Snapper, I., Marks, D., Schwartz, L., and Hollander, L.: Hemolytic anemia secondary to mesantoin. Ann. Int. Med., 37:619, 1953.
374. Swanson, M. A., Chanmougan, D., and Schwartz, R. S.: Immunohemolytic anemia due to antipenicillin antibodies. Report of a case. New England J. Med., 274:178, 1966.
375. Weiner, W.: To be or not to be an antibody: the "agent" in auto-immune hemolytic anemia. Blood, 14:1057, 1959.
376. Weiner, W., and Vos, G. H.: Serology of acquired hemolytic anemias. Blood, 22:606, 1963.
377. Welch, C. S., and Dameshek, W.: Splenectomy in blood dyscrasias. New England J. Med., 242:601, 1950.
378. Widal, F., Abrami, P., and Brulé, M.: Differentiation de divers types d'ictères hémolytiques par le procède des hématies deplastmatises. Presse Méd., 15:641, 1907.
379. Widal, F., Abrami, P., and Brulé, M.: Pleuralité d'origine des ictères hémolytiques recherchis cliniques et expérimentales. Bull. et Mém. Soc. Méd. Hôp. Paris, 24:1354, 1907.
380. Worlledge, S. M.: Immune drug-induced haemolytic anaemias. Semin. Hemat., 6:181, 1969.
381. Wurzel, H. A., and Silverman, J. L.: The effects of alpha-methyl-3, 4-dehydroxy-L-phenylalanine (methyldopa, Aldomet) on erythrocytes. Transfusion, 8:84, 1968.
382. Young, L. E., Miller, G., and Christian, R. M.: Clinical and laboratory observations on auto-immune hemolytic disease. Ann. Int. Med., 35:507, 1951.

PAROXYSMAL NOCTURNAL HEMOGLOBINURIA

383. Beal, R. W., Kronenberg, H., and Firkin, B. G.: The syndrome of paroxysmal nocturnal hemoglobinuria. Am. J. Med., 37:899, 1964.
384. Cartwright, G. E.: Diagnostic Laboratory Hematology. 4th Ed. Grune & Stratton, New York, 1968.
385. Crookston, J. H., Crookston, M. C., and Rosse, W. F.: Red cell membrane abnormalities in hereditary erythroblastic multinuclearity. Blood, 34:58, 1969 (Abstract).
386. Crosby, W. H.: Paroxysmal nocturnal hemoglobinuria. A classic description of Paul Strubing in 1882 and a bibliography of the disease. Blood, 6:270, 1951.
387. Dacie, J. V.: Transfusion of saline-washed red cells in nocturnal hemoglobinuria (Marchiafava-Micheli disease). Clin. Sci., 7:65, 1948.
388. Dacie, J. V.: Paroxysmal nocturnal haemoglobinuria: an acquired disorder of the red-cell membrane. Plenary Session Papers. XII Congress, International Society of Hematology, New York, 1968.
389. Dacie, J. V., and Gilpin, A.: Refractory anaemia (Fanconi type). Its incidence in three members of one family, with one case a relationship to chronic haemolytic anemia with nocturnal haemoglobinuria (Marchiafava-Micheli disease or "nocturnal haemoglobinuria"). Arch. Dis. Child., 19:155, 1944.
390. Dacie, J. V., and Mollison, P. L.: Survival of transfused erythrocytes from a donor with nocturnal hemoglobinuria. Lancet, 1:390, 1949.
391. Dameshek, W.: Riddle: what do aplastic anemia, paroxysmal nocturnal hemoglobinuria (PNH) and "hypoplastic" leukemia have in common? Blood, 30:251, 1967.
392. Firkin, F., Goldberg, H., and Firkin, B. G.: Glucocorticoid management of paroxysmal nocturnal haemoglobinuria. Aust. Ann. Med., 17:127, 1968.
393. Gaither, J. C.: Paroxysmal nocturnal hemoglobinuria. New England J. Med., 265:421, 1961.
394. Hartmann, R. C., Auditore, J. V., and Holland, W. C.: Erythrocyte acetylcholinesterase defect in paroxysmal nocturnal hemoglobinuria. J. Clin. Invest., 37:900, 1958.
395. Hartmann, R. C., and Jenkins, D. E., Jr.: Paroxysmal nocturnal hemoglobinuria: current concepts of certain pathophysiologic features. Blood, 25:850, 1965.
396. Hartmann, R. C., and Jenkins, D. E., Jr.: The "sugar-water" test for paroxysmal nocturnal hemoglobinuria. New England J. Med., 275:155, 1966.
396a. Hartmann, R. C., Jenkins, D. E., Jr., and Arnold, A. B.: Diagnostic specificity of sucrose hemolysis test for paroxysmal nocturnal hemoglobinuria. Blood, 35:462, 1970.
397. Hinz, C. F., Jr., Hurley, T. H., and Weisman, R., Jr.: Relation of anemia to in vitro and in vivo hemolysis in three patients with paroxysmal nocturnal hemoglobinuria. Clin. Res., 3:7, 1955. (Abstract.)
398. Holden, D., and Lichtman, H.: Paroxysmal nocturnal hemoglobinuria with acute leukemia. Blood, 33:283, 1969.
399. Jenkins, D. E., Jr., and Hartmann, R. C.: Paroxysmal nocturnal hemoglobinuria terminating in acute myeloblastic leukemia. Blood, 33:274, 1969.

400. Johns, R. J.: Familial reduction in red-cell cholinesterase. New England J. Med., *267*:1344, 1962.
401. Kan, S. Y., and Gardner, F. H.: Life span of reticulocytes in paroxysmal nocturnal hemoglobinuria. Blood, *25*:759, 1965.
402. Kaufman, R. W., Schecter, G. P., and McFarland, W.: Paroxysmal nocturnal hemoglobinuria terminating in acute granulocytic leukemia. Blood, *33*:287, 1969.
403. Lewis, S. M., and Dacie, J. V.: The aplastic anemia-paroxysmal nocturnal hemoglobinuria syndrome. Brit. J. Haematol., *13*:236, 1967.
404. Meriwether, W. D., and Mengel, C. E.: Peroxidation of lipid from normal and paroxysmal nocturnal hemoglobinuria erythrocytes. Nature, *210*:91, 1966.
405. Metz, J., Stevens, K., van Rensburg, N. J., and Hart, D.: Failure of in-vivo inhibition of acetylcholinesterase to affect erythrocyte life-span: the significance of the enzyme defect in paroxysmal nocturnal haemoglobinuria. Brit. J. Haematol., *7*:458, 1961.
406. Quagliana, J. M., Cartwright, G. E., and Wintrobe, M. M.: Paroxysmal nocturnal hemoglobinuria following drug-induced aplastic anemia. Ann. Int. Med., *61*:1045, 1964.
407. Rosse, W. F., and Dacie, J. V.: Immune lysis of normal human and paroxysmal nocturnal hemoglobinuria (PNH) red blood cells. I. The sensitivity of PNH red cells to lysis by complement and specific antibody. J. Clin. Invest., *45*:736, 1966.
408. Rosse, W. F., and Dacie, J. V.: Immune lysis of normal human and paroxysmal nocturnal hemoglobinuria red blood cells. II. The role of complement components in the increased sensitivity of PNH red cells to immune lysis. J. Clin. Invest., *45*:749, 1966.
408a. Rosse, W. F., and Gutterman, L. A.: The effect of iron therapy in paroxysmal nocturnal hemoglobinuria. Blood, *36*:559, 1970.
409. Sirchia, G., Ferone, S., and Mercuriali, F.: The action of two sulfhydryl compounds on normal human red cells: relationship to red cells of paroxysmal nocturnal hemoglobinuria. Blood, *25*:502, 1965.
410. Yachnin, S.: Studies on hemolysis of red cells from patients with paroxysmal nocturnal hemoglobinuria. J. Clin. Invest., *43*:1240, 1964.
411. Yachnin, S.: The hemolysis of red cells from patients with paroxysmal nocturnal hemoglobinuria by partially purified subcomponents of the third complement component. J. Clin. Invest., *44*:1534, 1965.
412. Yachnin, S., and Ruthenberg, J. M.: The initiation and enhancement of human red cell lysis by activators of the first component of complement and by first component esterase, studies using normal red cells and red cells from patients with paroxysmal nocturnal hemoglobinuria. J. Clin. Invest., *44*:518, 1965.

MECHANICAL HEMOLYSIS

413. Brain, M. C.: Microangiopathic hemolytic anemia. New England J. Med., *281*:833, 1969.
414. Brain, M. C.: The hemolytic-uremic syndrome. Semin. Hemat., *6*:162, 1969.
415. Brain, M. C., Dacie, J. V., and Hourihane, D. O'B.: Microangiopathic haemolytic anemia: the possible role of vascular lesions in pathogenesis. Brit. J. Haemat., *8*:358, 1962.
416. Brain, M. C., Esterly, J. R., and Beck, E. A.: Intravascular haemolysis with experimentally produced thrombi. Brit. J. Haemat., *13*:868, 1967.
417. Brain, M. C., and Hourihane, D. O'B.: Microangiopathic hemolytic anemia: the occurrence of haemolysis in experimentally produced vascular disease. Brit. J. Haemat., *13*:135, 1967.
418. Bull, B. S., and Kuhn, I. N.: The production of schistocytes by fibrin strands (a scanning electron microscope study). Blood, *35*:104, 1970.
419. Chaplin, H., Perkoff, G. T., Frisbie, J. H., Tateishi, S., and Haynes, C. R.: March hemoglobinuria. J.A.M.A., *208*:1700, 1969.
420. Dacie, J. V.: Secondary or Symptomatic Haemolytic Anaemias. Part III in The Hemolytic Anaemias, Congenital and Acquired. 2nd Ed. Grune & Stratton, New York, 1967.
421. Davidson, R. J. L.: Exertional haemoglobinuria: a report on three cases with studies on the haemolytic mechanism. J. Clin. Path., *17*:536, 1964.
422. Davidson, R. J. L.: March or exertional haemoglobinuria. Semin. Hemat., *6*:150, 1969.
423. Eyster, E., Mayer, K., and McKenzie, S.: Traumatic hemolysis with iron deficiency anemia in patients with aortic valve lesions. Ann. Int. Med., *68*:995, 1968.
424. Hollingsworth, J. H., and Mohler, D. N.: Microangiopathic hemolytic anemia caused by purpura fulminans. Ann. Int. Med., *68*:1310, 1968.
425. Marsh, G. W., and Lewis, S. M.: Cardiac haemolytic anaemia. Semin. Hemat., *6*:133, 1969.
426. Nevaril, C. G., Lynch, E. C., Alfrey, C. P., and Hellums, J. D.: Erythrocyte damage and destruction induced by shearing stress. J. Lab. & Clin. Med., *71*:784, 1968.
427. Pirofsky, B.: Hemolysis in valvular heart disease. Ann. Int. Med., *65*:373, 1966.

428. Rubenberg, M. L., Regoeczi, E., Bull, B. S., Dacie, J. A., and Brain, M. C.: Microangiopathic haemolytic anemia: the experimental production of haemolysis and red cell fragmentation by defibrination in vivo. Brit. J. Haemat., *14*:627, 1968.
429. Spicer, A. J.: Studies on march hemoglobinuria. Brit. Med. J., *1*:155, 1970.
430. Streeton, J. A.: Traumatic hemoglobinuria caused by karate exercises. Lancet, 2:191, 1967.
431. Venkatachalam, M. A., Jones, D. B., and Nelson, D. A.: Microangiopathic hemolytic anemia in rats with malignant hypertension. Blood, *32*:278, 1968.
432. Walinsky, P., Spitzer, S., Brodsky, I., Kasparian, H., and Mason, D.: Hemolytic anemia with a Cross-Jones prosthesis. Am. J. Med. Sci., *254*:831, 1967.
433. Ziperovich, S., and Paley, H. W.: Severe mechanical hemolytic anemia due to valvular heart disease without prosthesis. Ann. Int. Med., *65*:342, 1966.

VIII / Anemia Resulting from Other Disorders

Anemia Associated with Chronic Disease

Anemia, generally without neutropenia or thrombocytopenia, often develops in patients with chronic disease, particularly in infections, neoplasms, and the so called "connective tissue" or "collagen" disorders. In most patients the anemia is the result of hypofunction of the marrow associated with a mild shortening of the life span of the erythrocytes, a decrease that would be compensated for by a normally functioning marrow. In some debilitating diseases folate deficiency is a factor, and in others, particularly the collagen diseases and the lymphomas, abnormal antibodies are important.

The mild, non-progressive anemia occurring in chronic infection, cancer, and rheumatoid arthritis has been studied extensively.[1] The anemia is usually normochromic and normocytic or normocytic and hypochromic; occasionally it is slightly hypochromic and microcytic. It is characterized by low serum levels of both iron and transferrin, reduced saturation of transferrin, decreased sideroblasts in the marrow, normal or increased reticuloendothelial iron, and an increase in free erythrocyte protoporphyrin. The response of the marrow to the shortened erythrocyte survival time is subnormal. When erythropoietin production is stimulated, the response is less than expected;[2] in addition, the marrow response to the administration of erythropoietin is less than normal.[1] Neither the factors responsible for the abnormal marrow response to anemia nor those concerned in the trapping of iron in the reticuloendothelial cells, which produces an unusual type of iron deficiency, are understood.

262

Anemia Associated with Myxedema

The occurrence of anemia in myxedema was first noted by Charcot in 1881,[6] and in 1883 Kocher reported that anemia appeared gradually following surgical removal of the thyroid gland.[10] Since that time anemia has been recognized as a frequent development in patients with spontaneous myxedema and also in those who develop thyroid deficiency following surgery. The incidence of anemia was reported as 52 per cent in one series of patients[13] and was 43 per cent in a series of 100 patients seen at the University of Virginia Hospital.

Mechanism of the Anemia

Several different types of anemia occur singly or in combination in patients with myxedema. They are: the uncomplicated anemia of hypothyroidism, anemia caused by vitamin B_{12} deficiency, and anemia of iron deficiency.

The uncomplicated anemia of hypothyroidism, which is normochromic and normocytic or slightly macrocytic, is rarely if ever severe; usually the red count is over 3.0 mil. per cu.mm. and the hematocrit is over 30 per cent. The weight of evidence supports the concept advanced by Wälchli[20] and Bomford[4] that the anemia in myxedema is an adaptation to a condition of relative oxygen surfeit in the tissues rather than the consequence of an illness associated with partial failure of bone marrow function that is the result of the lack of thyroid factor. Clinical observation has shown that patients with myxedema and anemia associated with a deficiency of vitamin B_{12} or iron can respond at least partially to vitamin B_{12} or iron without treatment with thyroid hormone. Experiments have demonstrated that the hematopoietic response of hypothyroid rats subjected to bleeding or exposure to low pressure chambers is the same as that of normal rats.[9, 16] Clinical investigations in patients with myxedema and anemia have revealed that erythropoiesis is stimulated by phlebotomy and by dinitrophenol, a preparation which increases oxygen consumption without increasing thyroid function (Fig. 8–1).[11, 18] These clinical and experimental observations demonstrate that the marrow in the hypothyroid state is able to respond to an appropriate stimulus without the administration of thyroxin, and they support the concept that the anemia is the result of an adaptation to the hypometabolic state.

Pernicious anemia and myxedema may coexist in the same patient and the incidence of this association, variously estimated from 1 to 12 per cent, appears to be increased.[5] The cause of the increased frequency of vitamin B_{12} deficiency in myxedema is not apparent. Although there may be occasional instances of an effect of the thyroid hormone on the absorption of vitamin B_{12},[12] the absorption of vitamin B_{12} is normal in most patients with myxedema and the administration of thyroid preparation does not lead to an increase in the absorption or in the serum level of vitamin B_{12} in hypothyroid patients with vitamin B_{12} deficiency.[18, 19] The increased incidence of antibodies to thyroglobulin, 25 to 50 per cent, that has been found in patients with pernicious anemia suggests that auto-immunity may be a mechanism in the production of myxedema and pernicious anemia in the same patient.[7, 8]

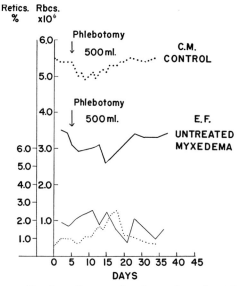

Figure 8–1. Response to bleeding of a normal patient and a patient with untreated myxedema. The restoration of the erythrocyte count to the pre-phlebotomy level within the normal period of time indicates that the bone marrow of patients with untreated myxedema is capable of responding to a stimulus for erythropoiesis. (From Leavell, Thorup, and McClellan: Tr. Am. Clin. & Climatol. A., vol. 68, 1956.)

Iron deficiency occurs in some patients with myxedema. Although the possible importance of a defective absorption of dietary iron that has been reported[17] has not been determined, it is likely that in most patients with myxedema the causes of iron deficiency are the same as in other individuals. One possible difference is an increased frequency of excessive menstrual flow in premenopausal women with hypothyroidism.[5]

Clinical Manifestations

The onset of the symptoms in myxedema is often insidious, with increasing weakness, muscular aches, lack of energy, and increased tolerance to heat and intolerance to cold. Severe constipation is often a troublesome symptom. Puffiness of the eyelids and swelling of the face and extremities are often apparent to the patient. Contrary to the popular lay opinion, weight gain is by no means a universal symptom in thyroid deficiency.

When the patient is examined the diagnosis may be suggested by the appearance of the patient's face, which is often pale, puffy, dull, and expressionless. The trunk and extremities frequently appear edematous, but the edema does not pit on pressure. Much of the hair normally present on the head and body may be lost and that which remains is coarse in texture. In severe cases the skin is dry and scaly and has a pale yellow tinge. The voice is usually hoarse and deep, and speech is slow and deliberate. In many patients the tongue is enlarged. The recovery phase of the deep tendon reflexes is sluggish. In addition to the signs characteristic of myxedema, the patient may have the signs of associated cardiovascular disturbance such as edema, ascites, and pericardial effusion.

Laboratory Examinations

The anemia is not severe in the uncomplicated case of myxedema. The lowest erythrocyte count observed in the authors' series was 3.0 mil. per cu.mm. The MCV ranged from 81 to 110 cu. microns and was over 94 cu. microns in 60 per cent. The blood smears showed little or no poikilocytosis or anisocytosis. There was no instance of hypochromic microcytic anemia in this group but the serum iron level was found reduced in four of 10 patients in whom it was measured. The values ranged from 32 to 99 μg. per 100 ml. (normal 60 to 150). Three of the patients with low serum iron levels were women who had mild normocytic anemia and the fourth was a man with a hematocrit of 40 per cent in whom no chronic blood loss could be demonstrated. Whether these values indicate undetected blood loss or the poor absorption of food iron that has been reported to occur in myxedema is uncertain. Leukocyte counts varied from 3400 to 13,000 per cu.mm. but were usually normal. The platelet counts were also normal. Although bone marrow hypoplasia has been reported to be a feature of myxedema,[3] bone marrow aspiration in this series revealed the cellularity of the marrow to be within normal limits in slightly more than one-half the patients and hypocellular in the remainder. Erythropoiesis was normoblastic in every instance.

The results of the other laboratory tests are similar to those that are usually found in any patient with myxedema, such as a low basal metabolic rate, elevation of the serum cholesterol, decreased uptake of radioactive iodine, and low plasma bound iodine. The plasma bilirubin is normal although the plasma may appear slightly icteric because of carotinemia.

Diagnosis and Prognosis

If myxedema is considered in the differential diagnosis, its presence can usually be established or excluded without difficulty by a consideration of the clinical features and by means of appropriate laboratory tests. Myxedema is sometimes mistaken for pernicious anemia because the pallor and yellowish tint of the skin of patients with myxedema suggest pernicious anemia, as does the macrocytosis. An incorrect diagnosis of aplastic anemia is also made at times because of the failure of the anemia to respond to treatment with iron, vitamin B_{12}, and other preparations.

The anemia of myxedema generally responds to the administration of thyroid substance in the usual dosage (desiccated thyroid 0.03 to 0.1 gm. per day) by a gradual rise in the hemoglobin and erythrocytes to normal levels in from 3 to 9 months. The prognosis is excellent as long as the patient continues treatment. If there is an associated deficiency of iron or vitamin B_{12} the appropriate preparation must be given in addition to desiccated thyroid in order to restore the blood to normal.

Anemia Associated with Acute Blood Loss

Anemia that is due to the sudden loss of a large volume of blood may occur in a variety of circumstances. Among these are trauma, postoperative hemorrhage, ruptured ectopic pregnancy, ruptured aneurysm, ruptured esophageal varices, and ulcerative lesions of the gastrointestinal tract. Massive bleeding occurs spontaneously or after minor trauma in patients with the various hemorrhagic disorders. The clinical picture that the patient presents depends on the amount, location, and acuteness of the bleeding as well as the nature of the underlying disorder and the previous condition of the patient. The usual symptoms of an acute hemorrhage are sudden weakness, dizziness, pallor, and sweating. The marked variability in the manifestations is shown by the fact that in some patients syncope is the initial symptom but in others the passage of bloody or tarry stools may be the only indication that a hemorrhage has occurred.

The changes in the peripheral blood depend on the time that has elapsed since the hemorrhage, the size and location of the hemorrhage, and the nature of the underlying disease. The amount of blood that is lost can be measured better by a determination of the blood volume than by the hematocrit reading because the latter may not reach its lowest point until 48 or 72 hours after the hemorrhage.[21] Unless preceding iron deficiency or a brisk reticulocytosis is present the anemia is usually of the normocytic type. Thrombocytosis and leukocytosis accompanied by an increase in the younger forms occur after a few hours. Reticulocytosis begins in 2 or 3 days and reaches a peak in from 4 to 7 days.[22] Reticulocyte counts as high as 12 or 14 per cent often follow an acute hemorrhage severe enough to reduce the red blood count to about 3.0 mil. per cu.mm. (Fig. 8–2). Hemorrhage into the tissues or body cavities may be followed by rises in both reticulocytes and serum bilirubin. If bleeding has ceased, an increase in the erythrocyte count becomes evident by the time the reticulocytosis reaches its maximum; the count continues to rise, even without treatment, until the normal level is reached, usually in from 4 to 6 weeks. The erythrocyte count is reported to return to a level of 4.5 mil. per cu.mm. within about 33 days after an acute episode irrespective of the size of the hemorrhage.[23]

There are two important aspects in the diagnosis of the patient with an acute hemorrhage. These are the recognition of acute blood loss as the cause of anemia and the determination of the cause of the bleeding. Recognition of the hemorrhage usually presents no difficulties but at times its severity may not be appreciated unless it is remembered that the hematocrit reading may give little or no indication of the amount of blood that has been lost. If the stool has not been examined for occult blood, an elevated reticulocyte count associated with a normocytic anemia or an elevation of the blood urea level may be the first clue to a recent hemorrhage. In order to determine the cause of the hemorrhage, roentgenographic study of the gastrointestinal tract, liver function tests, special studies for blood dyscrasias, and even surgical exploration may be necessary.

Treatment of acute hemorrhage is often the treatment of shock by means of intravenous fluids, vasopressor agents, and blood transfusions. Other treatment is directed toward the underlying disease. Unless the patient's iron stores have become depleted because of previous bleeding or some other factor, the hemo-

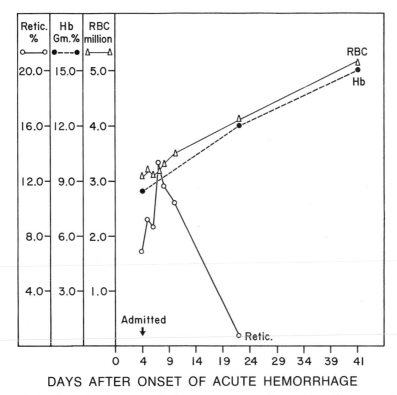

Figure 8–2. Chart showing hematologic response to acute hemorrhage. The peak reticulocyte response of 13 per cent occurred on the seventh day. The hemoglobin level and erythrocyte counts returned to normal during the fifth week.

globin and red cell count will return to normal levels after a moderate-sized hemorrhage without therapy with iron.

Anemia Associated with Pregnancy

During normal pregnancy reductions in the hematocrit, hemoglobin, and erythrocyte count are found. The maximal decrease occurs during the last trimester when the reduction may amount to 15 or 25 per cent.[25, 27, 30] These changes are due at least in part to hemodilution since the plasma volume increases by 800 to 1300 ml. while the red cell volume increases by only about 300 ml.[24] Because of these disproportionate changes, decreases in hematocrit, erythrocytes, and hemoglobin levels can be considered to be physiologic to a certain extent.

Not all changes that occur in the blood during pregnancy can be explained by hemodilution because the level of the serum iron falls while the values for the free erythrocyte protoporphyrin and the latent iron binding capacity rise.[27-29] In non-pregnant patients elevations of the free erythrocyte protoporphyrin and latent iron binding capacity are most often seen in iron deficiency. More direct evidence of the frequent development of actual iron deficiency during pregnancy is the observation that the serum iron level fell in about 80 per cent of a group of patients who received no supplemental iron during pregnancy but remained normal in 80 per cent of those who received iron salts orally.[30, 31]

The mother loses iron to the fetus and also with bleeding during delivery. The iron requirements for the fetus, which will be met at the expense of the mother, amount to about 400 mg. As the absence of menstruation during pregnancy allows the mother to conserve 325 mg. of iron that would ordinarily be lost through menstruation, the net added requirement of pregnancy is about 75 mg. However, the loss of iron in the placenta and in bleeding at the time of parturition has been estimated to average about 325 mg. Calculations from these figures therefore indicate that the net additional iron necessary for pregnancy is 400 mg. or more.

There is disagreement concerning the normal range of the blood values during pregnancy. The following values have been said to represent the lower normal limits of hemoglobin and erythrocytes during pregnancy: hemoglobin 10 gm. per 100 ml.; erythrocytes 3.5 mil. per cu.mm.;[34] hemoglobin 11.3 to 11.5 gm. per 100 ml.; red cells 3.7 mil. per cu.mm.; hematocrit 35 per cent.[25, 29] The reported frequency of anemia in pregnancy varies from 30 per cent to 80 per cent.[30, 34]

Types of Anemia

Iron deficiency is the commonest cause of anemia during pregnancy. It occurred in about 75 per cent of one series of patients.[30] In many instances some degree of iron deficiency antedates the pregnancy.[25, 30, 34] Severe iron deficiency is evidenced by the occurrence of a hypochromic microcytic type of anemia, but a milder degree of iron deficiency may be associated with only minor changes in the indices and in the appearance of the erythrocytes. When iron deficiency is present, the serum iron level is reduced to less than 60 micrograms per 100 ml., and the latent iron binding capacity is increased; erythropoiesis is normoblastic in type.

Other types of anemia are much less common than that due to iron deficiency. Macrocytic anemia, attributed to dietary deficiency, was observed in 8.4 to 25.7 per cent of the patients in one series.[26] The higher incidence of this type of anemia occurred in a group of 70 patients of a low economic status. Anemia associated with a megaloblastic type of erythropoiesis sometimes occurs during pregnancy or the puerperium. In one series of 45 patients with megaloblastic erythropoiesis indistinguishable from that seen in pernicious anemia, the mean corpuscular volume was greater than 100 cu. microns in only one-half the patients. The changes in the blood smears were similar to those seen in pernicious anemia but were less marked. Free hydrochloric acid was present in the gastric secretion in three-fourths of the patients.

The megaloblastic anemia of pregnancy is nearly always the result of folate deficiency. Megaloblastic maturation in the bone marrow, hypersegmented granulocytes in the peripheral blood, thrombocytopenia, and low serum folate levels occur. Multiple factors, such as increased need during pregnancy, inadequate intake, and malabsorption may be responsible. Evidence of intestinal malabsorption, as measured by xylose absorption, serum carotene levels, and fecal excretion of fat, is found in some pregnant patients.[36] The thrombocytopenia which occurs in folate deficiency may be responsible for serious vaginal bleeding during or after delivery;[32] its influence on increased susceptibility to toxemia, infection, and premature delivery has also been suspected but not established. Serum vitamin B_{12} levels have been variously reported as normal or slightly reduced in pregnancy, but vitamin B_{12} deficiency rarely is responsible for the megaloblastic anemia of pregnancy, probably because large reserve stores of the vitamins are normally present.

Recognition of the factors responsible for anemia during pregnancy is not always easy because iron deficiency occurs in association with normal indices and megaloblastic anemia occurs with normal indices or even with microcytosis. Determination of the serum iron level, which is reduced in iron deficiency and normal or elevated in other types of anemia, measurement of the serum folate level, and a study of the bone marrow usually enable one to establish the diagnosis. Even with the benefit of the bone marrow examination recognition of the type of anemia may be difficult if the patient has taken multivitamin tablets. These often contain amounts of folic acid that may be sufficient to convert a megaloblastic type of erythropoiesis to the normoblastic type and yet be inadequate to correct the anemia.

When the patient with anemia is seen for the first time during pregnancy, the possibility that the anemia may be the result of some coexisting disease rather than the pregnancy must be considered. Leukemia, diseases of the lymphoma group, renal disease, or almost any other cause of anemia may be recognized for the first time during pregnancy. The occurrence of pregnancy in a patient with one of the hemoglobinopathies may be serious because of the high incidence of complications in the mother or the child. When one of the hemoglobinopathies is considered in the diagnosis it is important to differentiate the benign combination of a trait condition and an anemia of pregnancy from the more serious homozygous or doubly heterozygous abnormalities.

Treatment and Prognosis

The best therapy for the anemia of pregnancy is preventive. In most patients iron deficiency anemia can be prevented by the ingestion of an adequate diet or by supplementation with 0.3 gm. of ferrous sulfate three times a day. A single 0.3 gm. tablet taken at bedtime is also effective. Most macrocytic anemias can be prevented by a liberal daily diet which contains one quart of milk, one-fourth pound of lean meat, and one egg a day or by supplementing the diet with 5 mg. of folic acid.[34] When multivitamin preparations are used to supplement the diet of pregnant patients, it is important to be sure that the multivitamin preparation includes at least 400 micrograms of folic acid.[32] If an iron deficiency anemia has developed it can generally be corrected by the administration of 0.3 gm. of ferrous sulfate three times a day. In the occasional patient who does not tolerate oral iron because of gastrointestinal symptoms, parenteral iron may be required. Most patients with megaloblastic anemia do not respond to vitamin B_{12} but usually respond to folic acid in a dose of from 5 to 20 mg. a day. The unusual occurrence of a response to the combination of vitamin B_{12} and ascorbic acid after the failure of each preparation singly has been reported.[28] As is true in other circumstances, the pregnant patient who is seriously ill with a severe degree of anemia may need blood transfusions before the diagnosis of the type of anemia can be established. Even in this situation it is rare that the necessary hematologic studies cannot be initiated or the necessary specimens obtained before the therapy is started.

The prognosis of the patients who develop anemia during pregnancy is excellent when proper treatment is given, if no serious complicating disorders are present. If iron deficiency develops, therapy with iron may be necessary for some months after the pregnancy in order to replenish the iron stores. Megaloblastic anemia rarely relapses after adequate therapy but may recur in subsequent pregnancies.[35]

Anemia Associated with Chronic Renal Disease

The majority of patients with chronic renal insufficiency develop anemia. In patients with severe renal disease, the hematocrit is usually in the range of 15 to 30 vol. per cent. Numerous studies have shown that the anemia is a result of one or more of the following factors: diminished erythropoiesis, hyperhemolysis, or bleeding. At times a deficiency of iron or folate is important.[37, 42a, 47]

The anemia associated with chronic renal disease is nearly always normochromic and normocytic in type but a macrocytic anemia occurs occasionally. In one series of patients with uremia secondary to various types of renal disease the hemoglobin levels ranged from 5.6 to 8.4 gm. per 100 ml. and the erythrocyte counts ranged from 1.5 to 3.5 ml. per cu.mm.[47] In the same series varying degrees of reticulocytosis, 2.4 to 22.5 per cent, occurred irregularly. The leukocyte and platelet counts are usually normal. Examination of the bone marrow reveals erythrocytic hypoplasia, normal cellularity, or erythrocytic hyperplasia. The serum iron level and the unsaturated iron binding capacity are usually normal or slightly decreased unless significant blood loss has occurred. The antiglobulin (Coombs) test, hypotonic saline fragility test, mechanical fragility test, and serum bilirubin levels are usually normal. The fecal urobilinogen excretion is increased when hyperhemolysis is present.

For many years the anemia of uremia was ascribed to an accumulation in the blood of poisons secondary to defective renal function.[38] It was noted that whatever the nature of these "poisons" might be, the action on the marrow appeared to be selective because erythrocyte precursors seemed to be depressed although activity was normal or increased in the other marrow elements.[39] Histologic evidence of hypoplasia of the erythroid series was found on examination of the marrow only when the non-protein nitrogen level of the blood was above 150 mg. per 100 ml. Complete aplasia was not found and it was suggested that a defect in the delivery of red blood cells to the peripheral blood from the bone marrow might be a factor in the anemia.

The diminished erythropoiesis in uremia has been demonstrated in several ways. It has been reported that in patients with uremia there is a decreased rate of utilization of radioactive iron[43, 47] and an increased storage of iron in the liver and spleen.[45] In vitro studies of bone marrow cells suspended in culture media containing uremic serum have revealed a decrease in the rate of maturation of erythrocyte precursors[48] and a diminished rate of removal of iron from the culture media.[50] The depression of erythropoiesis is probably due mainly to faulty erythropoietin production by the diseased kidneys. That there is an additional factor, an impaired response of the bone marrow to appropriate stimulation, is shown by observations made on patients being treated by chronic dialysis;[37] with this treatment erythropoiesis improved and erythropoietin levels rose, the latter probably coming from extra-renal sources.

In 1949 Emerson and Burroughs[41] published the first of a series of reports indicating that hyperhemolysis, manifested by a rapid fall in the hematocrit, difficulty in maintaining a hematocrit level of 15 vol. per cent, and an absolute rise in reticulocyte count, contributes to the production of anemia in uremia in some circumstances. When the survival time of erythrocytes was measured by the Ashby technique of differential agglutination, it was found that normal donor cells were destroyed in the recipient uremic patient at one and a half to three times the normal rate. Erythrocytes from uremic patients survived normally in the normal recipient. It was concluded that some extracorpuscular factor present in the plasma of uremic patients was responsible for the premature destruction of red blood cells. Other investigators demonstrated that this hemolytic activity was not found in all patients and was not constant in the same patient.[46] The occurrence of hemolysis appeared to coincide with the periods of rapid progression of the underlying renal disease. Nevertheless, hyperhemolysis is not the only mechanism concerned in the anemia of uremia. Even during periods of increased hemolytic activity the decrease in the life span of the red blood cells is not sufficient to produce anemia if the marrow responds normally.[40] Thus, although hemolysis contributes to the anemia in certain patients, it appears that depression of erythropoiesis is the most important and most common factor.

Another aspect of this complex problem has been indicated by the studies of Rees et al., which suggest that a disorganization of metabolism occurs in red blood cells that are suspended in uremic serum.[49] The transfer of iron into the developing erythrocyte seems to be energy dependent and it is possible that a metabolic dysfunction which alters energy output interferes with iron uptake in vivo and in vitro.

Patients being treated by chronic dialysis sometimes develop other hematologic complications. Some develop folate depletion, which may result in a megaloblastic anemia, and others develop iron deficiency anemia, probably the result of loss of red cells in the dialyzer. Iron overload from repeated transfusions of patients treated with chronic dialysis has not proved to be the problem that it was expected to be.

Figure 8–3 summarizes the various factors thought to play a role in the production of anemia in decompensated renal disease.

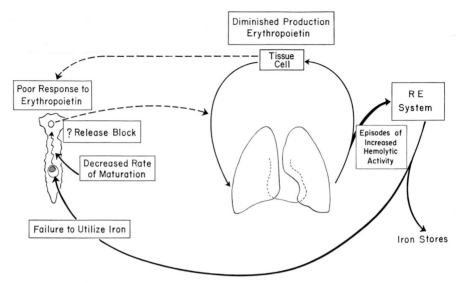

Figure 8–3. Schematic representation of the factors thought to be concerned in the production of anemia in chronic renal disease. Despite the presence of anemia and the reduced oxygen-carrying capacity of the blood there is a failure of the factors which normally operate to compensate for this deficiency.

Anemia Associated with Chronic Liver Disease

Anemia occurs often in patients with chronic liver disease. In one series of 132 patients with different types of liver disease, anemia was found in 78 per cent. The incidence is even higher in patients with atrophic cirrhosis.[58, 59, 63, 66] The degree of anemia, which is rarely severe unless complicated by a deficiency of iron or folic acid, cannot be correlated with the duration of the liver disease or with the clinical outcome. The morphologic characteristics of the anemia, which may be macrocytic, normocytic, or hypochromic microcytic, depend on what mechanisms are responsible for the anemia. Blood loss, increased hemolysis, or deficient erythropoiesis may be the most important factor in a particular individual.

Hypochromic microcytic anemia was present in 12 per cent of one series.[66] Its occurrence indicates iron deficiency, chronic blood loss from the gastrointestinal tract, the result of repeated severe hemorrhages from ruptured esophageal varices or mild chronic blood loss from irritation of the gastrointestinal tract. Increased pressure in the portal circulation and a defect in blood coagulation may be contributing factors.

In chronic liver disease the anemia is usually macrocytic, but is sometimes normocytic. The mean corpuscular volume has been found to range from 95 to 160 cu.microns, but is usually between 100 and 120.[58, 66] The marked anisocytosis and poikilocytosis which are usually seen in pernicious anemia are often absent in chronic liver disease but target cells are often numerous; nucleated red cells rarely appear in the peripheral circulation. Although significant poikilocytosis is rarely seen in the peripheral blood smear, a severe deformity "burr poikilocytosis" and a severe hemolytic anemia occur occasionally. In addition, examination of wet preparations of peripheral blood reveals a higher incidence of acanthoid cells. All these are reversible morphologic abnormalities that appear to be related to a serum factor.[53] Erythropoiesis is usually normoblastic in type and the reticulocytes are often slightly increased. Leukocyte and platelet counts are usually normal but they may be greatly reduced if "hypersplenism" or folate deficiency is present.

The mechanisms responsible for the macrocytic anemia of cirrhosis of the liver have been clarified by the studies of Jandl.[58] Sixteen of 20 patients with cirrhosis and anemia who were studied were found to have a definite hemolytic anemia, evidenced by the triad of elevated excretion of fecal urobilinogen, persistent reticulocytosis, and increased concentration of the erythrocyte precursors in the bone marrow. The extracorpuscular nature of the hemolytic process was shown by the survival times of transfused normal cells that were determined by the Ashby differential agglutination method. The exponential type of survival curve that was found suggested a random destruction of the red cells in a local site, such as the liver or spleen. Additional studies that utilized erythrocytes tagged with Cr^{51} indicated that the spleen is the major site of destruction. A correlation was found between the rate of red cell destruction and the degree of anemia. The presence of hemolytic anemia in liver disease was also indicated by the animal experiments of Higgins and Stasney.[56] They exposed rats to carbon tetrachloride by inhalation for short periods each day for 12 weeks. At the end of this time the rats developed "typical" atrophic cirrhosis of the liver and macrocytic anemia. In addition there was associated evidence of increased hemolysis in the form of icterus, increased hemosiderin in the organs, erythroid hyperplasia in the bone marrow, and an increase in reticulocytes.

Zieve's syndrome, first reported in 20 patients, consists of hemolytic anemia, hyperlipemia, and liver disease;[66a] the patients are usually alcoholic and often have pancreatitis. The hyperhemolysis was originally attributed to hyperlipemia, particularly lysolecithin, but later studies have failed to confirm that the hyperlipemia is responsible for the hyperhemolysis.[50a]

Although demonstration of the hemolytic nature of the anemia in cirrhosis of the liver affords the best explanation of the anemia in the majority of patients who have a macrocytic anemia associated with a normoblastic marrow, factors other than hyperhemolysis are important in the patients with the megaloblastic type of bone marrow.[58, 61, 62] The anemia in most of these patients has been more severe than that usually seen in cirrhosis. The erythrocyte count has been in the neighborhood of 1.0 mil. per cu.mm. in most patients and less than 2.0 mil. per cu.mm. in nearly all; the mean corpuscular volume usually has been over 130 cu. microns. In such patients hematologic recovery has followed the administration of folic acid,[58] vitamin B_{12},[62] liver extract,[52] and ascorbic acid. The possibility of a coexisting pernicious anemia can be excluded if the gastric analysis and determinations of the serum vitamin B_{12} level are normal. Patients with cirrhosis often have grossly deficient diets for long periods. In the majority of patients with chronic alcoholism and liver disease, the macrocytic anemia is related to a deficiency in folic acid; borderline or low serum folate concentration has been found in 80 per cent of a group of patients of this type.[55, 60] Herbert has shown that in normal conditions the storage of folate represents about a month's reserve supply.[54] The recognition of at least two types of macrocytic anemia, that associated with hyperhemolysis and that caused by a specific deficiency, in cirrhosis of the liver probably explains the conflicting reports of the presence and absence of vitamin B_{12} in livers of patients who died with cirrhosis.

Alcohol may be an important factor in the anemia of chronic liver disease. Reticulocytosis occurred in patients with cirrhosis kept on a diet deficient in erythropoietic factors if ingestion of alcohol was prevented,[58, 65] which suggested that alcohol depressed marrow activity. A dimorphic anemia associated with megaloblastic and sideroblastic changes in the bone marrow (including ringed sideroblasts), folate deficiency, hypomagnesemia, and hypokalemia was observed in a group of patients with severe alcoholism and liver disease; the megaloblastosis and sideroblastic changes disappeared within a few days when alcohol was withdrawn and a standard hospital diet was eaten.[57] Ingestion of alcohol, folate deficiency, and hypersplenism all may be important in the anemia, thrombocytopenia, or leukopenia that occurs in some patients with chronic liver disease.

Increased plasma volume and hemodilution may be responsible for reduction in the hematocrit and other blood values in some patients with chronic liver disease and splenomegaly.

Hypersplenism and Big Spleen Disease

Hypersplenism is the term used to denote a syndrome characterized by the following: splenomegaly; anemia, leukopenia, thrombocytopenia, singly or in combination; a marrow that has normal or increased cellularity; correction of the blood picture by splenectomy.

This syndrome occurs in a variety of disorders that are associated with splenomegaly. Among these are: congestive splenomegaly associated with portal hypertension of either the intrahepatic or extrahepatic variety; chronic infections, such as tuberculosis, kala-azar, malaria, subacute bacterial endocarditis, syphilis, brucellosis, fungus diseases; diseases of the lymphoma group, particularly lymphosarcoma, giant follicle lymphoma, and Hodgkin's disease; diseases of lipid metabolism (Gaucher's disease); diseases of uncertain etiology such as rheumatoid arthritis, sarcoidosis, and collagen diseases, particularly disseminated lupus erythematosus; and splenomegaly of undetermined origin. Usually hypersplenism is simply one aspect of an underlying disease that is not confined to the spleen.

Various mechanisms have been suggested to explain the changes that occur in the peripheral blood in hypersplenism. Doan and his group, largely as the result of supravital staining of splenic material, have considered that sequestration and destruction of the cellular elements by the abnormal spleen are the important factors.[70] A different concept, offered by Dameshek, was that the enlarged spleen exerts an inhibiting effect on the bone marrow by means of an unidentified humoral factor,[69] but no convincing evidence to support such a mechanism has been presented. Others consider that leukocyte antibodies are important in many splenic neutropenia syndromes.[77] It has been estimated that in some patients with greatly enlarged spleens 1000 ml. of red cells and 800 ml. of plasma have been sequestered in the congested spleen, probably to fill the increased vascular space.[73] Considerable increase in the plasma volume occurs often, but not invariably, in a number of different disorders and produces a low hematocrit value without a reduction in the total red cell mass. At present the mechanism involved in "hypersplenism" cannot be considered as definitely established and it is not certain that the same mechanism is the responsible one in every patient with the syndrome.

When hypersplenism is suggested by the occurrence of splenomegaly, cytopenia, and an apparently active marrow, the first objective becomes the recognition of the disease responsible for the splenomegaly. The clinical features of a disease may or may not suffice for a diagnosis. Usually the most direct evidence is afforded by biopsy: surgical removal of an enlarged lymph node or an aspiration biopsy of the liver or spleen often provides a definite diagnosis. Material obtained by biopsy should be cultured for infectious agents as well as studied histologically. When a definite diagnosis cannot be established, sometimes a presumptive diagnosis can be made on indirect evidence. A diagnosis of congestive splenomegaly associated with portal hypertension is suggested by a history of liver disease and abnormalites such as hepatomegaly, palmar erythema, or spider angiomata; abnormal liver function tests and the demonstration of esophageal varices by a barium study of the esophagus also favor this diagnosis. If lymphosarcoma is suspected but not proved by biopsy, a study of the bone marrow for lymphocytic infiltration, careful fluoroscopy of the chest for enlarged nodes, lymphangiograms, and barium study of the stomach and small bowel for involvement of these areas may give additional support for the suspected diagnosis. If chronic bacterial or fungal infection is suspected the possibility should be explored further by means of skin tests, blood cultures, agglutination tests, and complement fixation tests. If a disease of uncertain etiology, such as sarcoidosis or a connective tissue or collagen disorder, is suggested by the clinical feature but not established by biopsy of skin and muscle or other tissue, serologic tests, tests for LE cells, serum calcium determinations, and serum electrophoresis may be helpful. Some of the storage diseases, such as Gaucher's disease, may be diagnosed by the marrow aspiration but others are so ill defined that even study of the spleen after its removal serves only to place the disease in this group without a more specific diagnosis. In a small percentage of the patients the cause of the splenomegaly remains obscure even after histologic study of the spleen and other biopsy material removed at operation. Such cases may be termed "idiopathic" or "primary;" such a label does not dispel the suspicion that the subsequent course of the patient will disclose a more definitive diagnosis at a later time.

The decision regarding the advisability of splenectomy can be made only after careful consideration of the individual patient. Splenectomy relieves only one aspect of the underlying disorder and rarely if ever effects a cure of the primary disease.[76] In addition, splenectomy in very young children, particularly those with a reticuloendothelial system loaded from hyperhemolysis or other causes, may be followed by a lowered resistance to infection, particularly that caused by the pneumococcus.[71] In areas where malaria occurs, splenectomy in children or adults may impair the body's reaction to this infection. If the underlying disease is amenable to more definitive treatment, splenectomy may not be necessary because the hypersplenism syndrome may disappear after such therapy. When the nature and course of the underlying disease are such that an early fatal outcome is expected, splenectomy is rarely a justifiable procedure. If the nature of the underlying process cannot be diagnosed, or if it is identified as one for which no satisfactory therapy is available, splenectomy is a justifiable form of treatment if the presence of anemia, neutropenia, or thrombocytopenia is disabling or hazardous to the patient; an increase in the plasma volume of 50 per cent has been considered an indication for splenectomy, particularly if combined with evidence of red cell pooling, which can occur without increased destruction of the cells.[73] In such circumstances gratifying results occur often but not invariably. Clinical improvement in the patient often continues even though a partial hematologic relapse not infrequently develops some months after splenectomy.

"Big spleen disease" (tropical splenomegaly) has been studied extensively in Uganda.[72, 75] Most of these patients have pancytopenia. Study has revealed that the anemia is due in part to hyperhemolysis but in larger part to an expanded plasma volume with hemodilution; sequestration of red cells in the spleen appears to be of minor importance. This disorder is characterized by hyperplasia of the Kupffer cells in the liver accompanied by varying degrees of lymphocytic infiltration of the liver; considerable hyperplasia of the lymphoid tissue is evident in the spleen and sometimes in the marrow. Although repeated studies for malarial parasites in these patients have been negative, the presence of antibodies to quartan malaria and the distribution of the cases in Uganda suggest that the disorder is related to quartan malaria infection. Splenectomy is usually followed by a decrease in the plasma volume, which is not accounted for by removal of the plasma contained in the spleen, and improvement in the hematological values. In some patients, long-term antimalarial therapy, particularly with Paludrine, has been followed by a decrease in the size of the spleen and improvement in the hematologic values.

The clinical manifestations of patients with "non-tropical idiopathic splenomegaly" are similar to those seen in the tropics. In a group of such patients, splenomegaly, leukopenia, and neutropenia of a severe degree, moderate thrombocytopenia and slight to moderate reticulocytosis were present: all the patients who were studied were "anemic," although in only two was the total red cell volume subnormal.[68] Splenectomy produced a sustained and striking hematological improvement in most patients. Two patients later died with illnesses unconnected with splenomegaly and one died of lymphosarcoma and auto-immune hemolytic anemia.

Whether these patients have (1) an abnormal response to some infection, which appears to be the case when tropical splenomegaly occurs in certain patients with malaria, (2) an auto-immune disorder of uncertain origin, the main feature being exaggerated lymphoreticular cell proliferation, or (3) some atypical or "premalignant" early form of lymphoma is uncertain. It is possible that the presence of lymphoma is a late manifestation of, or a response to, one of the other disorders.

Felty's Syndrome

Felty's syndrome, characterized by the triad of arthritis, splenomegaly, and neutropenia, was described first in 1924.[78] The syndrome is more likely to occur in middle aged or older persons who have had arthritis, which may or may not be disabling, for 15 years or more. Enlargement of the superficial lymph nodes and lymphoid proliferation in some areas of the marrow are common. Some patients with the syndrome have repeated bacterial infections and chronic leg ulcers attributable at least in part to the neutropenia. Anemia occurs in over half of the patients.

Treatment with corticosteroids rarely produces any improvement in the neutrophil levels. Although the mechanisms responsible for the neutropenia are not understood, splenectomy is followed by a return of the neutrophil count to normal and a decrease in the incidence of infection in about two-thirds of the patients.[79] In some patients the immediate post-splenectomy rise in neutrophils partially relapses after several months, but some resistance to infections often persists.

Leukoerythroblastic Anemia

Leukoerythroblastic anemia, characterized by anemia, the presence of immature cells of the granulocytic series, and nucleated red cells in the peripheral circulation associated with low, normal, or elevated leukocyte and platelet counts, is most often a manifestation of involvement of the bone marrow by metastatic malignancy. A similar picture is sometimes seen in patients who are severely ill with bleeding or disseminated infecton. The hematological findings resemble those seen in myeloid metaplasia or myelofibrosis except for the appearance of the red cells; in leukoerythroblastic anemia the erythrocytes are usually normal, whereas in myelofibrosis there is considerable poikilocytosis and many "tear drop" forms. Careful study of the patient and examination of the bone marrow usually clarifies the diagnosis.

References

ANEMIA ASSOCIATED WITH CHRONIC DISEASE

1. Cartwright, G. E.: The anemia of chronic disorders. Semin. Hemat., 3:351, 1966.
2. Ward, P., Gordon, B., and Pickett, J. C.: Serum Levels of Erythropoietin in Rheumatoid Arthritis. J. Lab. & Clin. Med., 74:93, 1969.

ANEMIA ASSOCIATED WITH MYXEDEMA

3. Axelrod, A. R., and Berman, L.: The bone marrow in hyperthyroidism and hypothyroidism. Blood, 6:436, 1951.
4. Bomford, R.: Anaemia in myxoedema and the role of the thyroid gland in erythropoiesis. Quart. J. Med., 7:495, 1938.
5. Carpenter, J. T., Mohler, D. N., Thorup, O. A., and Leavell, B. S.: Anemia in myxedema. In Crispell, K. R.: Current Concepts in Hypothyroidism. Pergamon Press, New York, 1963.

6.   Charcot, M.: Myxoedème, cachexie pachydermique ou état crétinoïde. La Lancette française Gazette des Hôpitaux. January 25, 1881.
7.   Doniach, D., Roitt, I. M., and Taylor, K. B.: Autoimmune phenomena in pernicious anaemia. Serologic overlap with thyroiditis, thyrotoxicosis and systemic lupus erythematosus. Brit. M. J., 1:1374, 1963.
8.   Fisher, J. M., and Taylor, K. B.: A comparison of autoimmune phenomena in pernicious anemia and chronic atrophic gastritis. New England J. Med., 272:499, 1965.
9.   Gordon, A. S., Kadow, P. C., Finkelstein, G., and Charipper, H. A.: The thyroid and blood regeneration in the rat. Am. J. M. Sc., 212:385, 1946.
10. Kocher, T.: Ueber Kropf Extirpation and ihre Folgen. Arch. Chir., 29:254, 1883.
11. Leavell, B. S., Thorup, O. A., and McClellan, J. E.: Observations on the anemia in myxedema. Tr. Am. Clin. & Climatol. A., 68:137, 1956.
12. Leithhold, S. L., David, D., and Best, W. R.: Hypothyroidism with anemia demonstrating abnormal vitamin B_{12} absorption. Am. J. Med., 24:535, 1958.
13. Lerman, J., and Means, J. H.: Treatment of the anemia of myxedema. Endocrinology, 16:553, 1932.
14. McClellan, J. E., Donegan, C., Thorup, O. A., and Leavell, B. S.: Survival time of the erythrocyte in myxedema and hyperthyroidism. J. Lab. & Clin. Med., 51:91, 1958.
15. Muldowney, F. P., Crooks, J., and Wayne, E. J.: The total red cell mass in thyrotoxicosis and myxedema. Clin. Sc., 16:309, 1957.
16. Myer, O. O., Thewlis, E. W., and Rusch, H. P.: The hypophysis and hemopoiesis. Endocrinology, 27:932, 1940.
17. Pirzio-Biroli, G., Bothwell, T. H., and Finch, C. A.: Iron absorption. II. The absorption of radioiron administered with a standard meal in man. J. Lab. & Clin. Med., 51:37, 1958.
18. Tudhope, G. R., and Wilson, G. M.: Anemia in hypothyroidism. Quart. J. Med., 29:513, 1960.
19. Tudhope, G. R., and Wilson, G. M.: Deficiency of vitamin B_{12} in hypothyroidism. Lancet, 1:703, 1962.
20. Walchli, E.: Hypo- und athyreosis und blutbild. Folia haemat., 27:135, 1922.

ANEMIA ASSOCIATED WITH ACUTE BLOOD LOSS

21. Ebert, R. V., Stead, E. A., Jr., and Gibson, J. G., II: Response of normal subjects to acute blood loss. Arch. Int. Med., 68:578, 1941.
22. Gordon, A. S.: Quantitative nature of the red cell response to a single bleeding. Proc. Soc. Exper. Biol. & Med., 31:563, 1934.
23. Schiødt, E.: Observations on blood regeneration in man. I. The rise in erythrocytes in patients with hematemesis or melena from peptic ulcer. Am. J. M. Sc., 193:313, 1937.

ANEMIA ASSOCIATED WITH PREGNANCY

24. Berlin, N. I., Goetsch, C., Hyde, G. M., and Parsons, R. J.: The blood volume in pregnancy as determined by P-32 labelled red blood cells. Surg., Gynec. & Obst., 97:173, 1953.
25. Bethell, F. H.: The blood changes in normal pregnancy and their relation to the iron and protein supplied by the diet. J.A.M.A., 107:564, 1936.
26. Bethel, F. H., and Blecha, E.: Diet in pregnancy. Clinics, 1:346, 1936.
27. Fay, J., Cartwright, G. E., and Wintrobe, M. M.: Studies on free erythrocyte protoporphyrin, serum iron, serum iron-binding capacity and plasma copper during normal pregnancy. J. Clin. Invest., 28:487, 1949.
28. Holly, R. G.: Megaloblastic anemia in pregnancy. Remission following combined therapy with ascorbic acid and vitamin B_{12}. Proc. Soc. Exper. Biol. & Med., 78:238, 1951.
29. Holly, R. G.: The iron and iron-binding capacity of serum and the erythrocyte protoporphyrin in pregnancy. Obst. & Gynec., 2:119, 1953.
30. Holly, R. G.: The value of iron therapy in pregnancy. Journal-Lancet, 74:211, 1954.
31. Holly, R. G.: Anemia in pregnancy. Obst. & Gynec., 5:562, 1955.
32. Lawrence, C., and Klipstein, F. A.: Megaloblastic anemia of pregnancy in New York City. Ann. Int. Med., 66:25, 1967.
33. Streiff, R. R., and Little, A. B.: Folic acid deficiency in pregnancy. New England J. Med., 276:776, 1967.
34. Sturgis, C. C.: Hematology. Charles C Thomas, Springfield, Ill., 1948, pp. 74–90.
35. Thompson, R. B., and Ungley, C. C.: Megaloblastic anaemia of pregnancy and the puer-

perium. A review of forty-five cases with special reference to their response to treatment. Quart. J. Med., *20*:187, 1951.

36. Whitfield, C. R., and Love, A. H. G.: Intestinal malabsorption in megaloblastic pregnancy anemia. J. Obst. & Gynec. Brit. Commonwealth, *75*:844, 1968.

ANEMIA ASSOCIATED WITH CHRONIC RENAL DISEASE

37. Adamson, J. W., Eschbach, J., and Finch, C. A.: The kidney and erythropoiesis. Am. J. Med., *44*:725, 1968.
38. Brown, G. E., and Roth, G. M.: The anemia of chronic nephritis. Arch. Int. Med., *30*:817, 1922.
39. Callen, I. R., and Limarzi, L. R.: Blood and bone marrow studies in renal disease. Am. J. Clin. Path., *20*:3, 1950.
40. Chaplin, H., and Mollison, P. L.: Red cell life-span in nephritis and in hepatic cirrhosis. Clin. Sc., *12*:351, 1953.
41. Emerson, C. P., Jr., and Burroughs, B. A.: The mechanism of anemia and its influence on renal function in chronic uremia. J. Clin. Invest., *28*:779, 1949.
42. Erslev, A. J.: Erythropoietic function in uremic rabbits. Clin. Res. Proc., *5*:141, 1957.
42a. Erslev, A. J.: Anemia of chronic renal disease. Arch. Int. Med., *126*:774, 1970.
43. Finch, C. A., Gibson, J. G., III, Peacock, W. C., and Fluharty, R. G.: Iron metabolism, utilization of intravenous radioactive iron. Blood, *4*:905, 1949.
44. Jacobson, L. O., Goldwasser, E., Fried, W., and Plzak, L.: Role of the kidney in erythropoiesis. Nature, *179*:633, 1957.
45. Kaye, M.: The anemia associated with renal disease. J. Lab. & Clin. Med., *52*:83, 1958.
46. Loge, J. P., Lange, R. D., and Moore, C. V.: Characterization of the anemia of chronic renal insufficiency. J. Clin. Invest., *29*:830, 1950.
47. Loge, J. P., Lange, R. D., and Moore, C. V.: Characterization of the anemia associated with chronic renal insufficiency. Am. J. Med., *24*:4, 1958.
48. Markson, J. L., and Rennie, J. B.: The anaemia of chronic renal insufficiency. Scottish M. J., *1*:320, 1956.
49. Rees, S. B., et al.: Effect of dialysis and purine ribosides upon the anemia of uremia. J. Clin. Invest., *36*:923, 1957.
50. Thorup, O. A., Jr., Strole, W. E., and Leavell, B. S.: The rate of removal of iron from culture medium by human bone marrow suspension. J. Lab. & Clin. Med., *52*:266, 1958.

ANEMIA ASSOCIATED WITH CHRONIC LIVER DISEASE

50a. Blass, J. P., and Dean, H. M.: The relation of hyperlipemia to hemolytic anemia in an alcoholic patient. Am. J. Med., *40*:283, 1966.
51. Brown, A.: Megaloblastic anemia associated with adult scurvy: Report of a case which responded to synthetic ascorbic acid alone. Brit. J. Haem., *1*:345, 1955.
52. Goldhamer, S. M., Isaacs, R., and Sturgis, C. C.: The role of the liver in hematopoiesis. Am. J. M. Sc., *188*:193, 1934.
53. Grahn, E. P., Dietz, A. A., Stefani, S. S., and Donnelly, W. J.: Burr cells, hemolytic anemia and cirrhosis. Am. J. Med., *45*:78, 1968.
54. Herbert, V.: Minimum daily adult folate requirement. Arch. Int. Med., *110*:649, 1962.
55. Herbert, V., Zalusky, R., and Davidson, C. S.: Correlation of folate deficiency with alcoholism and associated macrocytosis, anemia, and liver disease. Ann. Int. Med., *58*:977, 1963.
56. Higgins, G. M., and Stasney, J.: The peripheral blood in experimental cirrhosis of the liver. Folia haemat., *54*:129, 1936.
57. Hines, J. D.: Reversible megaloblastic and sideroblastic marrow abnormalities in alcoholic patients. Brit. J. Haemat., *16*:87, 1969.
58. Jandl, J. H.: The anemia of liver disease: Observations on its mechanism. J. Clin. Invest., *34*:390, 1955.
59. King, R. B.: The blood picture in portal cirrhosis of the liver. New England J. Med., *200*:482, 1929.
60. Klipstein, F. A., and Lindenbaum, J.: Folate deficiency in chronic liver disease. Blood, *25*:443, 1965.
61. Koszewski, B. J.: The occurrence of megaloblastic erythropoiesis in patients with hemochromatosis. Blood, *7*:1182, 1952.
62. Movitt, E. R.: Megaloblastic erythropoiesis in patients with cirrhosis of the liver. Blood, *5*:468, 1950.

63. Rosenberg, D. H.: Macrocytic anemia in liver disease, particularly cirrhosis. Observations on the incidence, course and reticulocytosis with a correlated study of the gastric acidity. Am. J. M. Sc., *192*:86, 1936.
64. Schiff, L., Rich, M. L., and Simon, S. D.: The "haematopoietic principle" in the diseased human liver. Am. J. M. Sc., *196*:313, 1938.
65. Sullivan, L. W., and Herbert, V.: Suppression of hematopoiesis by ethanol. J. Clin. Invest., *43*:2048, 1964.
66. Wintrobe, M. M.: Relation of disease of the liver to anemia. Arch. Int. Med., *57*:289, 1936.
66a. Zieve, L.: Jaundice hyperlipemia and hemolytic anemia: a heretofore unrecognized syndrome associated with alcoholic fatty liver and cirrhosis. Ann. Int. Med., *48*:471, 1958.

HYPERSPLENISM AND BIG SPLEEN DISEASE

67. Bird, R. M., Clement, T., Jr., and Joel, W.: Primary splenic panhematopenia. Southern M. J., *48*:345, 1955.
68. Dacie, J. V., Brain, M. C., Harrison, C. V., Lewis, S. M., and Worlledge, S. M.: Non-tropical idiopathic splenomegaly ("primary hypersplenism"): a review of ten cases and their relationship to malignant lymphomas. Brit. J. Haemat., *17*:317, 1969.
69. Dameshek, W.: Hypersplenism. Bull. N.Y. Acad. Med., *31*:113, 1955.
70. Doan, C. A., and Wright, C. S.: Primary congenital and secondary acquired splenic panhematopenia. Blood, *1*:10, 1946.
71. Eraklis, A. J., Kevy, S. V., Diamond, L. K., and Gross, R. E.: Hazard of overwhelming infection after splenectomy in childhood. New England J. Med., *276*:1225, 1967.
72. Hamilton, P. J. S., Richmond, J., Donaldson, G. W. K., Williams, R., Hutt, M. S. R., and Lugumba, V.: Splenectomy in "big spleen disease." Brit. Med. J., *3*:823, 1967.
73. Prankerd, T. A. J.: The spleen and anaemia. Brit. Med. J., *2*:517, 1963.
74. Rambach, W. A., and Alt, H. L.: A revaluation of hypersplenism (an autoimmune concept). M. Clin. North America, *46*:3, 1962.
75. Richmond, J., Donaldson, G. W. K., Williams, R., Hamilton, P. J. S., and Hutt, M. S. R.: Hematologic effect of idiopathic splenomegaly seen in Uganda. Brit. J. Haemat., *13*:348, 1967.
76. Sandusky, W. R., Leavell, B. S., and Benjamin, B. I.: Splenectomy: indications and results in hematologic disorders. Ann. Surg., *159*:695, 1964.
77. Tullis, J. L.: Prevalence, nature and identification of leukocyte antibodies. New England J. Med., *258*:569, 1958.

FELTY'S SYNDROME

78. Felty, A. R.: Chronic arthritis in the adult associated with splenomegaly and leukopenia. Bull. Johns Hopkins Hosp., *36*:16, 1924.
79. Sandusky, W. R., Rudolf, L. E., and Leavell, B. S.: Splenectomy for control of neutropenia in Felty's syndrome. Ann. Surg., *167*:744, 1968.

IX / Polycythemia

An increase in red blood cell count above normal may be *relative* or *absolute*. If the volume of fluid in which the red blood cells are suspended is reduced, an increase in their concentration results. The number of cells per unit volume of whole blood is increased and this increase is reflected in the red blood cell count and the hematocrit. The total red cell mass remains unchanged. Such a condition of *relative* polycythemia exists in any situation in which the plasma volume is reduced without a concomitant reduction in red cell mass. Acute relative polycythemia is most frequently associated with a shift or loss of body water, and in such circumstances the red cell count and hematocrit determination are valuable aids in the recognition and quantification of such changes. A careful history will generally lead to a correct interpretation of the laboratory findings. In interpreting the hematocrit it must be remembered that osmotic changes associated with alterations of fluid volume may alter the volume of the red cell. Ingress or egress of water from the red cell in response to altered osmotic forces outside the cell may be sufficient to affect the hematocrit. *Chronic relative polycythemia* (erythrocytosis) is believed to be secondary to an abnormally low plasma volume. The factors responsible for the low plasma volume are not understood but the majority of these patients are white males in early middle age of somewhat stocky build and moderately overweight. Leukocytosis, thrombocytosis, and splenomegaly are absent. Many have been found to be tense and anxious and the condition has been referred to as *stress polycythemia*.[64, 76]

An *absolute* increase in red blood cell mass may occur either as the result of a physiologic response to tissue hypoxia or in the pathologic state known as polycythemia vera. In the first instance the polycythemia is secondary to some recognized inciting cause; in the second the polycythemia is classified as "primary" since no inciting cause has been identified.[5, 112]

The various conditions which cause an increase in red cell mass are classified in Table 9–1.

Table 9–1.   *Classification of Polycythemia*

   I. Polycythemia vera: a proliferative disorder involving all elements of the bone marrow.
  II. Secondary polycythemia: an increase in red cell mass with no involvement of other marrow
      elements.
      A. Associated with known hypoxic stimulus.
          1. Cardiovascular disease with right to left shunt.
          2. Pulmonary disease with decreased arterial oxygen saturation.
          3. Low barometric pressure.
          4. Abnormal hemoglobin.
      B. Associated with inappropriate erythropoietin production.
      C. Associated with excess adrenocortical steroids or androgens.
 III. Benign familial polycythemia: a familial disorder of unknown etiology manifested by an
      increase in red cell mass.

Polycythemia Vera
Synonyms: Primary Polycythemia, Vaquez's Disease, Osler's Disease, Polycythemia Rubra Vera, Erythremia

Historical.   Vaquez in 1892 described the first instance of polycythemia that was not associated with pulmonary or cardiac disease.[94] The second description of such a patient was published by Cabot in 1899.[20] In 1903 Osler collected eight cases, four from the literature and four of his own, and pointed out many features of the disease.[94] In 1908 he clearly defined the disorder and discussed the course and prognosis as well as the therapeutic use of bleeding, oxygen, and irradiation of the spleen.[95] Excellent comprehensive reviews of the disease have been written by Harrop,[49] Lawrence, Berlin, and Huff,[77] Pike,[99] Modan,[88] and Jepson.[62]

Pathogenesis

The etiology of polycythemia vera is unknown. Because of the proliferation of all the cell lines in the bone marrow and the frequent transformation of polycythemia vera into leukemia, myelofibrosis, and other related syndromes, polycythemia vera has been considered to be a myeloproliferative disorder.[20, 30, 69, 81, 124]

Because of the known development of polycythemia in response to hypoxia, numerous attempts have been made to explain polycythemia vera by a marrow hypoxia mechanism of some sort, but none has been satisfactory.[10, 110] The greater frequency of leukocytosis and thrombocytosis as well as the finding of normal arterial oxygen saturation in polycythemia vera serve to differentiate it from hypoxic polycythemia.[38]

The increased level of erythrocytes in polycythemia vera is due to increased production of cells rather than to an increased life span of the cells. Studies with radioactive iron showed that the plasma iron turnover in this disease is five times normal.[100] Studies on the life span of the cells have shown that it is normal,[82] or that there is a dual population of cells with a normal span together with cells that have a very short life span.[12] The stimulus for the increased erythropoiesis in this disease has not been identified. Extracts of plasma from patients with polycythemia vera have been reported by some to stimulate erythropoiesis when injected into test animals;[28, 81] others have been unable to confirm these results.[33, 65, 96] These conflicting data indicate the need for a more sensitive technique by which to assay plasma erythropoietin. There is no evidence that the marrow cells of patients with polycythemia are hypersensitive to erythropoietin or consume more erythropoietin than normal. The defect appears to reside in the stem cell.[72]

Most of the clinical manifestations of polycythemia vera can be explained by the alterations in the peripheral blood. There is a definite increase in total blood volume to two or three times the normal value that is due almost entirely to an increase in the total mass of circulating red cells. Associated with this increase in erythrocytes there is an increase in blood viscosity that may be five to eight times normal.[49, 84] The increased blood volume and the slowed circulation in the congested capillaries are responsible for the plethoric appearance of the patient and the ruddy cyanosis which appears when the level of the non-oxygenated hemoglobin in the capillaries rises above 5 gm. per 100 ml.[5, 112] The increased blood volume and viscosity place an added load on the heart which may result in cardiac decompensation and thrombosis of pulmonary vessels.[19] The consistently increased stroke volume with a normal or elevated cardiac output is thought to result from increased central blood volume and increased diastolic filling.[26] Recent studies have shown that the increase in cardiac output more than compensates for the increased viscosity and that oxygen transport is actually increased.[22] These patients frequently have vascular disease, however, and the vessels are unable to carry an increased flow of blood. For this reason the effect of viscosity may not be offset and local tissue ischemia may occur. This often improves markedly when the underlying disease is treated effectively. The frequent occurrence of thrombosis in this disorder appears to be related to the presence of the vascular disease in association with the increased blood viscosity, decreased blood flow, and increased number of the blood platelets.

One of the puzzling features of polycythemia, a disease characterized by thrombosis, is the frequent occurrence of abnormal bleeding. The distention of the blood vessels has been considered a possible explanation.[77] In addition, abnormalities in the quality of the blood clot and in clot retraction have been demonstrated. It has also been demonstrated that the presence of very large numbers of platelets interferes with the early stages of blood coagulation.[68] Several qualitative platelet defects have been studied.[68, 92, 120] The reported decrease in platelet factor III availability is not corrected by sonication of the platelets. Still another factor that may be important is the occurrence of increased fibrinolysis that has been demonstrated in polycythemia vera but not in secondary polycythemia.[13, 120]

Clinical Manifestations

Polycythemia vera occurs more often in males than in females, the ratio being about 1.3:1 or 2:1.[24, 69, 77, 98, 124] The disease appears to be more common in whites than in blacks; in a series of 50 patients with polycythemia vera seen at the University of Virginia Hospital the ratio of whites to blacks was 24:1, although in the total hospital admissions the ratio of whites to blacks was 4.5:1.[98] Clinical manifestations of the disease appear most often between the ages of 40 and 60, though the disease has been reported in children.[32, 77] In the authors' series the age at onset ranged from 21 to 88 years, but only 10 per cent of the patients were below the age of 40.[98]

Most of the symptoms of polycythemia vera are related to the increased red cell mass, the associated vascular disease, and the tendency to hemorrhage and thrombosis.

The onset is usually insidious and the manifestations variable. Weakness, easy fatigue, irritability, and dizziness are common early complaints. At other times the onset is abrupt and the first indication of the presence of the disease is the occurrence of a catastrophe such as a gastrointestinal hemorrhage, myocardial infarction, thrombosis of a retinal vessel, or the development of hemiplegia.

The most common clinical manifestations are referable to the cardiovascular system. Complaints such as dyspnea on exertion, ankle edema, angina pectoris, palpitation, headache, dizziness, and intermittent claudication are present in about two-thirds of the patients when first seen.[98]

In about one-third of the patients, gastrointestinal symptoms such as epigastric pain, nausea, bloating, vomiting, and constipation are prominent. The incidence of duodenal ulcer demonstrable by x-ray is reported to be 10 to 19 per cent.[77, 98, 99] Both hematemesis and melena occur not infrequently, and either may be the first manifestation of the disease. On occasion the patient's history of severe bleeding may be doubted because of the failure of the laboratory tests to demonstrate the degree of anemia suggested by the history.

Other symptoms occur much less often in polycythemia vera but are recognized as part of the disease. In some patients severe pruritus, particularly after a hot bath, and night sweats constitute the main complaints. Patients are sometimes treated for "conjunctivitis" for a time before the underlying disease is recognized. Other less common complaints are those due to hyperuricemia and those related to the genitourinary system, such as hematuria, dysuria, and frequency.

Often the most striking feature of the physical examination is the appearance of the patient—a ruddy and florid face, telangiectasia of the cheeks and nose, and purplish cyanosis of the lips and ears. The appearance frequently suggests the diagnosis, but the countenance of the middle-aged man who has spent most of his life out of doors and indulged freely in alcohol may be virtually indistinguishable. Marked reddening is often evident in the palms, conjunctivae, pharynx, and vaginal mucous membranes. Examination of the fundus frequently reveals retinal veins that are distended and dark purple in color. Hypertension is present in about half of the patients. The spleen is enlarged in about three-fourths of the patients; it is usually firm and rarely extends as low as the umbilicus unless the disease has been present for some years;[117] late in the course of the disease, especially when leukemia or myelofibrosis has developed, the spleen may become greatly enlarged and fill most of the abdominal cavity. Hepatomegaly occurs in about one-third to one-half of the patients.

Laboratory Findings

The laboratory data in patients with polycythemia vera illustrate the involvement of the granulocytic and megakaryocytic series and not the red cells alone.[31, 77, 105] The untreated patient typically has an erythrocyte count in the range of 6 to 10 million, a hemoglobin between 18 and 24 gm. per 100 ml., and a hematocrit that ranges from 55 to 80 per cent.[99] The total red cell mass is increased, but the plasma volume may be normal, slightly elevated, or even decreased.[1, 11] (Normal values: R.B.C. vol., ml./kg., men 28.27 ± 4.11, women 24.24 ± 2.59; plasma vol., ml./kg., men 33.45 ± 5.18, women 34.77 ± 3.24.[57]) The leukocyte count is usually elevated. In our series of 50 patients a range of 5400 to 88,000 per cu.mm. was found; 70 per cent of patients had counts higher than 10,000 per cu.mm.,[98] a figure comparable to that of 74 per cent found in a much larger series.[77] The total blood granulocytic pool in patients with polycythemia vera has been shown by studies of granulocytic kinetics to be increased.[85]

The leukocyte alkaline phosphatase score is usually high when there is leukocytosis; rarely it will be elevated when the leukocyte count is in the normal range.[6] Myelocytes and metamyelocytes are often present on the blood smear, and nucleated red blood cells occur not infrequently. Platelet counts range from 100,000 to 1.5 mil. per cu.mm.[98] In one series 50 per cent of the platelet counts were above 400,000 per cu.mm.[98] and in another, 65 per cent were over 300,000 per cu.mm.[77]

Study of fixed sections of bone marrow is reported to show a characteristic pattern consisting of clumps of stem cells and early normoblasts in about 85 per cent of patients.[14] Study of smears made from material obtained by aspirations was rarely helpful in our series, since about half the marrows appeared to be normal and the remainder showed varying degrees of hyperplasia;[98] a stain for iron usually indicates that storage iron is greatly reduced or absent.

Ferrokinetic studies indicate that as the disease progresses, an uncompensated shortening of the red cell life span occurs and produces progressive decrease in red cell mass. This happens regardless of therapy and appears to be part of the natural history of the disease.[100] Associated with this are increases in erythrocyte glutamic oxaloacetic transaminase, glucose-6-phosphate dehydrogenase, and hexokinase, which reflect a young red cell population.[9] Splenic sequestration of the red cells increases as the red cell survival decreases.

Other laboratory features of the disease are an increased basal metabolic rate, an increased level of uric acid,[83, 110] increased plasma iron turnover,[56] and normal arterial oxygen saturation.[38]

Course and Prognosis

It has been pointed out that the natural history of polycythemia vera is virtually unknown, since some form of therapy has always been available.[99] Developments such as thrombosis, hemorrhage, and the occurrence of other myeloproliferative syndromes are so frequent that it is difficult to decide whether they should be considered as complications of the disorder or as incidents in its natural history.

A high incidence of vascular thrombosis is to be expected in a disease characterized by an increased red cell mass, increased viscosity of the blood, and elevated numbers of platelets when the disease occurs in an age group in which vascular disease is common. The incidence of thrombosis is reported to be 22 per cent,[124] 28 per cent,[119] and was found to be as high as 40 per cent in our own series.[98] Thrombosis probably occurs in any of the vessels, but appears to be most common in the coronary, cerebral, mesenteric, pulmonary, retinal, and peripheral arteries and in the leg, retinal, and portal veins.[25] The episodes of thrombosis are seen more often when there is inadequate control of the red cell mass and platelet level by therapy.

Hemorrhage is a frequent occurrence in polycythemia vera. An incidence of 16 per cent,[124] 59 per cent,[119] and 30 per cent[98] has been observed. In our experience the most serious hemorrhages have been intracranial, gastrointestinal, and those occurring after various surgical procedures, but extensive ecchymoses, hemarthroses, epistaxis, bleeding after dental extractions, and bleeding after minor technical procedures have also proved extremely troublesome (Fig. 9–1).[25, 104, 126]

Peptic ulcer is not uncommon in this disease and the incidence has been found to be from 10 to 14 per cent,[99] 12 per cent,[98] and 19 per cent.[75] The incidence of gastrointestinal symptoms is higher, from 17 per cent[98] to 25 per cent,[77] and severe gastrointestinal hemorrhage occurs not infrequently. The rare association of polycythemia vera and pregnancy has been noted.[52, 107] The platelets, leukocytes, and hemoglobin fell progressively during the first two trimesters followed by a sharp rise in these elements in the seventh month. Fetal salvage was low.

The median survival time in polycythemia vera has been reported[77] to be 13.2 years in patients treated with radiophosphorus and 6.7 years in patients

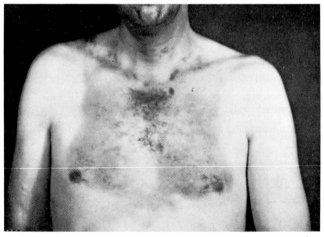

Figure 9–1. Extensive subcutaneous hemorrhage following dental extraction in a patient with polycythemia vera.

treated with various methods other than P[32]. Survival times in individual patients vary from a few months to 25 years.[36] The commonest causes of death are thrombotic episodes, hemorrhage, leukemia, and other myeloproliferative states. In one series, 30 per cent died from thrombosis and 30 per cent from leukemia or some allied disorder.[36] In Lawrence's series, the causes of death in 57 patients treated with P[32] were as follows: chronic myelogenous leukemia, 11 (6 were acute terminally); cerebral hemorrhage, 7; coronary thrombosis, 8; congestive heart failure, 9; carcinoma, 8; postoperative deaths, 5; miscellaneous, 4; unknown, 5.[77] In our own series of 24 patients who died, 12 had received no form of irradiation therapy and 12 had received treatment with P[32] or x-ray. The causes of death in the 12 who had received no irradiation were: heart failure or cerebrovascular accident, 8; postoperative hemorrhage, 1; carcinoma, 1; miscellaneous (peritonitis, multiple sclerosis, renal insufficiency), 3. The cause of death in 12 who had received P[32] or x-ray were: heart failure or thromboses, 3; myelogenous leukemia (acute), 3; myeloid metaplasia, 2; miscellaneous (hepatic cirrhosis, unknown), 3.[98]

Although the complications of thrombosis and hemorrhage are the most common serious developments in most patients with polycythemia vera, it is definitely established that leukemia, myelofibrosis, or some other myeloproliferative disorder develops in an appreciable number, perhaps 20 to 30 per cent. These complications are more likely to develop in patients with long survival times. If the incidence of these disorders is higher in patients treated with P[32], it is possible that the increased incidence is related to the longer survival of the patients so treated as well as to their exposure to some form of radiation.

Diagnosis

In most patients with polycythemia vera the diagnosis is made without difficulty. The appearance of the patient, the splenomegaly, and the increases in the erythrocyte, leukocyte, and platelet counts are characteristic. Occasionally it is difficult to decide if polycythemia is present in plethoric-appearing middle-aged hypertensive men with borderline blood counts, and it is not easy to determine whether a well established polycythemia is primary or secondary. Another problem arises when the leukocyte values are such that the distinction from chronic myelocytic leukemia is not easily made.

If the hematocrit is 55 per cent and erythrocyte count is elevated to 5.8 to 6.0 mil. per cu.mm., the possibility of an early polycythemia vera cannot be excluded in a middle-aged man simply because splenomegaly, leukocytosis, and thrombocytosis are absent. In such circumstances a determination of the red cell mass is often helpful.

The distinction between primary and secondary polycythemia is rarely a problem because leukocytosis, thrombocytosis, and splenomegaly do not usually occur in secondary polycythemia. In addition, the presence of a cardiovascular abnormality or chronic lung disease is usually evident in the secondary type. In obscure problems determination of the arterial oxygen saturation is often decisive, as the arterial oxygen saturation is almost invariably over 90 per cent in polycythemia vera and is often below this figure when polycythemia is secondary to some condition that produces anoxia. Recent reports[16, 17, 66] have emphasized the value of ferrokinetic studies, particularly the plasma iron turnover rate in the differential diagnosis of primary and relative polycythemia and in determining the need for treatment of polycythemia vera.

Although the presence of frank myelocytic leukemia, either acute or chronic, is easily recognized, a decision when polycythemia vera with a markedly elevated leukocyte count becomes transformed into chronic myelocytic leukemia may be virtually impossible without special techniques, since young cells of the myelocytic series appear in the peripheral blood in both circumstances. Metabolic differences are demonstrable between the leukocytes in chronic myelocytic leukemia and those seen in polycythemia vera.[118] These consist of differences in alkaline phosphatase activity, myeloid leukocyte glycogen, and blood histamine. The Philadelphia chromosome (Ph[1]), formerly thought to be diagnostic of chronic myelocytic leukemia, has now been reported in preparations from a small percentage of patients with polycythemia vera, myelofibrosis, granulocytic leukemia with high leukocyte alkaline phosphatase, and acute myelocytic leukemia.[109] Further studies of the Ph[1] chromosome and its significance in these disorders are needed.[80] Nevertheless, the finding of the Ph[1] chromosome almost invariably means that the patient has chronic myelocytic leukemia.[37a]

Treatment

At the present time there is no cure for polycythemia vera. Therapy is directed toward reducing the increased blood volume, increased viscosity, and increased platelet counts. Since it has been recognized for many years that these abnormalities are responsible for the clinical manifestations of the disease, numerous methods of treatment have been introduced. One author lists 24 methods or agents that have been tried.[36] Among these are many that were once considered to be the treatment of choice, such as benzol, Fowler's solution, phenylhydrazine, spray roentgen radiation, roentgen irradiation of the spleen and bones, phlebotomy, and a low iron diet. Some forms of therapy such as splenectomy, thyroidectomy, and oxygen inhalation never enjoyed much popularity because they were impractical, ineffective, and even dangerous. Numerous chemotherapeutic agents have been tried in polycythemia, and some such as nitrogen mustard, TEM, demecolcine, pyrimethamine, and 6-mercaptopurine have been found to be inferior to radiophosphorus. Bleeding, radioactive phosphorus, and chemotherapeutic agents are the therapeutic methods that are used most widely at the present time.

Venesection

Venesection is the oldest form of therapy for polycythemia vera. It is a means of reducing the blood volume promptly and often provides prompt symptomatic relief. Because of the development of undesirable symptoms when the blood volume is reduced too rapidly in middle-aged and elderly patients, it is desirable to remove only 500 ml. of blood once or twice a week if the blood volume is to be reduced to normal by this method. If the hematocrit is very high and more frequent bleedings are necessary, the use of plasma expanders[22] or the reinfusion of the patient's separated plasma reduces side effects and decreases viscosity. Although phlebotomy is an effective means of reducing the red cell mass in these patients, sometimes it is not a satisfactory method of treatment when used alone because high platelet levels are not reduced; also symptoms resulting from a state of chronic iron deficiency may develop.[33]

Radioactive Phosphorus

Radioactive phosphorus, P^{32}, was introduced as a method of treatment for polycythemia vera by Lawrence in 1938[73] and has many advantages for therapy. It can be administered orally or intravenously. It has a half-life of 14.3 days and emits only beta rays which travel less than 0.7 cm. in tissue.[36] It is concentrated in tissues that have a high rate of phosphorus turnover, particularly the bone marrow, liver, spleen, and lymph nodes. In these tissues it produces ionization within the cells and halts cell division. Radioactive phosphorus depresses erythropoiesis, granulocytopoiesis, and platelet production, which results in a reduction of these elements in the circulating blood. Since radioactive phosphorus does not cause any significant increase in the destruction of mature erythrocytes, a significant decrease in the red cell count does not occur for 2 or 3 months.

The effectiveness of therapy with radioactive phosphorus is indicated by reports of the reduction in the incidence of thromboses in several large series from 14.8 to 27.4 per cent in patients treated with conventional means exclusive of radiation to 2.7 to 4.2 per cent in patients with P^{32}.[128] In another series the incidence of thromboses was 50 per cent in 32 patients treated with other forms of therapy and less than 5 per cent in 148 patients treated with P^{32}.[115] Comparison of the life expectancy revealed an increase from 7 years in patients treated with drugs, phlebotomy, and roentgen ray to 13.3 years in patients treated with P^{32}.[75] Splenomegaly and hepatomegaly also often respond in a gratifying manner to this form of therapy.

Radioactive phosphorus is administered either intravenously or orally. If given intravenously, about 40 per cent of the dose is lost in the urine in 6 days, and if given orally, about 20 per cent is lost in the feces and an additional 15 per cent is lost in the urine in the same period.[36] It has been found that intravenous or oral doses of 1.5 millicuries do not alter the erythrocyte count in normal individuals.[36] The total dose that has been required to effect a remission has ranged from 2.3 to 21.3 millicuries. The initial dose is usually from 3.0 to 7.0 millicuries, and most often from 4.0 to 4.5 millicuries.[99] In about one-half the patients a satisfactory remission follows the initial dose, but 40 per cent require a second treatment and 10 per cent require three treatments.[1, 102] In one series the duration of remissions averaged about 2.5 years but sometimes they lasted as long as 10 years.[36] In another report, the average interval between courses was about 15 months; however, the greatest number of re-treatments occurred in the first 6 to 10 months. After the patient had a satisfactory remission the interval between treatments increased to about 33 months.[77]

It has been strongly suspected that therapy with P^{32} and other forms of radiation is associated with an increased incidence of leukemia, particularly the acute variety, and other myeloproliferative disorders.[25, 89, 93, 102, 111] The evaluation of survival data of retrospective case-control studies of patients with polycythemia vera has been challenged recently. Studies of the effects of P^{32} therapy in this disorder are being carried out.[47, 48, 79, 87, 125, 127]

Chemotherapy

Nitrogen mustard (HN_2), triethylenemelamine (TEM), demecolcine, and pyrimethamine have been used in the treatment of polycythemia vera.[35, 36, 59] All have a suppressive effect on the marrow, but the short duration of the remissions that occur and the difficulty in avoiding undesired toxic effects on the marrow have prevented their gaining an important place in therapy.

The recent concern over the use of P^{32} has prompted the use of the alkylating agents chlorambucil, cyclophosphamide, and busulfan. All are effective in about 80 per cent of patients, but there is a long latent period during which the patient must be controlled with phlebotomy. Although chlorambucil and cyclophosphamide may be given in maintenance doses, busulfan should be used intermittently, because long-term therapy has been associated with pulmonary fibrosis and other complications.[67, 121, 125]

Plan of Treatment

In the treatment of polycythemia vera it is important that the patient be kept ambulatory if possible. If the disease is even moderately severe, bed rest is dangerous for these patients because of the increased likelihood of thrombosis. For this reason patients with the disease should be treated without hospitalization whenever possible. Because of the tendency to both hemorrhage and thrombosis that exists in polycythemia vera, surgical procedures should be performed only if absolutely necessary. Prior treatment of the polycythemia reduces the likelihood of these complications but does not prevent them in all cases.[104, 126]

A divergence of opinion regarding the preferred therapy of polycythemia vera is evident in a review of the literature and has been emphasized in a symposium on this subject.[39a] Because of the lack of more definite data concerning the late complications of treatment with radioactive phosphorus, many hematologists treat the patients with phlebotomy, or a combination of phlebotomy and busulfan; radioactive phosphorus is employed if satisfactory control is not obtained with the other methods. The value of treatment with cytotoxic agents, which may have the same hazards as radioactivity, has not been established.

The aim of treatment in our clinic is to keep the hematocrit below 50 per cent and the platelet count below 500,000 per cu.mm. Patients are treated initially by phlebotomy, 500 ml. once or twice a week. If the platelet count is over 700,000, if thromboses occur, or if bleeding occurs in association with thrombocythemia, busulfan is used as found necessary to control the platelet count; this often requires three weeks or more and anticoagulants are used if thrombosis is a problem. When control is established treatment by phlebotomy or busulfan is given when necessary.

If control is not obtained by the method outlined above, the patient is given a dose of 3.5 to 5 millicuries of radioactive phosphorus orally. The patient is observed at monthly intervals, and if the hematocrit rises appreciably during this interval a phlebotomy is performed; phlebotomies are also performed if the initial hematocrit is at a dangerously high level. At the end of four months if the desired results have not been obtained a second dose of 2 to 4 millicuries of radiophosphorus is administered.

It is unusual for a patient to need more than two doses of treatment to obtain an initial remission but if necessary, 2 to 3 millicuries further can be given after four months' observation. After remission has been produced, the patients are followed at regular intervals and treatment repeated as necessary. Should it be established conclusively that radiotherapy does not significantly increase the incidence of leukemia and myelofibrosis, even in younger patients, or that the risk of these disorders is small compared to the other benefits of the therapy, treatment with radioactive phosphorus would be employed more widely. Therapy with roentgen rays is rarely used in polycythemia at the present, but local therapy over the spleen may be a helpful adjunct in patients in advanced stages who have symptoms of marked splenomegaly.

The complication of hyperuricemia and high urate excretion secondary to increased nucleoprotein turnover may be effectively treated with the xanthine oxidase inhibitor allopurinol while myelosuppression is being effected.

Secondary Polycythemia

A remarkable increase in total red cell mass may occur in any situation which results in tissue hypoxia. Oxygen deprivation leads to an increase in the level of erythropoietin, a humoral substance believed to be primarily responsible for the regulation of erythropoiesis.[37, 43, 44, 103] Although it is not the sole source, the kidney is the chief site of production or activation of erythropoietin. Erythropoietin appears to mediate the response of the bone marrow to hypoxia by increasing the number of pluri-potential stem cells which become erythroblasts and by increasing the rate at which they develop their full complement of hemoglobin.[4, 41, 55, 97]

The increase in red cell mass found in polycythemia vera is not accompanied by an increase in erythropoietin, whereas high levels are found in that which is secondary to hypoxia. In addition, there are forms of erythrocytosis associated with high levels of erythropoietin unrelated to hypoxia or other known stimuli. In secondary polycythemia the increase in the red cell mass is often accompanied by a decrease in plasma volume; in primary polycythemia vera the plasma volume is usually normal.[12, 46] Excessive elevations of the red blood cell mass may produce sufficient alterations of the viscosity of the blood to cause circulatory embarrassment and increase the danger of thrombosis.[84]

Associated with Known Hypoxic Stimulus

Cardiac and Vascular Malformations

Any cardiac or vascular lesion which results in a high grade veno-arterial shunt may produce polycythemia. As the result of the mixing of venous and arterial blood, inadequately oxygenated arterial blood reaches the peripheral tissues. An increase in erythropoietin is thought to occur and stimulate erythropoiesis. The subsequent polycythemia increases the oxygen-carrying capacity of the blood and affords a measure of relief to the patient.

Pulmonary Disorders

Polycythemia occurs in some chronic pulmonary disorders where it appears to be a physiologic response to the decreased arterial oxygen saturation. The commonest pulmonary abnormalities that lead to hypoxemia are:
1. Perfusion of non-aerated or poorly aerated alveoli.
2. Altered alveolar membrane characteristics interfering with gaseous exchange.
3. Direct pulmonary arteriovenous fistulas.

One end result of each of these conditions is decreased arterial oxygen saturation.[112] In the first instance the blood flow is through poorly aerated or non-aerated segments and there is inadequate exposure of the blood to oxygen. In the second instance the pulmonary segments are well aerated but the alveolar membranes have been so altered as to interfere with gaseous exchange between the alveoli and the capillaries. Direct pulmonary arteriovenous fistulas cause anoxia because the blood by-passes vessels in which gaseous exchange takes place.[18] A large reduction in the red cell mass of patients with polycythemia secondary to hypoxic lung disease was achieved by continuous oxygen administration. The effects lasted from 6 to 15 months.[23]

Low Barometric Pressure

Persons who reside at high altitude with lowered barometric pressure have a decreased alveolar oxygen tension which leads to incomplete arterial oxygen saturation. The polycythemia which occurs in response to the hypoxia appears to bear a direct relationship to the severity of the oxygen deficit.[58] If an individual is already compromised by lowered barometric pressure, the occurrence of any chronic pulmonary disorder may be catastrophic. Marked polycythemia, severe cyanosis, pulmonary hypertension, and right heart strain may result.[86] Some degree of improvement usually follows removal to sea level.[18, 91, 112]

Abnormal Hemoglobin

Several abnormal hemoglobin molecules have been reported to be associated with erythrocytosis.

Hemoglobin "M." Several abnormal hemoglobins have been described with structural anomalies which result in persistance of the oxidized form (methemoglobin) of the molecule. Since methemoglobin cannot transport oxygen there is a hypoxic stimulus and erythrocytosis. Several types of abnormality have been reported to produce hemoglobin M; some are located in the alpha chain, some in the beta chain.

Hemoglobins Chesapeake, Yakima, Rainer, and Ypsilanti have been found to have an abnormal oxygen dissociation curve. The shift of the dissociation curve to the left results in a reduction of tissue oxygen tension, a hypoxic stimulus, and erythrocytosis.[24, 40]

Associated with Inappropriate Erythropoietin Production

In the preceding conditions polycythemia appears to be the result of decreased arterial oxygen saturation which in some fashion causes the release of a humoral substance capable of stimulating erythropoiesis. Secondary polycythemia occurs in other conditions where the oxygen saturation is normal and the mechanism is unexplained. Among these are hypernephroma,[39, 51] polycystic kidney disease,[71] hydronephrosis,[29, 61, 78] renal tuberculosis,[115] cerebellar hemangioblastoma,[26, 53] hydrocephalus,[101] ovarian tumors,[42] uterine myomata,[50, 54, 116] pheochromocytoma,[15, 122] renal adenoma,[34] and hepatic carcinoma.[21, 65]

Fluid obtained from renal cysts,[106] a cystic cerebellar hemangioblastoma,[123] and extracts of hypernephroma and pheochromocytoma tissue[51, 122] have been demonstrated to have erythropoietin activity. However, the erythropoietin activity could not always be correlated with elevated plasma or urine erythropoietin levels and was not consistently associated with a secondary polycythemia.[106]

The mechanism by which these lesions may stimulate erythrocytosis remains unclear and their direct association with secondary polycythemia must rest on the demonstration of a return to normal hematologic values following their removal.

Associated with Excess Adrenocortical Steroids or Androgens

Secondary polycythemia may be seen in patients with Cushings syndrome if they have androgen as well as corticosteroid production. Both androgens and corticosteroids have been used successfully in the treatment of bone marrow failure. The mechanism of action of these steroid compounds is unknown.

Benign Familial Polycythemia

Recently the rare syndrome known as benign familial polycythemia or primary erythrocytosis has received further attention. In these patients, mostly children, there is an increase in total red cell mass without leukocytosis or thrombocytosis. There may be slight splenomegaly. Careful studies have revealed none of the recognized causes of secondary polycythemia. Reports have emphasized the familial nature of the disorder and its persistence into adult life. Some have noted an increased incidence of thromboembolic events, but the prognosis is better than it is in polycythemia vera.[2, 7, 70, 90]

The finding of plethora, vascular disease, labile hypertension, and obesity in a patient with elevated hematocrit, red cell count and hemoglobin, without splenomegaly, thrombocytosis, or leukocytosis, has been referred to as Gaisböck's syndrome. The red cell mass has been variously reported to be increased or normal, associated with a reduced plasma volume. Whether or not there is any relationship between this syndrome and benign familial polycythemia is uncertain.[45, 64, 108] Other studies, however, have shown that Gaisböck's syndrome can result from temporary hypoxia which develops during sleep and when the patient is in the recumbent position.[123a] Studies on a group of seven patients indicated that in the recumbent position the arterial PO_2 decreased significantly; in addition, during sleep the erythropoietin level increased significantly in five of six patients. All had normal ventilatory function tests. The hematocrits in the patients who were studied varied from 68 to 54 (normal is 42 to 49) and the red cell volume was increased in every patient. Oxygen therapy at night controlled the erythrocytosis in one patient and weight reduction produced the same result in another. The observed results are similar to those produced by hypoxia from exposure to low barometric pressure for only a few hours of the day.

Illustrative Cases

CASE 1

This 53 year old white housewife enjoyed good health until 12 months prior to admission when she had a single profuse nosebleed. Six months later she had a fall, and examining herself to ascertain its effects noted a non-tender mass in the left upper quadrant of her abdomen. One month prior to admission she developed dyspnea and ankle edema. Examination by her family physician revealed splenomegaly, and the patient was referred for investigation.

Physical examination. The spleen extended almost to the level of the umbilicus and was moderately firm. The liver was palpable two fingerbreadths below the right costal margin. The remainder of the physical examination was non-contributory.

Laboratory studies. Erythrocyte count 5.2 mil. per cu.mm., hematocrit 47 per cent, leukocyte count 15,000 per cu.mm., reticulocytes 0.2 per cent. Differential count (per cent) myelocytes 1, juvenile 1, bands 10, segmented 79, lymphocytes 4, monocytes 1, eosinophils 3, basophils 1. Platelet count was 426,000 per cu.mm. Bone marrow examination revealed the marrow to be hypercellular with hyperplasia of all cell lines.

It was thought that this patient had either an early polycythemia vera or chronic myelocytic leukemia. Treatment was withheld pending further periodic examinations.

Treatment and course. Six months later the diagnosis of polycythemia vera was evident. She had a very florid complexion; the spleen and liver were unchanged. The hematocrit was 59 per cent, leukocyte count 14,000 per cu.mm., platelets 580,000 per cu.mm. The hematocrit was reduced to 55 per cent after three phlebotomies over the next 8 days and she was given 4.0 millicuries of P^{32} orally.

Four months later the hematocrit had risen to 65 per cent, erythrocyte count was 7.3 mil. per cu.mm., and platelets 772,000 per cu.mm. Five hundred ml. of blood was removed by phlebotomy on two occasions to reduce the red cell count and the patient was given an additional 6.0 millicuries of P^{32} by the oral route. For the next 18 months the patient's hematocrit remained between 48 and 50 per cent, platelets less than 500,000 per cu.mm., and leukocyte count between 9000 and 13,000 per cu.mm. and the spleen edge was at the costal margin. At the end of that period, however, it was found that her hematocrit had risen and the spleen edge reached the level of the umbilicus. The patient was given another 4 millicuries of P^{32} by the oral route and 4 months later the hematocrit was 51 per cent and platelet count 500,000 per cu.mm.

Two and one-half years after the third dose of P^{32} the hematocrit had risen to 58, erythrocyte count had risen to 7.4 mil. per cu.mm., platelets were 1,200,000 per cu.mm. and the spleen had once again increased in size. At this juncture it was decided to institute therapy with busulfan. Phlebotomy once again reduced her hematocrit and the administration of busulfan 2 mg. twice a day was initiated. The levels of the cellular elements in her peripheral blood were followed at weekly intervals and were satisfactory. After 50 days the busulfan was stopped, and 3 months later the hematocrit was 46 per cent, platelet count 300,000, leukocyte count 9800 per cu.mm. The spleen was still at the level of the umbilicus.

Comments. As is true of the majority of patients with polycythemia vera, this patient's initial symptoms appeared in middle age. The evidence of increased red blood cell mass, the presence of a markedly enlarged spleen, and generalized marrow hyperplasia suggested the possibility of chronic myelogenous leukemia or polycythemia vera. The diagnosis could not be made with certainty on the initial visit. The first remission required 10 millicuries of P^{32} and lasted 18 months. Following the administration of an additional 4 millicuries of P^{32} the patient's hematocrit returned to normal levels and she remained free of symptoms for 36 months longer despite the fact that her platelet count was not adequately controlled. When the hematocrit values once again rose to abnormal levels it was decided to use the chemotherapeutic agent busulfan in an attempt to obtain a satisfactory reduction of erythrocytes, leukocytes, and platelets. This was successful. This patient's course has now extended over 12 years during which time she has had no complications and has lived a normal life.

CASE 2

A 69 year old white housewife with known diabetes mellitus of 15 years' duration was admitted with a history of passing tarry stools for 4 days. The most significant abnormalities on physical examination were splenomegaly and hepatomegaly. On this admission the hemoglobin was 7.5 gm. per 100 ml., erythrocyte count was 2.8 mil. per cu.mm., and the leukocyte count was 22,000 per cu.mm. Differential count (per cent): myelocytes 1, juvenile 1, bands 3, segmented 58, lymphocytes 15, monocytes 21, eosinophils 1. No nucleated red cells were seen. Occult blood was present in the stool, but barium studies of the entire gastrointestinal tract revealed no intrinsic lesion. The sternal marrow was markedly hypercellular and the myeloid-erythroid ratio was 3:1.

It was thought that the patient probably had chronic myelocytic leukemia with gastrointestinal hemorrhage. She was treated with blood transfusions and had a satisfactory response. Follow-up examinations for several months revealed normal hemoglobin and red count values, leukocyte counts of about 17,000 per cu.mm., and a differential count similar to that noted in the hospital. Six months later the patient again had a severe gastrointestinal hemorrhage with melena and hematemesis. Following this episode the hemoglobin was 10.5 gm. per 100 ml., red count 3.3 mil. per cu.mm., and leukocyte count 36,000 per cu.mm.

After recovery from this hemorrhage the red count rose to 6.3 million and hemoglobin to 17 to 18 grams, and it was apparent that the diagnosis of polycythemia vera was the correct one. Her leukocyte count varied from 12,000 to 36,000 per cu.mm. Because of the discomfort from the size of the spleen she received several courses of roentgen therapy over the spleen which resulted in a reduction of the splenic size as well as reduction in the leukocytes, hematocrit, and red cell count.

When she was 73 years of age, she had angina pectoris and intermittent claudication. During the next 5 years the erythrocyte cell count rose to 7.7 mil. per cu.mm. on several occasions and phlebotomies were performed as indicated. She fell and suffered an intertrochanteric fracture of the hip. During the operation to pin the fracture there was considerable bleeding; 2 days later a cerebral vascular accident occurred. The patient improved slowly and returned home. Six months later the patient's hematocrit was 45 per cent, erythrocyte count 4.7 mil. per cu.mm., but the leukocyte count had risen to 102,000 per cu.mm. Differential count (per cent): myelocytes 5, juveniles 8, bands 7, segmented 70, monocytes 8, eosinophils 1. It was the clinical impression that the patient had developed leukemia. Three weeks later the patient was admitted to the hospital after an episode of mental confusion followed by unconsciousness. She remained unconscious and died a few hours after admission. Death was attributed to an intracranial hemorrhage.

Autopsy showed extensive intracranial hemorrhage. There was evidence of old infarction of the myocardium and generalized arteriosclerosis. Marked splenomegaly and hepatomegaly were present. Microscopic examination of the liver, spleen, and bone marrow disclosed chronic myelocytic leukemia.

Comment. The patient died at the age of 78, some 10 years after the onset of her symptoms. Earlier in her illness she was thought to have myelocytic leukemia rather than polycythemia vera because the hematologic values were obtained after a massive gastrointestinal hemorrhage. Later in her course the diagnosis of polycythemia vera appeared to be well established. Subsequently the patient had many complications of this disease, such as angina pectoris, intermittent claudication, cerebral thrombosis, and postoperative bleeding. Her final episode was an intracranial hemorrhage. As is often the case it was difficult to determine whether these episodes were due to her blood dyscrasia or to the diabetes mellitus and arteriosclerosis which were present. It appeared likely, however, that the blood dyscrasia was a factor. The incidence of complications of this type has been reduced by treatment with radioactive phosphorus, and had this agent been used the course of her illness might have been altered. Late in her course this patient also developed chronic myelocytic leukemia which was evident at autopsy. This development illustrates the unsettled problem of the relationship between polycythemia vera and myelocytic leukemia and the important question as to whether there is any relationship between radiation therapy of polycythemia and the development of the leukemia.

References

1. Abbatt, J. D., Chaplin, H., Darte, J. M. M., and Pitney, W. R.: Treatment of polycythaemia vera with radiophosphorus: Haemological studies and preliminary clinical assessment. Quart. J. Med., *23*:91, 1954.
2. Abildgaard, C. F., Cornet, J. A., and Schulman, I.: Primary erythrocytosis. J. Pediat., *63*:1072, 1964.
3. Abraham, J. P., Ulutin, O. N., Johnson, S. A., and Caldwell, M. J.: A study of the defects in the blood coagulation mechanisms in polycythemia vera. Am. J. Clin. Path., *36*:7, 1961.
4. Adamson, J. W., and Finch, C. A.: Erythropoietin and the polycythemias. Ann. N.Y. Acad. Sci., *149*:560, 1968.
5. Altschule, M. D., Volk, M. C., and Henstell, H.: Cardiac and respiratory function at rest in patients with uncomplicated polycythemia vera. Am. J. M. Sc., *200*:478, 1940.
6. Anstey, L., Kemp, N. H., Stafford, J. L., and Tanner, R. K.: Leukocyte alkaline-phosphatase activity in polycythaemia rubra vera. Brit. J. Haem., *9*:91, 1963.
7. Auerback, M. L., Wolff, J. A., and Mettier, S. R.: Benign familial polycythemia in childhood. Pediatrics, *21*:54, 1958.
8. Bader, R. A., Bader, M. E., and Duberstein, J. L.: Polycythemia vera and arterial oxygen saturation. Am. J. Med., *34*:435, 1963.
9. Bartos, H. R., and Desforges, J. F.: Erythrocyte enzymes in polycythemia vera. Blood, *29*:916, 1967.
10. Berk, L., Burchenal, J. H., Wood, T., and Castle, W. B.: Oxygen saturation of sternal marrow blood with special reference to the pathogenesis of polycythemia vera. Proc. Soc. Exper. Biol. & Med., *69*:316, 1948.
11. Berlin, N. I., Lawrence, J. H., and Gartland, J.: Blood volume in polycythemia as determined by P^{32} labeled red blood cells. Am. J. Med., *9*:747, 1950.
12. Berlin, N. I., Lawrence, J. H., and Lee, H. C.: The life span of the red blood cell in chronic leukemia and polycythemia. Science, *114*:385, 1951.
13. Bjorkman, S. E., Laurell, C-B., and Nilsson, I. M.: Serum proteins and fibrinolysis in polycythemia vera. Scandinav. J. Clin. & Lab. Invest., *8*:304, 1956.
14. Block, M., and Bethard, W. F.: Bone marrow studies in polycythemia. J. Clin. Invest., *31*:618, 1952.

15. Bradley, J. E., Young, J. D., Jr., and Lentz, G.: Polycythemia secondary to pheochromocytoma. J. Urol., 86:1, 1961.
16. Brodsky, I.: The use of ferrokinetics in the evaluation of busulphan therapy in polycythemia vera. Brit. J. Haem., 10:291, 1964.
17. Brodsky, I., Kahn, S. B., and Brady, L. W.: Polycythemia vera: differential diagnosis by ferrokinetic studies and treatment with busulphan (Myleran). Brit. J. Haem., 14:351, 1968.
18. Burchell, H. B., and Clagett, O. T.: The clinical syndrome associated with pulmonary arterio-venous fistulas, including a case report of a surgical cure. Am. Heart J., 34:151, 1947.
19. Burgess, J. H., and Bishop, J. M.: Pulmonary diffusing capacity and its subdivisions in polycythemia vera. J. Clin. Invest., 42:997, 1963.
20. Cabot, R. C.: A case of chronic cyanosis without discoverable cause ending in cerebral hemorrhage. Boston Med. and Surg. J., 141:574, 1899.
21. Cannon, P., and Penington, D. G.: Erythropoietin and hepatoma. Lancet, 2:1276, 1967.
22. Castle, W. B., and Jandl, J. H.: Blood viscosity and blood volume: opposing influence upon oxygen transport in polycythemia. Semin. Hemat., 3:193, 1966.
23. Chamberlain, D. A., and Millard, F. J. C.: The treatment of polycythemia secondary to hypoxic lung disease by continuous oxygen administration. Quart. J. Med., 32:341, 1963.
24. Charache, S., Weatherall, D. J., and Clegg, J. B.: Polycythemia associated with a hemoglobinopathy. J. Clin. Invest., 45:813; 1966.
25. Chievitz, E., and Thiede, T.: Complications and causes of death in polycythaemia vera. Acta med. scandinav., 172:513, 1962.
26. Clinicopathologic Conference: Polycythemia and neoplastic disease. Am. J. Med., 33:942, 1962.
27. Cobb, L. A., Kramer, R. J., and Finch, C. A.: Circulatory effects of chronic hypervolemia in polycythemia vera. J. Clin. Invest., 39:1722, 1960.
28. Contopoulos, A. N., McCombs, R., Lawrence, J. H., and Simpson, M. E.: Erythropoietic activity in the plasma of patients with polycythemia vera and secondary polycythemia. Blood, 12:614, 1957.
29. Cooper, W. M., and Tuttle, W. B.: Polycythemia associated with a benign kidney lesion: Report of a case of erythrocytosis with hydronephrosis with remission of polycythemia following nephrectomy. Ann. Int. Med., 47:1008, 1957.
30. Dameshek, W.: Some observations on polycythemia vera. Bull. New England Med. Center, 16:53, 1954.
31. Dameshek, W., and Henstell, H. H.: The diagnosis of polycythemia. Ann. Int. Med., 13:1360, 1940.
32. Damon, A., and Holub, D. A.: Host factors in polycythemia vera. Ann. Int. Med., 49:43, 1958.
33. DeGowin, R. L., and Gurney, C. W.: Hemopoiesis in polycythemia vera after phlebotomy and iron therapy. Arch. Int. Med., 114:424, 1964.
34. DeMarsh, Q. B., and Warmington, W. J.: Polycythemia associated with a renal tumor. North-west Med., 54:976, 1955.
35. Ellison, R. R., Ginsberg, V., and Watson, J.: Triethylene melamine in polycythemia vera. Cancer, 6:327, 1953.
36. Erf, L. A.: Radioactive phosphorus in the treatment of primary polycythemia (vera). In Tocantins, L. M.: Progress in Hematology. Vol. 1. Grune & Stratton, New York, 1956, p. 153.
37. Erslev, A.: Humoral regulation of red cell production. Blood, 8:349, 1953.
37a. Ezdinli E. Z., Sokal, J. E., Crosswhite, L., and Sandberg, A. A.: Philadelphia chromosome—positive and negative—chronic myelocytic leukemia. Ann. Int. Med., 72:175, 1970.
38. Fisher, J. M., Bedell, G. N., and Seebohm, P. M.: Differentiation of polycythemia vera and secondary polycythemia by arterial oxygen saturation and pulmonary function tests. J. Lab. & Clin. Med., 50:455, 1957.
39. Forssell, J.: Polycythemia and hypernephroma. Acta med. scandinav., 150:155, 1954.
39a. Gardner, F. H.: Polycythemia (conclusion). Semin. Hemat., 3:232, 1966.
40. Glynn, K. P., Penner, J. A., Smith, J. R., and Rucknagel, D. L.: Familial erythrocytosis: a description of three families, one with hemoglobin Ypsilanti. Ann. Int. Med., 69:769, 1968.
41. Gordon, A. S., Cooper, G. W., and Zanjani, E. D.: The kidney and erythropoiesis. Semin. Hemat., 4:337, 1967.
42. Gottschalk, R. G., and Furth, J.: Polycythemia with features of Cushing's syndrome produced by luteomas. Acta haemat., 5:100, 1951.
43. Grant, W. C., and Root, W. S.: Fundamental stimulus for erythropoiesis. Physiol. Rev., 32:449, 1952.
44. Gurney, C. W., Goldwasser, E., and Pan, C.: Studies on erythropoiesis. VI. Erythropoietin in human plasma. J. Lab. & Clin. Med., 50:534, 1957.
45. Hall, C. A.: Gaisböck's disease. Redefinition of an old syndrome. Arch. Int. Med., 116:4, 1965.
46. Hallock, P.: Polycythemia of morbus caeruleus (cyanotic type of congenital heart disease). Proc. Soc. Exper. Biol. & Med., 44:11, 1940.

47. Halnan, K. E., and Russell, M. H.: Polycythemia vera. Comparison of survival and causes of death in patients managed with and without radiotherapy. Lancet, 2:760, 1965.

48. Harman, J. B., Ledlie, E. M.: Survival of polycythemia vera patients treated with radioactive phosphorus. Brit. Med. J., 2:146, 1967.

49. Harrop, G. A., Jr.: Polycythemia. Medicine, 7:291, 1928.

50. Hertko, E. J.: Polycythemia (erythrocytosis), associated uterine fibroids and apparent surgical cure. Am. J. Med., 34:288, 1963.

51. Hewlett, J. S., Hoffman, G. C., Senhauser, D. A., and Battle, J. D., Jr.: Hypernephroma with erythrocythemia. Report of a case and assay of the tumor for an erythropoietic-stimulating substance. New England J. Med., 262:1058, 1960.

52. Hochman, A., and Stein, J. A.: Polycythemia and pregnancy. Report of a case. Obst. & Gynec., 18:230, 1958.

53. Holmes, C. R., Kredel, F. E., and Hanna, C. B.: Polycythemia secondary to brain tumor. South. M. J., 45:967, 1952.

54. Horwitz, A., and McKelway, W. P.: Polycythemia associated with uterine myomas. J.A.M.A., 158:1360, 1955.

55. Huff, R. L., Elmlinger, P. J., Garcia, J. F., Oda, J. M., Cockrell, M. C., and Lawrence, J. H.: Ferrokinetics in normal persons and in patients having various erythropoietic disorders. J. Clin. Invest., 30:1512, 1951.

56. Huff, R. L., et al.: Plasma and red cell iron turnover in normal subjects and in patients having various hematopoietic disorders, J. Clin. Invest., 29:1041, 1950.

57. Huff, R. L., and Feller, D. D.: Relation of circulating red cell volume to body density and obesity. J. Clin. Invest., 35:1, 1956.

58. Hurtado, A., Merino, C., and Delgado, E.: Influence of anoxemia on the hematopoietic activity. Arch. Int. Med., 75:284, 1945.

59. Isaacs, R.: Treatment of polycythemia vera with Daraprim. J.A.M.A., 156:1491, 1954.

60. Jandl, J. H., Davidson, C. S., Abelmann, W. H., and MacDonald, R. A.: Hemochromatosis terminating in polycythemia and hepatoma with observations on the natural history of hemochromatosis. New England J. Med., 269:1054, 1963.

61. Jaworski, Z. F., and Wolan, C. T.: Hydronephrosis and polycythemia. A case of erythrocytosis relieved by decompression of unilateral hydronephrosis and cured by nephrectomy. Am. J. Med., 34:523, 1963.

62. Jepson, J. H.: Polycythemia: diagnosis pathophysiology and therapy Canad. Med. Assoc. J., 100:271, 327, 1969.

63. Jones, N. F., Payne, R. W., Hyde, R. D., and Price, T. M. L.: Renal polycythemia. Lancet, 1:299, 1960.

64. Kaung, D. T., and Peterson, R. E.: "Relative polycythemia" or "pseudopolycythemia." Arch. Int. Med., 110:456, 1962.

65. Keighley, G., Hammond, D., and Lowy, P. H.: The sustained action of erythropoietin injected repeatedly into rats and mice. Blood, 23:99, 1964.

66. Kiely, J. M., Stroebel, C. F., Hanlon, D. G., and Owen, C. A., Jr.: Clinical value of plasma iron turnover rate in diagnosis and management of polycythemia. J. Nucl. Med., 2:1, 1961.

67. Killmann, S. A., and Cronkite, E. P.: Treatment of polycythemia vera with Myleran. Am. J. Med. Sc., 241:218, 1961.

68. Klein, E., Farber, S., Freeman, G., and Fiorentino, R.: The effects of varying concentrations of human platelets and their stored derivatives on the recalcification time of plasma. Blood, 11:910, 1956.

69. Klemperer, P.: Reticuloendotheliosis. Bull. N. Y. Acad. Med., 30:526, 1954.

70. Knock, H. L., and Githens, J. H.: Primary erythrocytosis of childhood. Am. J. Dis. Child., 100:189, 1960.

71. Kurrle, G. R.: A case of Gaisböck's disease (polycythaemia hypertonica). M. J. Australia, 1:777, 1954.

72. Krantz, S. B.: Application of the in vitro erythropoietin system to the study of human bone marrow disease: polycythemia vera. Ann. N. Y. Acad. Sci., 149:430, 1968.

73. Lawrence, J. H.: Nuclear physics and therapy: Preliminary report on a new method for the treatment of leukemia and polycythemia. Radiology, 35:51, 1940.

74. Lawrence, J. H.: The control of polycythemia by marrow inhibition. J.A.M.A., 141:13, 1949.

75. Lawrence, J. H.: Polycythemia: Physiology, diagnosis, and treatment based on 303 cases. Grune & Stratton, New York, 1955.

76. Lawrence, J. H., and Berlin, N. I.: Relative polycythemia—polycythemia of stress. Yale J. Biol. & Med., 24:498, 1952.

77. Lawrence, J. H., Berlin, N. I., and Huff, R. L.: The nature and treatment of polycythemia vera. Medicine, 32:323, 1953.

78. Lawrence, J. H., and Donald, W. G., Jr.: Polycythemia and hydronephrosis or renal tumors. Ann. Int. Med., *50*:959, 1959.
79. Lawrence, J. H., Winchell, H. S., and Donald, W. G.: Leukemia in polycythemia vera. Ann. Int. Med., *70*:763, 1969.
80. Levin, W. C., Houston, E. W., and Ritzmann, S. E.: Polycythemia vera with PH-l chromosomes in two brothers. Blood, *30*:503, 1967.
81. Linman, J. W., Bethell, F. H., and Long, M. J.: Studies on the nature of the plasma erythropoietic factor(s). J. Lab. & Clin. Med., *51*:8, 1958.
82. London, I. M., Shemin, D., West, R., and Rittenberg, D.: Heme synthesis and red blood cell dynamics in normal humans and in subjects with polycythemia vera, sickle cell anemia and pernicious anemia. J. Biol. Chem., *179*:463, 1949.
83. Lynch, E. C.: Uric acid metabolism in proliferative diseases of the marrow. Arch. Int. Med., *109*:639, 1962.
84. Martin, W. J., and Bayrd, E. D.: Erythroleukemia, with special emphasis on the acute or incomplete variety. Blood, *9*:321, 1954.
85. Mauer, A. M., and Jarrold, T.: Granulocyte kinetic studies in patients with proliferative disorders of the bone marrow. Blood, *22*:125, 1963.
86. Mendlowitz, M.: The effect of anemia and polycythemia on digital intravascular blood viscosity. J. Clin. Invest., *27*:565, 1948.
87. Modan, B.: Computing survival in long-term disease. J.A.M.A., *192*:609, 1965.
88. Modan, B.: Polycythemia: a review of epidemiological and clinical aspects. J. Chron. Dis., *18*:605, 1965.
89. Modan, B., and Lilienfeld, A. M.: Leukemogenic effect of ionising-irradiation treatment in polycythemia. Lancet, 2:439, 1964.
90. Modan, B., and Modan, M.: Benign erythrocytosis. Brit. J. Haem., *14*:375, 1968.
91. Monge, C.: High altitude disease. Arch. Int. Med., *59*:32, 1937.
92. Niewiarowski, S., Zywicka, H., and Latallo, Z.: Coagulation disorders in thrombocythaemia; a study of seven cases. Thromb. et. Diath. Haemorrh., *7*:114, 1962.
93. Osgood, E. E.: Contrasting incidence of acute monocytic and granulocytic leukemias in P[32] treated patients with polycythemia vera and chronic lymphocytic leukemia. J. Lab. & Clin. Med., *64*:560, 1964.
94. Osler, W.: Chronic cyanosis, with polycythemia and enlarged spleen: a new clinical entity. Am. J. M. Sc., *126*:187, 1903.
95. Osler, W.: A clinical lecture on erythraemia. Lancet, *1*:143, 1908.
96. Penington, D. G.: Red-cell regulators. Letter to editor. Lancet, *1*:975, 1960.
97. Penington, D. G.: The relation of erythropoietin to polycythemia. Proc. Roy. Soc. Med., *59*:1091, 1966.
98. Personal observation.
99. Pike, G. M.: Polycythemia vera. New England J. Med., *258*:1250, 1297, 1958.
100. Pollycove, M., Winchell, H. S., and Lawrence, J. H.: Classification and evolution of patterns of erythropoiesis in polycythemia vera as studied by iron kinetics. Blood, *28*:807, 1966.
101. Primrose, D. A.: Polycythemia in association with hydrocephalus. Lancet, 2:1111, 1952.
102. Reinhard, E. H., and Hahneman, B.: The treatment of polycythemia vera. J. Chronic Dis., *6*:332, 1957.
103. Reissmann, K. R.: Studies on the mechanism of erythropoietic stimulation in parabiotic rats during hypoxia. Blood, *5*:372, 1950.
104. Rigby, P. G., and Leavell, B. S.: Polycythemia vera. A review of fifty cases with emphasis on the risk of surgery. Arch. Int. Med., *106*:622, 1960.
105. Rosenthal, N., and Bassen, F. A.: Course of polycythemia. Arch. Int. Med., *62*:903, 1938.
106. Rosse, W. F., Waldmann, T. A., and Cohen, P.: Renal cysts, erythropoietin and polycythemia. Am. J. Med., *34*:76, 1963.
107. Ruch, W. A., and Klein, R. L.: Polycythemia and pregnancy. Obst. & Gynec., *23*:107, 1964.
108. Russel, R. P., and Conley, C. L.: Benign polycythemia: Gaisböck's syndrome. Arch. Int. Med., *114*:734, 1964.
109. Sandberg, A. A., Ishihara, T., Crosswhite, L. H., and Hauschka, T. S.: Comparison of chromosome constitution in chronic myelocytic leukemia and other myeloproliferative disorders. Blood, *20*:393, 1962.
110. Schwartz, B. M., and Stats, D.: Oxygen saturation of sternal marrow blood in polycythemia vera. J. Clin. Invest., *28*:736, 1949.
111. Schwartz, S. O., and Ehrlich, L.: The relationship of polycythemia vera to leukemia; a critical review. Acta haemat., *4*:129, 1950.
112. Selzer, A.: Chronic cyanosis. Am. J. Med., *10*:334, 1951.
113. Shullenberger, C. C.: Long-range treatment of polycythemia vera with 6-mercaptopurine. Cancer Chemother. Rep., *16*:251, 1962.

114. Silverstein, A., Gilbert, H., and Wasserman, L. R.: Neurologic complications of polycythemia. Ann. Int. Med., *57*:909, 1962.

115. Stroebel, C. F., Hall, B. E., and Pease, G. L.: Evaluation of radiophosphorus therapy in primary polycythemia. J.A.M.A., *146*:1301, 1951.

116. Thompson, A. P., and Marson, F. G. W.: Polycythaemia with fibroids. Lancet, *2*:759, 1953.

117. Tinney, W. S., Hall, B. E., and Griffin, H. Z.: The liver and spleen in polycythemia vera. Proc. Staff Meet. Mayo Clin., *18*:46, 1943.

118. Valentine, W. N., Beck, W. S., Follette, J. H., Mills, H., and Lawrence, J. S.: Biochemical studies in chronic myelocytic leukemia, polycythemia vera and other idiopathic myeloproliferative disorders. Blood, *7*:959, 1952.

119. Videbaek, A.: Polycythemia vera: Course and prognosis. Acta med. scandinav., *138*:179, 1950.

120. Vries, S. I. de, Braat-Van Straaten, M. A. J., Müller, E., and Wettermark, M.: Antiplasmin deficiency in polycythaemia: a form of thrombopathy. Thromb. et Diath. Haemorrh., *6*:445, 1961.

121. Wald, N., Hoshino, T., and Sears, M. E.: Therapy of polycythemia vera with Myleran. Blood, *13*:757, 1958.

122. Waldman, T. A., and Bradley, J. E.: Polycythemia secondary to a pheochromocytoma with production of an erythropoiesis stimulating factor by the tumor. Proc. Soc. Exper. Biol. & Med., *108*:425, 1961.

123. Waldman, T. A., Levin, E. H., and Baldwin, M: The association of polycythemia with cerebellar hemangioblastoma. The production of an erythropoiesis stimulating factor by the tumor. Am. J. Med., *31*:318, 1961.

123a. Ward, H. P., Bigelow, D. B., and Petty, T. L.: Postural hypoxemia and erythrocytosis. Am. J. Med., *45*:880, 1968.

124. Wasserman, L. R.: Polycythemia vera — its course and treatment; relation to myeloid metaplasia and leukemia. Bull. N. Y. Acad. Med., *30*:343, 1954.

125. Wasserman, L. R., and Gilbert, H. S.: The treatment of polycythemia vera. Med. Clin. N. Amer., *50*:1501, 1966.

126. Wasserman, L. R., and Gilbert, N. S.: Surgery in polycythemia vera. New England J. Med., *269*:1226, 1963.

127. Watkins, P. J., Fairley, G. H., and Bodley-Scott, R.: Treatment of polycythemia vera. Brit. Med. J., *2*:664, 1967.

128. Wiseman, B. K., Rohn, R. J., Bouroncle, B. A., and Myers, W. G.: The treatment of polycythemia vera with radioactive phosphorus. Ann. Int. Med., *34*:311, 1951.

X / Hemostasis: Theory and Clinical Applications

Introduction

It is not surprising that the events responsible for hemostasis have been studied so extensively. The process by which fluid blood becomes a solid clot has stirred the curiosity of many, and the dreadful consequences of failure to maintain hemostasis in a variety of disorders have lent further impetus to the study. New techniques for the investigation of these problems have recently become available. Application of these techniques has made possible the development of a useful concept of blood coagulation and led to a better understanding of many of the blood dyscrasias which result in abnormal bleeding. Advances in therapy have occurred as the result and the clinician is now better able to cope with these distressing disorders.

Normal Hemostasis

Hemostasis is the end result of a series of related but not necessarily interdependent events. Damage to a vessel wall is followed by immediate but temporary reflex vasoconstriction and platelets are attracted to the site of injury and form a plug within seconds. The initial phase of hemostasis is followed by the formation of a fibrin clot which effectively seals the vessel and facilitates repair. The fibrin clot undergoes dissolution after repair of the vessel is complete. The defense mechanism of hemostasis can conveniently be divided into two phases, the initial vascular-platelet phase and the biochemical response.[192]

302

The Vascular-Platelet Phase of Hemostasis

The response of the vessel wall to injury, the role of the vascular endo-thelium in repair, and the factors responsible for the maintenance of the functional efficiency of the vascular wall are little understood. The importance of the vessel wall in hemostasis is evidenced by the fact that the platelets may be greatly reduced and the blood made biochemically incoagulable without the occurrance of purpura or hemorrhage. This remains a promising area for research.[321]

The platelet and its role in hemostasis have been extensively investigated in recent years.[121, 329] The vast majority of platelets are produced by the mega-karyocytes in the bone marrow.[10, 24, 125, 357] However, small numbers of mega-karyocytes are found to circulate in the blood of normal persons and larger numbers have been demonstrated in the venous blood of patients with malig-nancy.[147] The majority of these circulating megakaryocytes are trapped in the lungs, where they continue to release significant numbers of platelets.[156]

Some correlation of structure with function is now possible as the result of recent studies of the fine structure of the platelet. The marginal bundle of microtubules appears to be composed of microfilaments which have a periodic substructure similar to that of isolated thrombosthenin.[349, 360, 361] Granules con-taining serotinin, numerous glycogen particles, mitochondria and vacuoles have been identified.[349, 350] The hyaloplasm is penetrated by a vast canalicular system which is in continuity with the surface. Such a system provides the platelet with a large surface area and may bring the interior of the cell into closer proximity to the enveloping medium.

The platelets are metabolically active and require a constant supply of ATP. Glucose is the principal source of energy and is metabolized anaerobically or aerobically. The platelet contains all of the enzymes of the glycolytic pathway, citric acid cycle, and the hexose monophosphate shunt; there is abundant glycogen which is available to the glycolytic pathway.[292] Marked stimulation of glucose oxidation occurs when the platelet is exposed to thrombin.[343]

Associated with the platelet are at least 15 different proteins, most of which are found in the plasma as well, i.e., fibrinogen, albumin, prealbumin, globulins, plasminogen, and the coagulation factors II, V, VIII, IX, X, XI, XII, and XIII.[162] Platelet fibrinogen appears to be different from plasma fibrinogen.[76] Specific platelet proteins are the contractile protein, thrombosthenin, a glyco-protein (the role of which is unclear), and platelet clotting factors.[32, 111, 234, 236]

Protein synthesis has recently been demonstrated in young platelets.[45, 46] Labeled amino acids may be incorporated into the contractile protein for at least 72 hours of the platelet life span.[359] The platelet contains no DNA and it has been postulated that stable m-RNA is responsible for this activity; there is no RNA turnover.[46] Fatty acid synthesis is carried on by platelets which have a complete fatty-acid synthesizing system; it is not certain that synthesis of phos-pholipid is possible.[203]

Platelets have classical D-type receptors which enable them to bind sero-tonin, which they incorporate against a concentration gradient.[225] The role of serotonin in hemostasis, if it has any, is unknown.[229] The amine appears to be concentrated in the electron dense granules of the platelet and is released on

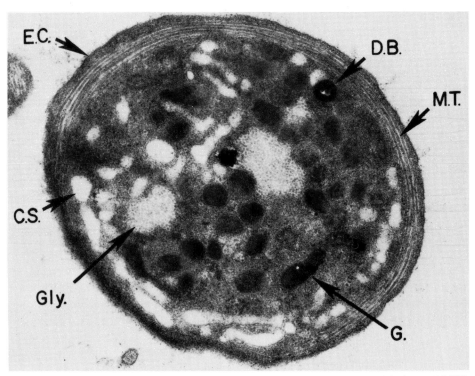

Figure 10–1. The appearance of a human platelet sectioned in the equatorial plane (×24,900). The structural elements noted include the exterior coat (EC), the circumferential band of microtubules (MT), granules (G), dense bodies (DB), the open canalicular system continuous with the cell surfaces (CS), and glycogen particles (Gly). (Reproduced by permission from White, J. G.: Blood, 32:324–335, 1968.)

exposure to thrombin, calcium, and reserpine.[140, 210, 225, 350] Acid phosphatase, B-glucuronidase, and cathepsin have been identified in the granules of the platelet; catalase and lactic dehydrogenase are present in the soluble fraction.[206, 318]

Platelets release 50 per cent of their adenine nucleotides in response to certain stimuli such as exposure to collagen or thrombin.[75, 140, 255] Inasmuch as platelets require the presence and resynthesis of ATP in order to function as a living cell, such a loss would be catastrophic unless the cell was protected against the effect of nucleotide loss. Recent work has demonstrated that the platelet has two different pools of adenine nucleotides; one is metabolically inert and is released and the other metabolically active pool participates in cellular metabolism.[139, 153]

Eighteen to twenty per cent of the extractable protein of the platelet is an actomyosin-like protein. Electron microscopy has revealed that the extracted protein (thrombosthenin) contains microfibrils; these microfibrils bear a striking resemblance to the myofibrils of the smooth muscle and may be responsible for the contractile properties of the platelet. Studies of the platelet under a variety of conditions have suggested that the microtubular structures represent

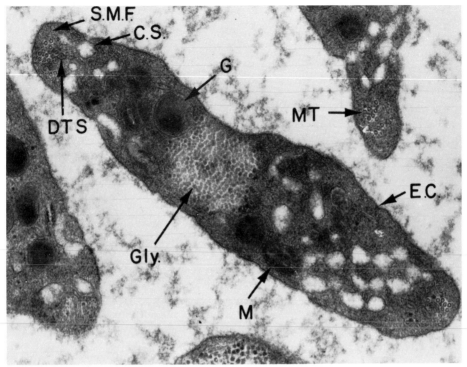

Figure 10-2. The anatomy of a human discoid platelet cut in cross section (×45,800). The structural elements noted include submembrane filaments (S.M.F.) and the dense tubular system (DTS), both of which are associated with the circumferential band of microtubules (MT), mitochondria (M), the exterior coat (E.C.), glycogen (Gly.), canalicular system (C.S.), and granules (G). (Reproduced by permission from White, J. G.: Blood, *31*:604–622, 1968.

different forms of the same substances.[349] The microtubules are formed when needed to maintain a rigid shape, whereas microfibrils are formed when contractile activity is needed.[361]

Platelet Clotting Factors

Platelet clotting factors are, by convention, identified by Arabic numerals, in contrast to the plasma clotting factors which are identified by Roman numerals.

Platelet factor 1 (PF-1). The "plasmatic atmosphere" of platelets has been shown to contain plasma clotting factors I, II, V, VII, VIII, IX, and XIII. Factors I and V are tightly bound and resist repeated washings. Factor V has been demonstrated to be identical with platelet factor 1.[80]

Platelet factor 2 (PF-2). This is a heat-stable, relatively low molecular weight protein which accelerates the conversion of fibrinogen (Factor I) to fibrin (Factor Ia) by thrombin (Factor IIa). This increase in the reactivity of fibrinogen to thrombin is associated with a release of non-protein nitrogen

suggesting that PF-2 has proteolytic activity. It will also produce platelet aggregation and neutralize antithrombin III.[242]

Platelet factor 3 (PF-3). A liproprotein found in association with both
the platelet membrane and the platelet granules, platelet factor 3 is required
for the activation of Factor VIII by activated Factor IX (IXa) and for the
conversion of prothrombin (Factor II) to thrombin (IIa) by activated X (Xa)
in the presence of Factor V. Both of these reactions require calcium ion.[80, 205]

There is increasing evidence to support the concept that the platelet
membrane serves as a surface catalyst locally at the site of vessel injury and
probably represents platelet factor 3 activity in vivo. The physiologic role of
soluble platelet phospholipids released during in vivo thrombus formation
is uncertain.

Platelet factor 4 (PF-4). Another low molecular weight, heat-stable
protein, PF-4, neutralizes heparin and the antithrombin activity of fibrinogen
breakdown products (antithrombin IV).[242, 234]

Function of the Platelet

There is evidence that the platelet, like other formed elements in the
blood, may serve as part of a transport system that carries enzymes or other
chemicals from one part of the body to another. The avidity of platelets for serotonin (5-hydroxytryptamine) is well known, but no essential role in platelet
metabolism or function has been identified for serotonin, and the platelet may
serve only as a storage site and transport mechanism for this amine.[225, 229]

Recently it has been noted that in the presence of polystyrene particles or
antigen-antibody complexes, aggregation is accompanied by phagocytosis of
the inducing agent by the platelet,[115, 255] and it has been suggested that platelets
may also have a role in rejection of organ transplants.

The platelet is chiefly important for the mechanical and chemical role it
plays in hemostasis and vascular repair.[191, 205] It acts mechanically to seal defects
in the vascular endothelium and to promote clot retraction by its interaction
with the strands of fibrin.[166, 333] It is important in blood coagulation because it
provides a phospholipid essential to blood coagulation.

Platelet Aggregation

The mechanism by which platelet aggregation is induced at sites of injury
in blood vessels has been extensively studied.[309] No aggregation of platelets
occurs in static blood in vitro. Agitation must be sufficient to produce a minimal
collision force before aggregation occurs and platelets must be numerous
enough for collisions to occur; little aggregation results if the concentration of
platelets falls much below 50,000 per cu.mm.[309] A wide variety of agents,
including long-chain saturated fatty acids, thrombin, collagen, adenosine
diphosphate (ADP), 5-hydroxytryptamine, and norepinephrine, are capable
of inducing platelet aggregation in vitro.[128, 161, 229, 232, 261, 354, 362]

Evidence has accumulated indicating that ADP may be the final common pathway by which these agents produce aggregation. Platelet aggregation is not induced by ADP in the absence of Ca^{++} and there is evidence that a protein co-factor is required[59, 62, 73, 215, 229, 235] (Fig. 10–3). If platelets are aggregated by minimal concentrations of ADP they will disperse after a period of time and appear unaltered. Removal of Ca^{++} will also result in dispersal of platelets from the aggregation.

There is much speculation as to the mechanism by which ADP induces platelet aggregation.[323] Serious objections have been raised to the suggestions that ADP-Ca^{++} complexes form an intercellular bridge, alter the charge of the platelet membrane, or act as an energy source.[295] It has been proposed that platelets require an active, constant source of energy to remain "unsticky" and that the source of this energy is ATP which is split by the ATPase on the platelet membrane. Addition of ADP would interfere with the reaction by product inhibition and would allow a change in the membrane resulting in aggregation.[294]

Recent evidence indicates that at any time part of the platelet population may be temporarily refractory and not equally responsive to ADP. This refractory state may be related to the function of the contractile protein.[201, 289] The aggregation of platelets in vitro by ADP is inhibited by adenosine monophosphate (AMP), adenosine, and most strongly by 2-chloroadenosine,[49] compounds that show vasodilator activity in the human forearm. The nature of the receptor sites on either platelets or smooth muscle is unknown.[51] The mechanism by which these compounds interfere with the action of ADP is unknown; it may relate to competition for bridging sites on the platelet or their participation in the synthesis of platelet ATP, which would favor the energy-producing reaction.[254, 294, 295]

Exposure to ADP results in remarkable changes in the fine structure of the platelet.[348] The platelet loses its discoid shape, becomes irregularly swollen, and develops multiple pseudopods. "Stickiness" of the platelet occurs at that

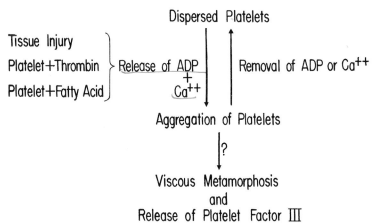

Figure 10–3. Adenosine diphosphate (ADP) appears to provide a common basis for the action of a variety of substances known to induce platelet aggregation. The action of ADP requires Ca^{++} and possibly a protein co-factor. Removal of Ca^{++} or ADP results in dispersion of platelets.

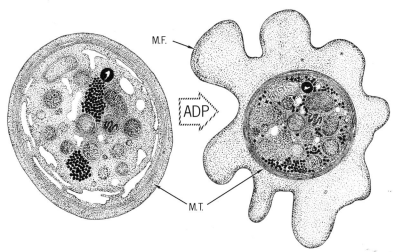

Figure 10–4. Schematic drawing showing the effect of ADP on an individual platelet. The circumferential band of microtubules contracts on exposure to ADP, forcing the organelles into close approximation. Swelling increases the cell size by some 15 per cent, and pseudopods containing microfilaments appear. These changes precede the platelet-release phenomena.

time, as aggregation is an associated phenomenon. The marginal bundle of microtubules crowd the organelles toward the center of the platelet so that the granules come to lie in close apposition; some of the microtubules appear to have been replaced by microfibrils.[360] The platelet canalicular system is altered and peripheral elements connected to the platelet surface become dilated and appear as deep clefts between the pseudopods.[348]

ADP may also be the stimulus responsible for platelet aggregation in vivo.[209, 309, 319] The formation of platelet plugs at the site of vessel damage in experimental animals is inhibited by a variety of enzyme poisons, suggesting dependence on metabolic activity. Anticoagulants do not inhibit platelet aggregation at the site of vessel injury, indicating probable independence of clotting factors.[141] The administration of ADP to experimental animals results in a fall in platelet concentration,[50] and the administration of adenosine and 2-chloroadenosine inhibits the formation of platelet thrombi and emboli in injured vessels.[52] The successful extraction of ADP from vessel walls lends further support to this hypothesis.[229] The finding that intravascular platelet aggregations disperse despite continued administration of ADP to experimental animals suggests the presence of a mechanism that can limit the size and extent of platelet aggregation. It has been proposed that an enzyme system in the platelets and plasma constantly re-establish AMP:ADP ratios capable of inhibiting platelet aggregation, thus preventing a self-extending process.[160, 290]

Prostaglandins, especially PGE, inhibit thrombin-induced platelet aggregation in vitro. Their role in vivo is not clear, but they may affect platelet aggregation through a regulatory effect on platelet levels of high-energy phosphates.

Aggregation by thrombin, collagen, and a variety of other biological agents differs from that induced by ADP alone in that viscous metamorphosis occurs and is irreversible.[139, 140, 150, 191, 247] During viscous metamorphosis, platelets selectively release part of the content of the intracytoplasmic storage system.

Serotonin, ADP, ATP, B-glucuronidase, platelet factor 3, and other substances appear in the surrounding medium or become active at the surface.[142, 192, 205] The precise event which initiates the "release phenomenon" is unknown. The reaction is inhibited by aspirin, sodium salicylate, fibrinogen degradation products, and other substances.[102]

Platelet Adhesion

In vivo, circulating platelets adhere to exposed collagen in the area of injury to vessel wall within one or two seconds. This platelet-collagen adhesion is dependent on the presence of the free amino groups of collagen; free carboxyl groups are not important for platelet adherence but are critical for activation of Factor XII.[248] The collagen effect is restricted essentially to one layer of platelets. Following adherence to the collagen, the platelets degranulate releasing ADP which results in further aggregation and a build up of the platelet mass. In the presence of collagen or thrombin the ADP induced aggregation is accompanied by degranulation and the release of several platelet constituents.

In vitro, platelets adhere to glass and a variety of methods have been developed to quantitate this phenomenon.[47, 132, 293, 296] Platelet adhesion to glass is different from platelet adherence to collagen. Platelets from patients with thrombasthenia, for example, fail to adhere to glass but adhere normally to collagen. The in vitro tests are useful clinically and have demonstrated decreased adhesion to glass by platelets of patients with von Willebrand's disease, thrombopathia, chronic renal failure, and afibrinogenemia. It has been abundantly demonstrated that ADP and fibrinogen influence adhesiveness of platelets to glass beads, but the precise mechanism underlying the phenomenon remains to be elucidated.

The Biochemical Phase of Hemostasis

Although much of our knowledge of blood coagulation is based on empiric laboratory tests, it has nonetheless found extensive clinical application. The theory of blood coagulation to be presented is but an expansion of the classic theory developed at the turn of the century. The various disorders of hemostasis will subsequently be presented within the same framework.

The system of nomenclature adopted by the International Committee for the Nomenclature of Blood Coagulation Factors.[174, 195] and the commonly used synonyms are as follows:

COMMITTEE	SYNONYMS
Factor I	Fibrinogen
Factor II	Prothrombin
Factor III	Thromboplastin (tissue) (extrinsic prothrombin activator)
Factor IV	Calcium

Factor V   Accelerator globulin, labile factor, pro-accelerin, co-factor of
               thromboplastin, AC globulin

Factor VI   No longer used

Factor VII   Serum prothrombin conversion accelerator (SPCA), pro-
               convertin, stable factor, co-thromboplastin, prothrombin
               accelerator, autoprothrombin I

Factor VIII   Antihemophilic globulin (AHG), antihemophilic factor (AHF),
               thromboplastinogen A, platelet co-factor I, antihemophilic
               factor A

Factor IX   Plasma thromboplastin component (PTC), Christmas factor,
               autoprothrombin II, antihemophilic factor B, beta thrombo-
               plastin

Factor X   Stuart-Prower factor, Stuart factor

Factor XI   Plasma thromboplastin antecedent (PTA)

Factor XII   Hageman factor, contact factor

Factor XIII   Fibrin stabilizing factor, L-L factor, Laki-Lorand factor

Historical Aspects

The current concepts of the process of coagulation are better understood when viewed in historical perspective. For details of the early history of the study of coagulation the reader is referred to the reviews by Gamgee in 1880[110] and Howell in 1935.[145]

In 1845 Buchanan[60] noted that a substance was formed during clotting which when extracted from the clot would cause the coagulation of serous fluids. The substance which Buchanan had discovered was thrombin. In 1859 Denis[110] demonstrated that a material which was the soluble precursor of the fibrin of the clot was present in the plasma. This protein was named fibrinogen. Schmidt[300] working along similar lines in 1872, concluded that the formation of fibrin was due to the interaction of fibrinogen and serum globulin in the presence of thrombin. He noted that the clot promoting substance, thrombin, could be extracted after a clot was formed, but no such substance could be demonstrated in the liquid state. From this observation he concluded that thrombin was present in the circulating blood in an inactive or precursor state, and the concept of prothrombin was evolved. In 1879 Hammarsten,[122] using a better method of preparation of fibrinogen, demonstrated that it could be converted to fibrin in the presence of thrombin without the participation of serum albumin or globulin.

In 1826, Joseph Jackson Lister, the father of Lord Lister, discovered that the spherical aberration of one lens could be neutralized by that of another and the potential of light microscopy was vastly increased. As a result, George Gulliver in 1841 and William Addison in 1842 discovered and described the platelet.[285]

Osler described his studies of shed blood in 1874; he called attention to the granular masses of platelets, their pseudopods, and their intimate association with the formation of fibrin. "Mucoid degeneration" was the term Osler used to describe the morphologic changes in platelets in the early stages of coagulation known today as "viscous metamorphosis."[251, 285]

In 1872, the French hematologist Hayem began his studies of the platelet which established the cell as an entity and its role in coagulation.[131] In 1890 Arthus and Pagés[18] proved that calcium was essential for the coagulation of blood. It was shown that substances which bind or remove calcium from the blood prevent coagulation.

At the turn of the century Morawitz[231] was able to formulate the classic therory of coagulation. It is summarized as follows:

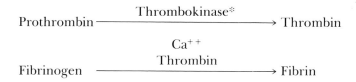

The classic theory, which was simple and agreed with the known facts, remained unaltered until recently. As additional factors essential to the process of coagulation were discovered expansion of the scheme became necessary, but the classic theory embodies the basic concept from which most of the modern theories of blood coagulation have evolved.

The most important contributions to the theory of coagulation have been concerned with the development of the substance activating prothrombin. For nearly 50 years after the introduction of the classic theory research was hampered by the failure to realize that "thrombokinase" could derive not only from a tissue source but from the blood itself. The exact nature of the material responsible for the conversion of prothrombin to thrombin is unknown and for purposes of discussion is designated as "thromboplastin activity."

Studies of patients with disorders of hemostasis have led to the discovery of new factors necessary for the development of normal thromboplastin activity. The general design of these investigations is simple. An in vitro test system is employed. The defect of the plasma, serum, or platelets of the patient under investigation is identified by successive substitutions of the corresponding fraction of normal blood until the coagulation defect is corrected. Thus localized to either the plasma, serum, or platelets, the defect is further identified by comparing the defective fraction with comparable fractions from patients with known defects. In this way it can be determined whether the defect under study is the result of the deficiency of a known or previously unknown factor.

The result of such studies has been an expansion of the classic theory of coagulation.[195]

Present Day Theories of Coagulation

For purposes of discussion the coagulation of blood may be considered to occur in three stages. During the first stage thromboplastin activity develops as

---

*Thromboplastin activity.

the result of both the coagulation factors in the blood and the admixture of tissue juices and plasma. The blood (intrinsic) and tissue (extrinsic) systems responsible for the development of thromboplastin activity may be separated in vitro and shown to be independent and equally potent. There seems little doubt that they both function in the physiologic defense of hemostasis. The second stage of blood coagulation is the conversion of prothrombin to thrombin. The evolution of thrombin from prothrombin will occur in the presence of thromboplastin activity and calcium ions. The third stage of blood coagulation is the conversion of fibrinogen to fibrin in the presence of thrombin. Each of these stages will be discussed separately.

The Development of Thromboplastin Activity

The first stage of blood coagulation may be outlined as shown in Figure 10–5.

This scheme indicates the factors unique to one or the other thromboplastin activity generating system and those common to both. Each develops potent thromboplastin activity though the rate of its development is more rapid in the extrinsic system.[35]

THE EXTRINSIC SYSTEM

Recent investigations have revealed that the formation of extrinsic thromboplastin activity involves two distinct steps.[89] The first reaction involves tissue

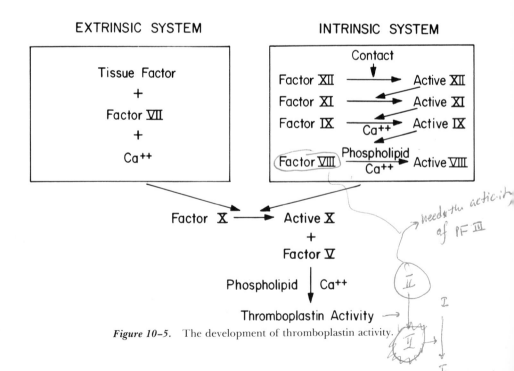

Figure 10–5. The development of thromboplastin activity.

factor (Factor III), Factor VII, Factor X, and calcium. The product of this reaction plus Factor V gives rise to thromboplastin activity.[326]

Tissue factor (Factor III). The extrinsic system requires a source of tissue factors. All tissues probably contain the factors essential to the development of thromboplastin activity and contribute to the physiologic defense of hemostasis. Brain or lung tissue is generally used as a tissue source in the performance of coagulation tests. For many years it was thought that these tissues contained one active principle but investigation has now revealed that they contain a complex of heat-stable and heat-labile fractions.[195] Removal of 95 per cent of tissue factor phospholipid results in a loss of 98 per cent of its biologic activity.[240] The activity can be restored to the extracted tissue by the addition of brain phospholipid or highly purified phospholipid. Phosphatidyl ethanolamine was the most active phospholipid tested. It is well to recognize that the nature of this complex is not completely understood and that it is in all probability the end result of a series of chemical and enzymatic reactions.

Marked quantitative and qualitative differences will appear in the results of laboratory tests if tissue extracts from various organs in the same species or from the same organ from different species are used. These results suggest that the mechanism of action of these materials is not the same and emphasizes the need for careful control of reagents in laboratory studies.

Factor VII. Factor VII is one of the plasma factors essential for the development of thromboplastin activity from a tissue source. This factor is apparently formed in the liver and like prothrombin is dependent on vitamin K for its continued production. It is stable on storage under blood bank conditions. Factor VII behaves as an enzyme in the formation of thromboplastin activity and is found in both plasma and serum. It is adsorbed by inorganic precipitating compounds and is relatively heat stable.[253] Factor VII behaves as a beta globulin on electrophoresis. It is not considered to play any role in the production of thromboplastin activity by the intrinsic system.[5, 165, 253] Recent evidence suggests that Factor VII and Factor II are similar chemically.[138]

The remaining factors necessary to the development of thromboplastin activity by the extrinsic system are essential to the intrinsic system as well. They will be discussed following a description of those factors unique to the intrinsic system.

THE INTRINSIC SYSTEM

The factors essential to the formation of intrinsic thromboplastin activity will be introduced in the order in which they are believed to react in vitro.

Factor XII (Hageman Factor). Factor XII was recognized when a patient was discovered whose blood did not coagulate in a normal period of time on contact with a glass surface.[208] The patient had no clinical disorder of hemostasis. Factor XII is not adsorbed by inorganic precipitating compounds nor is it consumed during coagulation;[197, 276] it behaves as a gamma globulin on electrophoresis and has a biologic half-time of between 50 and 70 hours.[337] It is activated on contact with glass and is thought to initiate clotting in vitro.[278] Activation of Factor XII is accompanied by a change in its physical properties[84] and is believed to be the result of unfolding of the molecule with exposure of reactive sites. Subsequent loss of activity marks a return to its prior conformation, from which it can again be activated.[283, 324] Not all of Factor XII is activated in glass, since it must compete for binding sites with other plasma proteins which have affinity for glass.[120] Factor XII is also activated by ellagic acid,[53] cellulose sulfate, and ℓ-homocystine.[159, 277] It has been suggested that the unusual frequency of thrombosis in patients with homocystinuria may be related to deposits of ℓ-homocystine in the walls of their blood vessels.[277]

Factor XII is also activated by collagen. Thermal denaturation or digestion of collagen blocks this effect, suggesting that the natural triple helical structure is important.[353] Esterification of 80 to 90 per cent of the free carboxyl groups of glutamic and aspartic acids reduced coagulant activity by over 90 per cent.[353] It appears that negatively charged sites are essential for the adsorption and activation of Factor XII and that inhibition of Factor XII activity will result from their neutralization.[247, 248]

Factor XII may play a role in inflammation either directly or through the activation of a plasma kinin similar to or identical with bradykinin.[118, 159]

Factor XI (Plasma thromboplastin antecedent, PTA). Factor XI[288] was discovered, as was Factor IX, during investigation of persons with hemophilia-like states. It is thought to be a globulin and migrates with the beta globulins electrophoretically.[287] Since it is not consumed during coagulation, it is present in both plasma and serum. Unlike Factor IX, it is not adsorbed by inorganic precipitating compounds and is present in $BaSO_4$ adsorbed plasma. Factor XI activity persists in fresh frozen plasma for at least 2 years, and for up to 4 months in plasma stored at room temperature.[69]

The activation of Factor XII and subsequent activation of Factor XI requires no Ca^{++} ions and is known as *the contact system*.[280]

Factor IX (Plasma thromboplastin component, PTC, Christmas factor). Factor IX was discovered during the investigation of persons with hemophilia-like bleeding disorders.[7, 8, 36, 37, 351] This factor, unlike Factor VIII, is not completely consumed in coagulation and is found in both plasma and serum. It is adsorbed by inorganic precipitating compounds and is not present in $BaSO_4$-adsorbed plasma. Though Factor IX is relatively heat labile it fares somewhat better on storage at 4° C than does Factor VIII.[7] Factor IX activity can still be demonstrated in near normal amounts after 2 weeks of storage at 4° C but may fall off rapidly thereafter.[55] Fresh frozen plasma retains its Factor IX activity for long periods.

Factor IX is thought to be activated as the result of the activation of Factor XI.[163, 279] Ca^{++} ions accelerate the reaction but it has been recently reported that activated Factor IX can develop slowly in the absence of Ca^{++} ions.[299] Inactive Factor IX is the substrate for active Factor XI and is proportionately reduced as active Factor IX develops.[246] The half-life of infused Factor IX has two phases; the first 15.1 hours and the second 8.4 days.[6]

Factor VIII (Antihemophilic factor, AHF, antihemophilic globulin, AHG). Among the factors essential for the intrinsic system is Factor VIII,[36, 340] originally termed antihemophilic factor because a deficiency of this factor is responsible for the bleeding diathesis in classic hemophilia. It is a globulin but the site of its production is unknown. Factor VIII is relatively short-lived in the body with a half-life on the order of 8 to 24 hours.[54, 264] Recently it was suggested that infused Factor VIII has a two phase survival in the body, the first with a half-time of 3.8 hours and assumed to represent equilibration with extracellular pools and the second with a half-time of 2.9 days.[6] It is consumed during coagulation and is therefore found only in the plasma.[35] Factor VIII is not adsorbed by the inorganic precipitating compounds and is present in BaSO$_4$-adsorbed plasma. The activity of Factor VIII in plasma or whole blood diminishes rapidly on storage under standard blood bank conditions, but will persist when fresh frozen plasma is stored at −30° C.[69] It is relatively heat stable. Factor VIII has not as yet been obtained in pure form but has been concentrated 6300 times by agarose gel filtration.[155, 224, 281]

New studies have revealed more than one molecular form of Factor VIII in fresh human plasma. The major fraction sediments in the region of a γ M immunoglobulin and has a molecular weight of approximately $2 \times 10.^6$ A minor component, which sediments more slowly, may be associated with fibrinogen;[42] the rapidly sedimenting component, which is found in cryoprecipitates, is not associated with fibrinogen.[345] Activation by thrombin results in a reduction in molecular size, suggesting that the more rapidly sedimenting components may be composed of subunits which are released and activated by thrombin.[345]

The activation of Factor VIII is believed to follow that of Factor IX and in turn activate Factor X. Although activated Factor IX can activate Factor VIII, trace amounts of thrombin profoundly alter the reaction. Thrombin appears to make Factor VIII more reactive to the action of active IX and may be responsible for the "autocatalytic reaction" in the blood clotting mechanism. The first traces of thrombin formed may catalyse the reaction of Factor VIII and speed more rapid generation of thromboplastin activity.[275] As the thrombin-activated Factor VIII is highly unstable, the process is self-limiting.[39] It has been suggested that the extrinsic system may be the source of the first traces of thrombin generated in physiologic clotting and thus would play an important role in the development of intrinsic blood coagulation.[39]

Platelet factor 3. The platelets play several important roles in hemostasis,[48, 124] among which is their contribution to the first stage of blood coagulation. The aggregation and fusion of platelets is known as viscous metamorphosis[27, 309] and is accompanied by the release of phospholipid which is probably unavailable until the platelets are disrupted[322] (Fig. 10–6). A number of phospholipids have been identified in the platelet but those possessing the most marked coagulant activity appear to be phosphatidyl serine and phosphatidyl ethanolamine. The activity of phosphatidyl serine is potentiated by lecithin but not dependent on it.[43] Mixtures of phospholipids containing one negatively charged phospholipid have the most marked clot promoting activity in vitro.[20, 74]

Additional factors. Reports suggesting the possibility of two additional factors important to the development of intrinsic thromboplastin activity have appeared in the literature. Further studies will be necessary before the significance of the Fletcher and Dynia clotting abnormalities can be assessed.[129, 258]

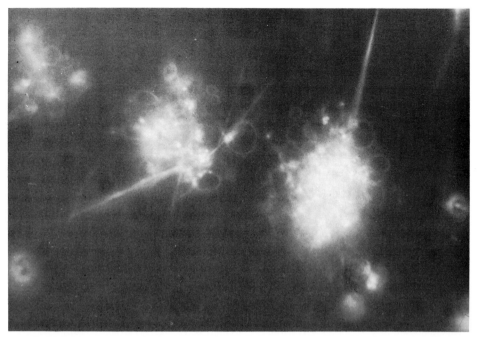

Figure 10–6. Viscous metamorphosis as observed through the phase microscope. Aggregation and fusion of platelets has occurred with formation of characteristic balloon-like structures. Needles of fibrin can be seen.

FACTORS COMMON TO BOTH THE EXTRINSIC AND INTRINSIC SYSTEMS

Factor V. Factor V is probably formed in the liver but is not vitamin K dependent. It is found only in the plasma as it is consumed during the coagulation of blood.[86] The time at which it enters the coagulation scheme has been investigated,[28, 36] and it seems to play an important part in the final phase of thromboplastin formation. Recent evidence indicates that Factor V acts as a co-factor with activated Factor X, phospholipid, and Ca^{++} to form the active prothrombin converting principle.[22, 103, 226] It has been suggested that Factor V has a dual role; phospholipid, Factor V and prothrombin form a colloidal (micellar) complex which is then acted upon by activated Factor X with Factor V as co-factor.[103] The question of whether Factor V is "activated" during coagulation is not yet settled,[23, 103, 265] but it is clear that even after prolonged exposure to activated Factor X, Factor V alone is not able to activate any significant amount of prothrombin.

Factor V is not adsorbed by inorganic precipitating compounds and remains in $BaSO_4$-adsorbed plasma. It migrates between the beta and gamma globulins on filter paper electrophoresis.[71] Factor V deteriorates rapidly on storage of blood under standard blood bank conditions.

Factor X (Stuart factor). Factor X[89, 117, 144, 241] is found in the plasma and serum as it is not consumed during coagulation. It is adsorbed by inorganic precipitating compounds and is stable on storage for 2 months under standard blood bank conditions. It migrates on electrophoresis as an alpha globulin.[78] Factor X has been confused in the past with Factor VII, since the two have many properties in common.

Activated Factor X (Xa) appears to be the prime activator of prothrombin. At normal concentrations of Factor X, the reaction requires Ca^{++}, phospholipid, and Factor V as co-factor.[133] In very high concentration, Xa alone can activate prothrombin.[22, 358] Factor X probably undergoes some reorientation as the result of exposure to Factor V and phospholipid, which increases its activity. In the laboratory, inactivated factor X is unaffected by perfusion through an isolated rabbit liver, whereas activated factor X is rapidly removed by such a procedure. Such a mechanism may function in vivo to aid in the control of the level of activated products of blood coagulation.[81, 83]

Calcium (Factor IV). Calcium ions are necessary for the development of thromboplastin activity in concentrations of between 5 and 20 mg. per 100 ml. Marked prolongation of coagulation time occurs only when the calcium is below 2.5 mg. per 100 ml., and these levels are not seen clinically.[72] The effectiveness of oxalates and citrates as anticoagulants depends on their ability to bind calcium.

The Conversion of Prothrombin to Thrombin

The second stage of blood coagulation may be outlined as follows:

$$\text{Prothrombin} \xrightarrow[\text{Ca}^{++}]{\text{Thromboplastin Activity}} \text{Thrombin}$$

The conversion of prothrombin to thrombin is brought about in the presence of thromboplastin activity and Ca^{++} ions.[94]

Prothrombin (Factor II). The existence of prothrombin was suspected by Schmidt in 1892, and since that time this material has been extensively studied.[178, 305] Prothrombin has a molecular weight of 62,700.[172] Eighteen amino acids and hexosamine have been identified in the molecule. Glutamic acid, aspartic acid, and arginine make up approximately 33 per cent of the protein nitrogen.[171] On electrophoresis, prothrombin behaves as an alpha-1 globulin. It is formed in the liver and is dependent on adequate intake of vitamin K for its production.

Thrombin is quite similar to prothrombin in its amino acid content, and the amount formed in the presence of thromboplastin activity and Ca^{++} varies directly with the amount of prothrombin available.[93, 228, 301] Thrombin is not present in circulating blood. It is the material found in shed blood which was shown capable of clotting fluid from serous cavities by Buchanan in 1842. The species specificity of thrombin-fibrinogen reactions suggests an evolutionary adaptation of the two molecules to yield the most effective possible clotting process.[85] Recent studies indicate that the bovine thrombin monomer has a molecular weight of approximately 8000.[301] A unit of thrombin is defined as that amount of thrombin necessary to clot 1 ml. of standard fibrinogen solution in 15 sec. at 28° C. Thrombin has been highly purified. Some of the preparations contain 12,000 units per mg. N.[306]

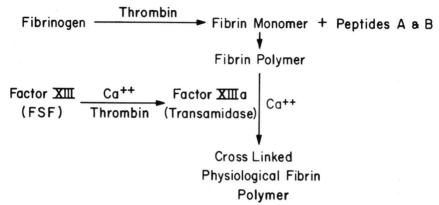

Figure 10–7. Final stage of blood coagulation.

The Conversion of Fibrinogen to Fibrin

The final stage of blood coagulation may be considered to occur as shown in Figure 10–7.

Fibrinogen (Factor I). It will be recalled that the conversion of fibrinogen to fibrin in the final phase of coagulation was recognized in 1859 by Denis when he demonstrated the existence of fibrinogen.

Fibrinogen is formed in the liver and is present in the blood in a concentration of 300 mg. per 100 ml. Its molecular weight is 450,000 and it is available in a highly purified form. The biologic half-life of fibrinogen determined by the I^{131} method is reported to be 109 ± 13 hrs.[127, 337] The clotting time of fibrinogen is inversely proportional to the concentration of thrombin.

Fibrin is formed when thrombin is added to fibrinogen.[94, 185, 195, 315] Thrombin has the ability to split arginylglycine bonds of the fibrinogen molecule to form a monomer of fibrin and two peptides A and B.[31, 169] Peptide A is apparently inert but peptide B has been found to potentiate the contraction of smooth muscle.[114]

Factor XIII (Fibrin stabilizing factor). End to end polymerization of the fibrin monomers with one-third molecular length overlap between laterally adjacent fibrils occurs independently of the presence of thrombin. There is evidence that polymerization may be delayed in the absence of Ca^{++}.[116, 157, 187, 207] Side to side bonding of these polymers occurs in the presence of activated Factor XIII (XIIIa). Factor XIII is activated in the presence of thrombin and Ca^{++}.[61, 167, 185, 188] XIIIa is a transpeptidase which produces covalent cross-linking of fibrin by selective formation of γ-glutamyl-ϵ-lysine bridges.[9, 186, 187] The reaction in human and bovine plasma releases glucosylamine and may account for the 20 per cent loss of carbohydrate from the clot if clotting takes place in the presence of Factor XIII.[57, 65, 182] No such release of carbohydrate has been found when rabbit blood is used, suggesting species variation.[271]

Factor XIII is found in plasma and platelets but is present in only trace amounts in the serum. It has a molecular weight of 350,000 and migrates in association with the α-2 globulins. Factor XIII is non-dialyzable and thermolabile, and requires Ca^{++} for activity.[183, 184, 297] Sulfhydryl inactivating compounds will inhibit its activity. It has a biologic half-life of between 4 and 7 days and very small amounts are required to cross-link fibrin. One milligram will stabilize 11,000 mgm. of insoluble fibrin.[9, 57]

Venom Coagulant System

Many snake venoms possess coagulant activity; of those tested, that of Russell's viper was the most potent.[158, 197] Study of the mode of action of this venom has contributed to the understanding of physiologic hemostasis and has led to its use as a local hemostatic agent. Russell's viper venom has recently been purified[352] and has been demonstrated to have esterase as well as coagulant activity. It behaves as an enzyme in the activation of a coagulation factor present in bovine serum. The bovine serum factor has a molecular weight of 36,000 and is activated as a portion of the molecule is removed by the enzymatic action of the venom. The activated serum factor then reacts with Factor V, phospholipid, and Ca^{++} to form a product which can convert prothrombin to thrombin.[100] As this reaction does not occur when serum from patients deficient in Factor X is used, it is believed that the serum substrate for the venom is Factor X.[196]

The venom of the Malayan pit viper is of great interest, as it has the capacity to convert fibrinogen to fibrin directly without activation of any early coagulation factors. The clot is friable since Factor XIII is not activated and cross-linking does not occur. Platelet counts are unaffected. Active fibrinolysis occurs locally and fibrin split products appear in the plasma. There are no massive clots and the small friable clots are removed by the reticuloendothelial system. The fibrinogen converting fraction has been successfully separated from whole venom and may prove useful in the future in anticoagulant therapy since the blood is effectively defibrinated in 2 to 4 hours. The effect can be stopped with antivenom.[282] Conversion of fibrinogen to fibrin by the active principles of the venom of the Malayan pit viper is not impeded by heparin.[99]

In light of recent evidence one may draw the tentative scheme of blood coagulation shown in Figure 10–8.

Factor X now appears to be the pivotal substance activated by each of the mechanisms noted. This scheme fits known facts and contributes additional insights into the intrinsic system. Macfarlane has likened the intrinsic system to an electronic amplifier and has pointed out that at each level a greater amount of proenzyme is activated, resulting in tremendous overall gain.[197] The rapid disappearance of coagulant enzymes may serve to stop the system, and protect the organism from widespread thrombosis.

No theory of blood coagulation may be considered fact until the chemical reactions responsible for the coagulation of blood are elucidated. The one presented is but an expansion of the classic theory and remains empiric. Deletions or additions must be made as old factors are reconsidered and new factors make their appearance. Despite its defects, this theory serves as a useful clinical and laboratory guide.

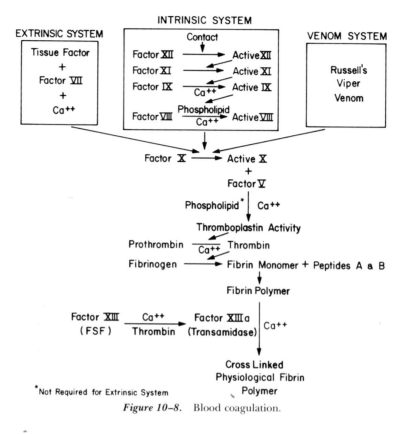

Figure 10–8. Blood coagulation.

Fibrinolysis

Physiologic Clot Dissolution

The fibrinolytic system serves to remove superfluous fibrin after repair of a vessel is complete and to protect the body from the effects of excess fibrin formation. Plasmin is the enzyme responsible for the digestion of fibrin. In health, only its precursor, plasminogen, is found in the plasma.[204]

PLASMINOGEN

Human plasminogen is a globulin found in plasma Factor III of Cohn.[286, 314] It is a glycoprotein with a molecular weight of 89,000 ± 1500. Activation to plasmin monomer is now believed to be due to cleavage of a single original valine bond by the activator. This cleavage results in a two-chain molecule held together by a single disulfide bond.[14, 284, 303] Sensitive radioimmunoassay has been developed to measure plasminogen and plasmin in the plasma.[269] Plasminogen has a strong affinity for fibrinogen and their concentrations in most body fluids vary directly.

ACTIVATORS OF PLASMINOGEN

Plasminogen is converted to plasmin in the presence of "activators." Activators have been found in the plasma and in a variety of tissues, notably the uterus, thyroid, lung, prostate, and in the urine.[200] It is interesting to note that by histologic techniques plasminogen activator was consistently found associated with the vascular endothelium, particularly veins, venules, and pulmonary arteries.[30, 331, 332, 341] There was none in normal liver. In the liver of patients with cirrhosis there was evidence of plasminogen activator around or in the veins.[331] Activator activity of the plasma is found to increase after exercise, and following the administration of epinephrine, nicotinic acid, or pyrogens.[63, 68, 170, 199, 327] Recent evidence suggests that Factor XII (Hageman factor) and other products of the coagulation system may play a role in the activation of these proteolytic enzymes.[96, 130, 149, 217]

Urokinase is an activator found in the urine.[164, 262] It is a colorless proteolytic enzyme with broad substrate specificity[314] and wide temperature and pH stability. The conversion of plasminogen to plasmin by urokinase proceeds as a first order reaction with an optimum of about pH 9.[164] Urokinase appears to be produced in the kidney[29] and has a molecular weight of 53,000.[176] Recent investigations using an antiserum against pure urokinase have demonstrated that it is not identical with the activator found in human milk or tissue activators.[168] Preparations of urokinase suitable for intravenous administration are presently available for clinical investigation. Recent studies have shown it to have predictable thrombolytic activity.[313] With continued improvement in purity and reduction in cost, urokinase may come to play an important role in thrombolytic therapy.[310]

Bacterial products capable of activating plasminogen have received intensive study.[67, 79] The best known is streptokinase, which has been highly purified in hopes of developing an effective thrombolytic agent. The mechanism of its action is not completely understood. Thus far no proteolytic or esterase activity of streptokinase has been reported. It requires an activator system in the plasma to function.[79, 121] Standardization of this agent has been difficult and pyrogenic reactions to its administration a frequent complication.[327] Streptokinase is antigenic and prior exposure to infection with streptococcus will alter the dose requirements. Care must be exercised lest a coagulation defect be induced in the course of treatment.[16, 338]

INHIBITORS OF THE ACTIVATION OF PLASMINOGEN

The existence of naturally occurring inhibitors of plasminogen activators has not been proved.[314] A variety of synthetic substances have been reported to have antiplasmin activity or inhibit the conversion of plasminogen to plasmin.[219]

The compound epsilon aminocaproic acid is worthy of special note as it has been demonstrated effective in inhibition of conversion of plasminogen to plasmin both in vitro and in vivo. As it has but a weak antiplasmin effect it is believed to inhibit the enzymatic conversion.[3, 88, 219, 310]

PLASMIN

Plasmin is the proteolytic enzyme that results from the enzymatic cleavage of the plasminogen molecule. It is an endopeptidase that can digest several proteins in the plasma, including a number of components of the coagulation and complement systems, certain trophic hormones, and others.[121, 303] Under normal circumstances the action of plasmin in vivo is effectively specific for fibrin. Plasmin belongs to the same group of proteinases as trypsin, chymotrypsin, and thrombin. Human plasmin has the same molecular weight as plasminogen 89,000 ± 1500[284] and has a half-life in the plasma on the order of 9.5 hours.[109]

ANTIPLASMIN

The plasma contains substances, which have not been adequately characterized, that appear to inhibit the action of plasmin.[314, 316, 317] Evidence for two inhibitors of plasmin in the plasma has been presented.[245] One substance was recently purified and found to be an α-1 globulin which has a molecular weight of 55,000. This inhibitor had both slow and immediate antiplasmin activity.[307] The other reacts immediately, is more stable at extremes of pH, and resists high temperature. It appears to be an α-2 macroglobulin which has the capacity to bind serine hydrolase enzymes like trypsin, thrombin, and plasmin to various degrees. The participation of plasma proteins in the fibrinolytic mechanism suggests that they function as a regulator and inhibitor of excessive fibrinolysis.[121]

Platelets also contain antiplasmin.[13] It has been shown that the antiplasmin of bovine platelets is separate from that of bovine plasma, though some of the latter may be adsorbed by the platelets.

PLASMINOGEN ACTIVATION

A schematic representation of the reactions believed to be responsible for the activation of plasminogen is shown in Figure 10–9.

The dual phase concept of plasminogen activation[15] as presented emphasizes the biologic importance of the affinity of plasminogen for fibrinogen. When plasminogen is slowly converted to plasmin in the plasma, antiplasmin neutralizes its action and no proteolytic activity can be detected. Fibrin clots, however, contain relatively little antiplasmin, and when activators diffuse into the clot the plasmin activated is unopposed and lysis of the clot results. There is therefore a dual response to the activation of plasminogen: plasmin which develops in the plasma is neutralized and plays little if any role in thrombolysis; plasmin which develops in the interstices of the clot is relatively unopposed and will effectively lyse the fibrin. In addition, certain tissues, especially the veins and pulmonary arteries, are rich in activator substances. The suggestion has been made that fibrin deposited on such tissues would lyse quickly and may

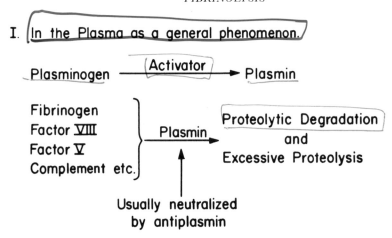

I. In the Plasma as a general phenomenon.

Plasminogen ——— Activator ——→ Plasmin

Fibrinogen
Factor VIII
Factor V   } —— Plasmin ——→   Proteolytic Degradation
Complement etc.   and
                                  Excessive Proteolysis

Usually neutralized
by antiplasmin

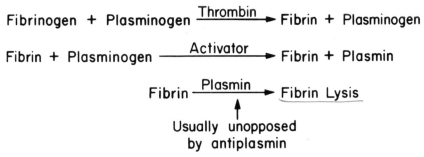

II. Within the Fibrin Clot or on the wall of a vessel as a local phenomenon.

Fibrinogen + Plasminogen ——— Thrombin ——→ Fibrin + Plasminogen

Fibrin + Plasminogen ——— Activator ——→ Fibrin + Plasmin

Fibrin ——— Plasmin ——→ Fibrin Lysis

Usually unopposed
by antiplasmin

Figure 10-9. Activation of plasminogen.

do so without significant change in circulating plasmin.[310] Thus, the action of this enzyme with broad digestive potential is limited by location and is biologically specific.[15]

Pathologic Coagulation and Proteolysis

RELATIONSHIP TO THROMBOTIC DISEASE

The possible relationship of some abnormality of the fibrinolytic mechanism to thrombotic disease remains of great interest.[298] Multiple thrombotic episodes were reported to be associated with an increase in an inhibitor of plasminogen activator in several patients.[56, 244] Thrombotic disorders have also been reported in two patients with high titers of antiplasmin and antiplasminogen.[237]

RELATIONSHIP TO ABNORMAL HEMOSTASIS

The mechanisms responsible for keeping the blood fluid within the vascular system have not been clearly defined. It seems reasonable that there must be a delicate balance between those forces tending to produce coagulation and those tending to inhibit it. The body must have a mechanism for disposing of a clot once repair of a vessel is complete.

THE HYPERCOAGULABLE STATE

Failure of the blood to remain fluid within the vascular system may result in a local thrombus, multiple thromboses, or diffuse intravascular coagulation (DIC).[233] Although thrombosis is an important defense mechanism, serious or fatal consequences may follow either a single thrombosis in an artery or vein or diffuse intravascular coagulation, which occurs in a number of different disorders.

When Virchow introduced the term thrombosis in 1856 he stated that stasis, changes in the walls of the vessels, and biochemical changes in the blood itself are the causes, concepts that have been extended since that time but have remained essentially valid.[320] Considerable effort has been devoted to the attempt to determine the factors that are responsible for non-physiologic thrombosis and coagulation. Factors such as changes in the vessel wall and stasis may be considered "local," whereas the biochemical aspect is a "general" one.

There is abundant clinical evidence that patients with certain conditions seem predisposed to intravascular thrombosis. The most often cited, but not uniformly supported, instance is that of the patient with malignancy.[179] The majority of reports indicate that the association is most common with mucin-producing tumors, particularly those arising in the body and tail of the pancreas, and have suggested a relationship between the frequency of thrombotic episodes and the grade of the malignancy.[213, 227, 320]

Other conditions thought to be associated with a hypercoagulable state appear to be examples of an inappropriate degree of response to a recognized stimulus rather than a response to an ill defined or unrecognized stimulus. Among these are pregnancy,[12] the postpartum and postoperative state,[342] prolonged bed rest,[346] atherosclerosis,[232] myocardial infarction, and congestive heart failure.[356] In each of these conditions, stasis, or vessel wall injury might well be the precipitating cause of the thrombus. It is often difficult to decide whether the response is appropriate or inappropriate to the stimulus.

Recently an association between oral contraceptives and thromboembolism has been recognized and various abnormalities have been found in the blood or vascular system of patients taking contraceptives. The risk of hospital admission for venous thromboembolism is nine-fold greater for women taking "the pill"[339] and a convincing relationship has been found between the use of oral contraceptives and an increased incidence of death from pulmonary embolism or cerebral thrombosis;[152, 336] no relationship to arterial thrombosis has been established. An increase in coagulation factors VII and X[263] and a decreased sensitivity to coumadin drugs have been reported.[97] There is an increase in platelet sensitivity to ADP,[98] which is thought to be secondary to an abnormality in the lecithin of the low density plasma lipoproteins.[44] An increased diameter of the veins at any given pressure has been clearly shown; this increased distensibility of the veins of the patient taking oral contraceptives results in a decrease in the velocity of venous blood flow, which is believed to be another factor contributing to thrombosis.[355] Oral contraceptives are contraindicated in patients with thromboembolism or a past history of any such disorder; their advantages must be carefully weighed against the dangers which have emerged from recent studies before prescribing them for any patient. Further studies of these agents are urgently needed.

Although the hypercoagulable state is recognized clinically, laboratory evidence to support the concept is sparse. The levels of the various blood coagulation factors have been reported to be elevated in pregnancy,[12, 257] in the postpartum and postoperative states,[342] and in patients with atherosclerosis.[232] Recently data which suggest that patients with a tendency to thrombosis have elevated levels of Factor VIII have been presented; in addition, experimental elevation of Factor VIII levels in the blood of dogs enhances intravascular coagulation.[259] Others have pointed out that it is not the absolute quantity of clotting factors present but whether they circulate in an active form that is important.[347] Large amounts of non-activated Factor X fail to produce a thrombus in a laboratory animal, but a small amount of activated Factor X will; the addition of a small amount of phospholipid further reduces the small quantity of activated X required.[23, 347] Of great importance in maintaining the blood in a fluid state is the rate at which activated clotting factors can be removed from the blood by the reticuloendothelial system.[81, 90]

A variety of diseases have been associated with disseminated intravascular coagulation. In most instances the mediating mechanism has been shown to be intravascular hemolysis, tissue extracts, bacterial endotoxins, antigen-antibody complexes, chemical or physical agents, hypoxia, endothelial damage, fibrinolysin inhibitors, or thrombocythemia.[312] Encouraging as the recent reports have been, much work remains to be done to understand the specific biochemical changes responsible for the hypercoagulable state.[70, 135, 212, 256]

EXCESSIVE PROTEOLYSIS

Study of iatrogenic proteolysis arising in the course of the therapeutic administration of thrombolytic agents has shed considerable light on the pathogenesis of these states.[109] If plasminogen is rapidly activated, antiplasmin cannot effectively neutralize the plasmin formed. Plasma fibrinogen, Factor VIII and Factor V levels fall and a hemorrhagic diathesis may develop.[108] Studies of the effect of plasmin on fibrin and fibrinogen have revealed that the proteolytic products retain the antigenic identity of fibrin or fibrinogen. Initially, they tend to be large and have a significant antithrombin effect; the products of further proteolysis do not have a strong antithrombin effect but are anticoagulent since they interfere with the polymerization of fibrin.[109] All interfere with platelet aggregation.[16, 19, 109, 173, 310] These products of proteolysis have also been found in patients with a hemorrhagic diathesis associated with fibrinolysis.[207, 239]

The Defibrination Syndrome (Disseminated Intravascular Coagulation, Consumptive Coagulopathy)

The defibrination syndrome occurs in a large number of clinical conditions.[211, 221] The patient usually presents with symptoms of the underlying disease and, in addition, associated anemia, hemorrhage, or thrombosis, singly or in combination.

There are two major mechanisms responsible for the syndrome of defibrination in clinical medicine. The vast majority of patients have been found to have intravascular coagulation with secondary activation of the fibrinolytic system. Depending on the severity of the process, there is more or less consumption of Factors I, V, VIII, and X and the platelets; rarely, Factors II, IX, and XIII are reduced as well. Activation of the fibrinolytic system results in further reduction of Factors I, V, and VIII as the result of proteolysis. Plasminogen is reduced and the products of proteolytic degradation of fibrinogen and fibrin appear in the circulating blood. Generally, little proteolytic activity can be demonstrated in the blood and the presence of split products suggests fibrinolytic activity at local sites of fibrin deposition.[222, 310] Since these split products are in themselves anticoagulant they contribute significantly to the hemorrhagic diathesis.

A minority of patients with defibrination syndrome have primary pathologic fibrinolysis which can occur as the result of several mechanisms. In the presence of large amounts of plasminogen activator, much of the available plasminogen may be converted to plasmin and overwhelm the antiplasmin system. This may occur as the result of the inadvertent administration of excessive amounts of exogenous plasminogen activator during the course of the treatment of thromboembolism. Large amounts of endogenous activator may be released from some activator-rich neoplastic tissue, such as metastatic carcinoma of the prostate, acute progranulocytic leukemia, or in the course of severe shock or hypoxia.[312] Impairment of the body's ability to remove plasminogen activator from the circulation will also result in hyperplasminemia which has been observed in cirrhosis of the liver and after portocaval shunting procedures.[106, 119] There is also the possibility that a fibrinolytic enzyme other than plasmin may gain access to the circulation.[107]

Despite the advances made in the past few years toward the understanding of the defibrination syndromes which occur in many and varied disorders, much work remains before these syndromes can be clearly delineated and more adequately treated.[105, 107, 220, 312]

The differential diagnosis between intravascular coagulation with secondary fibrinolysis and primary pathologic fibrinolysis is difficult because of overlapping findings and the lack of a definitive test. Factors I and V are reduced in both conditions; Factor VIII and blood platelets are reduced in intravascular coagulation but are usually unaffected in primary fibrinolysis. Excess circulating activator, reduced plasminogen level, and greatly increased fibrinolytic activity are more common in primary fibrinolysis. Clinical judgement and careful evaluation of the laboratory results will usually suffice to resolve the question.

Once the diagnosis is made, the underlying disease should be treated and therapy instituted to tide the patient over the defibrination. If the defibrination is secondary to disseminated intravascular coagulation with associated fibrinolysis, the treatment of choice is anticoagulation with heparin.[41, 220, 315] When primary pathologic fibrinolysis has resulted in defibrination the treatment of choice is epsilon aminocaproic acid (EACA).[214, 220, 310, 312]

Epsilon aminocaproic acid is one of several synthetic amino acids which are effective inhibitors of plasminogen activation.[177, 243, 310] It also inhibits the activation of plasminogen in the urine by urokinase[219] and has proved effective in the control of excessive hematuria following prostatectomy.[216, 291] The administration of EACA should not be considered a routine measure, for its use may allow obstructing fibrin clots to form and persist in the ureter or renal pelvis. There is always the potential hazard of further vascular occlusion as the result of inhibition of fibrinolysis if it is given to a patient with disseminated intravascular coagulation without first controlling the coagulation process.[104, 143, 218, 308]

Once the mechanism responsible for the fibrinolytic disorder is controlled the split products formed during digestion of fibrinogen and fibrin are removed from the circulation by the reticuloendothelial system over a period of several hours. Since the severity of the disorder is critically dependent on the presence of fibrinogen and fibrin split products, their rapid removal contributes to the control of the hemorrhagic diathesis.

Anticoagulants

Physiologic Anticoagulants

ANTITHROMBIN

Thrombin has been noted to be an extremely potent proteolytic enzyme and must be removed or in some manner neutralized following physiologic coagulation or all the blood in the body would soon be clotted.

A series of antithrombins have been described.[181, 193, 267, 304] In whole plasma the two major mechanisms for the removal of thrombin appear to be the immediate adsorption and inactivation of most thrombin by fibrin followed by a progressive inactivation of remaining thrombin by an antithrombin in the alpha globulin fraction of the serum.[193] Antithrombin III appears to be the main inactivator of thrombin. When it is present in physiologic amounts thrombin has a half-life of 40 seconds.[1] Some have suggested that antithrombin III and heparin co-factor are identical,[95] but there is controversy on this point.[112] An α_2-macroglobulin also contributes to a minor degree to the inactivation of thrombin.[2, 113]

Antithrombin activity has been recently reported to develop in the course of proteolysis of fibrinogen by plasmin in vitro.[167, 334]

Pharmacologic Anticoagulants

The major pharmacologic anticoagulants are heparin and the coumarin-indanedione drugs. Their use has doubtless prevented many deaths from thrombosis and embolism and has made possible the rapid development of cardiovascular surgery and extracorporeal by-pass procedures. However, they must be used with proper attention to laboratory control to prevent inadvertent hemorrhage.[11, 151]

Little or no controversy attends the use of pharmacologic anticoagulants to suppress the biochemical phase of blood coagulation in patients on cardiopulmonary by-pass, during renal dialysis, after vascular reconstructive surgery, and in those with thrombophlebitis. There remains considerable disagreement over the indications for their use to prevent further thrombosis following initial detrimental thrombosis as in myocardial infarction and cerebrovascular thrombosis. Further studies are needed to settle these issues.

Prior to the administration of these drugs the physician must determine by history, physical examination, and laboratory studies any actual or potential source of hemorrhage. He must then balance the risk of hemorrhage against that of thromboembolism for that particular patient under his care.

Anticoagulant therapy is usually contraindicated if the patient gives a history of hemorrhagic diathesis, active ulceration or bleeding from the gastrointestinal or genitourinary tract, recent trauma to the central nervous system, severe hepatic disease, or marked hypertension. The history of chronic ingestion of salicylates, phenylbutazone or other agents which potentiate the action of the coumarin-indanedione drugs, might indicate a need to reduce the dosage of anticoagulant.[11] Broad-spectrum antibiotics which alter the bacterial flora of the intestinal tract and reduce bacterial synthesis of vitamin K may profoundly augment the response to coumarin-indanedione anticoagulants. Malabsorption, biliary, or liver disease may also increase susceptibility to these medications.

Many drugs, such as phenobarbital, griseofulvin, and glutethimide, depress the effect of coumarin-like anticoagulants through their action as inducers of liver microsomal enzymes. Thus, the withdrawal of such drugs from patients stabilized on a given dose of these anticoagulants may precipitate a fall in prothrombin concentration to dangerous levels. Other drugs, such as salicylates, phenylbutazone, and sulfonamides, which potentiate the effect of coumarin-like anticoagulants, may act by competitively displacing the anticoagulant from plasma proteins, thus making available more active anticoagulant.[190a]

HEPARIN

Heparin is a mucopolysaccharide which is similar to the chondroitin-sulfuric acid of cartilage. It was isolated from the liver of dogs and contains large quantities of glucuronic acid (26 per cent) and glucosamine (23 per cent).[154] The natural occurrence of heparin in the tissues and circulating blood of man is disputed. Heparin is a direct anticoagulant. Its effect is due to its chemical properties and it affects coagulation directly in vivo or in vitro. The action of heparin is preventive; there is little evidence to indicate any significant effect on a formed thrombus other than the prevention of extension.[82]

Available evidence[34, 87, 202] indicates that heparin acts in vivo and in vitro by interfering with the development of thromboplastin activity. This is suggested by the fact that neither the Factor VIII nor Factor V is consumed in its presence. There is also direct interference with thromboplastin activity at higher concentrations.

Heparin combines with a co-factor in plasma to inhibit thrombin and at very high concentration can interfere with platelet aggregation.[267] Twenty per cent of heparin is eliminated by the kidneys while the rest is degraded by the liver. Heparin does not cross the placenta, nor does it appear in the milk of a nursing mother.[82] The half-life of the anticoagulent activity of heparin is 1.5 hours. Individuals vary widely in their response to the anticoagulant, however, and it is important to individualize control of heparin therapy.[101]

Heparin has several actions other than anticoagulation. It has a well recognized lipemia clearing activity mediated by its activation of endogenous lipoprotein lipase.[77] Severe metabolic bone disease with osteoporosis and vertebral collapse has occurred following prolonged administration of large doses of 10,000 units a day or more for more than a year. Interference with aldosterone production, occasional alopecia and transient thrombocytopenia have been reported.[82]

Administration. The intermittent intravenous administration of heparin is most satisfactory. Heparin is supplied in aqueous solution as the sodium salt. The initial dose is 70 to 100 mg. (7000 to 10,000 units USP) and subsequent doses of 50 mg. (5000 units USP) are given at 4 to 6 hourly intervals. A number of different dosage schedules have been suggested.[17, 82]

Control of anticoagulation is difficult as the administration of these drugs is largely on an empirical basis, and it is not accurately known how much the clotting time should be prolonged to provide successful anticoagulation. As a general rule, the whole blood clotting time should be more than one and a half but less than two and a half times the normal 3.5 hours following each dose of heparin. The whole blood clotting time has been the test most widely used to control heparin therapy. Recent studies indicate that the activated whole blood partial thromboplastin time is the best means of control when precision, information, and economy are considered.[40, 101, 363] Nevertheless, the whole blood coagulation time is still preferred by some.[261a]

Heparin may also be given subcutaneously and intramuscularly and concentrated solutions of heparin are available for this purpose. The intramuscular or subcutaneous injection of 100 mg. (10,000 units USP) alters the whole blood clotting time for approximately 8 hours. Long-acting "Depo" heparin preparations are also available. As the response to the administration of these preparations intramuscularly and subcutaneously is not as predictable as when heparin is given by the intravenous route and the occurrence of large hematoma at the site of injection is a serious risk, the intravenous route is preferred.

Aspirin should not be administered, as it interferes with platelet aggregation, which is one of the few hemostatic defenses left to the patient receiving heparin.

Antidote. The action of heparin may be quantitatively neutralized by protamine sulfate.[66] It is interesting that this reaction with protamine was discovered by investigators searching for a material to prolong the action of heparin. They chose protamine because of its action in slowing the release of insulin from subcutaneous depots.

COUMARIN AND INDANEDIONE DERIVATIVES

At the time when the original investigations of vitamin K were being conducted, a number of workers were investigating the hemorrhagic sweet clover disease in cattle. Although first thought to be of infectious origin, it was soon recognized to result from the ingestion of spoiled sweet clover. The agent in spoiled sweet clover responsible for the hemorrhagic tendency was identified[146, 325] as 3,3'-methylene-bis (4'-hydroxycoumarin), and its effect on the prothrombin time test demonstrated. This entire story is reviewed in excellent fashion by Link.[180]

A number of "coumarin drugs" have now been synthesized and are used in the prevention of thrombosis. The structural relationship between the coumarin drugs and synthetic vitamin K is striking, and it has been suggested that these anticoagulants may compete with vitamin K and substitute for it in reactions ordinarily leading to the formation of "prothrombin." They act as indirect anticoagulants. They do not alter clotting in vitro but will impair coagulation in vivo by depressing the plasma levels of the vitamin K-dependent coagulation Factors II, VII, IX, and X. The coagulation factors disappear at different rates, depending on the half-life of each one. Factor VII has the shortest half-life and disappears first, followed by IX, X, and finally II. A circulating anticoagulant protein has been noted in patients with vitamin K deficiency. It is believed to be an analogue of Factor X.[134]

A recent report has suggested that the coumarin drugs may act on an enzyme regulating the metabolism of vitamin K rather than at a binding site for the vitamin.[25]

Two groups of blood relatives have been reported in whom hereditary resistance to oral anticoagulant drugs has been documented. All were extremely sensitive to very small amounts of exogenous vitamin K. The abnormality is transmitted by a simple dominant effect on an autosomal chromosome.[250] The findings in these patients thus differ from those in the warfarin-resistant rats, which have been found to have 20 times the normal vitamin K requirement, suggesting a lowered binding capacity for both vitamin K and warfarin.[136]

Despite much study, the precise manner in which these drugs affect the synthesis or cellular release of these factors remains unknown.[21, 92, 189, 190, 249, 274, 328]

Coumarin and indanedione derivatives are different chemical compounds which are closely related in structure and action and may be considered together.[148] These compounds are generally completely absorbed from the gastrointestinal tract though in some individuals absorption is erratic. Peak plasma levels occur in from 2 to 13 hours and remain for variable periods. The duration of effect is related to persistence of the drug in the plasma but varies widely among various subjects.[252] The response to these drugs is apt to be more pronounced in elderly or febrile patients. Anything which interferes with the availability of vitamin K, such as poor nutrition, malabsorption syndrome, oral antibiotics which alter normal bacterial flora, and biliary or liver disease will increase susceptibility to these drugs. The administration of salicylate, phenyl-butazone, and oxyphenylbutazone may potentiate the effect of these anticoagulants. (Fig. 10–10).[302, 328, 344]

Increased resistance to the drugs has been noted following administration of barbiturates.[92]

The dosage schedule for these compounds must be developed for each patient. The figures given in Table 10–1 are intended only as general guide lines.

Control of therapy. In view of the variable effect of these drugs on hemostasis in different individuals, they cannot safely be used without access to a reliable laboratory in which their effect may be measured. The most widely used test to control anticoagulant therapy with the coumarin-indanedione derivatives is the Quick one-stage prothrombin time test. *PT*

The results of the test may be reported in a variety of ways, most of which relate the prothrombin time of the patient to that of a control plasma. The optimal range lies between one and a half and two and a half times normal, depending on the source of thromboplastin used.

The prothrombin and proconvertin (P and P) test and the thrombotest have also been used to control anticoagulant therapy with bishydroxycoumarin and indanedione drugs with good results.

Complications. The most serious side effect is hemorrhage. Microscopic hematuria, epistaxis, or bleeding from the gums or rectum occurs in approximately 5 per cent of patients on short-term treatment. As many of these patients

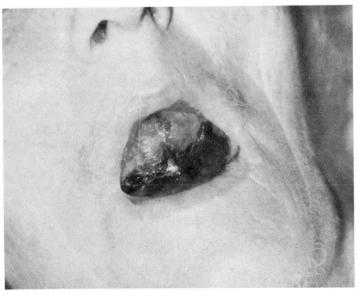

Figure 10–10. Large area of hemorrhage beneath the tongue of a patient who took salicylates for several days while on long-term anticoagulant therapy with coumarin compound.

Table 10–1. *Dosage Schedules for Coumarin and Indanedione Drugs*

Class	Generic Name	Initial	Daily Mainte-nance	Onset of Activity After Initial Dose	Return to Normal After Last Dose
			DOSE (mg.)*	RESPONSE (hrs.)	
Coumarin	Bishydroxycoumarin	First day 300 Second day 200	25–100	48–96	48–96
	Ethyl biscoumacetate	First day 900–1500 Second day 300–900	100–500	24–36	24–48
	Warfarin	First day 40–60 Second day 0–15	5–10	30–48	72–110
Indanedione	Phenindione	First day 200 Second day 100	25–100	24–48	48–72

*It is important to note that the doses given here represent a general approximation and that actual dosage required by an individual patient may vary widely in either direction from the figures given.

are not carried on long-term treatment, the incidence of hemorrhage is lower in the latter group. A rare complication is the occurrence of a sequence of petechiae, ecchymoses, and hemorrhagic infarcts in random sites usually between the third and sixth day. These lesions are believed to be due to a toxic reaction of the vascular system at the junction of the precapillary arteriole and capillary.[238] Of interest is the occasional patient who will have significant gastrointestinal or genitourinary hemorrhage while in the "therapeutic range," focusing attention on the possible presence of otherwise unsuspected disease in these areas. These drugs pass the placental barrier and also appear in the milk. As infants may already be deficient in those factors affected by these drugs, their use is contraindicated in pregnancy or lactation.

 Toxic reactions. Toxic reactions other than bleeding may occur but are quite rare. Nausea, vomiting, diarrhea, leukopenia, and thrombocytopenia, as well as hepatic and renal damage and leukemoid reactions, have been reported to be somewhat more common with the indanedione drugs than with those of the coumarin group.[11]

 Antidotes. Vitamin K administered intravenously, subcutaneously, intramuscularly, or orally, depending on the urgency, will reverse the effects of the coumarin-indanedione drugs. The most active preparation is aqua mephyton, 50 mg. I.V. or per os, which produces an effect in 6 hours, although the full effect is not apparent for 24 hours. Whole blood or plasma transfusion is used in addition to vitamin K if immediate correction is needed. The concentrate of vitamin K-dependent factors (factors II, VII, IX, and X) is effective, but its use is limited to those situations in which control can not be effected by the above measures, since it is derived from pooled plasma and may transmit hepatitis. The factors involved are relatively stable and ordinary bank blood or plasma will be effective. It should be noted that once vitamin K is given, the patient may be resistant to further anticoagulant therapy for a few days.

Examination of the Patient with Hemorrhagic Diathesis

The most accurate clinical diagnosis in the case of hemorrhagic diathesis is reached when a specific defect is demonstrated and its cause determined. To attain this goal, special laboratory techniques are often required in the course of the diagnostic examination which begins when the patient consults his physician because of abnormal bleeding. As with any diagnostic problem, however, the physician notes the character of the symptoms and signs, then proceeds in an orderly manner to a consideration of the various disorders known to produce such complaints. With constant review of the evidence collected during the course of his examination, the physician is able to exclude certain disorders while pursuing others with increased interest. Final identification of the cause of the complaint allows institution of rational therapy.

HISTORY

It is sometimes difficult to establish whether a particular patient has a hemorrhagic diathesis or not. The answer may be obvious if the patient presents with purpura or hemarthroses, but may be elusive when a patient with a history of "easy bruising" is to be evaluated prior to elective surgery. The presence of a hemorrhagic diathesis is best demonstrated by the history, as results of laboratory tests are often variable during the course of these disorders. A history of abnormal bleeding is far more significant than a battery of negative laboratory tests.

The history obtained from a patient suspected of having a bleeding diathesis should begin with a detailed review of the events of his birth and early childhood. Many disorders of hemostasis are familial and manifested soon after delivery. Specific inquiry should be made as to the occurrence of excessive bleeding from the umbilical cord or following circumcision. Prolonged bleeding or excessive bruising in the wake of minor trauma should be regarded with suspicion. Tonsillectomy and adenoidectomy are challenges to which many children are subjected and to which a child with a hemorrhagic diathesis may respond abnormally. Occasional epistaxis is not unusual in childhood but repeated or severe epistaxis is cause for concern. Loss of the first teeth during childhood is often accompanied by slight bleeding but persistent bleeding is evidence in favor of a hemorrhagic diathesis.

On reaching adult life, the hemostatic defenses of the patient continue to be challenged. The female patient may note excessive menstrual bleeding. Pregnancy and subsequent delivery further test hemostasis. In the event that excessive bleeding occurs with delivery or menstruation, efforts should be made to determine whether some obstetric or endocrine condition rather than a defect in hemostasis could be responsible for the bleeding. Minor cuts and scratches sustained in the kitchen or garden constantly test the efficiency of hemostasis. Operative procedures constitute important diagnostic trials of hemostasis and the result of each should be recorded. The oozing of blood from the gums after brushing the teeth occurs occasionally in normal persons but is of significance if severe or persistent. Men are daily exposed to minor razor nicks and will remember excessive bleeding because of the inconvenience it causes. It is clear that the most important tests of hemostasis are those afforded by the stress of day to day life about the home or while at work. The results of these tests are available to the physician for the asking.

A careful history of drug ingestion must be obtained. The importance of the anticoagulants is obvious but other drugs may also interfere with coagulation. Salicylates, phenylbutazone, and oxyphenylbutazone may potentiate anticoagulants, and salicylates alone can cause gastrointestinal hemorrhage; barbiturates may increase resistance to anticoagulants by induction of microsomal enzyme activity; Persantin and salicylates interfere with platelet aggregation and should be noted.

The family history is of paramount importance in determining if the defect is congenital or acquired. It is essential to discover whether any members of the patient's family are known to be "bleeders." If it appears likely that others do have a hemorrhagic diathesis, the physician should then examine as many members of the family as are available. This is important not only to the patient at hand but for purposes of counseling members of the family group. Such studies will allow the physician the opportunity of contributing to the general understanding of the genetic mechanisms involved.

The onset of abnormal bleeding at birth or during infancy is strong evidence that the disorder was genetically transmitted and a negative family history does not rule out the possibility. Some disorders of coagulation are transmitted by genes that are autosomal recessive, and the patient must be homozygous for the abnormal gene in order that its presence be clinically apparent. The child in question may be the first member of the family homozygous for the abnormal gene or may represent a mutation. The patient may be assumed to have an acquired hemorrhagic diathesis if he has reached adult life before the onset of abnormal bleeding and has a negative family history.

PHYSICAL EXAMINATION

Once it is established that the patient has a defect in hemostasis, it is important to determine what phase of hemostasis is defective and, if the hemorrhagic diathesis is of the acquired type, the nature of the underlying disease. The physical examination with particular reference to the characteristics of the abnormal bleeding will usually provide helpful information.

A disorder of the vascular phase of hemostasis is suggested by the finding of petechiae, ecchymoses, and superficial bruising. Characteristically these lesions are found in the skin of the extremities and over pressure points. The most common sites are the lower legs and ankles, but the forearms, wrists, and buttocks are frequently involved. Petechiae may also be seen in the mucous membranes of the mouth and on ophthalmoscopic examination of the retina. The ecchymotic lesions of senile purpura are located over the dorsum of the hands and feet where there is but scant subcutaneous tissue to provide support for the vessels. The occurrence of purpuric lesions only in the skin of the hands, feet, and ears suggests the presence of a cold precipitable protein or cold agglutinin, as these areas are most subject to exposure to the elements. Petechial hemorrhages widely scattered over the trunk as well as the extremities may be the result of a rickettsial, bacterial, or viral infection. A clue as to the etiology of the purpura may be found in the associated dermatologic lesions. The Schön-lein-Henoch syndrome is characteristically associated with a variety of skin lesions and erythema, edema, and necrosis of the skin have all been noted. The presence of eczema, hives, or wheals may indicate that an allergy is the inciting cause of the purpura; the finding of purplish-red infiltrations of the skin associated with petechiae and ecchymoses might point to a leukemic process.

A disorder of blood coagulation is suspected in the presence of joint hemorrhage, large hematomas, and post-traumatic hemorrhage. The joint into which bleeding has occurred is painful and swollen and the presence of fluid is usually demonstrable. Later there may be ankylosis and residual bone destruction. All joints should be carefully examined for evidence of prior hemorrhage. Hematomas may develop at any site but occur most frequently in those parts of the body exposed to trauma. Truly spontaneous hemorrhage is very rare but the amount of trauma necessary to produce hemorrhage may be slight indeed. It has been reported, for example, that hemorrhage into a vocal cord may occur while a patient is singing. Common locations of deep hematomas are the tongue, neck, buttocks, and extremities. The persistence of bleeding following operative or accidental trauma or its recurrence should alert the physician to the possibility of a bleeding dyscrasia.

Other details of the physical examination are also important. Ophthalmo-scopic examination of the retina may reveal retinopathy compatible with the presence of leukemia, thrombocytopenia, anemia, or polycythemia. Of these, only the lesions of leukemia are specific. The perivascular sheathing of the retinal veins seen in this disorder is thought to represent collections of leuko-cytes. Subhyaloid, flame-shaped, or punctate hemorrhages may be seen in patients with severe anemia or thrombocytopenia. Distention of the veins and a diffuse plethora of the retina are often present in polycythemia. The presence of hemorrhagic lesions with pale centers is suggestive of endocarditis, though similar lesions may occur in anemia and in tuberculosis.

The gums of patients with leukemia may be swollen and oozing blood. Ulcerations of the buccal mucosa and posterior pharynx are also commonly associated with this disease. The mouth is also a frequent site of the lesions of hereditary hemorrhagic telangiectasia.

LABORATORY EXAMINATION

Following completion of the clinical examination of the patient, the physician must turn to the laboratory for further information as to the nature of any defect in hemostasis which he has uncovered. It is important that he understand just what information laboratory tests do and do not afford. The tests which are used to identify defects in hemostasis are empiric. The reagents used in the performance of the tests are not pure and the reactions involved are largely unknown. Their usefulness is directly related to the experience of the technical staff who must perform the tests and the ability of the physician to interpret them.

The technical staff must be familiar with the range of normal results in their own laboratory. Results considered to be within the normal range in one laboratory may not be so considered in another. The constant use of normal controls is essential if meaningful results are to be obtained. The physician should become thoroughly familiar with the laboratory tests available to him. He should know something of the nature and purity of the reagents used, the technique of performing the tests, and the calculations used to derive the results recorded in the chart. He will then be able to interpret correctly the results of these empiric procedures and so obtain much useful information.

The platelet count, bleeding time, tourniquet test, and estimation of retraction all measure the adequacy of the vascular phase of hemostasis. The *platelet count* is quantitative and affords information as to the number of circulating platelets.[58] The factor used in calculating the result of the indirect count is from 2500 to 5000 and that used in the direct count from 1000 to 1500. A variation of 10 platelets counted by either method may result in a difference of 10,000 to 50,000 platelets per cubic millimeter being recorded in the chart. A careful examination of the peripheral blood smear often affords as much information as the quantitative enumeration of the platelets.

The *bleeding time* is designed to test the response of small vessels to injury.[91] It is immediately apparent that variations in the thickness of the skin and the distribution of the vessels combine to prevent uniformity of the test from patient to patient or indeed in the same patient from day to day. It is likely that the Ivy method of obtaining the average bleeding time of three uniform punctures of the skin of the inner surface of the forearm has some advantage over that obtained from the more commonly used single ear lobe puncture. Again it should be pointed out that the reliability of this test is directly related to the experience of the person doing it. False positive as well as false negative results may be obtained.

The *tourniquet test* is perhaps less reliable than either the platelet count or the bleeding time. Designed to test the response of the small vessels to stress, its reproducibility is depressingly rare. Minor variations from normal are unreliable and major variations can in many instances be predicted in advance. When it seems obvious that the tourniquet test will be positive, the performance of the test with the attendant discomfort to the patient is perhaps unwise.

Both the speed and completeness of *clot retraction* have been correlated with the quantity and quality of the platelets in the blood. In addition to reflecting alterations in platelet number and function, clot retraction is affected by the red blood cell volume. Clot retraction is also influenced by certain disease states, among which are multiple myeloma, pneumonia, and jaundice.[4, 194]

The *one stage prothrombin time* test is used to reveal deficiencies of those factors essential to the conversion of prothrombin to thrombin in the presence of *tissue* thromboplastin activity. The factors which influence the results of the test are Factor V, Factor X, Factor VII, and prothrombin. Since the end point of the test is the formation of a fibrin clot, a deficiency of fibrinogen will also be revealed. This test, despite its lack of specificity, is of great clinical importance.[266]

The *coagulation time* is another non-specific test which measures the overall effectiveness of blood coagulation.[175] It is a rather insensitive test and moderate abnormalities of the first stage of blood coagulation may go undetected. It is most accurately performed by the Lee and White four tube method. Care should be taken that an admixture of tissue juices with the blood does not occur during venipuncture.

The *partial thromboplastin time* is an excellent test which has proved valuable in the detection of deficiencies in the intrinsic system. It is simpler to perform and less time consuming than the thromboplastin generation test, and it has had widespread acceptance. The crucial aspect of this test is the use of a "partial" thromboplastin rather than a "complete" thromboplastin, as is used in the one stage prothrombin time test. The partial thromboplastin will not react with Factor VII of the extrinsic system but does allow activation of the intrinsic system, and clinically important clotting deficiencies of Factors XII, XI, IX, VIII, X, V, as well as II and I can generally be excluded if the results are normal. Defects in Factor VII, Factor XIII, and platelets will not be detected.

The test is sometimes difficult to interpret since mild deficiencies may not be detected. Usually deficiencies will be detected if the levels are below 35 per cent, but occasionally a patient with a deficiency at the 20 per cent level will have test results in the upper range of normal. Rarely, apparently normal individuals with no detectable clotting abnormality may have values slightly above the normal range.[26]

A number of methods have been developed for estimation of the products of proteolytic digestion of fibrinogen and fibrin.[64, 104, 107, 222, 260, 335] One of the most sensitive is the hemagglutination inhibition immunoassay. Serially diluted serum is incubated with antifibrinogenic rabbit serum. The quantity of split products present in the serum determines the residual antibody, which can be measured using tanned fibrinogen-coated red cells. Normal serum is found to contain up to 6 μg/ml.; that of patients with defibrination syndromes have up to 200 μg/ml.[223]

The thromboplastin generation test. The thromboplastin generation test has proved to be one of the most important tests of blood coagulation.[33] It will reveal any deficiency of the coagulation factors essential to the development of thromboplastin activity in the intrinsic (blood) system. The test is based on the fact that potent thromboplastin activity develops during the incubation at 37° C of normal Al(OH)$_3$ adsorbed plasma (containing Factor VIII, Factor XI, Factor XII, and Factor V), normal serum (containing Factor X, Factor XI, Factor XII and Factor IX), platelets or a cephalin substitute, together in the presence of calcium ions. The rate of development of the thromboplastin activity is measured by removing a sample of the incubation mixture at 1 minute intervals and measuring the time required for it to produce coagulation of normal platelet-free citrated plasma. The rate of development of thromboplastin activity in incubation mixtures using normal components is then compared to the rates obtained when the patient's plasma, serum, or platelets are substituted serially for their normal counterparts in three additional incubation mixtures. Each of the three mixtures contains two normal components and one from the patient. Thus the defect may be localized in the serum, adsorbed plasma, or platelets.

If the development of thromboplastin activity is abnormal when the patient's serum is substituted for the normal serum in the incubation mixture, the defect could be considered to be any one of the factors found in normal serum (Factor X, Factor XI, Factor XII, or Factor IX). Both Factor XI and

Factor XII are also present in Al(OH)$_3$ adsorbed plasma and, as they would be contributed by the normal adsorbed plasma in the mixture, their absence in the patient's serum would not be revealed. Thus the defect must be considered to be either of Factor IX or Factor X. As Factor X is essential to the one stage prothrombin time test and Factor IX is not, they can be separated by this test.

Should the development of thromboplastin activity be decreased when the patient's Al(OH)$_3$ adsorbed plasma is substituted for normal adsorbed plasma in the incubation mixture, the defect would be considered due to a deficiency of one of the factors contained in normal adsorbed plasma (Factor VIII, Factor V, Factor XI, or Factor XII). A deficiency of Factor XI or Factor XII is ruled out as they would be contributed by the normal serum in the incubation mixture. The defect must then be one of Factor VIII or Factor V. Once again the one stage prothrombin time test serves to differentiate the two, as Factor V is essential for the normal evaluation of thrombin in the test and Factor VIII is not.

Factor XI and Factor XII are present both in normal serum and in Al(OH)$_3$ adsorbed plasma. Should the patient have a deficiency of either factor it will not be revealed if normal adsorbed plasma or normal serum is in the incubation mixture. However, when the patient's serum and Al(OH)$_3$ adsorbed plasma are used together in the incubation mixture in place of their normal counterparts, the thromboplastin generation will be abnormal.[272, 273] There remains the task of separating Factor XII deficiency from that of Factor XI. This can usually be done on clinical grounds as patients with Factor XII deficiency have no hemorrhagic diathesis. Furthermore, the addition of Factor XI deficient plasma or serum will correct the clotting defect of Factor XII deficiency and vice versa. This, however, requires the availability of abnormal serum or plasma.

Circulating anticoagulants may produce abnormal results in the thromboplastin generation test when either the patient's serum or adsorbed plasma is substituted in the incubation mixture. If the titer of circulating anticoagulant is sufficiently high, both the patient's serum and adsorbed plasma will produce abnormal results. As circulating anticoagulants are not adsorbed by inorganic precipitating agents, the use of 50 per cent normal and 50 per cent patient's adsorbed plasma and normal serum in the incubation mixture will also produce abnormal results. As the results of the thromboplastin generation test in the case of Factor V or Factor VIII deficiency would be corrected by such an addition of normal adsorbed plasma, this maneuver may be used to identify the presence of circulating anticoagulants.

Should the platelets of the patient be deficient in factors necessary for the development of thromboplastin activity, it will be apparent when appropriate dilutions of platelets from the patient and from a normal donor are compared under conditions of the test.

Prothrombin, Factor VII, fibrinogen, Factor V, and Factor X are all essential for the normal evolution of thrombin from prothrombin in the presence of *tissue* thromboplastin activity. A deficiency of any of these factors results in a prolonged one stage prothrombin time. If a patient has a prolonged one stage prothrombin time and results of the thromboplastin generation test are normal, Factor V deficiency and Factor X deficiency are removed from consideration. A thrombin titer will determine whether a fibrinogen deficiency is responsible for the abnormal results of the test. To separate Factor VII deficiency from prothrombin deficiency a modification of the thromboplastin generation test may be employed. The patient's plasma is used as a substrate to test the thromboplastin activity of a normal incubation mixture. It has been shown that the substrate clotting time in the presence of normal intrinsic thromboplastin activity depends on the concentration in the substrate of prothrombin and fibrinogen. A normal clotting time precludes a prothrombin deficiency.[144, 270]

Fibrinogen concentration. The thrombin time and fibrinogen titer are used to estimate the concentration of fibrinogen in a patient's plasma. The thrombin used is that which is commercially available. It is made up according to the manufacturer's instructions and should be adjusted so that 0.1 ml. of thrombin will give a clotting time of 10 to 12 seconds when added to 0.25 ml. normal plasma. Platelet-free citrated plasma from the patient and a normal control are prepared by centrifuging citrated whole blood at 2000 rpm. for 15 minutes. Serial dilutions of both normal and patient's plasma are made and the highest dilution which contains a visible clot after addition of 0.1 ml. of thrombin is determined. Normal plasma should still contain a clot when diluted $1/64$ or $1/128$. The thrombin time is the thrombin clotting time of the $1/2$ dilution of patient's plasma compared to that of a normal. The objection to using whole blood for these determinations is that it is difficult to see the clot. This test also has the advantage over those which estimate the quantity of fibrinogen biochemically in that what is tested is reactive fibrinogen while the biochemical assay may include inert fibrinogen or other protein.[311]

Acquired hypofibrinogenemia often presents as an obstetrical or surgical emergency and the equipment necessary to perform the simple tests required for the diagnosis should be convenient to the operating theater and the delivery rooms. Failure of shed blood to form a firm clot should immediately alert the attending physician to this emergency. As acquired hypofibrinogenemia may be associated with Factor V and Factor VIII deficits as well, treatment must remedy these defects as well as replace the fibrinogen.

Choice of laboratory tests. These laboratory tests are sufficient to obtain the information needed to identify the particular defect responsible for disordered hemostasis in the vast majority of patients. There are many excellent laboratory procedures available which might serve to augment or extend the results obtained by those presented, but space does not permit their inclusion. For details of other methods the reader is referred to texts devoted entirely to the subject of blood coagulation.[38, 143, 268, 330]

The physician must determine which of these tests is necessary on the basis of his clinical findings. If the clinical examination gives no clue as to which phase of hemostasis is at fault, the platelet count, bleeding time, tourniquet test, partial thromboplastin time, and one stage prothrombin time should be obtained. This group of tests affords information concerning both phases of hemostasis, and if the results of each are normal it is unlikely that the patient has a disorder of hemostasis. The thromboplastin generation test will be needed to detect a mild abnormality of the first stage of coagulation.

Should the results of the clinical examination suggest a disorder of the vascular phase of hemostasis, the platelet count, tourniquet test, bleeding time, measurement of clot retraction, partial thromboplastin time, and one stage prothrombin time should be obtained. The partial thromboplastin time and one stage prothrombin time should be within normal limits if only the vascular phase of coagulation is abnormal. The tourniquet test should be positive and the bleeding time prolonged. The platelet count may be depressed and clot retraction may be poor or not occur at all. If the bleeding time alone is abnormal, a thromboplastin generation test should be obtained to be sure that no deficiency exists in the first stage of coagulation. If the platelet count is quantitatively normal but there is a prolonged bleeding time and poor clot retraction, special biochemical studies of the platelets may be necessary to identify the defect.[123] The platelet may also be at fault when, despite a strong history of abnormal hemostasis, all of the tests of coagulation are normal. Comparative dilution of the patient's platelets and platelets from a normal donor in the thromboplastin generation test may reveal a defect in platelet Factor III.

If the physician feels that the biochemical phase of hemostasis is at fault, the platelet count, bleeding time, one stage prothrombin time, and thromboplastin generation test should be obtained. The platelet count and bleeding time should be normal. If the one stage prothrombin time is prolonged and

Table 10-2. *Tests of Hemostasis*

Phase / Stage	NAME	SCREENING TESTS							SOME ADDITIONAL TESTS						
									THROMBOPLASTIN GENERATION				MODIFIED THROMBO-PLASTIN		
		PLATELET COUNT	BLEEDING TIME	CLOT RETRACTION	ONE STAGE PRO-THROMBIN	PTT	TOURNIQUET TEST	CLOTTING TIME	Serum	Plasma	Platelets	Serum and Plasma	MODIFIED THROMBOPLASTIN GENERATION TEST	FIBRINOGEN ASSAY	CLOT SOLUBILITY
Vascular Phase of Hemostasis	Thrombocytopenic Purpura	A	A	A	N	N	A	N	N	N	N	N	N	N	N
	Non-thrombocytopenic Purpura	N	A	N	N	N	A	N	N	N	N	N	N	N	N
	Hereditary Hemorrhagic Telangiectasia	N	N	N	N	N	N	N	N	N	N	N	N	N	N
First Stage of Clotting	Factor VIII Deficiency	N	N	N	N	A	N	N/A	N	A	N	A	N	N	N
	Factor IX Deficiency	N	N	N	N	A	N	N/A	A	N	N	A	N	N	N
	Factor XI Deficiency	N	N	N	N	A	N	N/A	N	N	N	A	N	N	N
	Factor XII Deficiency	N	N	N	N	A	N	A	N	N	N	A	N	N	N
	Circulating Anticoagulants	N	N	N	N/A	N/A	N	N/A	N/A	N/A	N	N/A	N/A	N	N
First and Second Stage of Clotting	Factor X Deficiency	N	N	N	A	A	N	N/A	A	N	N	A	N	N	N
	Factor V Deficiency	N	N	N	A	A	N	N/A	N	A	N	A	N	N	N
First or Second Stage of Clotting	Prothrombin Deficiency	N	N	N	A	A	N	N/A	N	N	N	N	A	N	N
	Factor VII Deficiency	N	N/A	N	A	N	N	N	N	N	N	N	N	N	N
Third Stage of Clotting	Congenital Afibrinogenemia	N	N	A	A	A	N	A	N	N	N	N	A	A	N
	Acquired Hypofibrinogenemia	N/A	N/A	A	A	A	N	A	N/A	N	N	N/A	A	A	N
	Factor XIII Deficiency	N	N	N	N	N	N	N	N	N	N	N	N	N	A
Vascular and Biochemical Phase of Hemostasis	von Willebrand's Disease	N	A	N	N	N/A	N	N	N	A	N	A	N	N	N

N = Normal.   A = Abnormal.   N/A = Inconstant.

the thromboplastin generation test reveals no deficiency of Factor V or Factor X, it must be determined if diminished prothrombin, fibrinogen, or Factor VII is responsible. A thrombin time and fibrinogen titer will establish the adequacy of fibrinogen concentration and a modification of the thromboplastin generation test will separate Factor VII and prothrombin.

Table 10–2 notes the results of various laboratory tests in disorders of hemostasis.

References

1. Abildgaard, U.: Inhibition of the thrombin-fibrinogen reaction by antithrombin III studied by N-terminal analysis. Scand. J. Clin. Lab. Invest., *20*:207, 1967.
2. Abildgaard, U.: Inhibition of the thrombin-fibrinogen reaction by α_2-macroglobulin studied by N-terminal analysis. Thromb. et Diath. Haemorrh., *21*:173, 1969.
3. Ablondi, F. B., Hagan, J. J., Philips, M., and DeRenzo, E. C.: Inhibition of plasmin, trypsin and streptokinase activated fibrinolytic system by epsilon aminocaproic acid. Arch. Biochem. & Biophys., *82*:153, 1959.
4. Ackroyd, J. F.: A simple method of estimating clot retraction with a survey of normal values and the changes that occur with menstruation. Clin. Sc., 7:231, 1949.
5. Ackroyd, J. F.: Function of Factor VII. Brit. J. Haem., *2*:397, 1956.
6. Adelson, E., Rheingold, J. J., Parker, O., Steiner, M., and Kirby, J. C.: The survival of factor VIII (antihemophilic globulin) and factor IX (plasma thromboplastin component) in normal humans. J. Clin. Invest., *42*:1040, 1963.
7. Aggeler, P. M., Spaet, T. H., and Emery, B. E.: Purification of plasma thromboplastin factor B (plasma thromboplastin component) and its identification as a beta globulin. Science, *119*:806, 1954.
8. Aggeler, P. M., White, S. G., Glendening, M. B., Pope, E. W., Leake, T. B., and Bates, G. B.: Plasma thromboplastin component (PTC) deficiency: a new disease resembling hemophilia. Proc. Soc. Exper. Biol. & Med., *79*:692, 1952.
9. Alami, S. Y., Hampton, J. W., Race, G. J., and Speer, R. J.: Fibrin stabilizing factor (factor XIII). Am. J. Med., *44*:1, 1968.
10. Albrecht, M.: Studies on the evolution of thrombocytes, experiences with megakaryocytes in vitro. Internat. Soc. Hem. Abstract 437, 1956, p. 346.
11. Alexander, B.: Anticoagulant therapy with coumarin congeners. Am. J. Med., *33*:679, 1962.
12. Alexander, B., Meyers, L., Kenny, J., Goldstein, R., Gurewich, V., and Grinspoon, L.: Blood coagulation in pregnancy. Proconvertin and prothrombin and the hypercoagulable state. New England J. Med., *254*:358, 1956.
13. Alkjaersig, N.: The antifibrinolytic activity of platelets. *In* Blood Platelets. Henry Ford Hospital Symposium. Little, Brown & Co., Boston, 1961.
14. Alkjaersig, N., Fletcher, A. P., and Sherry, S.: The activation of human plasminogen II. A kinetic study of activation with trypsin, urokinase and streptokinase. J. Biol. Chem., *233*:86, 1958.
15. Alkjaersig, N., Fletcher, A. P., and Sherry, S.: The mechanism of clot dissolution by plasmin. J. Clin. Invest., *38*:1086, 1959.
16. Alkjaersig, N., Fletcher, A. P., and Sherry, S.: Pathogenesis of the coagulation defect developing during pathological plasma proteolytic ("fibrinolytic") states. II. The significance, mechanism and consequences of defective fibrin polymerization. J. Clin. Invest., *41*:917, 1962.
17. "Anticoagulant drugs" (editorial). Brit. Med. J., *1*:365, 1969.
18. Arthus, M., and Pagés, C.: Nouvelle théorie chimique de la coagulation du sang. Arch. physiol. norm. et path., *2*:739, 1890.
19. Bang, N. U., Fletcher, A. P., Alkjaersig, N., and Sherry, S.: Pathogenesis of the coagulation defect developing during pathological plasma proteolytic ("fibrinolytic") states. III. Demonstration of abnormal clot structure by electron microscopy. J. Clin. Invest., *41*:935, 1962.
20. Bangham, A. D.: A correlation between surface charge and coagulant action of phospholipids. Nature, *192*:1197, 1961.
21. Barnhart, M. I., Anderson, R. F., and Bernstein, M. H.: Liver ultrastructure after coumadin and vitamin K. Fed. Proc., *23*:520, 1964.

22. Barton, P. G., Jackson, C. M., and Hanahan, D. J.: Relationship between factor V and activated factor X in the generation of prothrombinase. Nature, 214:923, 1967.

23. Barton, P. G., Yin, E. T., and Wessler, S.: Reactions of activated factor X-phosphatide mixtures in vitro and in vivo. J. Lipid Res., 11:87, 1970.

24. Bedson, S. P., and Johnston, M. E.: Further observations on platelet genesis. J. Path. & Bact., 28:101, 1925.

25. Bell, R. G., and Matschinger, J. T.: A possible mechanism for the action of warfarin. Fed. Proc., 29:381, 1970.

26. Bennington, J. L., Fonty, R. A., and Hougie, C.: Laboratory Diagnosis. The Macmillan Company, New York, 1970, pp. 669–670.

27. Bergsagel, D. E.: Viscous metamorphosis of platelets. Brit. J. Haem., 2:130, 1956.

28. Bergsagel, D. E., and Hougie, C.: Intermediate stages in the formation of blood thromboplastin. Brit. J. Haem., 2:113, 1956.

29. Bernik, M. B., and Kwaan, H. C.: Origin of fibrinolytic activity in cultures of the human kidney. J. Lab. Clin. Med., 70:650, 1967.

30. Bernik, M. B., and Kwaan, H. C.: Plasminogen activator activity in cultures from human tissues. An immunological and histochemical study. J. Clin. Invest., 48:1740, 1969.

31. Bettleheim, F. R.: The clotting of fibrinogen. II. Fractionation of peptide material liberated. Biochem. et Biophys. Acta, 19:121, 1956.

32. Bezkorvaing, A., and Rafelson, M. E., Jr.: Characterization of some proteins from normal human platelets. J. Lab. Clin. Med., 64:212, 1964.

33. Biggs, R., and Douglas, A. S.: The thromboplastin generation test. J. Clin. Path., 6:23, 1953.

34. Biggs, R., Douglas, A. S., and Macfarlane, R. G.: The action of thromboplastic substances. J. Physiol., 122:554, 1953.

35. Biggs, R., Douglas, A. S., and Macfarlane, R. G.: The formation of thromboplastin in human blood, J. Physiol., 119:89, 1953.

36. Biggs, R., Douglas, A. S., and Macfarlane, R. G.: The initial stages of blood coagulation. J. Physiol., 122:538, 1953.

37. Biggs, R., Douglas, A. S., Macfarlane, R. G., Dacie, J. V., Pitney, W. R., Merskey, C., and O'Brien, J. R.: Christmas disease. Brit. Med. J., 2:1378, 1952.

38. Biggs, R., and Macfarlane, R. G.: Human Blood Coagulation. 2nd Ed. Charles C Thomas, Springfield, Ill., 1957.

39. Biggs, R., Macfarlane, R. G., Denson, K. W. E., and Ash, B. J.: Thrombin and the interaction of factors VIII and IX. Brit. J. Haem., 11:276, 1965.

40. Blakely, A. A.: A rapid bedside method for the control of heparin. Canad. Med. Assoc., 99:1072, 1968.

41. Blix, S.: Anticoagulant treatment of the defibrination syndrome. Acta Med. Scand., 181:597, 1967.

42. Blomback, M., and Blomback, B.: Fractions rich in factor VIII. Biblio. Haematol., 29(part 4):1116, 1969.

43. Blomstrand, R., Nakayama, F., and Nilsson, I. M.: Identification of phospholipids in human thrombocytes and erythrocytes. J. Lab. & Clin. Med., 59:771, 1962.

44. Bolton, C. H., Hampton, J. R., and Mitchell, J. R. A.: Effect of oral contraceptive agents on platelets and plasma phospholipids. Lancet, 1:1336, 1968.

45. Booyse, F. M., Hoveke, T. P., and Rafelson, M. E., Jr.: Studies on human platelets. II. Protein synthetic activity of various platelet populations. Biochem. et Biophy. Acta, 157:660, 1968.

46. Booyse, F. M., and Rafelson, M. E., Jr.: Studies on human platelets. I. Synthesis of platelet protein in a cell free system. Biochem. et Biophy. Acta, 145:188, 1967.

47. Borchgrevink, C. F.: Platelet adhesion in vivo in patients with bleeding disorders. Acta Med. Scand., 170:231, 1961.

48. Bordet, D. J., and Delange, L.: La coagulation du sang et la genèse de la thrombine. Ann. Inst. Pasteur, 9:42, 1912.

49. Born, G. V. R.: Strong inhibition by 2-chloroadenosine of the aggregation of blood platelets by adenosine diphosphate. Nature, 202:95, 1964.

50. Born, G. V. R., and Cross, M. J.: Effect of adenosine diphosphate on concentration of platelets in circulating blood. Nature, 197:974, 1963.

51. Born, G. V. R., Haslam, R. J., Goldman, M., and Lowe, R. D.: Comparative effectiveness of adenosine analogues as inhibitors of blood-platelet aggregation and as vasodilators in man. Nature, 205:678, 1965.

52. Born, G. V. R., Honour, A. J., and Mitchell, J. R. A.: Inhibition by adenosine and by 2-chloroadenosine of the formation and embolization of platelet thrombi. Nature, 202:761, 1964.

53. Botti, R. E., and Ratnoff, O. D.: Studies on the pathogenesis of thrombosis: an experimental "hyper-coagulable" state induced by the intravenous injection of ellagic acid. J. Lab. Clin. Med., 64:385, 1964.

54. Bowie, E. J., Thompson, J. H., Jr., Didisheim, P., and Owen, C. A., Jr.: Disappearance rates

of coagulation factors: transfusion studies in factor-deficient patients. Transfusion, 7:174, 1967.

55. Brafield, A. J., Madras, M. B., and Case, J.: The stability of Christmas factor. A guide to the management of Christmas disease. Lancet, 2:867, 1956.

56. Brakman, P., Mohler, E. R., Jr., and Astrup, T.: A group of patients with impaired plasma fibrinolytic system and selective inhibition of tissue activator-induced fibrinolysis. Scand. J. Hemat., 3:389, 1966.

57. Bray, B. A., and Laki, K.: Glycopeptides from fibrinogen and fibrin. Biochemistry, 7:3119, 1968.

58. Brecher, G., and Cronkite, E. P.: Morphology and enumeration of human blood platelets. J. Appl. Physiol., 3:365, 1950.

59. Brinkhous, K. M., Read, M. S., and Mason, R. G.: Plasma thrombocyte-agglutinating activity and fibrinogen. Synergism with adenosine diphosphate. Lab. Invest., 14:335, 1965.

60. Buchanan, A.: On the coagulation of the blood and other fibriniferous liquids. J. Physiol., 2:158, 1879–1880.

61. Buluk, K., Januszko, T., and Olbromski, J.: Conversion of fibrin to desmofibrin. Nature, 191:1093, 1961.

62. Caen, J. P.: Is fibrinogen the plasma co-factor in ADP-induced human platelet aggregation? Nature, 205:1120, 1965.

63. Cash, J. D., and Woodfield, D. G.: Fibrinolytic response to moderate, exhaustive and prolonged exercise in normal subjects. Nature, 215:628, 1967.

64. Catt, K. J., Hirsh, J., Castelan, D. J., Niall, H. D., and Tregear, G. W.: Radioimmunoassay of fibrinogen and its proteolysis products. Thromb. et Diath. Haemorrh., 20:1, 1968.

65. Chandrasekhar, N., Osbahr, A., and Laki, K.: The mode of action of the Laki-Lorand factor in the clotting of fibrinogen. Biochem. & Biophys. Res. Commun., 15:182, 1964.

66. Chargaff, E., and Olson, K. B.: Studies on the chemistry of blood coagulation. VI. Studies on the action of heparin and other anticoagulants. J. Biol. Chem., 122:153, 1938.

67. Christensen, L. R.: Streptococcal fibrinolysis: A proteolytic reaction due to a serum enzyme activated by streptococcal fibrinolysin. J. Gen. Physiol., 28:363, 1944–1945.

68. Cohen, R. J., Epstein, S. E., Cohen, L. S., and Dennis, L. N.: Alterations of fibrinolysis and blood coagulation induced by exercise, and the role of beta-adrenergic-receptor stimulation. Lancet, 2:1264, 1968.

69. Collins, I. S.: The stability of coagulation factors in stored blood. Med. J. Australia, 2:718, 1955.

70. Conner, W. E.: The acceleration of thrombus formation by certain fatty acids. J. Clin. Invest., 41:1199, 1962.

71. Cox, F. M., Lanchantin, G. F., and Ware, A. G.: Chromatographic purification of human serum accelerator globulin. J. Clin. Invest., 35:106, 1956.

72. Crane, M. M., and Sanford, H. H.: The effect of variations in total calcium concentration upon the coagulation time of blood. Am. J. Physiol., 118:703, 1937.

73. Cross, M. J.: Effect of fibrinogen on the aggregation of platelets by adenosine diphosphate. Thromb. et Diath. Haemorrh., 12:524, 1964.

74. Daemen, F. J. M., van Arkel, C., Hart, H. C., van der Drift, C., and van Deenen, L. L. M.: Activity of synthetic phospholipids in blood coagulation. Thromb. et Diath. Haemorrh., 13:194, 1965.

75. Davey, M. G., and Lüscher, E. F.: Release reactions of human platelets induced by thrombin and other agents. Biochem. et Biophy. Acta, 165:490, 1968.

76. Davey, M. G., and Lüscher, E. F.: Platelet proteins. In Kowalski, E., and Niewiarowski, S. (Eds.): The Biochemistry of Blood Platelets. Academic Press, New York, 1967, p. 9.

77. Davis, H. L., and Davis, N. L.: Heparin and lipid metabolism. Lancet, 2:651, 1969.

78. Denson, K. W.: Electrophoretic studies of the Prower factor: A blood coagulation factor which differs from factor VII. Brit. J. Haem., 4:313, 1958.

79. DeRenzo, E. C., Boggiano, E., Barg, W. F., Jr., and Buck, F. F.: Interaction of streptokinase and human plasminogen. IV. Further gel electrophoretic studies on the combination of streptokinase with human plasminogen or human plasmin. J. Biol. Chem., 242:2428, 1967.

80. Deutsch, E., and Lechner, K.: Platelet clotting factors. In Kowalski, E., and Niewiarowski, S. (Eds.): The Biochemistry of Blood Platelets. Academic Press, New York, 1967, p. 23.

81. Deykin, D.: The role of the liver in serum-induced hypercoagulability. J. Clin. Invest., 45:256, 1966.

82. Deykin, D.: Current concepts: the use of heparin. New England J. Med., 280:937, 1969.

83. Deykin, D., Cochios, F., DeCamp, G., and Lopez, A.: Hepatic removal of activated factor X by the perfused rabbit liver. Am. J. Physiol., 214:414, 1968.

84. Donaldson, V. H., and Ratnoff, O. D.: Hageman factor: alterations in physical properties during activation. Science, 150:754, 1965.

85. Doolittle, R. F., Oncley, J. L., and Surgenor, D. M.: Species differences in the interaction of thrombin and fibrinogen. J. Biol. Chem., 237:3123, 1962.

86. Douglas, A. S.: Factor-V consumption during blood coagulation. Brit. J. Haem., 2:153, 1956.

87. Douglas, A. S.: The action of heparin in the prevention of prothrombin conversion. J. Clin. Invest., 35:533, 1956.

88. Douglas, A. S., and McNicol, G. P.: Thrombolytic therapy. Brit. M. Bull., 20:228, 1964.

89. Duckert, F., Flückiger, P., Matter, M., and Koller, F.: Clotting factor X. Physiologic and physiochemical properties. Proc. Soc. Exper. Biol. & Med., 90:17, 1955.

90. Duckert, F., and Streuli, F.: Role of coagulation in thrombosis. Thromb. et Diath. Haemorrh., Suppl. 21:185, 1966.

91. Duke, W. W.: The relation of blood platelets to hemorrhagic diseases. J.A.M.A., 55:1185, 1910.

92. Dulock, M. A., and Kolmen, S. N.: Influence of vitamin K on restoration of prothrombin complex proteins and fibrinogen in plasma of depleted dogs. Thromb. et Diath. Haemorrh., 20:136, 1968.

93. Eagle, H.: The role of prothrombin and of platelets in the formation of thrombin. J. Gen. Physiol., 18:531, 1934–1935.

94. Eagle, H.: The formation of fibrin from thrombin and fibrinogen. J. Gen. Physiol., 18:547, 1934–1935.

95. Egeberg, O.: Inherited antithrombin deficiency causing thrombophilia. Thromb. et Diath. Haemorrh., 13:516, 1965.

96. Eisen, V.: Fibrinolysis and formation of biologically active polypeptides. Brit. M. Bull., 20:205, 1964.

97. Elgee, N. T.: Medical aspects of oral contraceptives. Ann. Int. Med., 72:409, 1970.

98. Elkeles, R. S., Hampton, J. R., and Mitchell, J. R. A.: Effect of oestrogens on human platelet behavior. Lancet, 2:315, 1968.

99. Esnouf, M. P., and Tunnah, G. W.: The isolation and properties of the thrombin-like activity from Ancistrodon Rhodostoma venom. Brit. J. Haemat., 13:581, 1967.

100. Esnouf, M. P., and Williams, W. J.: The isolation and purification of a bovine-plasma protein which is a substrate for the coagulant fraction of Russell's-viper venom. Biochem. J., 84:62, 1962.

101. Estes, J. W.: Kinetics of the anticoagulant effect of heparin. J.A.M.A., 212:1492, 1970.

102. Evans, G., Packham, M. A., Nishizawa, E. E., Mustard, J. F., and Murphy, E. A.: Effect of acetylsalicylic acid on platelet function. J. Exper. Med., 128:877, 1968.

103. Ferguson, J. H., Ennis, E. G., Hitsumoto, S., and White, N. B.: Factor V and thrombin in the intrinsic clotting system. Thromb. et Diath. Haemorrh., 21:181, 1969.

104. Fisher, S., Fletcher, A. P., Alkjaersig, N., and Sherry, S.: Immunoelectrophoretic characterization of plasma fibrinogen derivatives in patients with pathological plasma proteolysis. J. Lab. Clin. Med., 70:903, 1967.

105. Fletcher, A. P., and Alkjaersig, N.: Plasma fibrinogen and hemostatic functions. Prog. Hemat., 5:246, 1966.

106. Fletcher, A. P., Biederman, O., Moore, D., Alkjaersig, N., and Sherry, S.: Abnormal plasminogen-plasmin system activity (fibrinolysis) in patients with hepatic cirrhosis: its cause and consequences. J. Clin. Invest., 43:681, 1964.

107. Fletcher, A. P., Alkjaersig, N., Fisher, S., and Sherry, S.: The proteolysis of fibrinogen by plasmin: the identification of thrombin clottable fibrinogen derivatives which polymerize abnormally. J. Lab. Clin. Med., 68:780, 1966.

108. Fletcher, A. P., Alkjaersig, N., and Sherry, S.: Fibrinolytic mechanisms and the development of thrombolytic therapy. Am. J. Med., 33:738, 1962.

109. Fletcher, A. P., Alkjaersig, N., and Sherry, S.: Pathogenesis of the coagulation defect developing during pathological plasma proteolytic ("fibrinolytic") states. I. The significance of fibrinogen proteolysis and circulating fibrinogen breakdown products. J. Clin. Invest., 41:896, 1962.

110. Gamgee, A.: Physiological Chemistry of the Animal Body. Vol. 1. Macmillan and Co., London, 1880.

111. Ganguly, P., and Moore, R.: Studies on human platelet proteins. Clin. Chim. Acta, 17:153, 1967.

112. Ganrot, P. O.: Electrophoretic separation of two thrombin inhibitors in plasma and serum. Scandinav. J. Clin. Lab. Invest., 24:11, 1969.

113. Ganrot, P. O., and Niléhn, J.-E.: Competition between plasmin and thrombin for α_2-macroglobulin. Clin. Chim. Acta, 17:511, 1967.

114. Gladner, J. A., Murtaugh, P. A., Folk, J. E., and Laki, K.: Nature of peptides released by thrombin. Ann. N.Y. Acad. Sc., 104:47, 1963.

115. Glynn, M. F., Movat, H. Z., Murphy, E. A., and Mustard, J. F.: Study of platelet adhesiveness and aggregation with latex particles. J. Lab. Clin. Med., 65:179, 1965.

116. Godal, H. C.: Delayed fibrin polymerization due to removal of calcium ions. Scand. J. Clin. Lab. Invest., *24*:29, 1969.
117. Graham, J. B., Barrow, E. M., and Hougie, C.: Stuart clotting defect. II. Genetic aspects of a "new" hemorrhagic state. J. Clin. Invest., *36*:497, 1957.
118. Graham, R. C., Ebert, R. H., Ratnoff, O. S., and Moses, J. M.: Pathogenesis of inflammation. II. In vivo observations of the inflammatory effects of activated Hageman factor and bradykinin. J. Exper. Med., *121*:807, 1965.
119. Grossi, C. E., Moreno, A. H., and Rousselot, L. M.: Studies on spontaneous fibrinolytic activity in patients with cirrhosis of the liver and its inhibition by epsilon amino caproic acid. Ann. Surg., *153*:383, 1961.
120. Haanen, C., Morselt, G., and Schoenmakers, J.: Contact activation of Hageman factor and the interaction of Hageman factor and plasma thromboplastin antecedent. Thromb. et. Diath. Haemorrh., *17*:307, 1967.
121. Hamberg, U.: The Fibrinolytic activation mechanism in human plasma. Proc. Roy. Society, Series B, Biol. Sci., *173*:293, 1969.
122. Hammarsten, O.: Über das Fibrinogen. Pflügers Arch. ges. Physiol., *19*:563, 1879.
123. Hardisty, R. M., Dormandy, K. M., and Hutton, R. A.: Thrombasthenia. Study of three cases. Brit. J. Haem., *10*:371, 1964.
124. Hardisty, R. M., and Pinniger, J. L.: Congenital afibrinogenaemia: Further observations on the blood coagulation mechanism. Brit. J. Haem., *2*:139, 1956.
125. Harker, L. A.: Megakaryocyte quantitation. J. Clin. Invest., *47*:452, 1968.
126. Harker, L. A.: Kinetics of thrombopoiesis. J. Clin. Invest., *47*:458, 1968.
127. Hart, H. C.: The biological half-life of I^{131}—fibrinogen. Thromb. et Diath. Haemorrh., Suppl., *17*:121, 1965.
128. Haslam, R. J.: Role of adenosine diphosphate in the aggregation of human blood platelets by thrombin and by fatty acids. Nature, *202*:765, 1964.
129. Hathaway, W. E., Belhasen, L. P., and Hathaway, H. S.: Evidence for a new plasma thromboplastin factor. I. Case report coagulation studies and physiochemical properties. Blood, *26*:521, 1965.
130. Hawkey, C.: Activation product and the fibrinolytic system. Nature, *197*:162, 1963.
131. Hayem, G.: Sur la formation de la fibrin du sang, études au microscope. Compt. rend. Acad. Sci., *86*:58, 1878.
132. Hellum, A. J.: The adhesiveness of human platelets in vitro. Scand. J. Clin. Lab. Invest., *12*: Suppl. 51, 1, 1960.
133. Hemker, H. C., Esnouf, M. P., Hemker, P. W., Swart, A. C. W., and Macfarlane, R. G.: Formation of prothrombin converting activity. Nature, *215*:248, 1967.
134. Hemker, H. C., and Muller, A. D.: Kinetic aspects of the interaction of blood-clotting enzymes. VI. Localization of the site of blood coagulation inhibition by the protein induced by vitamin K absence (PIVKA). Thromb. et Diath. Haemorrh., *20*:78, 1968.
135. Henderson, E. S., and Rapaport, S. I.: The thrombotic activity of activation product. J. Clin. Invest., *41*:235, 1962.
136. Hermodson, M. A., Suttie, J. W., and Link, K. P.: Warfarin metabolism and vitamin K requirement in the warfarin-resistant rat. Am. J. Phys. Med., *217*:1316, 1969.
137. Hiraki, K.: The function of the megakaryocyte: Observations both in idiopathic thrombocytopenic purpura and normal adults. Internat. Soc. Hem. Abstract 436, p. 345, 1956.
138. Hogenauer, E., Lechner, K., and Deutsch, E.: Isolation and characterization of blood clotting factors VII and X. Thromb. et Diath. Haemorrh., *19*:304, 1968.
139. Holmsen, H.: Adenine nucleotide metabolism in platelets and plasma. In Kowalski, E., and Niewiarowski, S. (Eds.): Biochemistry of Blood Platelets. Academic Press, New York, 1967, p. 81.
140. Holmsen, H., and Day, H. T.: Thrombin-induced platelet release reaction and platelet lysosomes. Nature, *219*:760, 1968.
141. Honour, A. J., and Mitchell, J. R. A.: Platelet clumping in injured vessels. Brit. J. Exper. Path., *45*:75, 1964.
142. Horowitz, H. I., and Papayoanou, M. F.: Release of nonsedimentable platelet factor 3 during coagulation. J. Lab. Clin. Med., *169*:1003, 1967.
143. Hougie, C.: Fundamentals of Blood Coagulation in Clinical Medicine. McGraw-Hill, New York, 1963.
144. Hougie, C., Barrow, E. M., and Graham, J. B.: Stuart clotting defect. I. Segregation of an hereditary hemorrhagic state from the heterogeneous group heretofore called "stable factor" (SPCA, proconvertin, Factor VII) deficiency. J. Clin. Invest., *36*:485, 1957.
145. Howell, W. H.: Theories of blood coagulation. Physiol. Rev., *15*:435, 1935.
146. Huebner, C. F., and Link, K. P.: Studies on the hemorrhagic sweet clover disease. VI. The synthesis of the δ-diketone derived from the hemorrhagic agent through alkaline degradation. J. Biol. Chem., *138*:529, 1941.

147. Hume, R., West, J. T., Malmgren, R. A., and Chu, E. A.: Quantitative observations of circulating megakaryocytes in the blood of patients with cancer. New England J. Med., *270*:111, 1964.

148. Hunter, R. B., and Shepherd, D. M.: Chemistry of coumarin anticoagulant drugs. Brit. M. Bull., *11*:56, 1955.

149. Iatridis, S. G., and Ferguson, J. H.: Effect of physical exercise on blood clotting and fibrinolysis. J. Appl. Physiol., *18*:337, 1963.

150. Inceman, S., Caen, J., and Bernard, J.: La "métamorphose visqueuse" des plaquettes de thrombasthénie de Glanzmann. Nouv. Rev. Franc. Hemat., *3*:575, 1963.

151. Ingram, G. I. C.: Anticoagulant therapy. Pharmacol. Rev., *13*:279, 1961.

152. Inman, W. H. W., and Vessey, M. P.: Investigation of deaths from pulmonary, coronary and cerebral thrombosis and embolism in women of child-bearing age. Brit. Med. J., *2*:193, 1968.

153. Ireland, D. M.: Effect of thrombin on the radioactive nucleotides of human washed platelets. Biochem. J., *103*:857, 1967.

154. Jorpes, J. E.: The origin and the physiology of heparin: The specific therapy in thrombosis. Ann. Int. Med., *27*:361, 1947.

155. Kass, L., Ratnoff, O. D., and Leon, M. A.: Studies on the purification of antihemophilic factor (factor VIII). J. Clin. Invest., *48*:351, 1969.

156. Kaufman, R. M., Airo, R., Pollack, S., Crosby, W. H., and Doberneck, R.: Origin of pulmonary megakaryocytes. Blood, *25*:767, 1965.

157. Kay, D., and Cuddigan, B. J.: The fine structure of fibrin. Brit. J. Haemat., *13*:341, 1967.

158. Kellaway, C. H.: Snake venoms. Bull. Johns Hopkins Hosp., *60*:1, 1937.

159. Kellermeyer, W. F., Jr., and Kellermeyer, R. W.: Hageman factor activation and kinin formation in human plasma induced by cellulose sulfate solutions. Proc. Soc. Exp. Biol. Med., *130*:1310, 1969.

160. Kerby, G. P., and Taylor, S. M.: The role of human platelets and plasma in the metabolism of adenosine diphosphate and monophosphate added in vitro. Thromb. et Diath. Haemorrh., *12*:510, 1964.

161. Kerr, J. W., Pirrie, R., MacAulay, I., and Bronte-Stewart, B.: Platelet-aggregation by phospholipids and free fatty acids. Lancet, *1*:1296, 1965.

162. Kiesselbach, T., and Wagner, R.: Fibrin stabilizing factor: a thrombin-labile platelet protein. Am. J. Phys. Med., *211*:1472, 1966.

163. Kingdon, H. S., and Davie, E. W.: Further studies on the activation of factor IX by activated factor XI. Thromb. et Diath. Haemorrh., Suppl., *17*:15, 1965.

164. Kjeldgaard, N. O., and Ploug, J.: Urokinase, an activator of plasminogen from human urine. II. Mechanism of plasminogen activation. Biochim. et biophys. Acta, *24*:283, 1957.

165. Koller, F., Loeliger, A., and Duckert, F.: Experiments on a new clotting factor (factor VII). Acta Haemat., *6*:1, 1951.

166. Kopéc, M., Budzynski, A. Z., Latallo, Z. S., Lipiński, B., Stachurska, J., Węgrzynowicz, Z., and Kowalski, G.: Interaction of platelet and fibrinogen degradation products in hemostasis. In Kowalski, E., and Niewiarowski, S. (Eds.): The Biochemistry of Blood Platelets. Academic Press, New York, 1967, p. 147.

167. Kowalski, E.: Fibrinogen derived inhibitors of blood coagulation. Thromb. et Diath. Haemorrh., Suppl., New blood clotting factors, *4*:211, 1960.

168. Kucinski, C. S., Fletcher, A. P., and Sherry, S.: Effect of urokinase antiserum on plasminogen activators: demonstration of immunologic dissimilarity between plasma plasminogen activator and urokinase. J. Clin. Invest., *47*:1238, 1968.

169. Kwaan, H. C., McFadzean, A. J. S., and Cook, J.: Plasma fibrinolytic activity in cirrhosis of the liver. Lancet, *1*:132, 1956.

170. Laki, K., Gladner, J. A., and Folk, J. E.: Some aspects of the fibrinogen fibrin transition. Nature, *187*:758, 1960.

171. Laki, K., Kominz, D. R., Symonds, P., Lorand, L., and Seegers, W. H.: The amino acid composition of bovine prothrombin. Arch. Biochem. & Biophys., *49*:276, 1954.

172. Lamy, F., and Waugh, D. F.: Certain physical properties of bovine prothrombin. J. Biol. Chem., *203*:489, 1953.

173. Latallo, Z. S., Fletcher, A. P., Alkjaersig, N., and Sherry, S.: Inhibition of fibrin polymerization by fibrinogen proteolysis products. Am. J. Physiol., *202*:681, 1962.

174. Laurell, C. B.: Synonyms for components influencing blood coagulation. Blood, *7*:555, 1952.

175. Lee, R. I., and White, P. D.: A clinical study of the coagulation time of blood. Am. J. M. Sc., *145*:495, 1913.

176. Lesuk, A., Terminiello, L., and Traver, J. H.: Crystalline human urokinase: some properties. Science, *147*:880, 1965.

177. Lewis, J. H., and Doyle, A. P.: Effects of epsilon aminocaproic acid on coagulation and fibrinolytic mechanisms. J.A.M.A., *188*:56, 1964.

178. Lewis, J. H., Ferguson, J. H., Spaugh, E., Fresh, J. W., and Zucker, M. B.: Acquired hypoprothrombinemia. Blood, *12*:84, 1957.
179. Lieberman, J. S., Borrero, J., Urdaneta, E., and Wright, I. S.: Thrombophlebitis and cancer. J.A.M.A., *177*:542, 1961.
180. Link, K. P.: The anticoagulant from spoiled sweet clover hay. Harvey Lect., *39*:162, 1944.
181. Loeliger, A., and Hers, J. F. P.: Chronic antithrombinemia (antithrombin V) with hemorrhagic diathiasis in a case of rheumatoid arthritis with hypergammaglobulinemia. Thromb. et Diath. Haemorrh., *1*:499, 1957.
182. Loewy, A. G., Dahlberg, J. E., Dorwart, W. V., Jr., Weber, M. J., and Eisele, J.: A transamidase mechanism for insoluble fibrin formation. Biochem. and Biophys. Research Comm., *15*:177, 1964.
183. Loewy, A. G., Dahlberg, A., Dunathan, K., Kriel, R., and Wolfinger, H. L., Jr.: Fibrinase. II. Some physical characteristics. J. Biol. Chem., *236*:2634, 1961.
184. Loewy, A. G., Veneziale, C., and Forman, M.: Purification of the factor involved in the formation of urea-insoluble fibrin. Biochim. et biophys. Acta, *26*:670, 1957.
185. Lorand, L.: Interaction of thrombin and fibrinogen. Physiol. Rev., *34*:742, 1954.
186. Lorand, L., Downey, J., Gotoh, T., Jacobsen, A., and Tokura, S.: The transpeptidase system which crosslinks fibrin by γ-glutamyl-ε-lysine bond. Biochem. Biophys. Res. Com., *31*:222, 1968.
187. Lorand, L., Urayama, T., Atencio, A. C., and Hsia, D. Y. Y.: Inheritance of deficiency of fibrin-stabilizing factor. Am. J. Hem. Genet., *22*:89, 1970.
188. Lorand, L., Urayama, T., deKiewiet, J. W. C., and Nossel, H. L.: Diagnostic and genetic studies on fibrin-stabilizing factor with a new assay based on amine incorporation. J. Clin. Invest., *48*:1054, 1969.
189. Lowenthal, J., and Birnbaum, H.: Vitamin K and coumarin anticoagulants: dependence of anticoagulant effect on inhibition of vitamin K transport. Science, *164*:181, 1969.
190. Lowenthal, J., and Macfarlane, J. A.: Nature of the antagonism between vitamin K and coumarin anticoagulants. Thromb. et Diath. Haemorrh., *19*:611, 1968.
190a. Lubran, M.: The effects of drugs on laboratory values. Med. Clin. N. Amer., *53*:211, 1969.
191. Lüscher, E. F.: Platelets in hemostasis and thrombosis. Brit. J. Haemat., *13*:1, 1967.
192. Lüscher, E. F.: Report of subcommittee on current concepts of hemostasis. Thromb. et Diath. Haemorrh., Suppl. 26:323, 1967.
193. Lyttleton, J. W.: The antithrombin activity of human plasma. Biochem. J., *58*:8, 1954.
194. Macfarlane, R. G.: A simple method for measuring clot retraction. Lancet, *1*:1199, 1939.
195. Macfarlane, R. G.: Blood coagulation with particular reference to the early stages. Physiol. Rev., *36*:479, 1956.
196. Macfarlane, R. G.: The coagulant action of Russell's viper venom; the use of antivenom in defining its reaction with a serum factor. Brit. J. Haem., *7*:496, 1961.
197. Macfarlane, R. G.: An enzyme cascade in the blood clotting mechanism, and its function as a biochemical amplifier. Nature, *202*:498, 1964.
198. Macfarlane, R. G., and Ash, B. J.: The activation and consumption of factor X in recalcified plasma. The effect of added factor VIII and Russell's viper venom. Brit. J. Haem., *10*:217, 1964.
199. Macfarlane, R. G., and Biggs, R.: Fibrinolysis: Its mechanism and significance. Blood, *3*:1167, 1948.
200. MacKay, A. C. P., Das, P. C., Myerscough, P. R., and Cash, J. D.: Fibrinolytic components of human uterine arterial and venous blood. J. Clin. Path., *20*:227, 1967.
201. Macmillan, D. C.: Secondary clumping effect in human citrated platelet rich plasma produced by adenosine diphosphate and adrenaline. Nature, *211*:140, 1966.
202. MacMillan, R. L., and Brown, K. W. G.: Heparin and thromboplastin. J. Lab. Clin. Med., *44*:378, 1954.
203. Majerus, P. W., Smith, M. B., and Clamon, G. H.: Lipid metabolism in human platelets. I. Evidence for complete fatty acid synthesizing protein. J. Clin. Invest., *48*:156, 1969.
204. Mann, R. D.: Effect of age, sex and diurnal variation on the human fibrinolytic system. J. Clin. Path., *20*:223, 1967.
205. Marcus, A. J.: Platelet function. N. England J. Med., *280*:1213, 1278, 1330, 1969.
206. Marcus, A. J., Zucker-Franklin, D., Safier, L. B., and Ullman, H. L.: Studies on human platelet granules and membranes. J. Clin. Invest., *45*:14, 1966.
207. Marder, V. J., and Shulman, N. R.: High molecular weight derivatives of human fibrinogen produced by plasmin. II. Mechanism of their anticoagulant activity. J. Biol. Chem., *244*: 2120, 1969.
208. Margolius, A., and Ratnoff, O. D.: Observations on the hereditary nature of Hageman trait. Blood, *11*:565, 1956.
209. Marr, J., Barboriak, J. J., and Johnson, S. A.: Relationship of appearance of adenosine diphos-

phate, fibrin formation and platelet aggregation in the haemostatic plug in vivo. Nature, *205*:259, 1965.

210. Maynert, E. W., and Isaac, L.: Uptake and binding of serotonin by platelet and its granules. Adv. Pharmacol., *6*:113, 1968.

211. McKay, D. G.: Disseminated intravascular coagulation: an intermediary mechanism of disease. Harper & Row, New York, 1965.

212. McKay, D. G.: Progress in disseminated intravascular coagulation. Calif. Med., *3*:186, 279, 1969.

213. McKay, D. G., Mansell, H., and Hertig, A.: Carcinoma of the body of the pancreas with fibrin thrombosis and fibrinogenopenia. Cancer, *6*:862, 1953.

214. McKay, D. G., and Müller-Bergnaus, E. G.: Therapeutic implication of disseminated intravascular coagulation. Am. J. Cardiol., *20*:392, 1967.

215. McLean, J. R., Maxwell, R. E., and Hertler, D.: Fibrinogen and adenosine diphosphate-induced aggregation of platelets. Nature, *202*:605, 1964.

216. McNicol, G. P.: Disordered fibrinolytic activity and its control. Scottish M. J., *7*:266, 1962.

217. McNicol, G. P.: The mechanism of fibrinolysis. Proc. Roy. Soc., Series B, Biol. Sci., *173*:285, 1969.

218. McNicol, G. P., and Douglas, A. S.: ϵ-Aminocaproic acid and other inhibitors of fibrinolysis. Brit. M. Bull., *20*:233, 1964.

219. McNicol, G. P., Fletcher, A. P., Alkjaersig, N., and Sherry, S.: Use of epsilon aminocaproic acid in management of postoperative hematuria. J. Urol., *86*:829, 1961.

220. Merskey, C.: Diagnosis and treatment of intravascular coagulation. Brit. J. Haemat., *15*:523, 1968.

221. Merskey, C., Johnson, A. J., Kleiner, G. J., and Wohl, H.: The defibrination syndrome: clinical features and laboratory diagnosis. Brit. J. Haem., *13*:528, 1967.

222. Mersky, C., Kleiner, G. J., and Johnson, A. J.: Quantitative estimation of split products of fibrinogen in human serum. Relation to diagnosis and treatment. Blood, *28*:1, 1966.

223. Mertins, B. F., McDuffie, F. C., Bowie, E. J. W., and Owen, C. A., Jr.: Rapid sensitive method for measuring fibrinogen split products in human serum. Mayo Clin. Proc., *44*:114, 1969.

224. Michael, S. E., and Tunnah, G. W.: The purification of factor VIII (antihaemophilic globulin). Brit. J. Haem., *9*:236, 1963.

225. Michal, F.: Blood platelets — platelet 5-HT receptors are of the classical D type. Nature, *221*:1253, 1969.

226. Milestone, J. H.: Thrombokinase as prime activator of prothrombin: historical perspectives and present status. Fed. Proc., *23*:742, 1964.

227. Miller, J. R., Baggenstoss, A. H., and Comfort, M. W.: Carcinoma of the pancreas: Effect of histological type and grade of malignancy on its behavior. Cancer, *4*:233, 1951.

228. Miller, K. D., Brown, R. K., Casillas, G., and Seegers, W. H.: The amino acid composition of thrombin preparations. Thromb. et Diath. Haemorrh., *3*:362, 1959.

229. Mitchell, J. R. A., and Sharp, A. A.: Platelet clumping in vitro. Brit. J. Haem., *10*:78, 1964.

230. Mitchell, J. S.: Metabolic effects of therapeutic doses of X and gamma radiations. Brit. J. Radiol., *16*:339, 1943.

231. Morawitz, P., Trans. by Hartmann, R. C., and Guenther, P. F.: The Chemistry of Blood Coagulation. Charles C Thomas, Springfield, Ill., 1958.

232. Murphy, E. A., and Mustard, J. F.: Coagulation tests and platelet economy in atherosclerotic and control subjects. Circulation, *25*:114, 1962.

233. Mustard, J. F., Murphy, E. A., Rowsell, H. C., and Downie, H. G.: Factors influencing thrombus formation in vivo. Am. J. Med., *33*:621, 1962.

234. Nachman, R. L.: Platelet proteins. Semin. Hemat., *5*:18, 1968.

235. Nachman, R. L.: Immunologic studies of platelet protein. Blood, *25*:703, 1965.

236. Nachman, R. L., Marcus, A. J., and Safier, L. B.: Platelet thrombosthenin, subcellular localization and function. J. Clin. Invest., *46*:1380, 1967.

237. Naeye, R. L.: Thrombotic disorders with increased levels of antiplasmin and antiplasminogen. New England J. Med., *265*:867, 1961.

238. Nalbardian, R. M., Mader, I. J., Barrett, J. L., Pearce, J. F., and Rupp, E. C.: Petechiae, ecchymoses, and necrosis of skin induced by coumarin congeners. J.A.M.A., *192*:107, 1965.

239. Nanninga, L. B., and Guest, M. M.: Preparation and properties of anticoagulant split product of fibrinogen and its determination in plasma. Thromb. et Diath. Haemorrh., *17*:440, 1967.

240. Nemerson, Y.: Phospholipid requirement of tissue factor in blood coagulation. J. Clin. Invest., *47*:72, 1968.

241. Niemetz, J.: Factors influencing the consumption of factor X (Stuart-Prower factor) during intrinsic coagulation. Thromb. et Diath. Haemorrh., *18*:332, 1967.

242. Niewiarowski, S., Farbiszewski, R., and Poplawski, A.: Studies on platelet factor 2 (PF_2-fibrinogen activating factor) and platelet factor 4 (PF_4-antiheparin factor). In: Kowalski,

E., and Niewiarowski, S. (Eds.): Biochemistry of Blood Platelets. Academic Press, New York, 1967, p. 35.

243. Nilsson, I. M., Anderson, L., and Bjorkman, S. E.: Epsilon-amino caproic acid (EACA) as a therapeutic agent based on 5 years clinical experience. Acta Med. Scand., Suppl. *448*:1, 1966.

244. Nilsson, I., Krook, H., Sternby, N.-H., Söderberg, E., and Söderström, N.: Severe thrombotic disease in a young man with bone marrow and skeletal changes and with a high content of an inhibitor in the fibrinolytic system. Acta med. scandinav., *169*:323, 1961.

245. Norman, P. S., and Hill, B. M.: Studies of the plasmin system. III. Physical properties of the two plasmin inhibitors in plasma. J. Exper. Med., *108*:639, 1958.

246. Nossel, H. L.: The activation and consumption of factor IX. Thromb. et Diath. Haemorrh., *12*:505, 1964.

247. Nossel, H. L., Drillings, M., and Hsieh, R.: Inhibition of Hageman factor activation. J. Clin. Invest., *47*:1172, 1968.

248. Nossel, H. L., Wilner, G. D., and LeRoy, E. C.: Blood polar groups important for initiating coagulation and aggregating platelets. Nature, *221*:75, 1969.

249. Olson, R. E., Li, L. F., Philipps, G., and Kipfer, R. K.: The mode of activation of vitamin K in stimulating prothrombin synthesis. Thromb. et Diath. Haemorrh., *19*:611, 1968.

250. O'Reilly, R. A.: The second reported kindred with hereditary resistance to oral anticoagulant drugs. New England J. Med., *282*:1448, 1970.

251. Osler, W.: On certain problems in the physiology of the blood corpuscles. Med. News, *48*:365, 393, 421, 1886. Abstract in Brit. Med. J., *1*:807, 861, 917, 1886.

252. Owen, C. A., and Bollman, J. L.: Prothrombin conversion factors of Dicumarol plasma. Proc. Soc. Exper. Biol. & Med., *67*:231, 1948.

253. Owren, P. A.: Proconvertin, the new clotting factor. Scandinav. J. Clin. & Lab. Invest., *3*:168, 1951.

254. Owren, P. A., Hellem, A. J., and Odegaard, A.: Linolenic acid for the prevention of thrombosis and myocardial infarction. Lancet, *2*:975, 1964.

255. Packham, M. A., Nishizawa, E. E., and Mustard, J. F.: Response of platelets to tissue injury. Biochem. Pharm., Suppl. *17*:171, 1968.

256. Pascuzzi, C. A., Spittel, J. A., Jr., Thompson, J. H., Jr., and Owen, C. A., Jr.: Thromboplastin generation accelerator. A newly recognized component of the blood coagulation mechanism present in excess in certain thrombotic states. J. Clin. Invest., *40*:1006, 1961.

257. Pechet, L., and Alexander, B.: Increased clotting factors in pregnancy. New England J. Med., *265*:1093, 1961.

258. Pechet, L., Cochios, F., and Deykin, D.: Further studies on the Dynia clotting abnormality. Thromb. et Diath. Haemorrh., *17*:365, 1967.

258a. Penick, G. D.: Blood States that Predispose to Thrombosis. *In* Thrombosis. Ed. by Sherry, S. et al. National Academy of Science, 1969, p. 553.

259. Penick, G. D., Dejanov, I. I., Reddick, R. L., and Roberts, H. R.: Predisposition to intravascular coagulation. Thromb. et Diath. Haemorrh., Suppl. *21*:543, 1966.

260. Perkins, H. A., and Rolfs, M. R.: Qantitative assay of fibrinogen and fibrinolytic activity. Blood, *22*:485, 1963.

261. Pilkington, T. R. E.: The effect of fatty acids and detergents on the calcium clotting time of human plasma. Clin. Sc., *16*:269, 1957.

261a. Pitney, W. R.: Heparin therapy and its laboratory control. Brit. J. Haemat., *18*:499, 1970.

262. Ploug, J., and Kjeldgaard, N. O.: Urokinase, an activator of plasminogen from human urine. I. Isolation and properties. Biochim. et biophys. Acta, *24*:278, 1957.

263. Poller, L., Tabiowo, A., and Thomson, J. M.: Effect of low-dose oral contraceptives on blood coagulation. Brit. Med. J., *3*:218, 1968.

264. Pool, J. G., Cohen, T., and Creger, W. P.: Biological half-life of transfused antihemophilic globulin (factor VIII) in normal man. Brit. J. Haem., *13*:822, 1967.

265. Prentice, C. R. M., and Ratnoff, O. D.: The action of Russell's viper venom on factor V and the prothrombin-converting principle. Brit. J. Haem., *16*:291, 1969.

266. Quick, A. J.: The prothrombin in hemophilia and in obstructive jaundice. J. Biol. Chem., *109*:73, 1935.

267. Quick, A. J.: The normal antithrombin of the blood and its relation to heparin. Am. J. Physiol., *123*:712, 1938.

268. Quick, A. J.: The Physiology and Pathology of Hemostasis. Lea & Febiger, Philadelphia, 1951.

269. Rabiner, S. F., Goldfine, I. D., Hart, A., Summaria, L., and Robbins, K. C.: Radioimmunoassay of human plasminogen and plasmin. J. Lab. Clin. Med., *74*:265, 1969.

270. Raccuglia, G., Duff, I. F., and Bethell, F. H.: The detection of defects of first stage of coagulation. J. Lab. & Clin. Med., *53*:789, 1959.

271. Raisys, V., Molner, J., and Winzler, R. J.: Study of carbohydrate release during the clotting of fibrinogen. Arch. Biochem., *113*:457, 1966.

272. Ramot, B., Angelopoulos, B., and Singer, K.: Plasma thromboplastin antecedent deficiency. Arch. Int. Med., 95:705, 1955.

273. Ramot, B., Singer, K., Heller, P., and Zimmerman, H. J.: Hageman factor (HF) deficiency. Blood, 11:745, 1956.

274. Ranhotra, G. S., and Johnson, B. C.: Vitamin K and the synthesis of factor VII by isolated rat liver cells. Proc. Soc. Exp. Biol., Med., 132:509, 1969.

275. Rapaport, S. I., Schippman, S., Patch, M. J., and Ames, S. B.: The importance of activation of anti-hemophilic globulin and proaccelerin by traces of thrombin in the generation of intrinsic prothrombinase activity. Blood, 21:22, 1963.

276. Ratnoff, O. D.: A familial trait characterized by deficiency of a clot-promoting fraction of plasma. J. Lab. & Clin. Med., 44:915, 1954.

277. Ratnoff, O. D.: Activation of Hageman factor by L-homocystine. Science, 162:1007, 1968.

278. Ratnoff, O. D., Botti, R. E., Crum, J. D., and Donaldson, V. H.: The activation of PTA (factor XI) and Hageman (factor XII). Thromb. et Diath. Haemorrh., 17:7, 1965.

279. Ratnoff, O. D., and Davie, E. W.: The activation of Christmas factor (factor IX) by activated plasma thromboplastin antecedent (activated factor XI). Biochemistry, 1:677, 1962.

280. Ratnoff, O. D., Davie, E. W., and Mallett, D. L.: Studies on the action of Hageman factor: evidence that activated Hageman factor in turn activates plasma thromboplastin antecedent. J. Clin. Invest., 40:803, 1961.

281. Ratnoff, O. D., Kass, L., and Lang, P. D.: Studies on the purification of antihemophilic factor VIII. J. Clin. Invest., 48:957, 1969.

282. Reid, H. A., and Chan, K. E.: The paradox in therapeutic defibrination. Lancet, 1:485, 1968.

283. Ridgway, H., and Speer, R. J.: The formation and "decay" of XIIa. Thromb. et Diath. Haemorrh., 18:259, 1967.

284. Robbins, K. C., Summaria, L., Hsieh, B., and Shah, R. J.: The peptide chains of human plasmin. J. Biol. Chem., 242:2333, 1967.

285. Robb-Smith, A. H. T.: Why the platelets were discovered. Brit. J. Haemat., 13:618, 1967.

286. Roberts, P. S., and Burkat, R. K.: Purification of human plasminogen. Thromb. et Diath. Haemorrh., 17:423, 1967.

287. Rosenthal, R. L.: Properties of plasma thromboplastin antecedent (PTA) in relation to blood coagulation. J. Lab. & Clin. Med., 45:123, 1955.

288. Rosenthal, R. L., Dreskin, O. H., and Rosenthal, N.: New hemophilia-like disease caused by deficiency of third plasma thromboplastin factor. Proc. Soc. Exper. Biol. & Med., 82:171, 1953.

289. Rozenberg, M. C., and Holmsen, H.: Adenosine nucleotide metabolism of blood platelets. IV. Platelet aggregation response to exogenous ATP and ADP. Biochim. Biophys. Acta, 157:280, 1968.

290. Rutty, D. A.: A mechanism to limit platelet aggregation in vivo. Nature, 206:1263, 1965.

291. Sack, E., Spaet, T. H., Gentile, R. L., and Hudson, P. B.: Reduction of postprostatectomy bleeding by epsilon-aminocaproic acid. New England J. Med., 266:541, 1962.

292. Salvidio, E.: Biochemical aspects of blood platelets. Acta haemat., 11:301, 1954.

293. Salzman, E. W.: Measurement of platelet adhesiveness. A simple in vitro technique demonstrating an abnormality in von Willebrand's disease. J. Lab. Clin. Med., 62:724, 1963.

294. Salzman, E. W., Chambers, D. A., and Neri, L. L.: Possible mechanism of aggregation of blood platelets by adenosine diphosphate. Nature, 210:167, 1966.

295. Salzman, E. W., Chambers, D. A., and Neri, L. L.: Incorporation of labelled nucleotides and aggregation of human blood platelets. Thromb. et Diath. Haemorrh., 15:52, 1966.

296. Salzman, E. W.: Measurement of platelet adhesiveness: progress report. Thromb. et Diath. Haemorrh., Suppl. 26:323, 1967.

297. Samih, Y. A., Hampton, J. W., Race, G. J., and Speer, R.: The relationship of plasma fibrinogen (factor I) level to fibrin stabilizing factor (factor XIII) activity. Blood, 31:93, 1968.

298. Sawyer, W. D., Fletcher, A. P., Alkjaersig, N., and Sherry, S.: Studies on the thrombolytic activity of human plasma. J. Clin. Invest., 39:426, 1960.

299. Schiffman, S., Rapaport, S. I., and Patch, M. J.: The identification and synthesis of activated plasma thromboplastin component (PTC). Blood, 22:733, 1963.

300. Schmidt, A.: Neue Untersuchungen über die Faserstoffgerinnung. Pflüegers Arch. ges. Physiol., 6:413, 1872.

301. Schrier, E. E., Broomfield, C. A., and Scheraga, H. A.: Molecular weight of bovine thrombin. Arch. Biochem. & Biophys. Suppl., 1:309, 1962.

302. Schulert, A. R., and Weiner, M.: The physiologic disposition of phenylindanedione in man. J. Pharmacol. & Exper. Therap., 110:451, 1954.

303. Schulman, S., Alkjaersig, N., and Sherry, S.: Physicochemical studies on human plasminogen (profibrinolysin) and plasmin (fibrinolysin). J. Biol. Chem., 233:91, 1958.

304. Seegers, W. H., Johnson, J. F., and Fell, C.: An antithrombin reaction related to prothrombin activation. Am. J. Physiol., 176:97, 1954.

305. Seegers, W. H., McClaughry, R. I., and Fahey, J. L.: Some properties of purified prothrombin and its activation with sodium citrate. Blood, 5:421, 1950.
306. Seegers, W. H., and McGinty, D. A.: Further purification of thrombin: Probable purity of products. J. Biol. Chem., 146:511, 1942.
307. Shamash, Y., and Rimon, A.: The plasmin inhibitors of human plasma. III. Purification and partial characterization. Biochim. Biophys. Acta, 121:35, 1966.
308. Sharp, A. A.: Pathological fibrinolysis. Brit. M. Bull., 20:240, 1964.
309. Sharp, A. A.: Present status of platelet aggregation. New England J. Med., 272:89, 1965.
310. Sharp, A. A.: The significance of fibrinolysis. Proc. Roy. Soc., Series B, Biol. Sci., 173:311, 1969.
311. Sharp, A. A., Howie, B., Biggs, R., and Methuen, D. T.: Defibrination syndrome in pregnancy. Value of various diagnostic tests. Lancet, 2:1309, 1958.
312. Sherry, S.: Fibrinolysis. Ann. Rev. Med., 19:247, 1968.
313. Sherry, S.: Urokinase, Ann. Int. Med., 69:415, 1968.
314. Sherry, S., Fletcher, A. P., and Alkjaersig, N.: Fibrinolysis and fibrinolytic activity in man. Physiol. Rev., 39:343, 1959.
315. Sherry, S., Troll, W., and Glueck, H.: Thrombin as a proteolytic enzyme. Physiol. Rev., 34:736, 1954.
316. Shulman, N. R.: Studies on the inhibition of proteolytic enzymes by serum. I. The mechanism of the inhibition of trypsin, plasmin and chymotrypsin by serum using fibrin tagged with I^{131} as a substrate. J. Exper. Med., 95:571, 1952.
317. Shulman, N. R.: Studies on the inhibition of proteolytic enzymes by serum. II. Demonstration that separate proteolytic inhibitors exist in serum; their distinctive properties and the specificity of their action. J. Exper. Med., 95:593, 1952.
318. Siegel, A., and Lüscher, E.: Non-identity of the α granules of human blood platelets with typical lysosomes. Nature, 215:745, 1967.
319. Silver, M. D., Stehbens, W. E., and Silver, M. M.: Platelet reaction to adenosine diphosphate in vivo. Nature, 205:91, 1965.
320. Sise, H. S., Moschos, C. B., and Becker, R.: On the nature of hypercoagulability. Am. J. Med., 33:667, 1962.
321. Spaet, T. H.: Vascular factors in the pathogenesis of hemorrhagic syndromes. Blood, 7:641, 1952.
322. Spaet, T. H., and Cintron, J.: Studies on platelet factor-3 availability. Brit. J. Haem., 11:269, 1965.
323. Spaet, T. H., and Lejnieks, I.: Studies on the mechanism whereby platelets are clumped by adenosine diphosphate. Thromb. et Diath. Haemorrh., 15:36, 1966.
324. Speer, R. J., Ridgway, H., and Hill, J. M.: Activated human Hageman factor (XII). Thromb. et Diath. Haemorrh., 14:1, 1965.
325. Stahmann, M. A., Huebner, C. F., and Link, K. P.: Studies on the hemorrhagic sweet clover disease. V. Identification and synthesis of the hemorrhagic agent. J. Biol. Chem., 138:513, 1941.
326. Straub, W., and Duckert, F.: The formation of extrinsic prothrombin activator. Thromb. et Diath. Haemorrh., 5:402, 1961.
327. Surgenor, D. M., et al.: Investigations of fibrinolysis and labeling changes in fibrinolysin products, J.A.M.A., 180:536, 1962.
328. Suttie, J. W.: Control of clotting factor biosynthesis by vitamin K. Fed. Proc., 28:1696, 1969.
329. Tocantins, L. M.: The mammalian blood platelets in health and disease. Medicine, 17:155, 1938.
330. Tocantins, L. M.: The Coagulation of Blood. Methods of Study. 1st Ed. Grune & Stratton, New York, 1955.
331. Todd, A. S.: The histological localisation of fibrinolysin activator. J. Path. & Bact., 78:281, 1959.
332. Todd, A. S.: Localisation of fibrinolytic activity in tissues. Brit. M. Bull., 20:210, 1964.
333. Tranzer, J. P., and Baumgartner, H. R.: Filling gaps in the vascular endothelium with blood platelets. Nature, 216:1126, 1967.
334. Triantaphyllopoulos, D. C.: Nature of thrombin-inhibiting effect of incubated fibrinogen. Am. J. Physiol., 197:575, 1959.
335. Triantaphyllopoulos, E., and Triantaphyllopoulos, D. C.: Fibrinogenolysis: the micromolecular derivatives. Brit. J. Haem., 15:337, 1968.
336. Truman, W. H. W., and Vessey, M. P.: Investigation of deaths from pulmonary, coronary and cerebral thrombosis and embolism in women of child-bearing age. Brit. Med. J., 2:193, 1968.
337. Veltkamp, J. J., Loeliger, E. A., and Hemker, H. C.: The biological half-time of Hageman factor. Thromb. et Diath. Haemorrh., 13:1, 1965.
338. Verstraete, M., Amery, A., and Vermylen, J.: Feasibility of adequate thrombolytic therapy

with streptokinase in peripheral arterial occlusions. I. Clinical and arteriographic results. Brit. M. J., *1*:1499, 1963.

339. Vessey, M. P., and Doll, R.: Investigation of the relation between use of oral contraceptives and thromboembolic disease. Brit. Med. J., *2*:199, 1968.

340. Wagner, R. H., Pate, D., and Brinkhous, K. M.: Further purification of antihemophilic factor (AHF) from dog plasma. Fed. Proc., *13*:445, 1954.

341. Warren, B. A.: Fibrinolytic activity of vascular endothelium. Brit. M. Bull., *20*:213, 1964.

342. Warren, R.: Postoperative thrombophilia. New England J. Med., *249*:99, 1953.

343. Warshaw, A. L., Laster, L., and Shulman, W. R.: The stimulation by thrombin of glucose oxidation in human platelets. J. Clin. Invest., *45*:1923, 1966.

344. Weiner, M., Shapiro, S., Axelrod, J., Cooper, J. R., and Brodie, B. B.: The physiological disposition of dicumarol in man. J. Pharmacol. & Exper. Therap., *99*:409, 1950.

345. Weiss, H. J., and Kochwa, S.: Molecular forms of antihaemophilic globulin in plasma, cryo-precipitate and after thrombin activation. Brit. J. Haem., *18*:89, 1970.

346. Wessler, S.: Thrombosis in the presence of vascular stasis. Am. J. Med., *33*:648, 1962.

347. Wessler, S., and Yin, E. T.: The experimental hypercoagulable state induced by factor X. A comparison of the non-activated and activated forms. J. Lab. Clin. Med., *72*:256, 1968.

348. White, J. G.: Five structure alterations induced in platelets by adenosine disphosphate. Blood, *31*:604, 1968.

349. White, J. G.: The substructure of human platelet microtubules. Blood, *32*:638, 1968.

350. White, J. G.: The dense bodies of human platelets: inherent electron opacity of the serotonin storage particles. Blood, *33*:598, 1969.

351. White, S. G., Aggeler, P. M., and Emery, B. E.: Plasma thromboplastin component (PTC) potency of plasma fractions. Proc. Soc. Exper. Biol. & Med., *83*:69, 1953.

352. Williams, W. J., and Esnouf, M. P.: The fractionation of Russell's-viper venom (vipera russellii) venom with special reference to the coagulant protein. Biochem. J., *84*:52, 1962.

353. Wilner, G. D., Nossel, H. L., and LeRoy, E. C.: Activation of Hageman factor by collagen. J. Clin. Invest., *47*:2608, 1968.

354. Wilner, G. D., Nossel, H. L., and LeRoy, E. C.: Aggregation of platelets by collagen. J. Clin. Invest., *47*:2616, 1968.

355. Wood, J. E.: Oral contraceptives, pregnancy and the veins. Circulation, *38*:627, 1968.

356. Wright, I. S.: Pathogenesis and treatment of thrombosis. Circulation, *5*:161, 1952.

357. Wright, J. H.: The histogenesis of the blood platelets. J. Morphol., *21*:263, 1910.

358. Yin, E. T., and Wessler, S.: Investigation of the apparent thrombogenicity of thrombin. Thromb. et Diath. Haemorrh., *20*:465, 1968.

359. Zieve, P. D., and Soloman, H. M.: Uptake of amino acids by the human platelet. Am. J. Phys., *214*:58, 1968.

360. Zucker-Franklin, D.: Microfibrils of blood platelets: their relationship to microtubules and the contractile protein. J. Clin. Invest., *48*:165, 1969.

361. Zucker-Franklin, D., Nachman, R., and Marcus, A. J.: Ultrastructure of thrombosthenin, the contractile protein of human blood platelets. Science, *157*:945, 1967.

362. Zucker, M. B., and Borrelli, J.: Platelet clumping produced by connective tissue suspensions and by collagen. Proc. Soc. Exper. Biol. & Med., *109*:779, 1962.

363. Zucker, S., Cathy, M. H., and Wylie, R. L.: Control of heparin therapy. Sensitivity of the activated partial thromboplastin time for monitoring the antithrombotic effects of heparin. J. Lab. Clin. Med., *73*:320, 1969.

XI / Disorders of Hemostasis

The various clinical syndromes which occur as the result of disordered hemostasis have been defined largely by application of a series of empiric laboratory tests.

Incomplete understanding of the biochemical reactions involved in these tests makes impossible a definitive classification of the disorders of hemostasis at this time. For purposes of discussion, they will be presented within the framework of the theory presented in Chapter X and grouped according to the results of the major laboratory tests in common use.

Classification

I. Vessel and/or platelet abnormalities
   A. Purpura
      1. Thrombocytopenic purpura
         a. Secondary
         b. Idiopathic
         c. Neonatal
         d. Thrombotic
      2. Non-thrombocytopenic purpura
         a. Allergic
         b. Infectious
         c. Other
   B. Hereditary telangiectasia
II. Abnormalities of blood coagulation
   A. Disorders affecting predominantly the first stage of blood coagulation and resulting in an abnormal thromboplastin generation test
      1. Factor XII deficiency (Hageman trait, Hageman deficiency)

    2. Factor VIII deficiency (antihemophilic factor deficiency, AHF deficiency)

    3. Factor IX deficiency (plasma thromboplastin component deficiency, PTC deficiency, Christmas disease)

    4. Factor XI deficiency (plasma thromboplastin antecedent deficiency, PTA deficiency)

    5. Circulating anticoagulants

B. Disorders affecting both the first and second stage of blood coagulation and resulting in an abnormality of both the thromboplastin generation test and the one stage prothrombin time

    1. Factor V deficiency

    2. Factor X deficiency (Stuart factor deficiency)

C. Disorders affecting predominantly the first or second stage of blood coagulation and resulting in an abnormal one stage prothrombin time with a normal thromboplastin generation test

    1. Factor VII deficiency

    2. Prothrombin deficiency (Factor II deficiency)

D. Disorders affecting the third stage of blood coagulation resulting in qualitative or quantitative changes in fibrinogen or fibrin

    1. Congenital afibrinogenemia (Factor I deficiency)

    2. Acquired hypofibrinogenemia

    3. Factor XIII deficiency (fibrin stabilizing factor deficiency)

III. Disorders affecting vessel and/or platelet function and blood coagulation

A. Von Willebrand's disease

B. Thrombasthenia, thrombocyopathy and thrombopathia

Vessel and/or Platelet Abnormalities

The Purpuras

The term purpura originated from the Greek work *porphyra*, which was the name of the mollusk from which a purple dye was obtained.[189] Prior to the eighteenth century, purpuric lesions were thought to occur only during the course of "fevers" such as plague or typhus. From that time, however, it has been recognized that purpura may occur in the absence of a febrile illness.

The conventional classification of the purpuras into those associated with thrombocytopenia and those with quantitatively normal platelets seems justified. The difference is striking. The significance of this difference is not at all clear, as will become apparent from the discussion.

Thrombocytopenic Purpura

The relationship between a decrease in the number of platelets in the peripheral blood and the occurrence of spontaneous bleeding is well known.

The level below which the platelets must fall before bleeding occurs varies from person to person. Bleeding is rare when the platelet count is above 50,000 per cu.mm., but it may not occur even when the platelets fall below this level. The life span of the platelet has been variously estimated at from 3 to 10 days. If a strict balance between production and destruction is to be maintained, 10 to 30 per cent of the circulating platelets must be replaced daily.

Thrombocytopenia, like anemia or fever, should be considered as a symptom of disease, not as a disease in itself. Every effort must be made to determine the cause.

PATHOLOGIC PHYSIOLOGY OF THROMBOCYTOPENIA

The physiologic function of the platelets has been extensively investigated and knowledge of their role in hemostasis continues to accumulate.[184, 191, 257, 304, 349, 368, 388, 392, 403] Platelets are known to participate in both the vascular and biochemical defense of hemostasis.[62, 63, 232] They mechanically plug rents in the wall of a vessel by their agglutination and thrombus formation. Evidence is growing that adenosine diphosphate (ADP) released from injured tissue or from the platelets themselves is the substance responsible for aggregation of platelets at the site of vessel injury.[26, 59, 130, 328, 420] The rate of removal or neutralization of ADP is likely to be important in the control of the extent of the thrombus.[168] Platelets are essential to the normal evolution of thromboplastin activity in the intrinsic or blood system, and in the final phase of coagulation they influence clot retraction by their interaction with fibrin. The capacity of the platelets to bring about clot retraction depends on their contractile protein which in turn is dependent on the presence of adenosine triphosphate as an energy source.[45, 152] They have also been demonstrated to contain a heparin-neutralizing factor.

It is apparent that a quantitative decrease in cells which play an important mechanical role in hemostasis and participate in at least two of the three major stages of blood coagulation would represent a serious hazard to the organism. It is not readily apparent, however, why relatively comparable degrees of thrombocytopenia are associated with such variability in clinical findings. It has been speculated that the plasma may contain a factor that is essential to the maintenance of vascular integrity and is complementary to the mechanical role of the platelet. The importance of such a factor in hemostasis would be enhanced if the platelets were diminished.[6]

The disturbed laboratory tests and clinical findings presented by patients with thrombocytopenic purpura may be ascribed to a defect in hemostasis resulting from a quantitative decrease in platelets in association with some as yet undefined change in the vascular endothelium.

CLINICAL EXAMINATION

Characteristically, the clinical manifestations of thrombocytopenic purpura from any cause develop over a period of several days or weeks, though the onset may on occasion be sudden, particularly in children. Bruising or prolonged bleeding from minor trauma, menorrhagia, or epistaxis may be noted before the appearance of petechiae which are the hallmark of the thrombocytopenic state. Petechiae vary in size from those too small to see with the unaided eye to approximately $\frac{1}{16}$ inch in diameter. They are the result of tiny extravasations of blood from the arteriolar end of the capillary loop in the skin or mucous membranes.[183] A coalescence of petechiae results in larger lesions of varied size which are referred to as ecchymoses.

Purpuric lesions may occur anywhere in the body. Those located in the mucous membranes are not as well supported as those in the skin, and free bleeding into the genitourinary tract or the gastrointestinal tract is common. The total amount of blood found in the urine or feces is more likely the result of multiple tiny hemorrhages than of a large hemorrhage from a single petechia. The occurrence of bleeding within the central nervous system presents the most serious threat. Once again it appears that the failure of the supporting tissues to contain the petechial hemorrhage allows its progression to serious proportions. The occurrence of bleeding in the optic fundus is not infrequent and may result in permanent impairment of vision.

The physical findings will vary, depending on the organ system involved and the magnitude of the blood loss.

LABORATORY EXAMINATION

Thrombocytopenia is the sine qua non of this condition. The degree of depression of the platelet count varies and is not always related to the severity of the clinical manifestations. If symptoms are present, however, the platelet count is usually below 40,000 to 50,000 per cu.mm. Anemia is not commonly noted in these patients. If present, the type and the degree of the anemia usually reflect the magnitude of the bleeding. The total and differential leukocyte counts are almost invariably normal in patients with idiopathic thrombocytopenic purpura; significant abnormalities occur in nearly all varieties of the secondary forms. The clotting time is normal. The bleeding time is prolonged, but may vary from day to day. The results of the test may return to normal during the course of the disease, though the platelet level remains depressed. Clot retraction is poor and, indeed, there may be no retraction of the clot after 24 hours. The degree of clot retraction is usually directly proportional to the number of platelets present. The tourniquet test is positive, but the performance of the test is usually unnecessary and unwarranted in the presence of thrombocytopenic purpura. Increased peripheral destruction of platelets may be detected by following their survival after tagging with Cr[51] or by measurement of plasma acid phosphatase value.[1, 274]

Examination of smears made from bone marrow aspirates may be valuable in establishing the diagnosis. The megakaryocytes in idiopathic thrombocytopenic purpura are often increased in number but immature. Many will contain but one, two, or four nuclei rather than the characteristic polyploid nucleus of the mature megakaryocyte (Fig. 11–1). The cytoplasm is reduced and contains few granules. Only rare platelets are seen forming at the edge of the cytoplasm. Similar findings are often present in thrombocytopenic purpura which occurs in certain susceptible persons on exposure to a particular drug, food, or chemical.

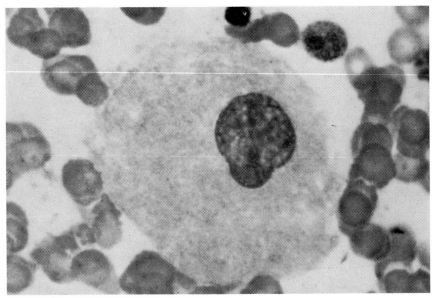

Figure 11–1. Megakaryocyte in bone marrow aspirate from a patient with idiopathic thrombocytopenic purpura. Note the immaturity of the nucleus, the reduction in cytoplasm, and the absence of platelets forming at the edge of the cytoplasm.

CLINICAL SYNDROMES

Four forms of thrombocytopenic purpura have been described: (1) secondary thrombocytopenic purpura; (2) idiopathic thrombocytopenic purpura; (3) neonatal thrombocytopenic purpura; and (4) thrombotic thrombocytopenic purpura.

As there is considerable variation in the etiology, course, prognosis, and treatment of these disorders, they will be discussed separately.

Secondary thrombocytopenic purpura. Secondary thrombocytopenic purpura bears a clear and identifiable relationship to some primary agent or disease. Some of the diseases and chemical and physical agents that may result in secondary thrombocytopenic purpura are listed in Table 11–1. Although thrombocytopenic purpura per se is a serious condition, the ultimate prognosis for any given patient depends largely on the underlying cause. Thrombocytopenic purpura following measles, threatening as it may be, does not carry so grave a prognosis as that associated with a malignancy.

Mechanisms. Thrombocytopenia is the end result of decreased production of platelets, increased destruction of platelets, or a combination of the two. The means through which this result is reached varies with the inciting cause.

A plasma factor required for normal platelet production has been described. Absence of this factor has been demonstrated to result in thrombocytopenia and thrombopoiesis is stimulated by infusions of normal plasma.[336, 337] The decrease in platelets which occurs as the result of the invasion of the bone marrow by tumor cells, granuloma, the reticuloendothelioses, lipidoses, and microorganisms is thought to be the result of (a) physical crowding of normal megakaryocytes, (b) competitive utilization of nutrient substrate by the invading cells, or

Table 11–1. *Causes of Secondary Thrombocytopenic Purpura*

1. Invasion of the marrow cavity with subsequent suppression or destruction of the normal marrow elements by:
   a. Malignant cells: carcinoma, sarcoma, leukemia, lymphoma
   b. Granuloma: sarcoid, tuberculosis
   c. Lipoidosis: Gaucher's disease, reticuloendotheliosis
   d. Microorganisms: bacteremia, viremia
2. Direct suppression of marrow elements by:
   a. Physical agents: roentgen rays, radioactive isotopes
   b. Chemical agents:
      (1) Universal susceptibility: urethan, alkylating agents (nitrogen mustard, busulfan, chlorambucil, TEM), benzol, antimetabolites (amethopterin, aminopterin, 6-MP)
      (2) Individual susceptibility:
         (a) Drugs: any from the group of analgesics, antipyretics, antibiotics, chemotherapy, antihistamines, hormones
         (b) Food
         (c) Insecticides: DDT
         (d) Dyes: organic
         (e) Other: any new agents to which the patient has been exposed must be suspected
3. Peripheral destruction of platelets by:
   a. Excessive demands from abnormal coagulation:
      (1) Widespread intravascular clotting
      (2) Burns
   b. Hypersplenism: enlarged spleen from any cause
   c. Hypothermia and heat stroke
   d. Hemangioendothelioma
   e. Blood transfusions:
      (1) Incompatible: immunologic incompatibility of platelets as well as red cells, trapping and stasis, intravascular coagulation
      (2) Compatible: after large numbers of transfusions; perhaps the result of immunologically incompatible platelets
   f. Viremia and bacteremia
   g. Collagen disorders

(c) production of metabolic end products by the invading cells which are toxic to the normal marrow elements. Thrombocytopenia that follows exposure to ionizing radiation and those chemicals which universally depress bone marrow function is believed due to the interference of those agents with cellular division, perhaps through inhibition of deoxyribonucleic acid synthesis.[100, 251] Vitamin B_{12}, folic acid, ascorbic acid, and severe iron deficiencies may result in thrombocytopenia. The possibility that the spleen may also produce a humoral factor which depresses megakaryocytic function has been considered.[164]

Increased destruction of platelets occurs when they are sequestered in hemiangioblastoma.[31, 142, 164] During hypothermia they are sequestered in the spleen, the liver, and possibly the intestinal tract and marrow; the sequestered platelets return to the circulation with rewarming.[397] Increased permeability of the capillaries during heat stroke is thought to be responsible for a decrease in the number of platelets.[419]

Several different platelet types have been demonstrated[164, 355] and thrombocytopenia may occur secondary to blood transfusions as the result of incompatibility of platelet types. Stasis due to sludging, or excessive utilization of platelets in those cases of incompatible transfusion accompanied by intravascular clotting, may result in thrombocytopenia.[164] The mechanism responsible for thrombocytopenia which may occur following massive transfusions is obscure;[206] dilution with platelet-poor bank blood and stimulation of an iso-antibody response by incompatible platelets may be factors. An enlarged spleen may trap large numbers of platelets. Normally the cardiovascular system contains approximately two-thirds of the platelets and one-third are in the spleen. Without any change in total numbers of platelets, a large spleen could harbor one-half of the platelets; a very large spleen might contain nine-tenths of the platelets. A large spleen may alter the peripheral platelet count without any deviation of total platelet mass, life span, or production.[27] An increased plasma volume and platelet dilution may be important.

Viremia and bacteremia are thought to cause agglutination and destruction of platelets in vivo.[164, 249] Megakaryocytes may appear inactive and diminished in number as well.[366] Thrombocytopenic purpura may be the presenting problem of patients with disseminated lupus erythematosus; the mechanism responsible is probably immunologic.[71]

The manner in which certain drugs, foods, or chemicals induce thrombocytopenia in susceptible individuals has been the subject of extensive investigations.[6, 22, 164, 370, 371] Thrombocytopenia in alcoholics has been attributed in the past to folic acid deficiency or hypersplenism, but there have been recent reports of thrombocytopenia in chronic alcoholics in the absence of cirrhosis, splenomegaly, or folic acid deficiency. The platelet counts returned to normal on withdrawal from alcohol. It has been suggested that alcohol acts directly on the megakaryocyte or platelet, as it affects erythropoiesis and leukopoiesis.[215, 294] Abnormal platelet aggregation also occurs in patients with cirrhosis of the liver.[387]

Whether increased destruction or decreased production is responsible for drug-induced thrombocytopenia has been for many years the subject of a lively debate. It is now known that immunologic factors can affect both the rate of destruction and production of platelets.[7, 8, 10] According to one concept a drug and platelet together act as a hapten and exhibit weakly antigenic properties. Antibodies may be formed which will destroy the platelets on the next exposure to that particular drug. The four factors necessary to demonstrate agglutination and lysis of platelets are: (1) platelets, (2) the drug, (3) serum from the drug sensitive patient, and (4) complement. Agglutination alone may occur without complement.[8] The factor responsible for the lysis of platelets is in the serum of the affected patient. Lysis and complement fixation may be demonstrated in vitro using serum from an affected patient, the drug, and his own or normal platelets, but will not occur if normal serum is used.

More recent evidence suggests that platelets, red cells, and leukocytes react with antibody because their membranes are capable of non-specific adsorption of certain drug-antibody complexes. According to this concept the complete antigen is not a cellular constituent but a non-cellular substance complexed with the drug. The antibody against the complete antigen is capable of reacting against the drug alone as well. The size, configuration, and charge on the antigen (drug)-antibody complex, rather than the characteristics of the antigen (drug) alone, determine the target cell with which it can react; the physical-chemical characteristics of the target cell determine its *accidental* participation in the reaction. The attachment of the antigen (drug)-antibody complex to the cell then leads to aggregation of the cells or complement fixation.[354] The site of destruction of the aggregated platelets appears to relate to the size of the aggregates; large aggregates are removed by the liver while smaller ones are trapped in the spleen.[28]

Whichever concept proves to be correct, the immunologic nature of the mechanism of this form of thrombocytopenia has been amply demonstrated,[8] and the sensitivity has been passively transferred.[44, 375] As the exhibition of minute amounts of the offending drug after recovery may cause severe thrombocytopenia to recur in these patients, it is best not to test the drug in vivo to confirm the suspicion of sensitivity.

Management.   It is clear in light of the foregoing discussion that a searching history must be obtained from any patient presenting with thrombocytopenia. Precipitating causes are legion. Exposure to any new drug, chemical, or foodstuff must be suspect and the possible association with recent infection should be kept in mind. Accidental as well as therapeutic exposure to ionizing radiation must be looked for in view of the widespread use of nuclear fission products in industry and medicine. A careful history and physical examination will often reveal the underlying disease.

Treatment of secondary thrombocytopenic purpura will depend in large measure on the nature of the underlying disorder. In addition to therapy directed at the precipitating cause, therapy to relieve the bleeding diathesis may be indicated and will be discussed under idiopathic thrombocytopenic purpura.

Idiopathic thrombocytopenic purpura.   The separation by Werlhof of the "morbus maculosus hemorrhagicus" from the infectious diseases in 1735 was the first recognition of this disorder as a distinct entity. It was not until 1883 that Krauss recognized that the platelets of these patients were deficient in number.[189] Kaznelson suggested the use of splenectomy in the treatment of these patients in 1916. As the term "idiopathic" indicates, knowledge of the etiology of this disorder is still incomplete and the diagnosis is made only after exclusion of the diagnosis of secondary thrombocytopenic purpura. Rare instances of hereditary and familial idiopathic thrombocytopenia have been reported.[55, 332, 340]

Incidence.   In a group of 50 patients with idiopathic thrombocytopenic purpura seen at the University of Virginia Hospital, one-half were under 20 years of age. Of the remaining 25 patients, 9 were past 50 and 3 were past 60 at the onset of their illness. Although other series[164, 165] indicate a similar preponderance in youth, the occurrence of the disease in so many patients beyond 50 years of age is unusual. There was no significant sex difference in our series, though idiopathic thrombocytopenic purpura has often been reported to be more common in females than in males.[164, 165]

Mechanism.   A great deal of effort has been made to elucidate the factors responsible for the development of idiopathic thrombocytopenic purpura. The finding that an altered immunologic response was the basis of some of the drug-induced secondary thrombocytopenic purpuras spurred efforts to demonstrate a similar mechanism in connection with the idiopathic variety.

The evidence indicates that an abnormal immunologic mechanism may be responsible for the low platelet count in many patients with this disorder.[163, 165, 166] The infusion of plasma from patients with this disorder will cause a transient thrombocytopenia in normal recipients. Infants born of mothers with idiopathic thrombocytopenic purpura may have neonatal thrombocytopenia. Normal platelets infused into patients with idiopathic thrombocytopenic purpura frequently have a short survival. The platelet-depressing factor in the serum of patients with idiopathic thrombocytopenic purpura has been found to affect autologous as well as homologous platelets, to be species specific, to be adsorbed by platelets, and to be present in the 7S immunoglobulin fraction of the plasma.[357] Despite such evidence for a humoral platelet-depressing factor, efforts to develop an in vitro test to demonstrate antiplatelet antibodies in the blood of these patients have been repeatedly frustrated.[95] The platelet-aggregating properties of serum from patients with idiopathic thrombocytopenic purpura, at first thought indicative of platelet antibodies,[165, 166, 370] appear now to be due to thrombin arising from the prothrombin remaining after coagulation of the thrombocytopenic blood.[187] The substrate for the action of thrombin is a clottable protein similar to or identical with fibrinogen which is adsorbed on the surface of the platelet.[333] The recently introduced new methods for the in vitro detection of platelet antibodies under conditions which rule out the possibility of thrombin or thrombin-generating agents being responsible appear promising. The antiplatelet factor measured by these techniques is an IgG immunoglobulin and was present in 85 per cent of patients with idiopathic thrombocytopenic purpura.[193]

It is not always possible to demonstrate increased platelet destruction; hence a decrease in the production of platelets may be responsible for thrombocytopenia in some instances,[296] although thrombopoietin activity is detectable.[85, 237] Sensitized platelets may be removed from the circulation by the spleen or the liver. The spleen has been demonstrated to be the major site for removal of platelets when they are lightly coated with antibodies, but when the disorder is more severe the liver also participates. The site of destruction therefore depends on the intensity of the immunologic process at any particular point in the course of the illness.[27, 29, 357] The spleen may also contribute to the production of platelet agglutinins and in some manner suppress megakaryocyte function in the bone marrow.[164]

Clinical examination. The disease may begin insidiously with an increased tendency to bruise followed in days or weeks by the appearance of petechiae on the skin or mucous membranes. In other patients, there may be a sudden onset with the appearance of petechiae and moderate to severe bleeding from the gastrointestinal or genitourinary tract. Neurologic defects or death may be the result if bleeding occurs in the central nervous system. The historical account of the illness and the results of the physical examination will depend largely on the site and extent of the bleeding.

Course and prognosis. The disease may pursue an unremitting and fulminant course to death in a few days or stop as suddenly as it began, within days or weeks of the onset. The designation of idiopathic thrombocytopenic purpura as being of the acute or chronic variety must be retrospective and is of little help in the handling of the new patient. The vast majority of patients with acute idiopathic thrombocytopenia have a complete and permanent recovery within 2 to 3 months. If they fail to recover within 6 months they are considered as having chronic idiopathic thrombocytopenic purpura. Death may result in either the acute or chronic type and recurrences may occur after many years of remission.

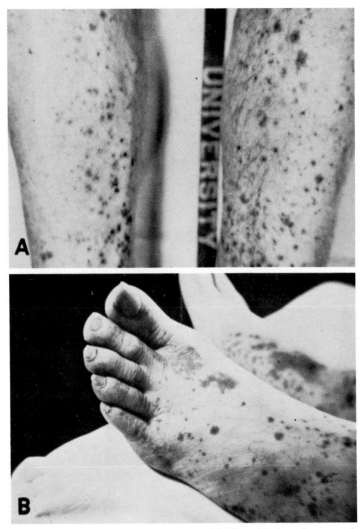

Figure 11-2.   Petechiae and ecchymoses in a patient with idiopathic thrombocytopenic purpura.

Treatment.   Evaluation of the various forms of treatment used in this disorder is made difficult by its unpredictable course.[88, 353, 367] The rationale for the use of adrenocortical steroids lies in the observation that they decrease antigen-antibody reactions and protect the vascular endothelium in some fashion as yet not understood.[205, 317] They also appear to inhibit the sequestration of sensitized platelets by the reticuloendothelial system of the spleen and liver.[357] This appears to be the most important mechanism concerned. Initially one of the adrenocortical steroids is administered in high doses and then gradually decreased as improvement occurs. A maintenance dose is continued for several weeks and the dose is gradually decreased under careful observation. Whole blood transfusions are withheld unless there is life-threatening hemorrhage. Platelet transfusions may be of value immediately prior to emergency splenectomy,[212, 258, 373] in retinal hemorrhage, and in suspected cerebral hemorrhage.

Platelet-rich plasma or platelet concentrates may be prepared from three to four units of freshly donated blood and should be administered within 6 hours of removal from donor to obtain maximal effect. Recent studies of the response of patients with malignancy have revealed that progressive resistance to repeated platelet transfusion is infrequently observed. Since the survival of transfused platelets is 1 to 3 days, the patients should be transfused repeatedly as needed; usually two to three times a week.[110, 211, 342, 371] Splenectomy is probably best reserved unless a life-threatening situation develops and bleeding cannot be controlled with adrenocortical steroids in adequate dosage. Recent reports, however, have emphasized the low percentage of sustained remission in patients treated with steroids as compared to those treated by splenectomy.[79, 83, 247, 266, 404, 414] The effect of splenectomy is to remove the major site of sequestration of lightly sensitized platelets. When it can be demonstrated that the spleen is the predominant site of platelet destruction, a rise in platelet count is to be expected after splenectomy and the long-term result is usually good. Splenic sequestration is found most commonly in children and in those who have responded to steroid therapy.[260] Failure of splenectomy occurs as the result of high titers of platelet-antibody with heavily coated platelets and more hepatic sequestration.[357] The high incidence of systemic lupus erythematosus following splenectomy in one series does not appear to be commonplace.[303]

In reviewing our experience it was apparent that failure of hormonal therapy did not prejudice the results of splenectomy nor did the failure to respond to splenectomy affect the future response to ACTH or adrenocortical steroids. Both ACTH and adrenocortical steroids produced similar results. When relapse occurred following cessation of hormonal therapy, remission was often obtained upon restarting therapy. Capillary fragility often diminished following institution of steroid therapy without a significant alteration of the platelet count. On the basis of these observations the following general plan of therapy seems indicated.

1. When first seen, these patients, whether "acute" or "chronic," are started on prednisone 60 to 80 mg. daily by mouth. Usually the dosage may be decreased over the next several days to 15 to 20 mg. daily. If there is no improvement in 1 or 2 weeks, it is unlikely to occur with further therapy.

It is pertinent to note that massive doses of steroids have been noted to produce a depression of the platelet count after an initial increase. As platelet survival is normal during the decline it has been assumed that the steroids suppress megakaryocyte activity.[86]

2. Splenectomy is employed in the event of failure to control bleeding with steroids after a reasonable period of trial.

3. Transfusions may be required to replace the blood lost. The use of platelet transfusions is limited because of the rapid destruction of platelets.

4. If remission obtained with steroid therapy is followed by relapse, the patient may be given another course. If failure recurs, splenectomy is carried out.

It is important to note that idiopathic thrombocytopenic purpura may recur weeks, months, or even years after splenectomy and may be related to the development of an accessory spleen.[166, 394] The question as to just when a splenectomy should be performed must be answered for each patient individually, depending on the course of disease.

There have been several encouraging reports of the use of azathioprine (Imuran) in the treatment of refractory idiopathic thrombocytopenic purpura. This immunosuppressive agent has been effective in many patients who relapsed after splenectomy or required large doses of steroids for maintenance.[64, 120, 380]

Neonatal thrombocytopenic purpura. Thrombocytopenic purpura occurring at the time of delivery may affect both the mother and baby, the baby alone, or the mother alone.[153, 164-166, 394] The infant usually appears normal at the time of delivery but develops purpura several hours later. The hemorrhagic manifestations may disappear after a few days but the thrombocytopenia often persists for weeks.

Mechanisms. Investigators have now established that several mechanisms may result in neonatal thrombocytopenia purpura.

Isoimmune neonatal thrombocytopenia. Isoimmune neonatal thrombocytopenia has been likened to that of Rh sensitization.[166, 284, 394] Several platelet types have now been identified and should the mother and fetus have different platelet types, maternal isoagglutinins may form, cross the placenta, and destroy the platelets of the fetus. Maternal immunization against antigens on fetal platelets has been demonstrated in both megakaryocytic and amegakaryocytic neonatal thrombocytopenic purpura. The antibody disappears from the infant's plasma in approximately 2 weeks and recovery ensues.[355]

A similar mechanism is believed to operate in instances of neonatal thrombocytopenic purpura occurring in infants of mothers with idiopathic thrombocytopenic purpura, though direct evidence for antibody is lacking. The platelet-depressing factor present in the mother's plasma is thought to gain access to the circulation of the fetus and thrombocytopenia results. The thrombocytopenia may persist longer than that seen in association with demonstrated maternal isoagglutinins.[355, 356] Most infants with isoimmune neonatal thrombocytopenic purpura recover without sequelae. However, severe complications or death may occur. In one review an immediate mortality of 12.7 per cent was noted. Intracranial hemorrhage was the most serious.[284]

Neonatal purpura and the rubella syndrome. Thrombocytopenic purpura may be one manifestation of the congenital rubella syndrome. It appears most commonly in those infants whose mothers were infected during the fourth to eighth week of gestation. Rubella virus was recovered from 83 per cent of infants with purpura in one study. The clinical picture may vary from that of an apparently healthy infant with a few scattered petechiae to that of a moribund infant with extensive purpuric lesions. Often platelets are but slightly reduced on the first day or two of life, but may drop over the next few days to low levels. Recovery occurs at a variable rate. Severe hemorrhage may occur but is unusual.[5]

Associated abnormalities may include retarded intrauterine growth, hepatomegaly, splenomegaly, congenital heart disease, eye defects, bone lesions, hepatitis, and anemia. Bone marrow specimens contain a reduced number of megakaryocytes.[92] A variety of mechanisms have been suggested to account for the occurrence of purpura in the course of viral illness. The virus may alter the platelets so that they become antigenic and stimulate antibody formation; a virus-antibody complex may "accidentally" attach to the platelet and cause their destruction; or the virus could damage the platelet directly and cause its destruction.[259] Vascular damage may result from direct virus attachment, the presence of virus-antibody complexes, or from the development of intravascular thrombi.[39] The damaged vessel walls may allow the escape of blood. The precise mechanism is not known.[39, 259]

Neonatal purpura and maternal ingestion of drugs. There have been recent reports of neonatal thrombocytopenic purpura occurring in infants delivered of mothers without platelet deficiency or detectable antiplatelet antibody in their serum. It was suggested but not proved that the thrombocytopenia in the infant was the result of the mother's having received one of the thiazides during the prepartum period. The precise mechanism or action by which these drugs may cause thrombocytopenia is not known, but there are reports of adults developing thrombocytopenia after taking thiazides.[135, 321]

Therapy. Most infants with isoimmune neonatal purpura recover without sequelae, but serious complications or death may occur. The aim of therapy is to tide the infant over the days or weeks until recovery occurs. Steroid therapy is used because it may suppress antibody formation and interfere with antigen-antibody complexes. Steroids also have a salutary effect on the vascular endothelium.

Blood transfusions should be used if indicated. Recent evidence suggests that platelet transfusions of the mother's platelets, washed with normal plasma to remove iso-antibody, are effective.[11] Exchange transfusions have been advocated in an effort to remove the circulating antibody.[284]

Splenectomy is not indicated unless there is a failure to control symptoms with steroids and platelet transfusions.

Infants born to mothers who have idiopathic thrombocytopenic purpura generally recover without serious sequelae. Steroid therapy may be very helpful. Once again, splenectomy is not indicated unless steroid therapy fails and the situation is life threatening.

Infants with the congenital rubella syndrome should be isolated because they shed virus and are contagious for a variable period of time. There is no specific therapy for congenital rubella and the thrombocytopenia is treated in the same manner as other forms of neonatal purpura.[5, 93, 182] The value of steroids in the treatment of the thrombocytopenia must be carefully weighed against their effect on the immunologic mechanism.

Thrombotic thrombocytopenic purpura (Thrombohemolytic thrombocytopenic purpura). Thrombotic thrombocytopenic purpura is an unusual malady first described by Moschowitz in 1925.[253] The syndrome is now being recognized more frequently prior to death.[328, 386] It occurs most commonly in the female in the 10 to 40 age group and may develop during pregnancy.[360] It has been reported in one neonatal infant.[252] The course of the disease is marked by the occurrence of hemolytic anemia, thrombocytopenic purpura, changing neurologic signs, and renal disease.[228]

Mechanism. The relationship of this disorder to the collagen diseases was pointed out quite early and the suggestion that it is primarily the result of a vascular lesion has recently received support.[138, 143, 211] The characteristic pathologic lesion of thrombotic thrombocytopenic purpura is partial or complete occlusion of many small arterioles and capillaries (rarely venules).[143] These lesions are widespread in the body, and any organ may be involved. The most commonly involved organs are the heart, adrenals, kidneys,[228] pancreas, and brain. The occlusive material is acidophilic, amorphous, and hyalin-like.[143, 386] Many believe that it is composed of platelets, but its exact nature is unknown. The thromboses may result in aneurysmal dilatation of the vessel and subsequent rupture.

The hemolytic anemia which occurs in patients with this disorder is of an extracorpuscular type. The Coombs antiglobulin test is usually negative. It has been suggested that the characteristic red cell distortion, shistocytes, helmet cells, burr cells, and fragmentation and the anemia may result from direct contact with fibrin of either the patient's or transfused normal red cells with diseased small blood vessels.[69]

The thrombocytopenic manifestations of the disorder are characteristic, but the mechanism by which the platelets are reduced has been the source of much debate.[138, 143] There is no evidence of diffuse intravascular coagulation.[211] A shortened survival time of normal platelets in these patients has been described, but infusions of plasma from patients with thrombotic thrombocytopenic purpura did not diminish the number of platelets in a normal recipient, indicating an absence of platelet antibodies. No platelet agglutinins have yet been described. There is evidence of alteration in megakaryocytic function in some patients, the megakaryocytes being immature.

The neurologic lesions are secondary to vascular lesions in the brain.

It has been pointed out that renal disease with hematuria, proteinuria, casts, and azotemia may be a prominent feature of thrombotic thrombocytopenic purpura;[228] azotemia may occur without demonstrable red cells, casts, or protein in the urine. The marked endothelial proliferation of the small arteries and arterioles of the kidney may be associated with thrombi and contain "foamy" macrophages.

Recently it has been suggested that thrombotic thrombocytopenic purpura is not a disease but a syndrome with diverse etiologies, including vasculitis and infection. Disseminated intravascular coagulation or extensive intravascular coagulation in a single organ was suggested as the probable mechanism by which the syndrome is produced.[386a, 390a, 397a]

Clinical aspects. Although there have been chronic or relapsing forms noted in the literature, most patients present with a dramatic and fulminating disease resulting in death in a few days or weeks.[138] The diagnosis is suspected in a young person critically ill with hemolytic anemia, thrombocytopenic purpura, and changing neurologic signs. Positive diagnosis has been made following the finding of characteristic lesions in small vessels removed by marrow aspiration and sectioned in paraffin block. Muscle biopsy may also be helpful.[94]

Occult vascular disease and infection with agents as varied as microtatobiotes,[245a] aspergillus,[390a] and meningococcus[269a] have been implicated in thrombotic thrombocytopenic purpura and should be searched for in any patient with the disorder.

Treatment. Recent reports of prolonged survival of patients with thrombotic thrombocytopenic purpura lend some urgency to the need for early diagnosis.[174, 228] Massive doses of steroids and splenectomy have been noted to prevent the rapid deterioration of these patients. Transfusions should be used to replace blood loss from hemorrhage or hemolysis. Anticoagulation has been used with variable success, but may prevent damage to vital organs.[44a, 201a]

Illustrative Cases

SECONDARY THROMBOCYTOPENIC PURPURA

A 14 year old white girl had been well until 3 or 4 days prior to admission when she contracted measles, which was epidemic in her community and present in her home. Eighteen hours before admission she had a sudden epistaxis and later vomited blood and passed tarry stools. Her mother, who had raised 14 children and "knew the measles," stated that she had noted a change in the character of the rash during the 24 hours prior to admission.

Careful questioning failed to reveal any history of a hemorrhagic diathesis in the patient or in her family. There had been no known exposure to chemicals, and she had received no drugs.

Physical examination. There were many petechiae over the lower legs and back and subconjunctival hemorrhages were noted in both eyes. There was a small amount of blood in the posterior pharynx and mild oozing from the nares. There were small nodes in both the posterior cervical triangles and the suboccipital area, but the spleen was not palpable. The remainder of the examination was non-contributory.

Laboratory examination. Laboratory examination revealed a hematocrit of 26 per cent and a white blood cell count of 11,000 per cu.mm. Urinalysis was negative but the stool examination was positive for occult blood. The bleeding time was 12 minutes, tourniquet test positive, and clot retraction poor after 2 hours. There were no platelets seen on examination of multiple smears. The prothrombin time and coagulation time were normal. Preparations made to demonstrate the lupus erythematosus cell phenomena were negative on three occasions. Bone marrow megakaryocytes were diminished in number and immature in appearance. Atypical lymphocytes and young plasma cells were seen on examination of the bone marrow smear and the smear of the peripheral blood. A diagnosis of thrombocytopenia secondary to measles was made.

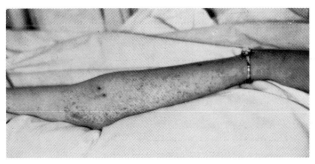

Figure 11–3. Positive tourniquet test in a patient with secondary thrombocytopenic purpura.

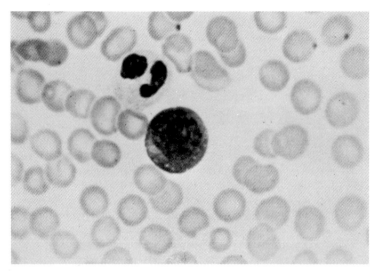

Figure 11-4. Pathologic lymphocyte in peripheral blood of patient with secondary thrombocytopenic purpura following measles.

Course. Because of continued bleeding and low hematocrit, the patient was transfused with 500 ml. of whole blood. Twenty-five mg. of ACTH was given intravenously over a 6 hour period, and prednisone was administered orally in a dosage of 25 mg. three times a day. The patient's nose was packed and bleeding was controlled adequately, though there was slight oozing for the first 4 days. Platelets, which were seen for the first time on a smear made on the sixth hospital day, numbered 216,000 by the eleventh hospital day. At that time the bleeding time had returned to 2½ minutes. The patient was discharged to be followed in the Hematology Clinic. Instructions were given to reduce the prednisone gradually. Her platelets remained at normal levels for the 4 months she was followed after steroid therapy had been discontinued.

Comments. This girl presents the classic clinical and laboratory findings of thrombocytopenic purpura. In addition to the failure to find platelets in the peripheral blood, the megakaryocytes which were seen in the marrow preparation were immature and did not seem to be forming platelets. L.E. preparations were obtained because purpuric lesions may be the presenting complaint of patients who are subsequently found to have disseminated lupus erythematosus. The presence of the atypical lymphocytes and young forms of plasma cells suggested the presence of a virus disease. In view of the history of measles it was felt that this represented *secondary thrombocytopenic* purpura occurring as the result of measles.

Thrombocytopenia is a rare sequela of measles. The appearance of the purpuric rash has been reported[166] as occurring from the third day of the measles rash to as long as 2 weeks subsequent to its disappearance. Contrary to popular opinion purpura does not follow only severe attacks of measles, and the accompanying infection may be but a mild one.

The use of blood transfusion was simply for blood replacement.

Steroids were used to sustain the patient through what proved to be self-limited acute thrombocytopenia secondary to an infectious viral disease.

The prognosis is good in this case, and it is doubtful if she will have a recurrence. However, the patient was instructed to return immediately if symptoms recurred.

IDIOPATHIC THROMBOCYTOPENIC PURPURA

History. A 24 year old white married mother had been in good health until 4 months prior to admission when she noted bruising without recognized trauma. Bruising continued, and when she sought medical attention 3 months prior to admission, she was told that "her platelets were less than 10,000." Intramuscular injections of ACTH gel were given with improvement. The platelets returned to normal levels and bruising ceased. After an interval of 2 or 3 weeks excessive bruising was again noted and upon examination platelets once more were found to be low. With the onset of excessive menstrual bleeding she was referred for further treatment. No significant family or personal history could be elicited. There had been no exposure to toxins nor had there been any recent infections.

Physical examination. The physical examination revealed many ecchymoses over the upper and lower extremities. Several petechiae were noted on the buccal mucosa. The remainder of the examination was negative. No lymph nodes were enlarged and the spleen was not palpable.

Laboratory examinations. Laboratory examinations revealed a hematocrit of 41 per cent and a white blood cell count of 10,300 per cu.mm. Differential white count was normal. Urinalysis was normal and examination of the feces was negative for occult blood. The platelet count was 22,000, the bleeding time 18 minutes, and the tourniquet test positive. The coagulation time and prothrombin time were both normal. A diagnosis of idiopathic thrombocytopenic purpura was made.

Course. Since the patient had responded once to adrenocortical steroid therapy, it was decided to attempt once again to control her bleeding with these compounds. Accordingly, oral prednisone 15 mg. every 6 hours (60 mg. a day) was begun. After 4 days the platelet count was 150,000 per cu.mm., and bruising had ceased. The dose of prednisone was reduced to 10 mg. every 6 hours (40 mg. a day), and improvement continued. On the sixth day the platelet count was 409,000 per cu.mm., and the dosage of prednisone was reduced to 5 mg. four times a day. The patient was discharged in the care of her physician and was instructed to take 5 mg. prednisone three times a day.

The dosage of prednisone was decreased gradually and after 2 months it was discontinued. Immediately her platelets fell to less than 10,000. In view of the two relapses following withdrawal of steroid therapy it was decided that splenectomy should be performed. Accordingly prednisone was restarted in preparation for operation and continued through the postoperative period. The platelet count at time of operation was 748,000 per cu.mm., and on the first postoperative day was 898,000. The patient was discharged with instruction to reduce the prednisone gradually over an 8 day period. She continued well during the following year without the support of adrenocortical steroid therapy.

Comment. Careful search failed to reveal any primary etiology, and a diagnosis of idiopathic thrombocytopenic purpura was made. Laboratory findings confirmed the diagnosis in that bleeding time and tourniquet test were both abnormal, and the finding of a low platelet count revealed the reason for the abnormal tests.

Splenectomy was performed because adrenocortical steroid administration could not be discontinued without relapse after a 6 month trial period. The increase in thrombocytes after splenectomy is but one of the characteristic changes in the peripheral blood after this operation. Others include the appearance of target cells, Howell-Jolly bodies, leukocytosis, and nucleated red blood cells. These changes have been thought to indicate that the spleen exerts some inhibitory effect on the bone marrow. Another explanation may be that removal of the spleen decreases the peripheral destruction of these particular elements. A relapse may occur in this patient as long as 20 to 25 years after splenectomy. Should this occur, a decision must then be made as to whether she may have developed an accessory spleen and warrants reexploration.

Non-Thrombocytopenic Purpura

Patients with non-thrombocytopenic purpura may have all of the hemorrhagic lesions noted for those with thrombocytopenic purpura. They differ in that their platelet count remains within the normal range. Characteristic lesions include petechiae, ecchymoses, hematoma, or spontaneous bleeding from the genitourinary tract or gastrointestinal tract. The hemorrhagic lesions may be present in the skin or mucous membranes.

ALLERGIC PURPURA

This disorder, known also as the Schonlein-Henoch syndrome, was extensively studied by Osler,[276] and his reports are the basis of much of our present day knowledge of the variability of the clinical findings. It occurs most commonly in children, usually males, but is also found in adults.[17, 25]

Clinical examination. The presenting complaints will depend on the site and extent of the involvement. Osler[276] remarked that the two outstanding clinical features were recurrence, at long or short intervals, and marked variability of the skin lesions. The syndrome characteristically recurs several times before final remission. The recurrences may appear over a period of weeks, months, or, in some cases, years. The underlying pathology allows the development of skin lesions of great variability. There may be only purpura, with petechiae and ecchymoses, or there may be associated effusion, erythema, or necrosis of the skin. Gastrointestinal involvement is marked by colicky abdominal pain which is often of great severity and occurs chiefly at night. Diarrhea and vomiting are frequent and both the vomitus and stools may contain blood.[7, 276] Intussusception or perforation may occur.[17, 320] Gastrointestinal x-rays will reveal edema of the mucosa early in the course of the illness and evidence of submucosal hemorrhage and mucosal ulceration later. These changes are reversible.[25] Hematuria and proteinuria occur in from 12 to 49 per cent of the reported series.[172] In most cases they are transient findings. In some the hematuria and proteinuria may persist for months or years unaccompanied by azotemia or hypertension. A few patients develop azotemia, hypertension and occasionally the nephrotic syndrome early in the course of their illness. These patients may die of rapidly progressive renal failure over a period of months or as the result of slowly developing renal failure over a period of years.[7, 108, 132, 172, 280] Joint symptoms may be the presenting complaint. Several joints are usually involved by pain at one time and there may or may not be associated swelling.

The prognosis for life is generally good unless the patient develops progressive renal disease, uncontrolled gastrointestinal hemorrhage, or unrecognized intussusception or perforation.[17] The disease is marked by repeated attacks which may extend over months or years, though most recover after a month or so.

There is no consistent laboratory finding. There may be an anemia if the bleeding has been extensive enough, but this is rare. Platelets, of course, are normal or only slightly reduced. The capillary fragility test is positive in only a portion of the cases.[7]

Mechanism. The etiology of this disorder remains unknown. There is increased capillary permeability which allows the escape of elements of the blood into the surrounding tissue but the nature of the capillary lesion is not clear. In some cases infection may play a role. Streptococcal infection of the throat has been implicated by some,[288] but the evidence is weak.[7, 32, 396] Hypersensitivity to certain foods has been implicated in some instances of this disorder and recovery has followed the avoidance of the offending agent. Some have pointed to a resemblance between the lesions of allergic purpura and those of the collagen diseases, but again the evidence is incomplete.[108]

Treatment. The treatment of this syndrome is largely supportive. A careful search should be made for an offending food in chronic cases. Throat culture should be made and dealt with as indicated. The frequency with which the syndrome is accompanied by nephritis makes it imperative to pay close attention to the cultures. Ackroyd feels the patients should be kept in bed in the hope of reducing the incidence and severity of nephritis.[7]

Steroids alone have not proven effective in the management of skin manifestations or renal involvement but are useful in the control of joint involvement, soft tissue swelling, and gastrointestinal symptoms.[17, 139, 374] The likelihood of intussusception or perforation should be kept in mind in order that surgical intervention can be performed immediately if it should become necessary.[17]

Recently, azathioprine and steroids were used in the successful management of progressive renal failure with the nephrotic syndrome.[139]

INFECTIOUS PURPURA

Purpura in association with infection has been known since ancient times.[189] It is a recognized and expected clinical finding in such disorders as Rocky Mountain spotted fever, typhus, meningococcemia, and bacterial endocarditis. In each of these disorders an escape of blood elements into the surrounding tissue follows damage to the vascular endothelium.

There are instances in which purpura is associated with severe forms of exanthems, such as chickenpox or smallpox. In these instances the purpura seems to occur because of the unusual severity of the disease, which causes damage to the vascular endothelium.[190]

Finally, purpura may be associated with infection in certain patients who exhibit what appears to be individual susceptibility. The purpura may be thrombocytopenic or non-thrombocytopenic. Both types have occurred in association with scarlet fever, varicella, measles, tuberculosis, infectious mononucleosis, and infectious hepatitis.[7] These diseases need not be particularly severe for purpura to be a complication. The natural history of the purpura in these instances is similar to that of idiopathic thrombocytopenic purpura.

The mechanism responsible for the purpura is not clear. No histologic change in the vascular system has yet been demonstrated.

Treatment. Although treatment is directed to the underlying disease with the use of appropriate antibiotics, care should be taken to tide the patient over the hemorrhagic episode. Adrenocortical steroids may be helpful, but caution must be observed in light of recent reports of the extraordinary severity and frequent deaths from varicella in children who have been on steroid therapy.[154] Adrenocortical steroids should be used with caution in varicella, if at all, and should be used with caution in other virus exanthems. In patients with thrombocytopenia the use of platelet transfusions should be considered. Splenectomy would not be indicated except possibly in chronic cases, for example, those associated with tuberculosis involving the spleen.

PURPURA FULMINANS

Purpura fulminans is a rare, severe, usually fatal illness which occurs most often in children and young adults. The disorder is marked by the sudden appearance of large areas of cutaneous gangrene and hemorrhage during the convalescent period of a variety of infectious diseases such as streptococcus pharyngitis, scarlet fever, varicella, meningococcemia, and rubella. Associated with the skin manifestations are chills, fever, shock, coma, and death. The mortality rate has been 90 per cent in the past. The pathogenesis of the disorder is not completely clear. There is extensive intravascular coagulation and stasis, and various abnormalities of coagulation have been demonstrated, including diminished platelets and reduced Factors V and VIII. There is a marked similarity to the Shwartzman phenomenon.

The Shwartzman reaction is produced in rabbits by two intravenous injections of toxin from gram-negative bacteria administered 24 hours apart. While each injection activates the clotting system, the reticuloendothelial system is able to clear the activated factors, fibrin, and endotoxin after the first injection.

The second injection finds the reticuloendothelial system blocked as a result of the first injection and produces massive precipitation of fibrin which results in severe vascular disturbances.[176] In recent years an increasing number of patients have been recognized with clinical course and laboratory studies resembling the generalized Shwartzman reaction.[318]

The Shwartzman reaction in the experimental animal can be blocked by the administration of anticoagulants[239, 318] and these agents have been successfully employed in the treatment of purpura fulminans. Heparin is the agent of choice.[24, 98, 318, 348] The use of low molecular weight dextran has been advocated and may reduce the tendency to thrombosis.[203, 282, 359] The administration of fibrinogen is usually contraindicated since the intravascular deposition of fibrin may be increased. Late in the course of the disorder enhancement of fibrinolysis may be indicated.[319] Since necrotic lesions resembling purpura fulminans may be seen in other conditions not involving intravascular coagulation the diagnosis of intravascular coagulation must be carefully substantiated prior to treatment.

OTHER TYPES

Non-thrombocytopenic purpura may occur following exposure to chemicals or drugs to which the individual is susceptible,[7] in vitamin C deficiency,[173] as the result of certain snake bites,[198] and in disorders characterized by the presence of abnormal serum proteins. In the last case deposition of abnormal proteins in the small vessels alters their permeability and allows escape of fluid content. This is seen in multiple myeloma in association with cryoglobulins or para-amyloid. Waldenstrom has described[400] a macroglobulinemia usually occurring in elderly men and characterized by the presence of abnormal lymphocytes in the bone marrow and a globulin of high molecular weight in the serum. In this disorder, purpura occurs particularly over the lower extremities.[344] Purpura may also occur in association with cold agglutinins, for example, following virus pneu-

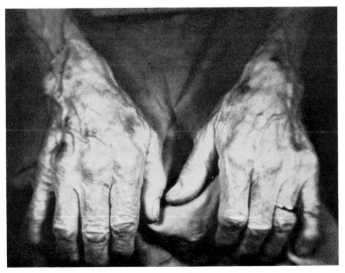

Figure 11–5.   Senile purpura.

monia. Non-thrombocytopenic purpura may be a feature of old age, presumably as the result of loss of support to the small vessels.

Ingestion of aspirin and other anti-inflammatory compounds can cause abnormal bleeding associated with a prolonged bleeding time in the presence of a normal number of platelets.[300a, 408a] These drugs interfere with platelet-collagen reaction and block the secondary wave of irreversible aggregation of platelets; aggregation after ADP or epinephrine, the release of serotonin, and activation of PF-3 are abnormal. These effects, which follow the ingestion of 1.8 gm. of aspirin, may be detected for from 4 to 7 days, although salicylate is no longer demonstrable in the plasma.[410]

Hereditary Hemorrhagic Telangiectasia

This hereditary vascular anomaly was first described in 1896 by Rendu.[275] In 1901 Osler[275] reported several cases in detail and noted most of the clinical findings known today. Weber[405] reported an extensive family study in 1907, and two years later Hanes[157] made further contributions on the subject and suggested the name by which the disorder is known today.

PATHOLOGIC PHYSIOLOGY

Hereditary hemorrhagic telangiectasia is genetically transmitted by either sex as an autosomal dominant. Often the disease may not become apparent until the second or third decade when the lesions develop and gradually increase in number. Abnormal bleeding may be delayed until middle or old age and often grows more severe with advancing years.[43] Some patients are unaffected by the presence of telangiectasia, and hemorrhage does not occur. These lesions are composed of greatly dilated, thin-walled vessels which are reported to have inadequate smooth muscle and elastic tissues.[157]

In recent years angiographic studies have provided evidence of extensive involvement of larger vessels of the vascular system in this disorder.[61] Pulmonary arteriovenous fistulas have been reported which may lead to erythrocytosis, cyanosis, and clubbing and have a significant incidence of central nervous system complications, including sterile embolism and brain abscess.[43, 112, 141] Shunting may be so extensive in the liver that portosystemic encephalopathy may occur in the absence of cirrhosis.[248] Vascular abnormalities have also been reported to involve the spleen, eye,[418] central nervous system, and bone.[155]

An interesting syndrome of calcinosis, Reynaud's phenomena, sclerodactyly, and telangiectasis (CRST) has been reported.[104, 416] The telangiectasis of these patients appears somewhat later and there is less tendency to episodes of hemorrhage. The gross and microscopic appearance of these lesions as well as their distribution is similar to that found in hereditary hemorrhagic telangiectasia, but the lack of a family history of hemorrhagic diathesis or similar telangiectases serves to distinguish this syndrome from hereditary hemorrhagic telangiectasia. The CRST syndrome is classified as a collagen disorder. It is slowly progressive as compared with diffuse systemic sclerosis.

CLINICAL EXAMINATION

The characteristic vascular lesions are pinpoint in size or several millimeters in diameter. They are red or purple in color and slightly raised from the surrounding surface. They may blanch slightly with pressure. The lesions, which may occur anywhere on the surface of the body or in any organ, are most frequently found on the skin of the face, the ears, or the hands and feet, at the base of the fingernails, or on the mucous membranes of the nose and mouth.

The diagnosis must be suspected in cases of recurrent hemorrhage associated with telangiectasia and a family history of abnormal bleeding. The most common complaints are those of hemorrhage and anemia. Hemorrhage may occur as the result of slight trauma to one of the vascular lesions anywhere on the body or may be spontaneous. Hemorrhage from the nose or mouth is common, but bleeding may occur from the respiratory tract, gastrointestinal tract, or genitourinary tract as well.

The importance of finding the lesions of hereditary hemorrhagic telangiectasia is enhanced by the recently established associations with significant large vessel abnormalities in various parts of the body.

The chief laboratory findings are those of anemia. There may be iron deficiency with low serum iron and high iron binding capacity if bleeding has been chronic. Coagulation studies are completely normal.

TREATMENT

The use of electrocoagulation and skin grafts has been successful in controlling some of the accessible lesions.[331] One of Osler's patients used a small balloon which he inserted into his nose in a deflated condition and then inflated to control nasal hemorrhage. This procedure is used with success today. The management of hemorrhage from the lesions of hereditary hemorrhagic telangiectasia presents a difficult problem when they are located in the gastro-

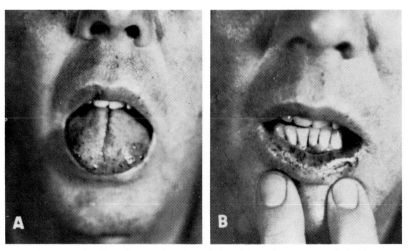

Figure 11-6. Hereditary telangiectasia involving (A) tongue and (B) lips.

intestinal tract. They are difficult if not impossible to localize by x-ray but occasionally may be demonstrated by endoscopy.[415] Although resection may remove one source of hemorrhage, the future development of similar lesions remains a constant threat.

The management of large vessel abnormalities must depend on individual evaluation of their hemodynamic significance, prognosis, and risk involved.

Abnormalities of Blood Coagulation

A genetically inherited deficiency of the appropriate activity of each of the clotting factors has been recorded. The deficiencies were all believed to be quantitative until recently, when it was demonstrated that the plasma of patients with a deficiency of Factor I, II, VIII, IX, or X may contain functionally inactive molecular forms of these factors. Additional qualitative defects will undoubtedly be detected. The familial occurrence of a deficiency of more than one clotting factor has also been noted.

Acquired deficiency of each of the clotting factors has also been reported. Such deficiencies may result from impaired synthesis, as in the course of liver disease, the development of circulating anticoagulants in association with any of a wide variety of disorders, as the result of the intended action of medicinal agents such as the anticoagulant drugs, or the toxic effect of a variety of drugs or chemical or physical agents. Deficiency of various clotting factors may also arise in the course of the defibrination syndrome as the result of over-utilization or proteolysis.

Disorders Affecting Predominantly the First Stage of Blood Coagulation

Factor XII Deficiency (Hageman Trait, Hageman Deficiency)

The existence of Factor XII was discovered as the result of studies undertaken to explain the unexpected finding of a greatly prolonged clotting time of the blood of a patient with no personal or family history of hemorrhagic diathesis.[306]

PATHOLOGIC PHYSIOLOGY

Hageman trait is the inherited deficiency of the specific plasma protein Factor XII.[194, 305] The disorder is transmitted as an autosomal recessive defect. Heterozygotes have from 25 to 60 per cent of the normal concentration of Factor XII, whereas the homozygotes have less than 1 per cent.[305, 310]

Factor XII circulates in an inert form, but once a sample of blood is removed from the body and placed in contact with glass it undergoes physical and chemical changes which initiate the intrinsic clotting sequence.[365] The mechanism of Factor XII activation in vivo is not completely understood, but contact with exposed collagen fibers may play a role.[307] Factor XII participates in a number of the biologic activities of the body. It plays a role in the process of inflammation and activation of the kallikrein-kinin system, the fibrinolytic system, and the complement system.[151, 235, 307, 309] It may also play a role in the pathogenesis of acute gouty arthritis.[199, 200, 383]

CLINICAL MANIFESTATIONS

With very few exceptions, these patients have no personal or family history of a hemorrhagic diathesis. The exceptions have included patients with menorrhagia or mild bleeding following significant trauma.[57, 127, 306] The clotting time is prolonged and the results of the thromboplastin generation abnormal. Direct comparison of the patient's plasma or serum with that of a patient known to have the defect is the only way to establish a firm diagnosis.

The several reports of thrombosis in patients with Factor XII deficiency[138a, 177a] may relate to the role of this factor in the initiation of fibrinolysis.

TREATMENT

There is no need to treat patients with classic Factor XII deficiency if they have no hemorrhagic diathesis. The atypical patient with hemorrhagic diathesis would probably respond to treatment with plasma.[53]

Disorders of Factors VIII, IX, and XI

The following disorders are grouped together because of the similarity of their clinical and laboratory findings. Each results in a delay in the development of blood thromboplastin activity to a greater or less extent[74, 363] but produces no alteration in the one stage prothrombin time.

"Hemophilia" is one of the oldest recognized bleeding disorders and affected members of several of the ruling houses in Europe.[327] It has been recognized in recent years that the clinical findings of classic "hemophilia" may result from any one of three distinct genetic defects or from acquired circulating anticoagulants. These disorders can be differentiated only by appropriate laboratory tests, since they present similar clinical findings. It is for this reason that accurate classification of the cases presented in the older literature as "hemophilia" is not possible. The three genetic disorders now recognized, with their relative incidence in two series,[126, 322, 323] are as follows:

1. Factor VIII (Antihemophilic factor, AHF) deficiency, 80 to 82 per cent

2. Factor IX (Plasma thromboplastin component, PTC) deficiency (Christmas disease), 11 to 15 per cent

3. Factor XI (Plasma thromboplastin antecedent, PTA) deficiency, 5 to 7 per cent

Factor VIII (Antihemophilic Factor, AHF) Deficiency

PATHOLOGIC PHYSIOLOGY

Factor VIII deficiency is passed from one generation to the next as a sex-linked recessive. Ordinarily the female is a carrier and manifests no clinical signs or symptoms of the disorder.

The genetic possibilities inherent in this and similar disorders are best indicated by the use of symbols and diagrams. By common usage the male is designated as XY, and the female is designated XX. In order for a male to be conceived, the male parent must contribute the Y chromosome; the female contributes the X. Specific genes are usually referred to by superscript letters. A dominant gene is designated by a capital letter and a recessive by a lower case letter.

The abnormal gene responsible for Factor VIII deficiency is recessive and is designated by the lower case letter h. The normal gene, which is dominant, is designated by a capital H. A normal female would thus be designated $X^H X^H$. The carrier female would be $X^H X^h$. In the case of the carrier female, expression will depend on which X chromosome is functional in the somatic cells. The carrier usually has no symptoms, since random distribution would result in at least 50 per cent of the X chromosomes being X^H in the somatic cells.[201] The Y chromosome of the male does not carry this gene and has neither H nor h. Whether a male child has Factor VIII deficiency or not depends entirely on the character of the X chromosome he must receive from the female. If the female carrier contributes the normal X^H to the male offspring, the male is normal. If, however, the X chromosome contributed by the female to her male offspring is that which carries the abnormal gene, it would find expression as there would be no normal gene (H) to suppress it.

The accompanying diagrams will illustrate the possibilities. The male in each instance is designated by the rectangle and the female by the circle.

Figure 11–7 represents a normal family with no factor deficiency. All offspring are normal.

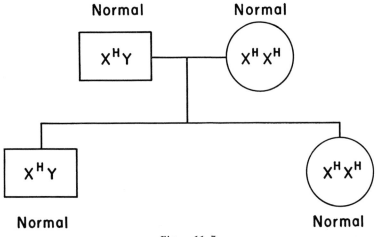

Figure 11–7.

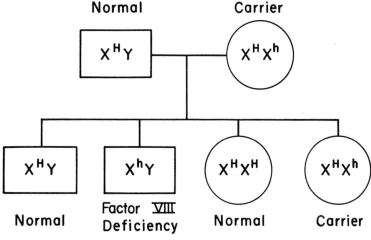

Figure 11–8.

Figure 11–8 indicates that a mating of a normal male and a carrier female may result in a hemophilic male or a carrier female as well as normal children of both sexes. Unfortunately, there is no way to establish with certainty whether a female is a carrier or not. There is evidence, however, that the degree of recessiveness may vary and that some carrier females may have depressed Factor VIII levels.

Figure 11–9 indicates the results of a mating of a Factor VIII deficient male with a normal female. All of their female children *must* be carriers, since the only X chromosome the male has to contribute carries the abnormal gene. On the other hand, none of the male offspring can have hemophilia, since a male must receive the lone X chromosome from the normal mother.

In Figure 11–10 we see the results of the mating of a Factor VIII deficient

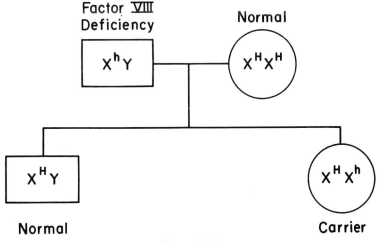

Figure 11–9.

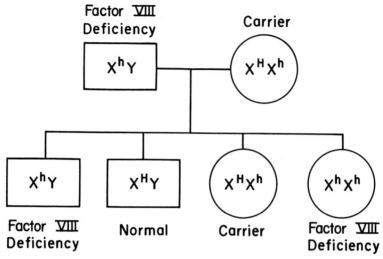

Figure 11–10.

male and a carrier female. For many years the possibility that a female could have a Factor VIII deficiency was not accepted, but several well documented cases have now been reported.[243, 413] The female offspring of the mating noted here would receive an X^h from the Factor VIII deficient male, and the second X^h from the carrier mother.

In Figure 11–11 we see the result of a mating between a normal male and a Factor VIII deficient female. All male progeny would receive X^h from the mother, and all female would receive an X^H from the father in addition to the X^h from the mother. All males would then be Factor VIII deficient and all females would be carriers.

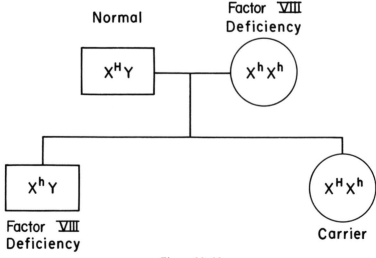

Figure 11–11.

The mating of a male and a female both deficient in Factor VIII has probably never occurred except in laboratory animals. All of the offspring of such a mating would be Factor VIII deficient (Fig. 11–12).

As there are patients with hemophilia who have no family history of the disorder, the rate of mutation is thought to be high.

Although the defect in classic hemophilia is transmitted as a sex-linked recessive mendelian characteristic, there is evidence that at least one and possibly two autosomal loci are involved in Factor VIII production as well. Von Willebrand's disease, characterized by a prolonged bleeding time and decreased Factor VIII level, is transmitted by an autosomal dominant gene and one report has appeared in which Factor VIII deficiency alone appears to have been transmitted as an autosomal dominant trait.[34, 171]

The result of the genetic defect is known to be the deficiency of the Factor VIII activity of a globulin first described by Patek and Taylor.[281] In the absence of this activity, the first phase of coagulation is impeded. Since the platelets and the capillaries are unaffected, the bleeding time is normal but the coagulation time is often prolonged. The more severe the deficiency of Factor VIII activity, the more severe the bleeding problem. Levels of below 3 per cent are usually found in symptomatic patients, though a bleeding diathesis may be found in patients with levels as high as 20 per cent. The level of Factor VIII activity in any one patient is remarkably constant throughout his life.

Recent data suggest that reduced Factor VIII activity may occur as the result of qualitative change in the Factor VIII molecule rather than a quantitative deficiency of the globulin.[119, 181] Using a naturally occurring human antibody against Factor VIII, investigators found that the plasma of a small percentage of patients with classic hemophilia would neutralize the antibody. Hemagglutination-inhibition tests using rabbit antibody to highly purified

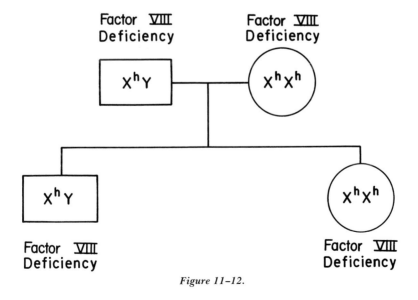

Figure 11–12.

Factor VIII from normal humans have revealed the presence of a protein antigenically related to, or identical with, Factor VIII in similar amounts in both normal and hemophilic plasma and serum.[375a] The evidence suggests the presence of a molecule with the same antigenic determinants as Factor VIII but lacking Factor VIII coagulant activity.[106] Similar information has been developed concerning Factor IX activity deficiency.[180, 314]

Factor VIII is one of the factors needed in the development of blood thromboplastin activity, and in its complete absence the only effective hemostatic defense left to the patient is that supplied by the vascular phase of hemostasis and the extrinsic system. In the event of a defect in the larger vessels, these defenses are not sufficient to maintain hemostasis and extensive bleeding may occur.

CLINICAL ASPECTS

In the past many born with Factor VIII deficiency died in infancy or in the first 5 years, but with modern therapy there has been marked improvement in the prognosis. The availability of adequate transfusion service has probably been the most important factor in the reduction of mortality from this disorder.

Mildly affected hemophiliacs may reach adult life before serious bleeding occurs. The more severely affected individuals may have repeated episodes of bleeding from the surface of the body, the serous surfaces, the gastrointestinal tract, the genitourinary tract, or into joint spaces. Bleeding does not often, if ever, occur in the absence of trauma. The hemarthroses which are suffered often result in permanent ankylosis and deformity.

Until recently conditions which made surgery imperative were catastrophic. Now it is possible to prepare for such emergencies with a good chance of success.[123, 227]

For many years the diagnosis of "hemophilia" was made when it could be demonstrated in vitro that plasma from the patient in question did not correct clotting defect of a patient with known "hemophilia." The diagnostic difficulties previously encountered are now recognized to have occurred because any one of several defects can produce clinical findings of classic hemophilia. These defects may be identified only by proper laboratory tests. The platelet count, tourniquet test, and bleeding time are unaffected, as they depend on capillary integrity and platelets, both of which are normal in Factor VIII deficiency.[301] Clot retraction is likewise normal, since there is adequate fibrin and normal platelet function. The prothrombin time is normal, since this test system bypasses the factor deficient in hemophilia.

The coagulation time may be prolonged owing to a decrease in the formation of thromboplastin activity. It is important to note, however, that the coagulation time may be normal despite relatively severe Factor VIII deficiency. The thromboplastin generation test can be used to identify the specific defect in any of these disorders.[49] Modifications may be made in the thromboplastin generation test which enable one to determine the percentage of Factor VIII activity present in the suspect plasma.

TREATMENT

The treatment of patients with hemophilia has improved considerably in recent years. Modern blood banking methods have made available large quantities of whole blood and plasma; high potency preparations of Factor VIII from animal blood are in use in Europe[226] and concentrates of human Factor VIII are available in this country and in Europe.[290] Although none of these materials provide "the answer" for hemophilia, as does vitamin B_{12} for pernicious anemia, they have nonetheless proved a great boon to the hemophiliac. Blood is more quickly replaced and hemostasis secured. If the patient is properly prepared, tooth extraction, so often denied these patients in the past despite desperate need, is now reasonably safe, and major surgery, though still hazardous, is feasible.

The use of human plasma as a source of Factor VIII has been successful in controlling most hemorrhage into soft tissues, hematuria, and the bleeding which follows tooth extraction in those hemophilic patients with a mild deficiency. It must be freshly prepared, for it loses over 50 per cent of its activity in 4 days if stored at usual blood bank temperatures of 2 to 4° C.[197] Plasma which has been quickly separated and frozen at −30° C retains its activity for as long as 30 days, however, and is an excellent product to have available. The relatively low concentration and short half-life of Factor VIII in normal plasma is an inherent limitation, and it is difficult to maintain patients free of bleeding following major surgery or severe trauma without the danger of overloading the circulatory system.

The need for a source of concentrated Factor VIII has long been recognized. The first successful preparation of high potency material was from animal blood[46, 226] and made it possible to give to the patient an amount of Factor VIII equivalent to that found in 8 liters of human blood in a single infusion of small volume. However, as these preparations are of heterologous protein, they are antigenic and are thus limited in their usefulness. It has proved possible to give a single course of therapy to a patient over 8 to 10 days, but the response to the infusions often progressively diminishes. A second course may be given but does carry the risk of anaphylactic reaction. Since there are only two animal preparations available (bovine and porcine), they are reserved for more serious episodes of bleeding and major surgery.

The rapid improvement in concentrates of human Factor VIII over the past few years has had a major impact on the treatment of patients with hemophilia. For many years, the only concentrate available was that prepared by a modification of the Cohn procedure of plasma fractionation.[197] Starting with pooled plasma, the final preparation contained a 10X concentration of Factor VIII.

This concentrate has not been widely accepted in the treatment of hemophilia because the use of pooled plasma as a starting material makes the risk of serum hepatitis high and the potency, although better than that of fresh plasma, is still low enough that circulatory overload may occur. Hemolysis has been noted during the administration of this material to some patients and has been attributed to the presence of high titer anti-A or -B isoantibodies contaminating the concentrate.[234]

An important breakthrough occurred when it was recognized that Factor VIII could be separated from plasma by cryoprecipitation.[121, 236, 284, 290, 295] When previously frozen plasma is thawed at icebox temperature, most Factor VIII remains as a gel and can be separated from the rest of the plasma by centrifugation.[292] After extraction of antihemophilic factor, the remaining plasma fraction may be used for other purposes.[271] This process results in a concentration of Factor VIII some 15 to 40 times that of normal plasma but the danger of transmitting serum hepatitis remains a problem.[91] The great advantage of this technique has been its practicality. Cryoprecipitated antihemophilic factor can be produced and stored in any well-equipped blood bank laboratory and its cost is well below that of other concentrates.[236]

A second major advance occurred when it was found that Factor VIII would precipitate in the presence of certain amino acids. One glycine-precipitated material has been developed which contains a 100-400X concentration of Factor VIII.[75]

The Factor VIII level of a patient with hemophilia may be brought to normal with a small volume of such material administered by syringe. If the cost of such preparations can be reduced and the possibility of the transmission of hepatitis is eliminated, continued improvement in the concentration of Factor VIII will make it practical to treat the patient with hemophilia prophylactically.[47, 195, 308, 316, 343]

Since the use of human plasma concentrates carried the risk of hepatitis, many make it a practice to administer prophylactic gamma gobulin while the Factor VIII level is being maintained.

The site of synthesis of Factor VIII is not known. The possibility that the spleen, liver, or bone marrow may play a role in the synthesis of Factor VIII has prompted exploration of the use of organ homografts to correct the deficiency. Transplantation of a spleen into dogs genetically deficient in Factor VIII has produced conflicting reports. One group found the procedure to be effective in increasing the levels of circulating Factor VIII.[267] Others have been unable to confirm the results obtained following spleen transplantation but were able to correct the deficiency by the transplantation of a liver. Bone marrow graft did not appear to influence the Factor VIII levels.[231]

A recent report of allogenic transplantation of a spleen into a young boy with severe Factor VIII deficiency indicated an initial effect on circulating Factor VIII levels. The spleen ruptured and had to be removed 5 days following the transplant; the cause of the rupture was not clear.[169] A great deal more investigative study must be done before it is known if there is any role for organ homografts in the treatment of hemophilia.

Proper dental hygiene should not be neglected. Dental extractions have been rendered more safe by the use of dental splints of acrylic resin.[417] These splints protect the gum and prevent the dislodgment of a clot once it has formed, thus avoiding the use of sutures. If gum margins are sutured there is a constant danger that bleeding may continue beneath the suture and dissect into the fascial planes of the neck, causing respiratory obstruction. Calcium-alginate gauze soaked in Russell viper venom may be placed between the splint and the gum to act as a local hemostatic agent. Fresh plasma or one of the available concentrates[75] is given these patients an hour before the extraction and thereafter as indicated. The use of high doses of steroids has been reported to reduce bleeding after dental extraction in patients with hemophilia.[389] Hemorrhage-free dental extraction, without the use of plasma or blood, using protective splints and carefully packing the sockets with the patient under hypnosis has been reported.[222]

Hemorrhage in the tissue of the throat, at the base of the tongue, or in the neck is usually controlled by the infusion of fresh plasma or concentrate. The possibility of respiratory obstruction should be appreciated in time to enable an endotracheal tube to be passed. Tracheostomy should be avoided if possible as it increases the danger of serious hemorrhage. The blood in these tissues does not localize and the surgeon should not attempt drainage, as such efforts result only in further bleeding and increased danger to the patient. The hemorrhage will cease and the blood will be absorbed quickly if an adequate concentration of Factor VIII is obtained. Superficial hemorrhage is controlled by the immediate application of local pressure while the infusion of fresh plasma or concentrate is started. After an elevation of the Factor VIII is obtained, the pressure should be released to allow blood with adequate Factor VIII to replace the Factor VIII deficient blood in the blocked vessels, and then reapplied.

With the increased availability of antihemophilic factor concentrates, hemophilic arthropathy is being treated more vigorously. Some have reported that synovectomy results in better joint function and reduces the frequency of hemorrhage.[197, 261, 376]

Joint hemorrhage continues to be treated as conservatively as possible. Infusion of fresh plasma or concentrates to raise the levels of Factor VIII is of great importance and, if started early, may abort the episode.[16] Bed rest, ice bags, and compression bandages on the affected joint during the acute phase all offer relief. Many feel that aspiration and lavage of the joint should be avoided as it may lead to further bleeding or infection;[372] others believe it to be of value.[107] Cautious activity with good physiotherapy as improvement occurs seems indicated. It is desirable to have the joint in the most functional position should ankylosis occur.

Surgery should be avoided if possible. Should major surgery be essential, a concentration of not under 35 per cent Factor VIII must be obtained. Since this is not possible using plasma alone, animal or human Factor VIII concentrates must be available. It is essential that surgery on these patients be carried out in centers where careful laboratory control can be exercised.[91, 123, 227]

Interpersonal problems may develop between the physician and the patient with hemophilia during long-term management. In a recent study, patients with hemophilia were found to complain most about delays in institution of infusion therapy, inadequate analgesia, and inept venipuncture by hospital staff personnel. These patients become quite expert at the diagnosis of bleeding and resent any delay in treatment.[16, 129]

Aspirin should not be given to patients with hemophilia. In some patients aspirin causes defective platelet function and the combination of this with the Factor VIII deficiency may aggravate the bleeding difficulty with serious or even catastrophic results.[190a]

Illustrative Case

HISTORY

An 18 year old white male was admitted for the first time because of continued bleeding for 6 days from the site of a tooth extraction. This young man stated that he had been told by his mother that he had been a "bleeder" since birth. He had always bled easily from minor cuts and abrasions, bruised quite easily, and had frequent nose bleeds. He had suffered "bluish" swelling of the right knee and painful hip joints. Because of his bleeding tendency, he had never been allowed to go to school. Six days prior to admission he had had a right lower molar extracted. The gum flaps were sutured as bleeding continued after the extraction. Several hours later a mass was noted at the angle of his jaw, and bleeding from the gum continued. He was seen by his physician, who referred him for treatment.

Family history revealed that his mother and father were cousins. One brother was known to have a bleeding dyscrasia. Two sisters and the other brother were normal.

PHYSICAL EXAMINATION

The patient was a thin, pale young man lying quietly in bed. Examination revealed a large clot in his mouth overlying the right gum from beneath which blood was still oozing. An indurated 3 × 4 cm. mass was palpable below the angle of the right ramus of the mandible. A large ecchymosis of the skin extended from the area occupied by the mass to the anterior chest wall on the right. There was no lymphadenopathy and no organs or masses were palpable in the abdomen.

LABORATORY EXAMINATION

Laboratory examination revealed a hematocrit of 28 per cent and white blood cell count of 5600 per cu.mm. Platelet count, bleeding time, and tourniquet test were normal. The coagulation time was 16 minutes and the prothrombin time normal. Thromboplastin generation test was abnormal when the patient's plasma was substituted for normal plasma in the incubation mixture. The patient's serum was normal. Assay revealed less than 1 per cent AHF activity. No circulating anticoagulants could be demonstrated.

Subchondral cystic change and irregularity of articulating surfaces of both hips and knees were noted by x-ray. These changes were felt to be consistent with hemophilic arthritis. A diagnosis of antihemophilic factor deficiency was made.

COURSE

The patient was transfused with 2000 ml. of fresh whole blood during the next 48 hours. The bleeding ceased and the clotting time returned to 11 minutes. A dentist removed the sutures from the gum flap and cleaned the area gently, after which a firm clot formed.

COMMENT

This case history demonstrates several features of importance. It is a classic example of the grave risks which are encountered when tooth extraction is attempted without proper preparation. The risks were compounded by the suturing of the gum flaps. This lad is fortunate to have escaped asphyxiation which might have resulted from continued bleeding *internally*—beneath the sutured flaps, with dissection of fascial planes of the neck.

The use of fresh whole blood (or plasma) or plasma concentrates to control bleeding of this sort is demonstrated to be of value. The amount of blood given would not have been expected to raise the Factor VIII concentration greatly but was adequate. It should be noted that the coagulation time returned to normal despite the fact that the Factor VIII concentration was still very low. This test may not reveal coagulation defects if they are not severe.

The social problem presented by this patient is quite apparent. His parents had been advised never to send him to school. He had had no education whatsoever and without his parents would be unable to support himself. These children should be protected from trauma, but they must not be denied an education.

The use of the thromboplastin generation test clearly separated this Factor VIII deficiency from the other defects in the first phase of coagulation.

The patient's brother was subsequently brought to the hospital and was demonstrated to have Factor VIII deficiency.

Factor IX (Plasma Thromboplastin Component, PTC) Deficiency (Christmas Disease, Hemophilia B)

The practice of comparing the coagulation characteristics of plasma from patients with undiagnosed hemorrhagic disease with those of plasma from clinically accepted cases of hemophilia in order to establish the diagnosis of hemophilia has in the past led to considerable confusion.[363] In 1947 Pavlosky[283] reported that the addition of blood from one hemophilic patient to that of another in vitro occasionally resulted in a normal coagulation time. Aggeler et al.[12] and Biggs et al.[50] later recognized that the existence of a heretofore unrecognized factor must be postulated and that the absence of this factor would produce a syndrome clinically indistinguishable from hemophilia. Factor IX has been extensively investigated. Many patients thought to have Factor VIII deficiency have now been recognized to have a deficiency of this factor.

PATHOLOGIC PHYSIOLOGY

This defect is transmitted as a sex-linked recessive with genetic possibilities similar to those described above under Factor VIII deficiency. The gene is not as recessive as that responsible for Factor VIII deficiency and symptoms may occur in female heterozygotes. Recent reports suggest that deficiency of Factor IX activity may result from qualitative as well as quantitative changes in Factor IX.[180, 314] In 90 per cent of patients with Factor IX deficiency the ability to neutralize an antibody against Factor IX was directly proportional to Factor IX activity (hemophilia$^-$). In the remaining 10 per cent the antibody neutralizing capacity was normal, indicating the presence of a molecule with the antigenic determinants of Factor IX but without Factor IX activity (hemophilia$^+$).[314]

Some of the patients with functionally inactive Factor IX have been shown to have a grossly prolonged prothrombin time if ox-brain thromboplastin is used. The functionally inactive Factor IX molecule interferes in some way with the reaction involving Factor VII and brain and provides a third way to classify patients with Factor IX deficiency (hemophilia B_m).[77, 180]

Like the Factor VIII, Factor IX takes part in the first phase of the coagulation of blood. A deficiency of this factor impedes the development of thromboplastin activity. The platelets and capillaries are unaffected and repair of small capillary rents proceeds normally.

The severity of the hemorrhagic diathesis appears to vary directly with the level of Factor IX activity. Variation in severity occurs more commonly between families than within the same family. Studies of large kindred have revealed an increase in the number of children born into those families whose members have a hemorrhagic diathesis.[401]

CLINICAL FINDINGS

These patients may present any of the problems found in Factor VIII deficiency. Manifestations of the hemorrhagic diathesis may appear at birth with bleeding from the umbilical cord, or following circumcision. Excessive bleeding will mark minor trauma and surgical procedures throughout the life of the patient.

The laboratory findings in this disorder follow the same general pattern as those in Factor VIII deficiency. The platelet count, capillary fragility, clot retraction, bleeding time, and prothrombin time are normal. The coagulation time is often prolonged, since the development of thromboplastin activity is impeded. As in Factor VIII deficiency, however, Factor IX deficient patients may have normal coagulation times. As Factor IX is not consumed during coagulation it is present in normal serum. As a consequence, the coagulation of Factor IX deficient plasma may be brought to normal in vitro by the addition of normal serum. The defect will not be corrected by the addition of $BaSO_4$-treated normal serum or plasma since $BaSO_4$ adsorbs Factor IX completely. This disorder may be identified by the thromboplastin generation test, which is based on these facts. Substitution in the incubation mixture of the patient's serum for the normal serum will prevent the normal evolution of thromboplastin activity.

Hemizygous males are most severely affected, but this gene appears to be less completely recessive than that responsible for Factor VIII deficiency and finds expression in some female heterozygotes. Female carriers may have symptoms of abnormal bleeding as well as depressed levels of Factor IX.

TREATMENT

Patients with Factor IX deficiency may have a clinical course as severe as that in patients with Factor VIII deficiency. Development of concentrated preparations of Factor IX has been needed for patients requiring therapy for control of hemorrhage since there is a constant danger of precipitating cardiac failure by infusion of massive quantities of plasma.[48, 52]

Recent reports of clinical trials of new commercially prepared concentrates have been encouraging.[136, 177] They have been recommended for management of those patients whose required level of Factor IX could not be maintained with infusions of plasma alone. Since the concentrates are prepared from pooled plasma they may transmit hepatitis.[73, 136, 177, 362, 390]

It is thought that Factor IX is stable on storage at blood bank temperatures for 2 or 3 weeks.[133, 150, 323] It has been reported that when acid-citrate dextrose plasma stored at 4° C is the source of Factor IX, the results of the thromboplastin generation test are abnormal within 14 days and normal during the first 4 days of storage only.[68] However, plasma stored at 4° C for 15 days and longer has been reported to raise the Factor IX level of patients with known Factor IX deficiency.[150] The results of plasma transfusions as measured by the assay of Factor IX are often disappointing and the clinical response can be better than expected from the assay level. Serum which can be shown to be a good source of Factor IX in vitro has been demonstrated to be ineffective in the treatment of Factor IX deficiency. The reason for this is not clear.[269] The comments that have been made on the clinical management of Factor VIII deficiency apply equally to the management of this disorder.

Factor XI (Plasma Thromboplastin Antecedent, PTA) Deficiency

Factor XI deficiency was described by Rosenthal in 1953.[325] The clinical findings are similar to those of Factor VIII and Factor IX deficiency but the hemostatic defect is usually less severe.

PATHOLOGIC PHYSIOLOGY

Factor XI deficiency is genetically transmitted as an autosomal dominant with incomplete expression.[210, 325] Reception of the abnormal gene from either parent will produce the disease. The disorder may occur in either sex, as the gene is not carried on the sex chromosome. The patient will have a 50 per cent chance of passing the disorder to his or her offspring. The gene has a high degree of penetrance and variable expression. This indicates that the gene will more than likely manifest itself if present but that the seriousness of the defect will vary.[324, 325]

Factor XI deficiency, like Factor IX or Factor VIII deficiency, interferes with the development of adequate thromboplastin activity during the first phase of coagulation. Factor XI activity has been reported to increase in the plasma 4 to 5 hours following a fat-rich meal.[114]

CLINICAL ASPECTS

Patients of either sex present with a bleeding diathesis similar to Factor VIII and Factor IX deficiency. The bleeding episodes are neither so frequent nor so severe as those encountered in patients with Factor VIII and Factor IX deficiency and there appear to be periods when bleeding does not occur despite major trauma. Menorrhagia may be a serious feature. The bleeding diathesis is usually of equal severity in various members of the family. Rarely epistaxis or post-traumatic bleeding may be life-threatening.[84] There is no absolute relationship between the Factor XI level and the occurrence of bleeding.[210] An asymptomatic patient with less than 1 per cent Factor XI activity has been reported.[113]

The laboratory findings follow the same general pattern as that described for Factor VIII or Factor IX deficiency. The platelet count, capillary fragility test, bleeding time, clot retraction, and fibrinogen assay are all normal. The coagulation time may reflect the impaired thromboplastin activity.[268]

Unlike Factor VIII, Factor XI is not consumed during coagulation, and with Factor IX is present in both plasma and serum. Factor XI, however, is not adsorbed from normal plasma by $BaSO_4$; Factor IX is adsorbed. Consequently, the clotting time of Factor XI deficient plasma is corrected by $BaSO_4$-treated normal plasma, which does not correct the clotting time of Factor IX deficient plasma. It is also corrected by the addition of normal serum, which would not correct the clotting time of Factor VIII deficient plasma. The three disorders may be separated by the thromboplastin generation test, the design of which makes use of these facts. No defect is apparent when the patient's adsorbed plasma or serum is incubated with normal serum or adsorbed plasma respectively. The defect is discovered when the patient's adsorbed plasma and serum are tested together.

TREATMENT

These patients are successfully treated with plasma stored up to 14 days since Factor XI fares well on storage. The effect of the administered plasma is gradually lost over a period of a week to 10 days. If surgery cannot be avoided, these patients should be carefully prepared. It has been suggested that levels of 50 per cent Factor XI are necessary to maintain hemostasis if extensive surgery is contemplated.[299] It was found that 4.5 ml. of fresh frozen plasma per kg. body weight raised the level of Factor XI by 10 per cent. The half-life of the infused activity was up to 60 hours.[299, 324, 326] There is a tendency for secondary bleeding to occur 2 to 3 days after surgery and smaller amounts of plasma may be indicated at intervals following surgery.[287]

Circulating Anticoagulants

Severe hemorrhagic symptoms may be caused by the development of circulating anticoagulants. They interfere with the development of thromboplastin activity and may produce any of the findings noted to occur as the result of deficiencies of those coagulation factors concerned with the development of thromboplastin activity. When circulating anticoagulants occur in patients with preexisting hemorrhagic diathesis, the treatment is made far more difficult. Although there may be no increase in the number of hemorrhagic episodes, the treatment of each episode is complicated by the need to overcome the effect of the circulating anticoagulant as well as treat the original defect. Circulating anticoagulants developing during or subsequent to pregnancy may produce a severe hemorrhagic diathesis which persists for months or years.[272] There have been reports of circulating anticoagulants occurring in association with a heterogeneous group of disorders including syphilis, disseminated lupus erythematosus,[72] chronic nephritis, tuberculous lymphadenopathy, and the collagen diseases.[127, 209, 221, 241] Rarely they may develop spontaneously in persons without known disease.

CLINICAL FINDINGS

These patients may have any of the physical findings associated with the other disorders affecting the formation of thromboplastin activity or its function. Once again it is in the laboratory that positive identification of the disorder is made. Since the vascular phase of hemostasis is unaffected, the platelet count, bleeding time, tourniquet test and, if fibrinogen is unaffected, clot retraction are normal. Fibrinogen assay is abnormal if the anticoagulant is directed against fibrinogen. Interference by the circulating anticoagulant with the formation of thromboplastin activity results in an abnormal thromboplastin generation test. Diminished formation of thromboplastin activity occurs when the patient's serum or adsorbed plasma is substituted in the incubation mixture. The use of 50 per cent normal and 50 per cent patient's adsorbed plasma with normal serum in the incubation mixture results in diminished formation of thromboplastin activity. The presence of a circulating anticoagulant is thereby identified, as any genetic defect likely to be confused with it would have been corrected by the addition of 50 per cent normal adsorbed plasma. Assays of specific factors before and after incubation will identify the factor which is the target of the inhibitor. Some of the antibodies are slow acting and the incubation period should be at least 1 hour.[42]

Heparin-like compounds may be differentiated from circulating anticoagulants by the addition to the plasma of protamine sulfate or toluidine blue which neutralizes the heparin-like compounds and leaves circulating anticoagulants unaffected.

PATHOLOGIC PHYSIOLOGY

The circulating anticoagulants have been shown to interfere with the reactions leading to the formation of thromboplastin activity in the intrinsic system.[58, 125, 178, 186] Others have suggested they may also interfere with the action of formed thromboplastin.[118, 127, 209, 241]

The circulating anticoagulants are believed to result from some immunologic mechanism.[97, 158, 178, 209, 402] They are present in the gamma fraction of the plasma and several recent reports have identified them in the IgG_4 subclass in acquired hemophilia.[23, 345, 379, 393] The finding of circulating anticoagulants in patients treated repeatedly with blood or blood products, following pregnancy, and in association with diseases known to have deranged immunologic mechanisms, particularly in disseminated lupus erythematosus, has lent substance to this theory. In one study the level of the inhibitor rose sharply 4 to 5 days after plasma infusion, peaked at 10 to 14 days, and slowly declined. The magnitude and timing of the inhibitor varied among the patients studied and was used as a guide in therapy.[377, 379] There are, however, instances in which such a mechanism does not seem to operate and the mechanism is unclear.[89, 178]

Circulating anticoagulants are relatively heat stable and fare well on storage at 0 to 4° for long periods of time. Circulating anticoagulants against Factor VIII are most common, but anticoagulants against Factor IX, Factor V, Factor VII, Factor XI, Factor XIII, and fibrinogen (Factor I) have been described, as well as those reportedly interfering with thromboplastin activity.[315] In those instances when circulating anticoagulants interfere with Factor V, Factor VII, or thromboplastin activity itself, the one stage prothrombin time will of course be prolonged.

TREATMENT

Treatment of these patients is the same as that employed in other disorders interfering with the formation of blood thromboplastin activity. Occasionally massive transfusions of fresh blood effect a response when smaller ones do not. The deficiency of specific clotting factors secondary to circulating anticoagulants should be treated with specific factor concentrates if they are available, using the level of inhibitor activity as a guide to therapy.[379]

Constant infusion of Factor VIII concentrates which takes advantage of the time dependent antigen-antibody reaction seen in acquired hemophilia has been shown to be helpful in some cases. However, porcine and bovine Factor VIII are probably the best therapy in life-threatening hemorrhages.[356a] Adrenocortical steroids have not been used with striking success but should be tried.[40]

A recent study noted one transient partial remission and two complete remissions following immunosuppressive therapy in the non-hemophilic patients with circulating anti-Factor VIII who were unresponsive to conventional therapy.[350]

Disorders Affecting Both the First and Second Stages of Blood Coagulation

The disorders to be discussed in this section affect both the first and second stages of blood coagulation. The thromboplastin generation test and the one stage prothrombin time test are abnormal. Both disorders may be hereditary or acquired.

Factor V Deficiency (Parahemophilia)

Factor V deficiency was first demonstrated to be a distinct clinical entity by Owren[277] in 1947. The young woman whose disorder he reported suffered from epistaxis, easy bruising, and excessive menstrual bleeding. The one stage prothrombin time was prolonged and was not shortened by the addition of prothrombin. It was corrected, however, by the addition of a prothrombin-free plasma fraction obtained from a normal source. Thus was it demonstrated that a deficiency of a factor other than prothrombin could not only prolong the one stage prothrombin time but could produce a serious clinical disorder as well.

PATHOLOGIC PHYSIOLOGY

Factor V deficiency may be congenital or acquired. The congenital form is thought to be transmitted as an autosomal recessive although the abnormal gene has a potency roughly equal to the normal counterpart. There is a high degree of variation in expressivity, which is thought responsible for the finding of some heterozygotes with hemorrhagic symptoms although in others the carrier state is not detectable.[202] Consanguinity has been noted to be a feature of some of the family pedigrees. Congenital Factor V deficiency has been reported to occur in association with congenital Factor VIII deficiency.[341]

The acquired form of the disorder has been reported in association with severe liver damage and a variety of other diseases.[278, 369] Notably the level of Factor V is depressed in association with fibrinolysis and certain instances of acquired fibrinogen deficiency. As Factor V is essential to the first phase of blood coagulation, its deficiency will result in the inadequate production of thromboplastin activity. Fantl[116] has reported that abnormal bleeding will occur when the level of Factor V falls below 30 per cent of normal. Serum does not contain Factor V because it is consumed during the process of blood coagulation.

Indirect evidence points to the liver as the normal source of Factor V and acquired deficiencies have been reported in severe liver disease. The factor is not vitamin K dependent and deficiency of Factor V does not occur in obstructive jaundice or during the administration of coumarin drugs.

A specific inhibitor of Factor V has been reported in the plasma and serum of an elderly female under treatment of tuberculosis.[217]

CLINICAL FINDINGS

In a review of the reported cases of congenital Factor V deficiency,[116] it was noted that bleeding occurs in the first few years of life. Bleeding from accidental or operative trauma was excessive and spontaneous bleeding into the genitourinary tract and the gastrointestinal tract was noted. Hemarthrosis was not common. Menstrual bleeding is found to be excessive and may be life-threatening. The clinical findings of the acquired form of the disorder are similar to those of the congenital variety, complicated of course by the underlying disease.

The vascular phase of hemostasis is unaffected. Platelets are normal in number and function and the bleeding time and tourniquet test are normal. There is no quantitative or qualitative defect in fibrinogen. Since Factor V deficiency affects the first stage of coagulation, it is reflected in an abnormal thromboplastin generation test. The one stage prothrombin time is prolonged since Factor V is essential for the normal evolution of thrombin from prothrombin under the conditions of the test. Inadequate formation of thromboplastin activity is responsible for the abnormal coagulation time.

The laboratory findings in the acquired form of the disorder will of course be modified by the associated disease.

TREATMENT

Treatment consists of the administration of fresh plasma by the intravenous route. Fantl[116] has reported that it is necessary in the case of complete deficiency to administer 10 ml. of fresh citrated human plasma per kilogram of body weight in order to attain adequate levels. The half-life of the Factor V is reported to be approximately 20 hours.

Factor X (Stuart Factor) Deficiency

In 1957, Hougie, Barrow, and Graham[179] restudied a patient thought to suffer from a deficiency of Factor VII. Their careful work established the heterogeneity of the coagulation defects in the patients in this group. A new blood clotting factor was uncovered and its properties detailed in their report.

PATHOLOGIC PHYSIOLOGY

Factor X deficiency is transmitted by an incompletely recessive autosomal gene.[147] Although most severe in the homozygote, bleeding tendencies have been noted in the heterozygote and carriers can often be detected with appropriate tests. Factor X deficiency, like that of Factors VIII and IX and fibrinogen, can result from a qualitative as well as a quantitative abnormality. The plasma of some patients with Factor X deficiency has been demonstrated to have a protein which is antigenically similar to Factor X though functionally inactive.[105]

Factor X deficiency is more commonly an acquired defect. With the other vitamin K-dependent factors (II, VII, and IX), Factor X will be reduced by anything which interferes with the metabolic function of vitamin K. It may also be one of a variety of proteins whose synthesis is affected by liver disease.

Rarely, an isolated deficiency of Factor X may develop. A temporary deficiency of Factor X developed in one patient presumably as the result of contact with a farm insecticide.[149] In another report, a 10 year old boy suddenly developed a severe hemorrhagic diathesis as the result of an acquired deficiency of Factor X. The defect persisted 6 months, after which Factor X reappeared. No inhibitor could be detected and no cause discovered despite extensive studies.[38]

Factor X is essential in the first phase of blood coagulation and a deficiency of the factor is demonstrated by the thromboplastin generation test. The defect is apparent when the patient's serum is substituted for normal serum in the incubation mixture. Factor X is adsorbed by $BaSO_4$ from normal plasma. As $BaSO_4$-treated plasma is used in performance of the test, the defect is not detectable when the patient's $BaSO_4$-treated plasma is substituted for normal. Both normal and patient plasma are deficient in Factor X under conditions of the test. Factor X is present in normal serum as it is not consumed in coagulation and substitution of the patient's serum for normal serum in the incubation mixture reveals the defect. The one stage prothrombin time is prolonged since Factor X, as well as Factors II, V and VII is essential for optimal development of thromboplastin activity from the usual tissue sources and platelets.[229]

Factor X has been shown to be vitamin K dependent and is reduced after several days of administration of coumarin drugs.[109] The average intravascular half-life of Factor X has been reported to be 32.5 hours. Extravascular diffusion occurs, as demonstrated by the appearance of the factor in the lymph of a patient with Factor X deficiency following transfusion of normal plasma.[145, 313]

CLINICAL FINDINGS

The patients described have had a moderate bleeding diathesis. Though hemorrhagic symptoms may occur in childhood, clinical manifestation of the disorder may not appear until later in life. Frequent epistaxis and hematoma have been most disturbing. Hemarthrosis has been reported but is mild and infrequent. Although the defect is most severe in the homozygote, it is important to note that heterozygotes with hemorrhagic symptoms have been reported. These patients, usually female, have been noted to be bad operative risks and to have persistent anemia presumably secondary to menorrhagia.

The bleeding time, tourniquet test, and platelets are normal. Fibrinogen is quantitatively and qualitatively normal. The whole blood clotting time and thromboplastin generation test are abnormal, owing to deficient formation of blood thromboplastin activity. One stage prothrombin time is prolonged, as Factor X is required for evolution of optimal tissue thromboplastin activity.

TREATMENT

Transfusion with whole blood or plasma is effective in relieving symptoms. As Factor X is relatively stable, it is not necessary to use freshly prepared material. The general management of these patients is similar to that of those with antihemophilic factor deficiency.

Recently a new concentrate of clotting Factors II, VII, IX, and X has become available and is effective in the treatment of Factor X deficiency. It should be used only if hemostatic levels of Factor X cannot be maintained with plasma alone, as some of the material is reported to transmit hepatitis.[73, 136, 362, 390]

Disorders Affecting Predominantly the First or Second Stage of Blood Coagulation

The following disorders affect predominantly the first or second stage of blood coagulation and result in an abnormal one stage prothrombin time test. Although congenital prothrombin deficiency is recognized, it is extremely rare. Many cases formerly thought to represent congenital deficiency of prothrombin have on retesting in light of present knowledge proved to be deficiencies of Factor V, Factor X, or Factor VII.

Factor VII Deficiency

In 1951, Alexander, Goldstein, Landwehr, and Cook reported the first patient recognized to have a congenital deficiency of Factor VII.[14, 140] The characteristic defect noted was a prolonged one stage prothrombin time corrected by normal plasma or serum but not by $BaSO_4$-treated plasma. Since the two stage prothrombin time was consistently normal, it was recognized that the defect could not be due to a prothrombin deficiency. As $BaSO_4$-treated plasma contains Factor V, its failure to correct the prolonged one stage prothrombin time established the syndrome as distinct from Owren's Factor V deficiency as well.

Since 1951, a number of case reports have appeared in the literature described as Factor VII deficiency. All had prolonged one stage prothrombin times uncorrected by $BaSO_4$-treated plasma, but results of other coagulation tests varied. A third factor (Factor X) has been shown to be necessary for optimum development of thromboplastin activity under the conditions of one stage prothrombin time test.[118] Some of the cases formerly designated Factor VII deficiency have now been reexamined and found to be deficient not in Factor VII but in Factor X. Much of the confusion in the literature prior to 1957 relative to Factor VII deficiency can now be resolved.

PATHOLOGIC PHYSIOLOGY

Factor VII deficiency is inherited co-dominantly. Homozygotes have a hemorrhagic diathesis and have Factor VII levels of 10 per cent or less. Heterozygotes usually have no clinical symptoms and have Factor VII levels of about 50 per cent.[144, 170]

It seems clear from the studies carried out on the blood of patients with Factor VII deficiency that this factor, although necessary for optimal development of extrinsic thromboplastin activity, is not required for the development of intrinsic thromboplastin activity. Normal clotting time and thromboplastin generation test are therefore understandable. The presence of hemorrhagic symptoms in these patients attests to the importance of the development of optimal extrinsic thromboplastin activity in the physiologic defense of hemostasis.[3]

Factor VII is thought to be formed in the liver and is vitamin K dependent. It may be diminished in severe liver disease and is rapidly reduced during the administration of coumarin drugs.[109] Recent studies indicate the half-life of Factor VII in normal man to be 7.2 to 10.8 hours.[128] A two component decay curve has been reported following rapid infusion of a Factor VII concentrate into patients with congenital Factor VII deficiency.[233] The first component, with a half-life of 35 minutes, probably represents equilibration with the extravascular space, and the second, with a half-life of 300 minutes, the metabolic decay phase. The clinical and laboratory findings in acquired Factor VII deficiency would of course reflect the primary disorder in addition to presenting those of the congenital deficiency.

CLINICAL FINDINGS

Patients with Factor VII deficiency may have the onset of abnormal bleeding in infancy and hemorrhage from the cord has been noted. Gastrointestinal hemorrhage, easy bruising, and frequent epistaxis are common. These patients may also have mild hemarthroses. The tourniquet test and platelets are normal. In the majority of the patients, bleeding time is normal; but in as many as one-third it may be prolonged. This finding cannot be explained at present. The thromboplastin generation test is normal in Factor VII deficiency but abnormal in Factor X deficiency. The one stage prothrombin time is prolonged and not corrected by the addition of $BaSO_4$-treated normal plasma (containing Factor V). In the Stypven time test the venom of the Russell's viper will correct the prothrombin time of Factor VII deficient plasma, but not that of Factor X deficient plasma. The laboratory findings of acquired Factor VII deficiency will of course reflect the underlying pathology in addition.

TREATMENT

Administration of fresh blood or plasma to patients with a congenital defect of Factor VII has been effective. The effects are short-lived and the prothrombin time returns to pre-transfusion levels within 24 hours.[140] Maintenance of a Factor VII concentration of 15 to 20 per cent by the infusion of plasma or plasma concentrates to patients with congenital Factor VII deficiency has been reported sufficient to control spontaneous as well as operative hemorrhage.[233]

Factor VII deficiency secondary to anticoagulant coumarin drugs will respond to vitamin K_1 administration.

It seems unlikely that the recently available concentrate of Factors II, VII, IX, and X would be needed in the treatment of patients with this defect.[73, 136, 177, 362, 390]

Factor II Deficiency (Prothrombin Deficiency)

In 1934 Dam and Schonheyder[20, 102] noted that chicks raised on an artificial diet had a hemorrhagic diathesis unaffected by ascorbic acid. The following year Dam[101] proposed the name vitamin K for the antihemorrhagic factor deficient in the diet and noted that it was fat soluble. Many compounds have been found to have vitamin K activity. All of these compounds are essentially derivatives of 2-methyl, 1, 4-naphthoquinone. They differ from the synthetic menadione by having a group substituted in the 3-position and from each other by the nature of the group. Vitamin K_1, which is 2-methyl, 3-phytyl, 1, 4-naphthoquinone, was isolated from alfalfa and Vitamin K_2 from putrefying fish meal.[18, 76] Vitamin K_1 and menadione are both used clinically.

PATHOLOGIC PHYSIOLOGY

Congenital hypoprothrombinemia exists but is extremely rare.[60, 196, 291] It is inherited as an autosomal trait and is usually a mild disorder. The level of prothrombin has varied and the severity of the symptoms seems to reflect the level of prothrombin. There has been one report of a structural disorder of the prothrombin molecule. The hereditary pattern was autosomal and all of the affected patients were heterozygotes. The immunologically detectable abnormal molecule underwent some change during the activation but was unable to release the active enzyme thrombin.[346]

The acquired form of the deficiency is vastly more common and usually the result of liver disease or some disturbance in vitamin K metabolism.

It is not possible to produce a significant dietary deficiency of vitamin K in man as the intestinal bacteria produce sufficient vitamin to cover the daily needs. A deficiency will become apparent in any situation wherein the vitamin cannot be absorbed from the intestinal tract, however. Vitamin K is fat soluble and its absorption from the intestinal tract is impaired by disorders which result in a decrease in bile acids and consequent decrease in fat absorption.[300] Loss of large quantities of fat in the stool will likewise lead to loss of the vitamin. The occurrence of vitamin K deficiency in patients receiving wide spectrum antibiotics over long periods of time with sterilization of the intestinal tract and loss of vitamin K-producing bacteria has been reported when associated with a vitamin K-deficient diet.

Severe liver disease may also result in an abnormal prothrombin time. In these cases there is an adequate amount of the vitamin, but the reactions in which it takes part in the liver are impaired.

The administration of anticoagulant drugs may produce the same effects as vitamin K deficiency. Anything which interferes with the availability of vitamin K, such as poor nutrition, malabsorption syndrome, oral antibiotics which alter normal bacterial flora, or biliary or liver disease, will increase susceptibility to these drugs. The administration of salicylate, phenylbutazone and oxyphenylbutazone, quinine, or quinidine can reduce the prothrombin complex of normal people or of patients with liver disease and can act to potentiate the effect of oral anticoagulants.[35, 204, 216, 382] Rarely, isolated prothrombin deficiency may be acquired.[192, 214]

Prothrombin, Factor VII, Factor IX, and Factor X levels are below normal during the first 6 weeks of life.[2, 3] Although most investigators have found a rise in these factors following the administration of vitamin K to the mother in labor or to the newborn infant, others[124] have failed to achieve this result. It has been suggested[196, 399] that the low concentration of these factors in the neonatal period could be responsible for some instances of hemorrhagic disease of the newborn.[2, 3] Though this point is not yet settled[124] it is common practice to administer a routine prophylactic dose of 1 or 2 mg. vitamin K to all infants at birth. Since human milk contains less vitamin K than cow's milk, this appears to be of particular importance to breast-fed infants.[381] Some types of soy bean protein formula have been found to have lower concentrations of vitamin K than others and may contribute to the problem.[256] Large doses of vitamin K (over 5 mg.) have been reported to increase serum bilirubin levels and the risk of kernicterus in premature infants and should be avoided.[246]

CLINICAL EXAMINATION

Hypoprothrombinemia may result in a hemorrhagic diathesis manifested by bleeding from the gums, nose, or gastrointestinal tract. Hemarthrosis, hematemesis, and soft tissue bleeding have been recorded. There may be severe hemorrhage after surgical trauma. Excessive menstrual flow is also a common finding.

A prolongation of the one stage prothrombin time is found in these disorders. The thromboplastin generation test should be normal and the modified thromboplastin generation test will indicate a deficiency of prothrombin. Fibrinogen assays are normal.

TREATMENT

Blood transfusions should be given in emergency situations and will serve to treat shock, correct anemia, and aid in restoration of missing coagulation factors. The new concentrate containing Factors II, VII, IX, and X is available and would serve to restore the missing coagulation factors. Since this material is prepared from pooled plasma there is the danger of the transmission of hepatitis.[136, 362]

It has been found,[302] contrary to the original report,[19] that natural vitamin K_1 (2-methyl, 3-phytyl, 1, 4-naphthoquinone) (phytonadione) is more effective than the synthetic vitamin K (menadione).

Vitamin K_1 may be given by the intramuscular, subcutaneous, or intravenous route. It is given slowly by the intravenous route in severe deficiencies when bleeding is imminent or has occurred. The time needed for a response to the drug to be demonstrable depends on the cause of the deficiency and the amount of vitamin administered. Generally bleeding is controlled in 3 to 6 hours. A 1 ml. ampule contains 10 mg. vitamin K_1. It is recommended that 25 to 50 mg. be administered slowly at a rate not exceeding 5 mg. per min. as severe toxic reactions have occurred with rapid intravenous administration.

Vitamin K_1 is also available in 5 mg. tablets for oral administration in non-emergency situations. Five to 10 mg. is given initially and the dosage adjusted depending on the clinical situation. In the presence of obstructive jaundice or biliary fistula the concomitant administration of bile salts is necessary when the drug is given by mouth.

Synthetic vitamin K (menadione), supplied as the sodium salt of 2 methyl, 1, 4-naphthohydroquinone, is a water soluble compound. It is supplied in 0.5 ml. ampules containing 2.5 mg. and in 1 ml. ampules containing 5 or 10 mg. It may be administered subcutaneously, intramuscularly, or intravenously. A 10 ml. ampule containing 72 mg. is available for intravenous administration in emergency situations.

Illustrative Case

This 10 year old child was admitted to the hospital for investigation of a hemorrhagic diathesis. At birth she had a severe hemorrhage from the umbilicus and over the succeeding years recurrent episodes of epistaxis, gastrointestinal hemorrhages, and multiple hematomas. Excessive bleeding often followed minor trauma but hemarthroses had not occurred.

Physical examination revealed only the presence of multiple bruises on the lower legs.

LABORATORY EXAMINATION

Erythrocyte count 4.58 mil. per cu.mm., leukocyte count 9880 per cu.mm., hemoglobin 10.5 gm. per 100 ml. Tourniquet test, bleeding time, clot retraction, and coagulation time were normal. Platelet count (indirect) 261,000 per cu.mm. Quick one stage prothrombin time was 54 seconds with a control of 14 seconds.

On her first admission at the age of 5 years, it was thought that she had idiopathic hypoprothrombinemia on the basis of the data then available.

During a subsequent admission, it was found that when normal plasma was mixed with that of the patient the prothrombin time was reduced but did not return to normal. The addition of "purified" prothrombin did not result in a normal one stage prothrombin time. One part of serum when mixed with three parts of the patient's plasma resulted in a normal one stage prothrombin time. On the basis of these studies it was felt that the patient probably had a Factor V deficiency.

The patient was then followed at another hospital where it was realized that she could not represent a Factor V deficiency since the one stage prothrombin time was corrected by the addition of normal serum and not by normal plasma. Factor VII was described at that time and it was noted that the clinical and laboratory findings of this patient fitted well with those of the Factor VII deficiency state. She was then carried as a Factor VII deficiency until the thromboplastin generation test became available. Once again the patient was reevaluated. It was concluded that a deficiency of Factor X was responsible for her hemorrhagic diathesis.

COMMENT

This case illustrates the growth of our knowledge of the first and second stage of blood coagulation. The patient was known to have abnormal bleeding which was not related to platelet or vessel factors. She was studied extensively with all of the tests available during each hospitalization. A diagnosis of idiopathic hypoprothrombinemia was made when she was first admitted on the basis of the Quick one stage prothrombin time test. It was not until the thromboplastin generation test became available and it was found that the substitution of this patient's serum for normal serum in the incubation mixture resulted in a reduction in thromboplastin activity that the patient could be identified as having a Factor X defect.

Disorders Affecting the Third Stage of Blood Coagulation

Fibrinogen deficiency may be either congenital or acquired. The congenital variety is quite rare. Acquired fibrinogen deficiencies are more common and usually present as complications of certain surgical procedures or obstetrical accidents and are of grave importance.

Congenital Quantitative Fibrinogen Deficiency

PATHOLOGIC PHYSIOLOGY

Congenital fibrinogen deficiency appears to be genetically transmitted as a non-sex-linked recessive. In many of the reported cases the family history revealed consanguineous marriages in parents or grandparents.[15, 137, 224, 297]

In these cases the absence of fibrinogen prevents the coagulation process from completing its final phase, i.e., the conversion of fibrinogen to the fibrin clot. Thus coagulation cannot occur. The arrest of small vessel hemorrhage is normal as it is brought about by vasoconstriction and platelet thrombi.[162] Menstrual bleeding is normal and seems to be controlled by vasoconstriction of endometrial arterioles.[213] These patients have been shown to have a decrease in synthesis of fibrinogen rather than an increase in its destruction. Minute traces of fibrinogen have been detected immunochemically in the blood and connective tissues of some of these patients and the defect may not be absolute in all instances.[137] Others have been unable to detect fibrinogen by any method.[162]

CLINICAL EXAMINATION

The disorder is often manifested at birth by the occurrence of bleeding from the umbilical cord.[162, 224, 297, 339] The condition resembles Factor VIII deficiency clinically but is usually less severe.[15] Persistent bleeding may occur, however, in the wake of minor trauma and spontaneous bleeding may occur into joint spaces or soft tissues. Crippling hemarthroses do not occur in this disorder.[224, 297] The thromboplastin generation test is normal since there is no defect in the early stage of clotting. Platelet count, tourniquet test, and bleeding time are likewise unaffected by the absence of fibrinogen. The whole blood clotting time, one stage prothrombin time, and thrombin time all require a fibrin clot as an end point and are abnormal in the absence of fibrinogen. Fibrinogen assay reveals only minute traces of fibrinogen or a complete absence.

TREATMENT

The hemostatic defect in patients with congenital fibrinogen deficiency can be corrected by the administration of fibrinogen. Half of the fibrinogen administered intravenously to patients with congenital afibrinogenemia has been reported to be lost in 48 hours and thereafter it disappears with a half-life of approximately 4 days.[213] The early loss of half of the administered fibrinogen is thought to represent equilibration with the extravascular compartment.[137] The mass of plasma protein located in extravascular spaces is approximately equal to the mass of plasma protein circulating within the blood vessels and the two are in dynamic equilibrium. As the extravascular deficit must be made up as well as that of the intravascular compartment, the first dose of fibrinogen administered will have less effect on the plasma fibrinogen level than will subsequent doses of comparable size. Transfusions of whole blood should be given to replace blood loss if need be.[297]

Congenital Qualitative Fibrinogen Abnormality

There have been several reports of inherited qualitative abnormalities in plasma fibrinogen.[122, 230, 242, 255, 398] Most of the reported individuals had no personal or family history of hemorrhagic diathesis. A few reports indicate a mild hemorrhagic diathesis and some of the reported patients had thrombosis.[122] The defect is characterized by delayed aggregation of fibrin monomers. It is transmitted as an autosomal dominant and in the heterozygotes a normal fibrinogen fraction can be identified.[398] A specific amino acid substitution has been identified in the plasma fibrinogen of one patient.[230]

Acquired Fibrinogen Deficiency

PATHOLOGIC PHYSIOLOGY

The mechanism by which the blood becomes depleted of fibrinogen in these conditions has been extensively studied. The fibrinogen level may be reduced as the result of deficient production (as in severe liver disease), excessive utilization (as in intravascular coagulation), increased destruction (as occurs in primary pathologic fibrinolysis), or some combination of these mechanisms.[37, 90, 298, 311, 312, 334, 351, 406] Separation of excessive utilization from excessive destruction is difficult but clinically important.

Liver injury has been known for many years to result in a decrease in plasma fibrinogen,[412] and some patients with severe hepatocellular disease have been found to have low levels of fibrinogen. It has been emphasized that the liver disease must be severe for the hypofibrinogenemia to occur and that when it occurs the association is seldom in doubt.[244]

Widespread intravascular coagulation may stimulate fibrinolysis, which further reduces clotting Factors I, V, VIII, and X as the result of proteolysis.[240, 290, 334, 348] Proteolytic digestion of fibrinogen and fibrin results in split products, which are in themselves anticoagulant since they interfere with thrombin activity, platelet function, and fibrin polymerization.[348]

The syndrome of primary pathologic fibrinolysis is now considered responsible for hypofibrinogenemia in just a minority of patients.[347] The disturbance in hemostasis is not so profound as that associated with diffuse intravascular coagulation. Primary pathologic fibrinolysis may occur as the result of the administration of excessive amounts of exogenous activator during thrombolytic therapy,[351] the release of excessive endogenous activator from neoplastic tissue[384] or severe shock or anoxia.[351] Failure of the liver to remove circulating activators may also result in excessive proteolysis.[37, 311, 312, 351, 406]

Sharp et al.[349] have noted that a portion of the plasma fibrinogen may be physiologically inert during the early phases of this syndrome. Laboratory methods which quantitatively measure the level of fibrinogen may not be adequate and a test which measures the reactivity of the fibrinogen to thrombin is preferred.

CLINICAL EXAMINATION

Acquired hypofibrinogenemia may be seen in association with diffuse hepatocellular disease, diffuse intravascular coagulation, or primary pathologic fibrinolysis. The clinical and laboratory findings are those of anemia, thrombosis, hemorrhage, and the underlying disease. The occurrence of hypocoagulable or incoagulable blood in a patient previously free of hemorrhagic diathesis is dramatic in the acute form and it is important to emphasize the suddenness with which the syndrome may arise. In the subacute or chronic form it may go on for days or weeks.[33, 244]

Severe hemorrhage has been noted primarily in obstetrical patients with the acute form of the syndrome. It may develop suddenly during labor or shortly thereafter and is manifested by generalized bleeding and incoagulability of the blood. The acute form has been seen most frequently following abruptio placenta,[245, 334, 406] in association with amniotic fluid emboli,[311] and in septic abortion.[245] The condition has also been reported following pulmonary resections, allergic reactions, purpura fulminans, incompatible blood transfusions, septicemia and severe burns.[30, 384, 385]

Patients with neoplastic disease and women with retained products of conception generally have the subacute or chronic form, with excessive bruising, bleeding from the gums and nose, and thrombosis of superficial or deep veins.

Reduced levels of fibrinogen may occur in the course of severe liver disease as the result of diminished production and increased fibrinolysis secondary to a reduction in the capacity of the liver to remove circulating plasminogen activator.[351]

Laboratory tests commonly used to demonstrate fibrinogen deficiency employ the fibrin clot. Observation of the clot can be of valuable assistance since the clot initially appears to form normally, then retracts rapidly to a small residual strand of fibrin; the clot may be disrupted easily. The fibrinogen titer is one of the most reliable tests. Normal plasma when diluted 1:64 with saline (and often in the 1:128 dilution) will clot following the addition of thrombin; plasma from patients with fibrinogen deficiency will fail to clot even at low dilutions. The thrombin clotting time of plasma is often prolonged (normal is 10 to 12 seconds) but is less sensitive than the fibrinogen titer.

Blood coagulation Factors V, VIII and X and platelets are frequently reduced during the acute phase of the syndrome.[335] Plasminogen levels are usually low and fibrinolytic split products can often be demonstrated immunologically.[244]

TREATMENT

Most defibrination is the result of a limited episode of coagulation or lysis and a spontaneous return of the blood to normal is expected. No specific therapy to replace fibrinogen, inhibit coagulation, or interfere with fibrinolysin is necessary in the absence of bleeding unless major surgery is anticipated.[352]

Usually heparin therapy will promptly reverse the manifestation of the syndrome of diffuse intravascular coagulation responsible for the reduction of fibrinogen levels in the vast majority of patients and tide the patient over while the underlying disease is being treated. Heparin interferes with intravascular coagulation and thereby reduces secondary fibrinolysis.[190, 240, 351]

If bleeding has been a major manifestation of the syndrome, transfusions may be necessary. Unless fresh whole blood is available, packed red cells from stored bank blood may be used to replace red cell loss. The volume is replaced by fresh frozen plasma which contains Factors V and VIII, which are often deficient in this syndrome and are in low concentration in the plasma of stored bank blood. Although thrombocytopenia rarely requires specific therapy, platelet transfusion is occasionally necessary.

Administration of fibrinogen may be indicated after the coagulation process is controlled if the patient continues to bleed due to the residual incoagulable blood. It is contraindicated if fibrinogen is still present and active, since it might theoretically increase the amount of thrombosis.[240] Since fibrinogen is prepared from pooled plasma, its administration is accompanied by a high risk of hepatitis.[286]

Primary pathologic fibrinolysis may be treated with ε-aminocaproic acid (EACA) which will inhibit activation of plasminogen and allow time for the treatment of the underlying disorders. This drug is contraindicated in the presence of diffuse intravascular coagulation since it will prevent the removal of locally deposited fibrin and may augment thrombus formation.[240, 262, 351, 395]

The clinical and hematological problems vary so much from patient to patient that no standard therapy is possible. Acquired hypofibrinogenemia is a manifestation of some underlying disorder that must be controlled to allow time to discover and treat the primary disease process. The differential diagnosis of the defibrination syndrome is often so difficult that the careful use of heparin and ε-aminocaproic acid together has been suggested.[240, 351]

Illustrative Case

History. In December, 1963, this 45 year old hosewife was admitted to the University Hospital for the second time because of migratory phlebitis of seven months' duration.

She first developed superficial thrombophlebitis in April, 1963, while in another hospital under observation for intermittent hypertension. Recurrent episodes of superficial and deep phlebitis over the next few weeks, despite the use of oral anticoagulants, prompted her first University Hospital admission in May, 1963. At that time her left leg was edematous to the buttock and there was induration of the skin over the calf. Homan's sign was negative. The leg was cool and pale and unaffected by position. Physical examination was otherwise negative. Laboratory studies at that time were: hematocrit 36 per cent, hemoglobin 10.1 gm. per cent, leukocyte count 12,200 per cm., and platelet count 377,000 per cu.mm.; stool examination for occult blood was negative three times. X-ray examination of the chest, gall bladder, and upper and lower gastrointestinal tract were negative. Consultation from the gynecologist and surgeon failed to reveal any evidence of malignancy. She was treated with butazolidine, ferrous sulfate, and coumadin and discharged to the care of her physician.

Anticoagulation was continued but in August, 1963, she again had thrombophlebitis in the right leg and required admission to her local hospital for five days.

Two weeks prior to the admission in December, 1963, the patient again developed swelling and redness with minimal pain in the calves of both legs despite continued oral anticoagulation and was readmitted to her local hospital. In the week prior to admission she noted mild epistaxis and painful areas over the dorsum of her left hand and left neck; the ends of her toes became black and very painful two days prior to transfer to this hospital.

Physical examination. Physical examination revealed a moderately obese female in moderate distress. Blood pressure was 130/80, pulse was 86, and temperature was 99.2° F. There was a superficial bleeding point in the anterior nares on the nasal septum on the left. The liver edge extended the width of two fingers below the right costal margin and the upper border was in the seventh interspace. The spleen was not palpable. There was a large, firm, non-tender, moveable, irregular mass arising from the left side of the pelvis and extending into the lower abdomen to the level of the umbilicus. A tender, firm cord was noted in the course of a superficial vein on the dorsum of the left hand and another on the left side of the neck, thought to be in the external jugular vein. Both legs were swollen. The skin was slightly erythematous over the dorsum of the feet and the distal portion of the toes was black. Blisters were noted on the dorsal surface of the great toes. The dorsalis pedis pulses were palpable bilaterally. Pelvic examination revealed a large, firm, irregular mass on the left which appeared to be attached to the fundus of the uterus.

Laboratory examination. Hematocrit was 32 per cent, leukocyte count was 9900 per cu.mm., and differential count normal. A thromboplastin generation test was performed using barium sulfate–absorbed plasma diluted 1/50 rather than 1/10 in order to delay the generation of thromboplastin activity; the minimal clotting time of 8 minutes with a control of 14 minutes suggested more rapid development of thromboplastin activity.

Course. The patient was transferred to surgery where a 10 x 15 cm. cystic tumor of the left ovary was removed. The tumor was not adherent to the surrounding structures, and there was no evidence of intraperitoneal metastatic disease. Intravenous and subcutaneous heparin therapy was begun and continued for the duration of her hospital stay. On the first postoperative day, 15 microcuries of radioactive chromic phosphate was installed intraperitoneally. Her toes were treated by careful debridement of necrotic tissue. A staphylococcus aureus infection of the abdominal lesion, which was discovered on the fourteenth day, was successfully treated with penicillin. On her twenty-first hospital day, oral anticoagulation with coumarin was

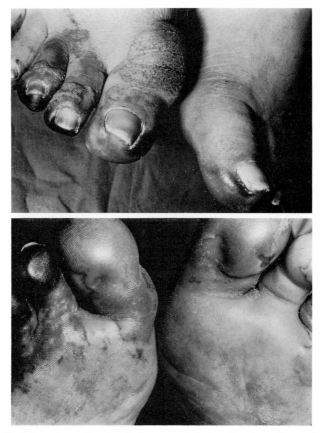

Figure 11–13. Two views of patient's feet on admission showing effects of vascular insufficiency, ranging from bleb formation to well demarcated areas of dry gangrene.

substituted for heparin therapy. Her feet continued to improve and
she was discharged to the care of her physician.

No evidence of accelerated generation of thromboplastin activity
could be detected in the patient's plasma when she returned in 3
months, and there was no clinical evidence of intravascular coagulation
before her death from metastasis 2 years later.

Comment. This patient demonstrates several points of interest.
She had migratory phlebitis for 7 months prior to the discovery of
her tumor despite extensive investigation for a malignant tumor.
Severe hemorrhage was not a feature of the illness but modest epistaxis had occurred. The gangrene of the toes appeared quite similar
to that seen with frostbite in which capillary circulation is by-passed by
shunting; the presence of microthrombi in the small vessels cannot
be excluded, however. Oral anticoagulants were not effective in
preventing the continual thrombotic process before treatment of
the malignancy.

Factor XIII (Fibrin Stabilizing Factor) Deficiency

The fibrin clot which is formed as the result of blood coagulation is insoluble in 5 M urea while the fibrin clot which is formed when fibrinogen in saline is exposed to thrombin is soluble in 5 M urea. This difference is due to the presence in whole blood and plasma of a factor capable of cementing the fibrin filaments together. Without this factor the fibrin clot is unstable and dissolves in a number of solvents resisted by normal clots. This factor is known as Factor XIII, the fibrin stabilizing factor (FSF), or the L-L factor.[111, 218]

CLINICAL ASPECTS

Reports of patients with congenital deficiency of Factor XIII have emphasized the occurrence of umbilical hemorrhage 12 to 14 days after birth, repeated hematoma, and slow wound healing.[36, 185] Bleeding generally occurs 24 to 36 hours after injury. Family studies are compatible with an autosomal incompletely recessive inheritance of the trait.[115]

The acquired form may occur in association with multiple myeloma, lead poisoning, pernicious anemia, or liver cirrhosis.[219, 220, 270]

New techniques for the identification of Factor XIII deficiency have been developed which have allowed the study of heterozygotes and the effect of transfusions. Following transfusion of fresh plasma, the level of Factor XIII fell to pre-transfusion levels in 5 or 6 days.[220, 250]

Fibrin stabilizing activity has been reported to be decreased in a variety of diseases.[270]

TREATMENT

The defect is corrected by the administration of transfusions of small amounts of whole blood. The half-time of the factor appears to be on the order of 3 days. The Pool cryoprecipitate is a good source of Factor XIII activity and has been used in the prophylactic treatment of patients with severe Factor XIII deficiency.[21]

Disorders Affecting Vessel and/or Platelet Function and Blood Coagulation

Von Willebrand's Disease (Inherited Autosomal Hemmorrhagic Diathesis with Antihemophilic Factor Deficiency and Prolonged Bleeding Time)

In 1926 von Willebrand described a hemorrhagic diathesis found in members of a family living on the Åland Islands off the coast of Finland. He designated the condition as pseudohemophilia and felt that it resulted from abnormal platelet function. A number of reports of cases of pseudohemophilia have since appeared in the literature. The patients reported generally have had clinical findings similar to those of the family described by von Willebrand but the results of the laboratory tests have been varied. It now seems apparent that the term pseudohemophilia as used in the literature is not specific. Reassessment of the patients originally described by von Willebrand has made clear the nature of their defect[264] and it seems reasonable to refer to their disorder as von Willebrand's disease.

PATHOLOGIC PHYSIOLOGY

Von Willebrand's disease is inherited and is transmitted as an autosomal dominant with varying degrees of expressivity.[65, 264, 265] Although the underlying cause of the defect in hemostasis is not understood, the disorder is manifested by a prolonged bleeding time and a decrease in Factor VIII. A defect in platelet function has been suspected since the original description of the disorder. Studies have indicated that Platelet Factor 3 (PF-3) is normal; the platelets have a normal surface charge[423] and adhere normally to connective tissue.[411] Release of ADP by the platelets and their aggregation proceeds normally.[364]

A marked decrease in platelet adhesiveness has been demonstrated in vivo[59] and to glass in vitro.[273, 329, 421] The relationship of this defect to the prolonged bleeding time is not clear. Family studies have revealed that asymptomatic relatives of patients with von Willebrand's disease may have normal bleeding time and Factor VIII levels with abnormal platelet adhesiveness in vitro.[378]

A recent report noted the association of intermittent thrombocytopenia with von Willebrand's disease.[261] In 1941 Macfarlane[225] demonstrated that the capillaries in the nail beds of some of these patients appeared bizarre and failed to constrict normally.

The abnormal bleeding time of these patients has been corrected by the infusion of normal or hemophilic plasma fraction 1–0.[96, 264, 285] This factor is labile and lost on contact with glass. It is reported to correct abnormal platelet adhesiveness in vitro.[330] The "bleeding time factor" is present in the Pool cryoprecipitate but not in commercially prepared Factor VIII concentrates.[285]

The Factor VIII level may be raised by the administration of fraction 1–0 of normal plasma and the bleeding time simultaneously corrected.[261] It is of great interest that the Factor VIII level may be raised and the bleeding time corrected by the administration of plasma fraction 1–0 from hemophilic patients. As plasma from hemophilic patients contains little Factor VIII the data suggest that patients with von Willebrand's disease have the capacity to produce Factor VIII.[56, 96] The substances responsible for stimulating patients with von Willebrand's disease to produce their own Factor VIII has not been completely identified. It appears to be concentrated in the fibrinogen fraction of the plasma, even in that prepared from "outdated" plasma. The serum contains this substance in good concentration and it is present in the cryoprecipitate prepared by the method of Pool.[41] Albumin and globulin contain no such activity.[54] It is not absorbed by $Ca_3(PO_4)_2$. The factor responsible for stimulation of Factor VIII synthesis appears to be physically distinct from the "bleeding time factor." The decrease in Factor VIII levels found in many patients with von Willebrand's disease indicates that the regulation of Factor VIII is controlled by at least two genes: the X-chromosome gene which is abnormal in classic hemophilia and an autosomal gene which is abnormal in von Willebrand's disease.[146, 148, 407]

CLINICAL FEATURES

This disorder is often apparent in the first few weeks of life when spontaneous bleeding from the nose or gums may occur. Excessive bleeding often follows minor trauma. Uterine bleeding may be excessive and pregnancy is often complicated by bleeding episodes.[78, 96, 208, 265] Mucosal bleeding from the gastrointestinal tract may occur.[70] Neither petechiae nor hemarthrosis is common in this disease. The great variability in the bleeding tendency in the same patient from time to time makes the clinical course difficult to anticipate, but it is rare for these patients to succumb during an episode of bleeding.

The hemorrhagic diathesis in these patients relates most clearly to the degree of Factor VIII deficiency,[54, 378] and adequate hemostatic control for surgery is usually maintained when adequate levels of Factor VIII are attained, though the Ivy bleeding time may not be shortened. In those patients with spontaneous bleeding, however, hemostatic control may not be adequate unless the Ivy bleeding time is also corrected.

The diagnosis of von Willebrand's disease can usually be established by the demonstration of a prolonged bleeding time and a decrease in Factor VIII level. The Ivy bleeding time has been shown to be more sensitive than the Duke bleeding time but both are useful.[4] Tests of platelet adhesiveness are under continuing study but are not yet standardized.[156, 167, 175, 289, 329] The laboratory findings in this group of patients are not consistent from patient to patient or indeed in the same patient from one examination to the next.[13, 51, 263, 265, 338] Repeated testing may be necessary in order to establish the diagnosis.[4]

There has been a report of acquired von Willebrand's disease occurring in the course of systemic lupus erythematosus.[358]

TREATMENT

The fact that more than one disorder has in the past been included under this name may be responsible for the wide variation reported in response to therapy.

Appropriate transfusion therapy can accomplish several important effects for these patients. The bleeding time may be corrected, Factor VIII levels restored, and the patient stimulated to produce his own Factor VIII. The stimulation of endogenous Factor VIII makes it easier to raise and maintain adequate levels of Factor VIII in these patients than in patients with classic hemophilia. The use of fresh plasma and fresh frozen plasma has been effective in the control of Factor VIII levels. The bleeding time is more difficult to correct, since the "bleeding time factor" is labile and lost on contact with glass. The finding that the "bleeding time factor" is present in the Pool cryoprecipitate makes it possible that Factor VIII levels and bleeding time can be corrected simultaneously.[41, 285] There has been one report of a patient who became unresponsive to plasma following a large number of transfusions necessitated by persistent gastrointestinal bleeding. Neither the bleeding time nor the Factor VIII level would respond any longer to infusions of fresh plasma. An anti-Factor VIII inhibitor could not be demonstrated.[70]

The natural history of this disorder is extremely variable and it is difficult to interpret the efficacy of a particular therapeutic maneuver. Surgery may be a major hazard to these patients and should be avoided if possible. If surgery is unavoidable the patient should be prepared by the administration of fresh or fresh frozen plasma or cryoprecipitate and these infusions should be repeated every second day until healing is complete.

Illustrative Case

History. A 50 year old white married woman was admitted to the hospital for the extraction of several teeth. She had been known to be a "bleeder" all her life. Minor cuts and abrasions were followed by excessive bleeding in childhood, and there had been repeated epistaxis, subcutaneous hemorrhages, and oozing from the gums. At 18 years of age she had a severe hemorrhage which continued for 2 to 3 days following the extraction of a tooth. Following a miscarriage at the age of 33 she had intermittent bleeding for 6 months. Bleeding was finally controlled by the administration of a number of whole blood transfusions. There were, however, long intervals of freedom from any evidence of bleeding tendency.

She began to have severe pain as the result of excessive dental caries while in her late thirties. Dental extractions were denied her on several occasions because of her history of a hemorrhagic diathesis. She was 42 years of age when Gelfoam and topical thrombin became available and an extraction was successfully carried out using these agents. She was now admitted for further dental work, having had but one nosebleed of any significance in 7 years and only rare vaginal spotting.

The patient's mother and father were first cousins. There was no history that either the parents or grandparents had had any abnormal bleeding. Two brothers had died following hemorrhage in infancy, another brother died following uncontrollable epistaxis, and a fourth brother bled to death during an appendectomy. A fifth committed suicide. The remaining five siblings were alive and well without historical evidence of abnormal bleeding.

A review of the old record revealed marked variability of the bleeding time and the fact that the coagulation time was somewhat prolonged occasionally. Prothrombin time, platelet counts, and clot retraction were consistently normal. The results of the tourniquet test varied and from time to time were slightly positive. On one occasion the bleeding time was noted to be 17½ minutes in one ear while at the same time it was 180 minutes in the other. There was also striking evidence that the infusion of whole blood affected the bleeding time. On one occasion the capillaries were visualized directly, and it was noted that they did not retract properly after being punctured with a needle.

Physical examination. In addition to dental caries for which she was admitted the only positive physical finding was very slight hepatomegaly.

Laboratory findings. The red blood cell count was 3.5 mil. per cu.mm.; hemoglobin 9.6 gm. per 100 ml., hematocrit 29 per cent, and platelets 364,000 per cu.mm. The bleeding time was discontinued at 15 minutes, the coagulation time was 13 minutes, and the thromboplastin generation test revealed a depression of Factor VIII.

Course. The patient was given prednisone and 3 units of fresh (4 to 6 hours old) blood. Her bleeding time and thromboplastin generation test returned to normal and she tolerated the removal of three teeth without excessive bleeding. Within 48 hours the bleeding time was again prolonged despite continued administration of prednisone. Five hundred ml. of fresh plasma in glass bottles was given, and once again the bleeding time was returned to normal. She tolerated the removal of two more teeth without excessive bleeding.

Comment. The history presented indicates the variability of the clinical manifestation of this disorder. There is clear evidence that the bleeding time was affected by both whole blood transfusions and plasma transfusions. The fact that plasma transfusions collected in and administered from glass bottles corrected the defect affords evidence against the possibility that platelets played any role in the correction of the bleeding time. The patient's platelets were normal in the thromboplastic generation test. The decreased Factor VIII and prolonged bleeding time indicates the similarity of this patient's disorder to those described by von Willebrand, though this patient's defect may have been inherited as an autosomal recessive. The clinical course of this patient was favorably altered by the administration of fresh plasma. The administration of adrenocortical steroids was not considered to have played a role in the correction of the bleeding time, since it was prolonged again 48 hours after administration of fresh whole blood despite their continued administration. In retrospect, the use of dental splints as described under the treatment of Factor VIII deficiency may have obviated some of this patient's difficulty with extraction.

Thrombasthenia, Thrombocytopathy, and Thrombopathia

Hemorrhagic diathesis has been attributed to qualitative as well as quantitative changes in the platelets.[103, 188, 207, 361, 391, 392] As the platelets play so broad a role in the defense of hemostasis, altered platelet function may affect the vascular or biochemical phase of hemostasis or both. It is not surprising to find a wide range of abnormal laboratory tests reported in the literature, since individual platelet functions are difficult to assess and more than one function may be altered.

The study of these disorders is complicated by confusing and overlapping terminology. In general, the term *thrombasthenia* is applied to platelet disorders characterized by abnormal clot retraction and platelet clumping but with adequate platelet phospholipid and normal clotting function. The term *thrombo-*

cytopathy is applied to those conditions in which Platelet factor 3 is quantitatively reduced or unavailable to the coagulation process. *Thrombopathia* indicates a condition in which the platelet fails to release normal amounts of ADP in response to aggregating agents.[232]

THROMBASTHENIA

Hereditary thrombasthenia (Glanzmann's disease) is a disorder characterized by a prolonged bleeding time, poor clot retraction, and the failure of platelets to aggregate in the presence of ADP. The disorder appears to be transmitted by an autosomal recessive defect and is manifested in childhood by easy bleeding from mucous membranes and skin. There is evidence of some improvement in hemostasis with age. Transfusions of fresh whole blood or platelets alone are usually helpful. Platelet life span is normal.[80] Two distinct groups of these patients have thus far been separated on the basis of the biochemical abnormalities of their platelets.

Patients have been reported[152] in whom a deficiency of glyceraldehyde-3-phosphate dehydrogenase and pyruvate kinase resulted in a 50 per cent reduction of platelet ATP. As the contractile protein of the platelet is dependent on ATP as an energy source,[45, 223] any interference with the formation or function of ATP might result in abnormal platelet function.

The second group of patients have a normal platelet glycolytic cycle and normal platelet ATP levels. It was suggested that reduced Mg^{++} and ATPase levels were perhaps responsible for non-utilization of platelet ATP. One report noted a failure of these platelets to release platelet phospholipid in vitro and suggested that the defects may be attributable to a single abnormality of the platelet membrane.[208]

Both groups had reduced levels of platelet fibrinogen.[411, 421] Recently, the report of a reduction in glutathione reductase activity in two patients with thrombasthenia has appeared.[254] Since no other enzyme defect could be demonstrated the suggestion was made that reduction in the availability of SH-groups might inferfere with platelet function in vivo. SH-group blocking agents have been shown to interfere with clot retraction in vitro.[117] Further studies may well separate other defects within the group with normal glycolytic enzymes and ATP levels.

THROMBOCYTOPATHY (Platelet Factor 3 Deficiency)

Platelet Factor 3 (PF-3) may be quantitatively reduced (thrombocytopathy) or unavailable to participate in hemostasis (thrombopathia). The specific nature of the defect is unknown in either.[66, 238, 409] Special studies are necessary to distinguish between these patients and those with thrombasthenia and von Willebrand's disease.[410]

Patients with thrombocytopathy have a mild to moderate hemorrhagic diathesis characterized by epistaxis, spontaneous bruising, menorrhagia, and an unpredictable amount of bleeding during surgery; in a few patients severe symptoms occur, but visceral hemorrhage and hemarthrosis are rarely seen.

Both primary and secondary forms of the disorder have been reported, but the primary form is rare.[67] The secondary or acquired disorder has been reported in multiple myeloma, idiopathic thrombocytopenic purpura, disseminated lupus erythematosus, uremia, chronic liver disease, and chronic lymphocytic leukemia. The defect in the acquired form is thought to be the result of a plasma factor which affects the release of PF-3 from the platelet and interferes with its clot-promoting function, possibly the release of platelet phospholipid.

THROMBOPATHIA

Thrombopathia is the term given to a disorder characterized by a failure to release normal amounts of ADP from the platelets in response to aggregating agents, although the platelets themselves can respond to ADP by normal aggregation.[82, 161, 232, 408b] Disaggregation is rapid; it occurs in 2 to 3 minutes.[99, 408, 410] Platelet aggregation is associated with an increase in PF-3 availability.[160] Failure to release platelet ADP and maintain aggregation reduces the availability of this important substance despite its presence in the platelets. Aggregation induced by thrombin, collagen, and epinephrine is absent or defective.

The disorder, which may be inherited or acquired, is characterized by mild bleeding, mainly spontaneous bruising, and a prolonged bleeding time in the presence of a normal number of platelets. The abnormalities found in this group of patients are similar to those which occur after the ingestion of aspirin.[410]

It is probable that various types of platelet dysfunction can arise from a number of different causes. Considerable work is needed to clarify these problems and, in view of studies on the ADP release phenomenon, to reassess much of the earlier work on platelet dysfunction.

References

1. Aas, K. A., and Gardner, F. H.: Survival of blood platelets labeled with Chromium[51]. J. Clin. Invest., *37*:1257, 1958.
2. Aballi, A. J., Banus, V. L., deLamerens, S., and Rozengvaig, S.: Coagulation studies in the newborn period. III. Hemorrhagic disease of the newborn. Am J. Dis. Child., *97*:524, 1959.
3. Aballi, A. J., Banus, V. L., deLamerens, S., and Rozengvaig, S.: Coagulation studies in the newborn period. IV. Deficiency of Stuart-Prower factor as a part of the clotting defect of the newborn. Am. J. Dis. Child., *97*:549, 1959.
4. Abildgaard, C. F., Simone, J. V., Honig, G. R., Forman, E. N., Johnson, C. A., and Seeler, R. A.: Von Willebrand's disease: a comparative study of diagnostic tests. J. Pediat., *73*:355, 1968.
5. Ackerman, B. D., Taylor, W. F., Ingman, M. J., and O'Loughlin, B. J.: Diagnosis and treatment of congenital rubella. G. P., *40*:137, 1969.
6. Ackroyd, J. F.: The pathogenesis of thrombocytopenic purpura due to hypersensitivity to Sedormid (allyl-isopropyl acetylcarbamide). Clin. Sc., *7*:249, 1949.
7. Ackroyd, J. F.: Allergic purpura, including purpura due to foods, drugs, and infection. Am. J. Med., *14*:605, 1953.
8. Ackroyd, J. F.: The role of Sedormid in the immunologic reaction that results in platelet lysis in Sedormid purpura. Clin. Sc., *13*:409, 1954.
9. Ackroyd, J. F.: Function of factor VII. Brit. J. Haem., *2*:397, 1956.
10. Ackroyd, J. F.: The immunological basis of purpura due to drug hypersensitivity. Proc. Roy. Soc. Med., *55*:30, 1962.
11. Adner, M. M., Fisch, G. R., Starobin, S. B., and Aster, R. N.: Use of compatible platelet transfusions in treatment of congenital iso-immune thrombocytopenic purpura. The New England J. Med., *280*:244, 1969.
12. Aggeler, P. M., White, S. G., Glendening, M. B., Pope, E. W., Leake, T. B., and Bates, G. B.

Plasma thromboplastin component (PTC) deficiency: A new disease resembling hemophilia. Proc. Soc. Exper. Biol. & Med., *79*:692, 1952.

13. Alexander, B., and Goldstein, R.: Dual hemostatic defect in pseudohemophilia. J. Clin. Invest. (abs.), *32*:551, 1953.

14. Alexander, B., Goldstein, R., Landwehr, G., and Cook, C. D.: Congenital SPCA deficiency: A hitherto unrecognized coagulation defect with hemorrhage rectified by serum and serum fractions. J. Clin. Invest., *30*:596, 1951.

15. Alexander, B., Goldstein, R., Rich, L., LeBolloc'h, A. G., and Diamond, L. K.: Congenital afibrinogenemia. Blood, *9*:843, 1954.

16. Ali, A. M., Gandy, R. H., Britten, M. I., and Dormandy, K. M.: Joint haemorrhage in haemophilia: is full advantage taken of plasma therapy? Brit. Med. J., *3*:828, 1967.

17. Allen, D. M., Diamond, L. K., and Howell, D. A.: Anaphylactoid purpura in children (Schönlein-Henoch syndrome). Am. J. Dis. Child., *99*:833, 1960.

18. Almquist, H. J.: Purification of the antihemorrhagic vitamin. J. Biol. Chem., *114*:241, 1936.

19. Almquist, H. J., and Klose, A. A.: Antihemorrhagic activity of 2-methyl-1,4-naphthoquinone. J. Biol. Chem., *130*:787, 1939.

20. Almquist, H. J., and Stokstad, E. L. R.: Hemorrhagic chick disease of dietary origin. J. Biol. Chem., *111*:105, 1935.

21. Amris, C. J., and Hilden, M.: Treatment of Factor XIII deficiency with cryoprecipitate. Throm. et Diath. Haemorr., *20*:528, 1968.

22. Ancona, G. C., Ellenhorn, W. J., and Falconer, E. H.: Purpura due to food sensitivity. J. Allergy, *22*:487, 1951.

23. Andersen, B. R., and Terry, W. D.: Gamma G4-globulin antibody causing inhibition of clotting Factor VIII. Nature, *217*:174, 1968.

24. Antley, M., and McMillan, C. W.: Sequential coagulation studies in purpura fulminans. New England J. Med., *276*:1287, 1967.

25. Arcomano, J. P., and Eskes, P. W. H.: "Schönlein-Henoch syndrome." Am. J. Dis. Child., *114*:674, 1967.

26. Ashford, T. P., and Freiman, D. G.: The role of the endothelium in the initial phases of thrombosis: electron microscopic study. Am. J. Path., *50*:257, 1967.

27. Aster, R. H.: Pooling of platelets in the spleen: role in the pathogenesis of "hypersplenic" thrombocytopenia. J. Clin. Invest., *45*:645, 1966.

28. Aster, R. H., and Jandle, J. H.: Platelet sequestration in man. I. Methods. II. Immunological and Clinical Studies. J. Clin. Invest., *43*:843, 856, 1964.

29. Aster, R. H., and Keene, W. R.: Site of platelet destruction in idiopathic thrombocytopenic purpura. Brit. J. Haemat., *16*:61, 1969.

30. Astrup, T.: Fibrinolysis in the organism. Blood, *11*:781, 1956.

31. Atkins, H. J., Wolff, J. A., and Sitarz, A.: Giant hemangioma in infancy with secondary thrombocytopenic purpura. Am. J. Roentgenol., *89*:1062, 1963.

32. Ayoub, E. M., and Hoyer, J.: Anaphylactoid purpura: Streptococcal antibody titers and B gammaglobulin levels. J. Pediat., *75*:193, 1969.

33. Baker, L. R. I., Rubenberg, M. L., Dalie, J. V., and Brain, M. C.: Fibrinogen catabolism in microangiopathic haemolytic anaemia. Brit. J. Haem., *14*:617, 1968.

34. Barrow, E. M., Heindel, C. C., Roberts, H. R., and Graham, J. B.: Heterozygosity and homozygosity in von Willebrand's disease. Proc. Soc. Exp. Biol. Med., *118*:684, 1965.

35. Barrow, M. V., Quick, D. T., and Cunningham, R. W.: Salicylate hypoprothrombinemia in rheumatoid arthritis with liver disease. Arch. Int. Med., *120*:620, 1967.

36. Barry, A., and Delâge, J. M.: Congenital deficiency of fibrin-stabilizing factor: Observation of a new case. New England J. Med., *272*:943, 1965.

37. Barry, A. P., Geoghegan, F., and Shea, S. M.: Acquired fibrinopenia in pregnancy. Brit. M. J., *2*:287, 1955.

38. Bayer, W. L., Dario, C. C., Szeto, I. L. F., and Lewis, J. H.: Acquired Factor X deficiency in a Negro boy. J. Pediat., *44*:1007, 1969.

39. Bayer, W. L., Sherman, F. E., Michaels, R. H., Szeto, I. L. F., and Lewis, J. H.: Purpura in congenital and acquired rubella. New England J. Med., *273*:1362, 1965.

40. Beck, P., Giddings, J. C., and Bloom, A. L.: Inhibitor of Factor VIII in mild haemophilia. Brit. J. Haem., *17*:283, 1969.

41. Bennett, E., and Dormandy, K.: Pool's cryoprecipitate and exhausted plasma in the treatment of von Willebrand's disease and Factor XI deficiency. Lancet, *2*:731, 1966.

42. Bennington, J. L., Fonty, R. A., and Haugie, C.: Laboratory Diagnosis. Collier-Macmillan, Ltd., London, 1970, p. 522.

43. Beresford, O. D.: Hereditary haemorrhagic telangiectasia with pulmonary arteriovenous fistula. Brit. J. Dis. Chest, *61*:219, 1967.

44. Berger, H.: Cause of drug-induced thrombocytopenic purpura identified by the passive transfer reaction. Ann. Int. Med., *56*:618, 1962.

44a. Bernstock, L., and Herson, C.: Thrombotic thrombocytopenic purpura. Remission on treatment with heparin. Lancet, *1*:28, 1960.

45. Bettex-Galland, M., and Lüscher, E. F.: Extraction of an actomyosin-like protein from human thrombocytes. Nature, *184*:276, 1959.

46. Bidwell, E.: The purification of bovine antihaemophilic globulin. Brit. J. Haem., *1*:35, 1955.

47. Biggs, R.: Fractions rich in Factor VIII. Biblio. Haemat., *29*:1122, 1968.

48. Biggs, R., Bidwell, E., Handley, D. A., Macfarlane, R. G., Trueta, J., Elliot-Smith, A., Dike, G. W. R., and Ash, B. J.: The preparation and assay of a Christmas-factor (factor IX) concentrate and its use in the treatment of two patients. Brit. J. Haem., 7:349, 1961.

49. Biggs, R., and Douglas, A. S.: The thromboplastin generation test. J. Clin. Path., *6*:23, 1953.

50. Biggs, R., Douglas, A. S., Macfarlane, R. G., Dacie, J. V., Pitney, W. R., Merskey, C., and O'Brien, J. R.: Christmas disease. Brit. Med. J., 2:1378, 1952.

51. Biggs, R., and Macfarlane, R. G.: Haemophilia and related conditions. Brit. J. Haem., *4*:1, 1958.

52. Biggs, R., and Macfarlane, R. G.: Christmas disease. Postgrad. Med. J., *38*:3, 1962.

53. Biggs, R., and Macfarlane, R. G.: Treatment of Haemophilia and Other Coagulation Disorders. F. F. Davis Co., Philadelphia, 1966, p. 246.

54. Biggs, R., and Matthews, J. M.: The treatment of haemorrhage in von Willebrand's disease and the blood level of factor VIII (AHG). Brit. J. Haem., *9*:203, 1963.

55. Bithell, T. C., Didisheim, P., Cartwright, G. E., and Wintrobe, M. M.: Thrombocytopenia inherited as an autosomal dominant trait. Blood, *25*:231, 1965.

56. Blombäck, M., Jorpes, J. E., and Nilsson, I. M.: Von Willebrand's disease. Am. J. Med., *34*:236, 1963.

57. Bok, J., Veltkamp, J. J., and Loeliger, E. A.: Moderate Factor XII deficiency. Throm. et Diath. Haemorr., *13*:8, 1965.

58. Bonnin, J. A., Cohen, A. K., and Hicks, N. D.: Coagulation defects in a case of systemic lupus erythematosus with thrombocytopenia. Brit. J. Haem., 2:168, 1956.

59. Borchgrevink, C. F.: Platelet adhesion in vivo in patients with bleeding disorders. Acta Med. Scandinav., *170*:231, 1961.

60. Borchgrevink, C. F., Egeberg, O., Pool, J. G., Skulason, T., Stormorken, H., and Waaler, B.: A study of a case of congenital hypoprothrombinemia. Brit. J. Haem., 5:294, 1959.

61. Borman, J. B., and Schiller, M.: Osler's disease with multiple large vessel aneurysms. Angiology, *20*:113, 1969.

62. Born, G. V. R.: Changes in the distribution of phosphorus in platelet-rich plasma during clotting. Biochem. J., *68*:695, 1958.

63. Born, G. V. R., and Esnouf, M. P.: Appearance of a phosphorous compound in platelet-rich plasma on clotting. Nature, *183*:478, 1959.

64. Bouroncle, B. A., and Doan, C. A.: Treatment of refractory idiopathic thrombocytopenic purpura. J.A.M.A., *207*:2049, 1969.

65. Bowie, E. J., Didisheim, P., Thompson, J. H., Jr., and Owen, C. A.: The spectrum of von Willebrand's disease. Thromb. et Diath. Haemorrh., *18*:40, 1967.

66. Bowie, E. J. W., and Owen, C. A., Jr.: Thrombopathy. Seminars Hemat., *5*:73, 1968.

67. Bowie, E. J. W., Thompson, J. H. Jr., and Owen, C. A. Jr.: The blood platelet (including a discussion of the qualitative platelet diseases). Proc. Mayo Clinic, *40*:625, 1965.

68. Brafield, A. J., Madras, M. B., and Case, J.: The stability of Christmas factor. A guide to the management of Christmas disease. Lancet, 2:867, 1956.

69. Brain, M. C., Dacie, J. V., and Hourihane, D. O'B.: Microangiopathic haemolytic anaemia: The possible role of vascular lesions in pathogenesis. Brit. J. Haem., *8*:358, 1962.

70. Brandstaetter, S., Scharf, J., Salomon, H., and Tatarsky, I.: Gastrointestinal bleeding in von Willebrand's disease. Arch. Int. Med., *118*:108, 1966.

71. Breckenridge, R. T., Moore, R. D., and Ratnoff, O.: A study of thrombocytopenia. New histologic criteria for the differentiation of idiopathic thrombocytopenia and thrombocytopenia associated with disseminated lupus erythematosus. Blood, *30*:39, 1967.

72. Breckenridge, R. T., and Ratnoff, O. D.: Studies on the site of action of a circulating anticoagulant in disseminated lupus erythematosus. Am. J. Med., *35*:813, 1963.

73. Breen, F. A., and Tullis, J. L.: Prothrombin concentrates in treatment of Christmas disease and allied disorders. J.A.M.A., *208*:1848, 1969.

74. Brinkhous, K. M., Langdell, R. D., Penick, G. D., Graham, J. B., and Wagner, R. H.: Newer approaches to the study of hemophilia and hemophilioid states. J.A.M.A., *154*:481, 1954.

75. Brinkhous, K. M., Shanbrom, E., Roberts, H. R., Webster, W. P., Fekete, L., and Wagner, R. N.: A new high potency glycine-precipitated antihemophilic factor (AHF) concentrate. J.A.M.A., *205*:613, 1968.

76. Brinkley, S. B., MacCorquodale, D. W., Thayer, S. A., and Doisy, E. A.: The isolation of vitamin K_1. J. Biol. Chem., *130*:219, 1939.

77. Brown, P. E., Hougie, C., and Roberts, H. R.: The genetic heterogeneity of hemophilia B. New England J. Med., *283*:61, 1970.
78. Buchanan, J. C., and Leavell, B. S.: Pseudohemophilia: Report of 13 new cases and statistical review of previously reported cases. Ann. Int. Med., *44*:241, 1956.
79. Bunting, W. L., Kiely, J. M., and Campbell, D. C.: Idiopathic thrombocytopenic purpura. Arch. Int. Med., *108*:733, 1961.
80. Caen, J., Castaldi, P. A., Leclerc, J. C., Inceman, S., Larrieu, M. J., Probst, M., and Bernard, J.: Congenital bleeding disorders with long bleeding time and normal platelet count. I. Glanzmann's thrombasthenia (report of 15 patients). Am. J. Med., *41*:4, 1966.
81. Caen, J., and Cousin, C.: Le trouble d'adhésivité "in vivo" des plaquettes dans la maladie de Willebrand et les thrombasthénies de Glanzmann. Nouv. Rev. Franc. Hemat., *2*:685, 1962.
82. Caen, J. P., Sultan, Y., and Larrieu, M. J.: New familial platelet disease. Lancet, *1*:203, 1968.
83. Carpenter, A. F., Wintrobe, M. M., Fuller, E. A., Haut, A., and Cartwright, G. E.: Treatment of idiopathic thrombocytopenic purpura. J.A.M.A., *171*:1911, 1959.
84. Cavins, J. A., and Wall, R. L.: Clinical and laboratory studies of plasma thromboplastin antecedent deficiency (PTA). Am. J. Med., *29*:444, 1960.
85. Choi, S. F., McClure, P. D., and Vranic, M.: Thrombopoietin activity in idiopathic thrombocytopenic purpura. Brit. J. Haem., *15*:345, 1968.
86. Cohen, P., and Gardner, F. H.: The thrombocytopenic effect of sustained high-dosage prednisone therapy in thrombocytopenic purpura. New England J. Med., *265*:611, 1961.
87. Coldwell, B. B., and Zawidzka, Z : Effect of acute administration of acetylsalicylic acid on the prothrombin activity of bishydroxycoumarin-treated rats. Blood, *32*:945, 1968.
88. Conley, C. L., Evans, R. S., Harrington, W. J., Schwartz, S. O., and Dameshek, W.: Panels in therapy. X. Treatment of acute ITP. Blood, *11*:384, 1956.
89. Conley, C. L., Rathbun, H. K., Morse, W. I., II, and Robinson, J. E., Jr.: Circulating anticoagulant as a cause of hemorrhagic diathesis in man. Johns Hopkins Hosp. Bull., *83*:288, 1948.
90. Connor, W. E., Hoak, J. C., and Warner, E. D.: Massive thrombosis produced by fatty acid infusion. J. Clin. Invest., *42*:860, 1963.
91. Cooke, J. V., Holland, P. V., and Shulman, N. R.: Cryoprecipitate concentrates of Factor VIII for surgery in hemophiliacs. Ann. Int. Med., *68*:39, 1968.
92. Cooper, L. Z., Green, R. H., Krugman, S., Giles, J. P., and Mirick, G. S.: Neonatal thrombocytopenia purpura and after manifestation of rubella contracted in utero. Am. J. Dis. Child., *110*:416, 1965.
93. Cooper, L. Z., Ziring, P. R., Ockerse, A. B., Fedun, B. A., Kiely, B., and Krugman, S.: Rubella: clinical manifestations and management. Am. J. Dis. Child., *118*:18, 1969.
94. Cooper, T., Stickney, J. M., Pease, G. L., and Bennett, W. A.: Thrombotic thrombocytopenic purpura. Am. J. Med., *13*:374, 1952.
95. Corn, M., and Upshaw, J. D.: Evaluation of platelet antibodies in idiopathic thrombocytopenic purpura. Arch. Int. Med., *109*:157, 1962.
96. Cornu, P., Larrieu, M. J., Caen, J., and Bernard, J.: Transfusion studies in von Willebrand's disease. Effect on bleeding time and Factor VIII. Brit. J. Haem. *9*:189, 1963.
97. Craddock, C. G., and Lawrence, J. S.: Hemophilia. Blood, *2*:505, 1947.
98. Cram, D. L., and Soley, R. L.: "Purpura fulminans." Brit. J. Dermatol., *80*:323, 1968.
99. Cronberg, S., and Nilsson, I. M.: Investigation of patients with mild thrombasthenia—a haemorrhagic disorder with prolonged bleeding time probably due to a primary platelet defect. Acta Med. Scandinav., *183*:163, 1968.
100. Cronkite, E. P.: Ionizing radiation injury: Its diagnosis by physical examination and clinical laboratory procedures. J.A.M.A., *139*:366, 1949.
101. Dam, H.: The antihemorrhagic vitamin of the chick. Biochem. J., *29*:1273, 1935.
102. Dam, H., and Schonheyder, F.: A deficiency disease in chicks resembling scurvy. Biochem. J., *28*:1355, 1934.
103. Davey, M. G., and Lüscher, E. F.: Actions of thrombin and other coagulant and proteolytic enzymes on blood platelets. Nature, *216*:857, 1967.
104. Dellipiani, A. W., and George, M.: Syndrome of sclerodactyly, calcinosis, Reynaud's phenomenon and telangiectasia. Brit. Med. J., *4*:334, 1967.
105. Denson, K. W. E.: Abnormal forms of Factor X. Lancet, *2*:1256, 1969.
106. Denson, K. W. E., Biggs, R., Borrett, H. R., and Cobb, K.: Two types of haemophilia (A+ and A−): a study of 48 cases. Brit. J. Haemat., *17*:163, 1969.
107. DePalma, A.: Hemophilic arthropathy. Clinical orthopedics and related research. *52*:145, 1967.
108. Derham, R. J., and Rogerson, M. M.: The Schönlein-Henoch syndrome and collagen disease. Arch. Dis. Childhood, *27*:139, 1952.

109. Dische, F. E.: Blood-clotting substances with "Factor VII" activity: A comparison of some congenital and acquired deficiencies, Brit. J. Haem., *4*:201, 1958.

110. Djerassi, I., Farber, S., and Evans, A. E.: Transfusions of fresh platelet concentrates to patients with secondary thrombocytopenia. New England J. Med., *268*:221, 1963.

111. Duckert, F., Jung, E., and Shmerling, D. H.: A hitherto undescribed congenital haemorrhagic diathesis probably due to fibrin stabilizing factor deficiency. Thromb. et Diath. Haemorrh., *5*:179, 1961.

112. Dyer, N. H.: Cerebral abscess in hereditary haemorrhagic telangiectasia: report of two cases in a family. J. Neurol. Neurosurg. Psychiat., *30*:563, 1967.

113. Edson, J. R., White, J. G., and Krivit, W.: The enigma of severe Factor XI deficiency without hemorrhagic symptoms. Thromb. et Diath. Haemorrh., *18*:342, 1967.

114. Egeberg, O.: Blood Factor XI after fat-rich meals. Thromb. et Diath. Haemorrh., *15*:390, 1966.

115. Egeberg, O.: New families with hereditary hemorrhagic trait due to deficiency of fibrin stabilizing factor (F. 13). Thromb. et Diath. Haemorrh., *20*:534, 1968.

116. Fantl, P.: Parahemophilia (proaccelerin deficiency) occurrence and biochemistry. In Brinkhous, K. M., Ed.: Hemophilia and Hemophilioid Diseases. University of North carolina Press, Chapel Hill, 1957, pp. 79–92.

117. Fantl, P.: Thiol groups of blood platelets in relation to clot retraction. Nature, *198*:95, 1963.

118. Fantl, P., and Nance, M. H.: An acquired haemorrhagic disease in a female due to an inhibitor of blood coagulation. Med. J. Australia, 2:125, 1946.

119. Feinstein, D., Chong, M. N. Y., Kasper, C. K., and Rapaport, S. I.: Hemophilia A: polymorphism detectable by a Factor VIII antibody. Science, *163*:1071, 1969.

120. Fontein, D. L., Waldring, M. C., Nieweg, H. O.: Management of idiopathic thrombocytopenic purpura. Brit. J. Haemat., *17*:301, 1969.

121. Forbes, C. D., Hunter, J., Barr, R. D., Davidson, J. F., Short, D. W., McDonald, G. A., McNicol, G. P., Wallace, J., and Douglas, A. S.: Cryoprecipitate therapy in haemophilia. Scottish Med. J., *14*:1, 1969.

122. Forman, W. B., Ratnoff, O. D., and Boyer, M. N.: An inherited qualitative abnormality in plasma fibrinogen: fibrinogen Cleveland. J. Lab. Clin. Med., *72*:455, 1968.

123. Fraenkel, G. J.: Surgery in haemophilia. J. Roy. Coll. Surgeons, Edinburgh, *3*:54, 1957.

124. Fresh, J. W., Ferguson, J. H., Stamey, C., Morgan, F. M., and Lewis, J. H.: Blood prothrombin, proconvertin and proaccelerin in normal infancy: Questionable relationships to vitamin-K. Pediatrics, *19*:241, 1957.

125. Frick, P. G.: Hemophilia-like disease following pregnancy. Blood, *8*:598, 1953.

126. Frick, P. G.: Relative incidence of anti-hemophilic globulin (AHG), plasma thromboplastin component (PTC), and plasma thromboplastin antecedent (PTA) deficiency. J. Lab. & Clin. Med., *43*:860, 1954.

127. Frick, P. G.: Acquired circulating anticoagulants in systemic "collagen disease;" autoimmune thromboplastin deficiency. Blood, *10*:691, 1955.

128. Frick, P. G.: Studies on the turnover rate of stable prothrombin conversion factor in man. Acta Haemat., *19*:20, 1958.

129. Frommer, E., and Ingram, G. I. C.: Haemophiliacs and their doctors. The Practitioner, *202*:413, 1969.

130. Gaarder, A., Jonsen, J., Laland, S., Hellem, A., and Owren, P. A.: Adenosine diphosphate in red cells as a factor in the adhesiveness of human blood platelets. Nature, *192*:531, 1961.

131. Ganguly, P.: Studies on human platelet proteins. II. Effect of thrombin. Blood, *33*:590, 1969.

132. Gary, N. E., Mazzara, J. T., and Holfelder, L.: The Schönlein-Henoch syndrome. Ann. Int. Med., *72*:229, 1970.

133. Geratz, J. D., and Graham, J. B.: Plasma thromboplastin component (Christmas factor, factor IX) levels in stored human blood and plasma. Thromb. et Diath. Haemorrh., *4*:376, 1960.

134. Genton, E., and Pechet, L.: Thrombolytic agents: a perspective. Ann. Int. Med., *69*:625, 1968.

135. Gesink, M. H., and Bradford, H. A.: Thrombocytopenic purpura associated with chlorothiazide therapy. J.A.M.A., *172*:556, 1960.

136. Gilchrist, G. S., Ekert, H., Shanbrom, E., and Hammond, D.: New concentrate for treatment of Factor IX deficiency. New England J. Med., *280*:291, 1969.

137. Gitlin, D., and Borges, W. H.: Studies on the metabolism of fibrinogen in two patients with congenital afibrinogenemia. Blood, *8*:679, 1953.

138. Gitlow, S., and Goldmark, C.: Generalized capillary and arteriolar thrombosis. Ann. Int. Med., *13*:1046, 1939.

138a. Glueck, H. I., and Roehll, W., Jr.: Myocardial infarction in patient with Hageman (Factor XII) defect. Ann. Int. Med., *64*:390, 1966.

139. Goldbloom, R. B., and Drummond, K. N.: Anaphylactoid purpura with massive gastrointestinal hemorrhage and glomerulonephritis. Am. J. Dis. Child., *116*:97, 1968.

140. Goldstein, R., and Alexander, B.: Further studies on proconvertin deficiency and the role of proconvertin. In Brinkhous, K. M., Ed.: Hemophilia and Hemophilioid Disease. University of North Carolina Press, Chapel Hill, 1957, pp. 93–110.

141. Gomes, M. R., Bernatz, P. E., and Dines, D. E.: Pulmonary arteriovenous fistulas. Amer. J. Thorac. Surgery, 7:582, 1969.

142. Good, T. A., Carnazzo, S. F., and Good, R. A.: Thrombocytopenia and giant hemangioma in infants, Am. J. Dis. Child., 90:260, 1955.

143. Gore, I.: Disseminated arteriolar and capillary platelet thrombosis. A morphologic study of its histogenesis. Am. J. Path., 26:155, 1950.

144. Graham, J. B.: Genetic problems: Hemophilia and allied diseases. In Brinkhous, K. M., Ed.: Hemophilia and Hemophilioid Diseases. University of North Carolina Press, Chapel Hill, 1957, pp. 137–162.

145. Graham, J. B.: Stuart clotting defect and Stuart factor. Thromb. et Diath. Haemorrh., Suppl., 1:22, 1960.

146. Graham, J. B.: Biochemical genetic speculations provoked by considering the enigma of von Willebrand's disease. Thromb. et Diath. Haemorrh., Suppl., 11:119, 1963.

147. Graham, J. B., Barrow, E. M., and Hougie, C.: Stuart clotting defect. II. Genetic aspects of a "new" hemorrhagic stage. J. Clin. Invest., 36:497, 1957.

148. Graham, J. B., Barrow, E. M., and Roberts, H. R.: Possible implications of the autosomal and x-linked hemophilia phenotypes. Thromb. et Diath. Haemorrh., Suppl., 17:151, 1965.

149. Graham, J. B., Barrow, E. M., and Wynne, T. R.: Stuart clotting defect III: An acquired case with complete recovery. In Brinkhous, K. M., Ed.: Hemophilia and Other Hemorrhagic States. University of North Carolina Press, Chapel Hill, 1959, Chapter 18.

150. Graham, J. B., and Geratz, J. D.: Recent experiences with transfusion therapy in PTC-deficiency. In Holländer, L. (Ed.): Trans. VII Congr. Internat. Soc. of Blood Trans., Base., 1959.

151. Graham, R. C., Jr., Ebert, R. H., Ratnoff, O. S., and Moses, J. M.: Pathogenesis of inflammation. II In vivo observations of the inflammatory effects of activated Hageman factor and bradykinin. J. Exp. Med., 121:807, 1965.

152. Gross, R.: Metabolic aspects of normal and pathological platelets. Blood Platelets, Little, Brown & Co., Boston, 1961, p. 407.

153. Gröttum, K. A., and Solum, N. O.: Congenital thrombocytopenia with giant platelets: a defect in the platelet membrane. Brit. J. Haem., 16:277, 1969.

154. Haggerty, R. J., and Eley, R. C.: Varicella and cortisone. Pediatrics, 18:160, 1956.

155. Halpern, M., Turner, A. F., and Citron, B. P.: Angiodysplasias of the abdominal viscera associated with hereditary hemorrhagic telangiectasia. Am. J. Roent., 102:783, 1968.

156. Hampton, J. R.: The study of platelet behaviour and its relevance to thrombosis. J. Atherosclerosis Res., 7:729, 1967.

157. Hanes, F. M.: Multiple hereditary telangiectases causing hemorrhage. Bull. Johns Hopkins Hosp., 20:63, 1909.

158. Hardisty, R. M.: Acquired haemophilia-like disease. J. Clin. Path., 7:26, 1954.

159. Hardisty, R. M., Dormandy, K. M., and Hutton, R. A.: Thrombasthenia. Brit. J. Haemat., 10:371, 1964.

160. Hardisty, R. M., and Hutton, R. A.: Platelet aggregation and the availability of platelet Factor 3. Brit. J. Haema., 12:764, 1966.

161. Hardisty, R. M., and Hutton, R. A.: Bleeding tendency associated with "new" abnormality of platelet behaviour. Lancet, 1:983, 1967.

162. Hardisty, R. M., and Pinniger, J. L.: Congenital afibrinogenaemia: Further observations on the blood coagulation mechanism. Brit. J. Haemat., 2:139, 1956.

163. Harrington, W. J.: The clinical significance of antibodies for platelets. Sang, 25:712, 1954.

164. Harrington, W. J.: The Purpuras. Disease-a-Month. Year Book Publications, Chicago, July, 1957.

165. Harrington, W. J., Minnich, V., and Arimura, G.: The autoimmune thrombocytopenias. In Tocantins, L. M., Ed.: Progress in Hematology. Grune & Stratton, New York, 1956.

166. Harrington, W. J., Sprague, C. C., Minnich, V., Moore, C. V., and Dubach, R.: Immunologic Mechanisms in idiopathic and neonatal thrombocytopenic purpura. Ann. Int. Med., 38:433, 1953.

167. Hartman, R. C.: Tests of platelet adhesiveness and their clinical significance. Seminars Hemat., 5:60, 1968.

168. Haslam, R. J.: Role of adenosine diphosphate in the aggregation of human blood platelets by thrombin and by fatty acids. Nature, 202:765, 1964.

169. Hathway, W. E., Mull, M. M., Githens, J. H., Groth, C. G., Marchioro, T. L., and Starzl, T. E.: Attempted spleen transplant in classical hemophilia. Transplantation, 7:73, 1969.

170. Heikinheimo, R., and Reinikainen, M.: Congenital Factor VII deficiency—two cases in children of cousins. Thromb. et Diath. Haemorrh., *21*:245, 1969.
171. Hensen, A., Mattern, M. J., and Loeliger, E. A.: Hemophilia A with apparently autosomal dominant inheritance—evidence for a second autosomal locus involved in Factor VIII production. Thromb. et Diath. Haemorrh., *14*:341, 1965.
172. Heptinstall, R. H.: Pathology of the Kidney. Little, Brown and Co., Boston, 1966, pp. 335–344.
173. Hess, A. F., and Fish, M.: Infantile scurvy: the blood, the blood-vessels and the diet. Am. J. Dis. Child., *8*:385, 1914.
174. Hill, J. M., and Loeb, E.: Massive hormonal therapy and splenectomy in acute thrombotic thrombocytopenic purpura. J.A.M.A., *173*:778, 1960.
175. Hirsh, J., and McBride, J. A.: Increased platelet adhesiveness in recurrent venous thrombosis and pulmonary embolism. Brit. Med. J., *2*:797, 1965.
176. Hjort, P. F., and Rapaport, S. I.: The Shwartzman reaction: pathogenic mechanisms and clinical manifestations. Am. Rev. Med., *16*:135, 1965.
177. Hoag, M. S., Johnson, F. F., Robinson, J. A., and Aggeler, P. M.: Treatment of hemophilia B with a new clotting-factor concentrate. New England J. Med., *280*:581, 1969.
177a. Hoak, J. C., Seanson, L. W., Warner, E. D., and Connor, W. E.: Myocardial infarction associated with severe Factor XII deficiency. Lancet, 2:884, 1966.
178. Hougie, C.: Circulating anticoagulants. Brit. M. Bull., *11*:16, 1955.
179. Hougie, C., Barrow, E. M., and Graham, J. B.: Stuart clotting defect. I Segregation of an hereditary hemorrhagic state from the heterogeneous group heretofore called "stable factor" (SPCA, proconvertin, Factor VII) deficiency. J. Clin. Invest., *36*:485, 1957.
180. Hougie, C., and Twomey, J. J.: Hemophilia B in a new type of Factor IX deficiency. Lancet, *1*:698, 1967.
181. Hoyer, L. W., and Breckenridge, R. T.: Immunologic studies of antihemophilic factor (AHF, Factor VIII): cross reacting material in a genetic variant of hemophilia A. Blood, *32*:962, 1968.
182. Hughes, D. W. O. G., Parkinson, R., Beveridge, J., Reid, R. R., and Murphy, A. M.: The expanded congenital rubella syndrome: report of two cases with neonatal purpura and review of the recent literature. Med. J. Aust., *1*:420, 1967.
183. Humble, J. G.: The mechanism of petechial hemorrhage function. Blood, *4*:69, 1949.
184. Iatridis, P. G., and Ferguson, J. H.: The plasmatic atmosphere of blood platelets. Evidence that only fibrinogen, AcG, and activated Hageman factor are present on the surface of platelets. Thromb. et Diath. Haemorrh., *13*:114, 1965.
185. Ikkala, E., and Nevanlinna, H. R.: Congenital deficiency of fibrin stabilizing factor. Thromb. et Diath. Haemorrh., *7*:567, 1962.
186. Ingram, G. I. C.: Observations in a case of multiple hemostatic defects. Brit. J. Haem., *2*:180, 1956.
187. Jackson, D. P., Schmid, H. J., Zieve, P. D., Levin, J., and Conley, C. L.: Nature of a platelet-agglutinating factor in serum of patients with idiopathic thrombocytopenic purpura. J. Clin. Invest., *42*:383, 1963.
188. Johnson, S. A., Monto, R. W., and Caldwell, M. J.: A new approach to the thrombocytopathies. Thrombocytopathy A. Thromb. et Diath. Haemorrh., *2*:279, 1958.
189. Jones, H. W., and Tocantins, L. M.: The history of purpura hemorrhagica. Ann. M. History, 5:349, 1933 (N.S.).
190. Jorpes, J. E.: The origin and the physiology of heparin: the specific therapy in thrombosis. Ann. Int. Med., *27*:361, 1947.
190a. Kaneshiro, M. M., Mielke, C. H., Jr., Kasper, C. K., and Rapaport, S. I.: Bleeding time after aspirin in disorders of intrinsic clotting. New England J. Med., *281*:1039, 1969.
191. Karpatkin, S.: Heterogeneity of human platelets. II. Functional evidence suggestive of young and old platelets. J. Clin. Invest.,*48*:1083, 1969.
192. Karpatkin, S., Ingram, F. I. C., and Graham, J. B.: Severe isolated prothrombin deficiency: an acquired state with complete recovery. Thromb. et Diath. Haemorrh., *8*:221, 1962.
193. Karpatkin, S., and Siskind, G. W.: In vitro detection of platelet antibody in patients with idiopathic thrombocytopenic purpura and systemic lupus erythematosus. Blood, *33*:795, 1969.
194. Kasper, C. K., Buechy, D. Y. E. W., and Aggeler, P. M.: Hageman factor (Factor XII) in an affected kindred and in normal adults. Brit. J. Haemat, *14*:543, 1968.
195. Kass, L, Ratnoff, O. D., and Leon, M. A.: Studies on the purification of antihemophilia factor (Factor VIII). J. Clin. Invest., *48*:351, 1969.
196. Kattlove, H. E., Shapiro, S. S., and Spivack, M.: Hereditary prothrombin deficiency. New England J. Med., *282*:57, 1970.

197. Kekwick, R. A., and Wolf, P.: A concentrate of human antihaemophilic factor — its use in six cases of haemophilia. Lancet, *1*:647, 1957.
198. Kellaway, C. H.: Snake venom. Bull. Johns Hopkins Hosp., *60*:1, 1937.
199. Kellermeyer, R. W.: Inflammatory process in acute gouty arthritis. III. Vascular permeability-enhancing activity in normal human synovial fluid: induction by Hageman factor activators; and inhibition by Hageman factor antiserum. J. Lab. Clin. Med., *70*:365, 1967.
200. Kellermeyer, R. W.: Hageman factor and acute gouty arthritis. Arth. Rheum., *11*:452, 1968.
201. Kerr, C. B., Preston, A. E., Barr, A., and Biggs, R.: Inheritance of Factor VIII. Thromb. et Diath. Haem., Suppl., *17*:173, 1965.
201a. Kibel, M. A., and Barnard, P. J.: Treatment of acute hemolytic-uremic syndrome with heparin. Lancet, 2:259, 1964.
202. Kingsley, C. S.: Familial Factor V deficiency: The pattern of heredity. Quart. J. Med., *23*:323, 1954.
203. Kisker, C. T., Glueck, H., and Kander, E.: Anaphylactoid purpura progressing to gangrene and its treatment with heparin. J. Pediat., *73*:748, 1968.
204. Koch-Weser, J.: Quinidine-induced hypoprothrombinemic hemorrhage in patients on chronic warfarin therapy. Ann. Int. Med., *68*:511, 1968.
205. Kramar, J.: Stress and capillary resistance (capillary fragility). Am. J. Physiol., *175*:69, 1953.
206. Krevans, J. R., and Jackson, D. P.: Hemorrhagic disorder following massive whole blood transfusions. J.A.M.A., *159*:171, 1955.
207. Kurstjens, R., Bolt, C., Vossen, M., and Haanan, C.: Familial thrombopathic thrombocytopenia. Brit. J. Haem., *15*:305, 1968.
208. Larrieu, M. J., Caen, J., Lelong, J. C., and Bernard, J.: Maladie de Glanzmann. Nouv. Rev. Franc. Hemat., *1*:662, 1961.
209. Lee, S. L., and Sanders, M.: A disorder of blood coagulation in systemic lupus erythematosus. J. Clin. Invest., *34*:1814, 1955.
210. Leiba, H., Ramot, B., and Many, A.: Heredity and coagulation studies in ten families with Factor XI (plasma thromboplastin antecedent) deficiency. Brit. J. Haem., *11*:654, 1965.
211. Lerner, R. G., Rapaport, S. I., and Meltzer, J.: Thrombotic thrombocytopenic purpura. Ann. Int. Med., *66*:1180, 1967.
212. Levin, R. H., Pert, J. H., and Freireich, E. J.: Response to transfusion of platelets pooled from multiple donors and the effects of various technics of concentrating platelets. Transfusion, *5*:54, 1965.
213. Lewis, J. H., and Ferguson, J. H.: Afibrinogenemia. Report of a case. Am. J. Dis. Child., *88*:711, 1954.
214. Lewis, J. H., Ferguson, J. H., Spaugh, E., Fresh, J. W., and Zueker, M. B.: Acquired hypoprothrombinemia. Blood, *12*:84, 1957.
215. Lindenbaum, J., and Hargrave, R. L.: Thrombocytopenia in alcoholics. Ann. Int. Med., *68*:526, 1968.
216. Link, K. P.: The anticoagulant from spoiled sweet clover hay. Harvey Lect., *39*:162, 1944.
217. Lopez, V., Pflugshaupt, R., and Bütler, R.: A specific inhibitor of human clotting Factor V. Acta. Haemat., *40*:275, 1968.
218. Lorand, L.: Properties and significance of the fibrin stabilizing factor (FSF). Thromb. et Diath. Haemorrh. 7(Suppl. I):238, 1962.
219. Lorand, L., Urayama, T., Atencio, A. C., and Hsia, D. Y-Y.: Inheritance of deficiency of fibrin-stabilizing factor. Amer. J. Hem. Genet., *22*:89, 1970.
220. Lorand, L., Urayama, T., deKiewiet, J. W. C., and Nossel, H. L.: Diagnostic and genetic studies on fibrin-stabilizing factor with a new assay based on amine incorporation. J. Clin. Invest., *48*:1054, 1969.
221. Lozner, E. L., Jolliffe, L. S., and Taylor, F. H. L.: Hemorrhagic diathesis with prolonged coagulation time associated with a circulating anticoagulant. Am. J. Med. Sci., *199*:318, 1940.
222. Lucas, O. N., Finkelman, A., and Tocantins, L. M.: Management of tooth extraction in hemophiliacs by the combined use of hypnotic suggestion, protective splints and packing of sockets. J. Oral Surg., *20*:488, 1962.
223. Lüscher, E. F.: Retraction activity of the platelets: biochemical background and physiological significance. In Blood Platelets. Henry Ford Hospital Symposium. Little, Brown & Co., Boston, 1961, p. 445.
224. Macfarlane, R. G.: A boy with no fibrinogen. Lancet, *1*:309, 1938.
225. Macfarlane, R. G.: Critical review: The mechanism of haemostasis. Quart. J. Med., *10*:1, 1941 (N.S.).
226. Macfarlane, R. G., Biggs, R., and Bidwell, E.: Bovine antihaemophilic globulin in the treatment of haemophilia. Lancet, *1*:1316, 1954.
227. Macfarlane, R. G., Mallan, P. C., Wills, L. J., Bidwell, E., Biggs, R., Fraenkel, F. J., Honey, G. E., and Taylor, K. B.: Surgery in haemophilia. Lancet, *2*:251, 1957.

228. MacWhinney, J. B., Jr., Packer, J. T., Miller, G., and Greendyke, R. M.: Thrombotic thrombo-cytopenic purpura in childhood. Blood, *19*:181, 1962.
229. Malhotra, O. P., and Carter, J. R.: Prothrombin in Factor X deficiency. J. Lab. Clin. Med., *75*:120, 1970.
230. Mammen, E. F., Prasad, A. S., Barnhart, M. I., and Au, C. C.: Congenital dysfibrinogenemia: fibrinogen Detroit. J. Clin. Invest., *48*:235, 1969.
231. Marchioro, T. L., Hougie, C., Ragde, H., Epstein, R. B., and Thomas, E. D.: Hemophilia: role of organ homografts. Science, *163*:188, 1968.
232. Marcus, A. J.: Platelet function. New England J. Med., *280*:1213, 1278, 1330, 1969.
233. Marder, V. J., and Shulman, N. R.: Clinical aspects of congenital Factor VII deficiency. Am. J. Med., *37*:182, 1964.
234. Marder, V. J., and Shulman, N. R.: Major surgery in classic hemophilia using Fraction I. Am. J. Med., *41*:56, 1966.
235. Margolis, J.: Hageman factor and capillary permeability. Australian J. Exp. Biol. Med. Sci., *37*:239, 1959.
236. Masure, R.: Human Factor VIII prepared by cryoprecipitation. Vox Sanguinis, *16*:1, 1969.
237. McClure, P. D., and Choi, S. I.: Thrombopoietin and erythropoietin levels in idiopathic thrombocytopenic purpura and iron-deficiency anaemia. Brit. J. Haem., *15*:351, 1968.
238. McClure, P. D., Ingram, G. I. C., Stacey, R. S., Glass, U. H., and Matchett, M. O.: Platelet function tests in thrombocythemia and thrombocytosis. Brit. J. Hemat., *12*:478, 1966.
239. McKay, D. G.: Progress in disseminated intravascular coagulation. II. California Medicine, *3*:186, 279, 1969.
240. McKay, D. G., and Müller-Berghaus, G.: Therapeutic implications of disseminated intra-vascular coagulation. Am. J. Cardiol., *20*:392, 1967.
241. Meacham, G. C., and Weisberger, A. S.: Unusual manifestations of disseminated lupus erythematosus. Ann. Int. Med., *43*:143, 1955.
242. Ménaché, D.: Constitutional and familial abnormal fibrinogen. Thromb. et Diath. Haemorrh., *10*:Suppl. 13, 173, 1963.
243. Merskey, C.: The occurrence of haemophilia in the human female. Quart. J. Med., *20*:299, 1951 (N.S.).
244. Merskey, C.: Diagnosis and treatment of intravascular coagulation. Brit. J. Haemat., *15*:523, 1968.
245. Merskey, C., Johnson, A. J., Kleiner, G. J., and Wohl, H.: The defibrination syndrome: clinical features and laboratory diagnosis. Brit. J. Haemat., *13*:528, 1967.
245a. Mettler, N. E.: Isolation of a microtatobiote from patients with hemolytic-uremic syndrome and thrombotic thrombocytopenic purpura and from mites in the United States. New England J. Med., *281*:1023, 1969.
246. Meyer, T. C., and Angus, J.: The effect of large doses of "Synkavit" in the newborn. Arch. Dis. Child., *31*:212, 1956.
247. Meyers, M. C.: Results of treatment in 71 patients with idiopathic thrombocytopenic pur-pura. Am. J. Med. Sci., *242*:295, 1961.
248. Michaeli, D., Ben-Bassat, I., Miller, H. I., and Deutsch, V.: Hepatic telangiectasis and porto-systemic encephalopathy in Osler-Weber-Render disease. Gasteroenterology, *54*:929, 1968.
249. Mills, S. D.: Purpuric manifestations occurring in measles in childhood. J. Pediatrics, *36*:35, 1950.
250. Miloszewski, K., Walls, W. D., and Losowsky, M. S.: Absence of plasma transamidase activity in congenital deficiency of fibrin stabilizing factor (Factor XIII). Brit. J. Haemat., *17*:159, 1969.
251. Mitchell, J. S.: Metabolic effects of therapeutic doses of X and gamma radiations. Brit. J. Radiol., *16*:339, 1943.
252. Monnens, L. A. H., and Retera, R. J. M.: Thrombotic thrombocytopenic purpura in a neo-natal infant. J. Pediatrics, *71*:118, 1967.
253. Moschowitz, E.: An acute febrile pleiochromic anemia with hyaline thrombosis of the terminal arterioles and capillaries. An undescribed disease. Arch. Int. Med., *36*:89, 1925.
254. Moser, K., Lechner, K., and Vinazzer, H.: A hitherto not described enzyme defect in throm-basthenia: glutathionreductase deficiency. Thromb. et Diath. Haemorrh., *19*:46, 1968.
255. Mosesson, M. W., and Beck, E. A.: Chromatographic, ultracentrifugal, and related studies of fibrinogen "Baltimore." J. Clin. Invest., *48*:1656, 1969.
256. Moss, M. H.: Hypoprothrombinemic bleeding in a young infant. Am. J. Dis. Child., *117*:540, 1969.
257. Mürer, E. H.: Thrombin-induced release of calcium from blood platelets. Science, *166*:623, 1969.
258. Mustard, J. F.: Platelets in stored blood. Brit. J. Haem., *2*:17, 1956.
259. Myllylä, G., Vaheri, A., Vesikari, T., and Penttinen, K.: Interaction between human blood platelets, viruses and antibodies. Clin. Exp. Immunol., *4*:323, 1969.

260.   Najean, Y., Ardaillou, N., Dresch, C., and Bernard, J.: The platelet destruction site in throm-
       bocytopenic purpuras. Brit. J. Haemat., *13*:409, 1967.
261.   Nilsson, I. M.: Treatment of haemophilia A and von Willebrand's disease. Biblio. Haemat.,
       23:1307, 1965.
262.   Nilsson, I. M., Anderson, L., and Bjorkman, S. E.: Epsilon-aminocaproic acid (EACA) as a
       therapeutic agent based on 5 years clinical experience. Acta Med. Scandinav., Suppl.
       448:1, 1966.
263.   Nilsson, I. M., and Blombäck, M.: Von Willebrand's disease in Sweden. Occurrence, patho-
       genesis and treatment. Thromb. et Diath. Haemorrh., *9*(Suppl. 2):102, 1963.
264.   Nilsson, I. M.: Blombäck, M., Jorpes, E., Blombäck, B., and Johansson, S.-A.: Von Wille-
       brand's disease and its correction with human plasma fraction 1-0. Acta Med. Scandinav.,
       159:179, 1957.
265.   Nilsson, I. M., Blombäck, M., and von Francken, I.: On an inherited autosomal hemorrhagic
       diathesis and antihemophilic globulin (AHG) deficiency and prolonged bleeding time.
       Acta Med. Scandinav., *159*:35, 1957.
266.   Norcross, J. W., and Cyr, D. P.: Treatment of chronic idiopathic thrombocytopenic purpura
       in the adult. Postgrad. Med., *33*:74, 1963.
267.   Norman, J. C., Covelli, V. H., and Sise, H. S.: Transplantation of the spleen: experimental
       cure of hemophilia. Surgery, *64*:1, 1968.
268.   Nossel, H. L., Niemitz, J., Mibashan, R. S., and Schulze, W. G.: The measurement of Factor
       XI (plasma thromboplastin antecedent): diagnosis and therapy of the congenital deficiency
       state. Brit. J. Haemat., *12*:133, 1966.
269.   Nour-Eldin, F., and Wilkinson, J. F.: Changes in the blood-clotting defect in Christmas
       disease after plasma and serum transfusions. Clin. Sc., *17*:303, 1958.
269a. Nussbaum, M., and Dameshek, W.: Transient hemolytic and thrombocytopenic episode
       (? acute transient thrombohemolytic thrombocytopenic purpura) with probable menin-
       gococcemia. New England J. Med., *256*:448, 1957.
270.   Nussbaum, M., and Morse, B. S.: Plasma fibrin stabilizing factor activity in various diseases.
       Blood, *23*:669, 1964.
271.   Oberman, H. A., and Penner, J. A.: Utilization of residual plasma following preparation of
       Factor VIII cryoprecipitate. J.A.M.A., *205*:819, 1968.
272.   O'Brien, J. R.: An acquired coagulation defect in a woman. J. Clin. Path., 7:22, 1954.
273.   O'Brien, J. R., and Heywood, J. B.: Some interactions between human platelets and glass:
       von Willebrand's disease compared with normal. J. Clin. Path., *20*:56, 1967.
274.   Oski, F. A., Naiman, J. L., and Diamond, L. K.: Use of the plasma acid phosphatase value in
       the differentiation of thrombocytopenic states. New England J. Med., *268*:1423, 1963.
275.   Osler, W.: On a family form of recurring epistaxis, associated with multiple telangiectases of
       the skin and mucous membranes. Johns Hopkins Hosp. Bull., *12*:333, 1901.
276.   Osler, W.: The visceral lesions of purpura and allied conditions. Brit. M. J., *1*:517, 1914.
277.   Owren, P. A.: The coagulation of blood-investigation on a new clotting factor. Acta Med.
       Scandinav., Suppl. 194, 1947.
278.   Owren, P. A.: The diagnostic and prognostic significance of plasma prothrombin and factor
       V levels in parenchymatous hepatitis and obstructive jaundice. Scandinav. J. Clin. & Lab.
       Invest., *1*:131, 1949.
279.   Packham, M. A., Nishizawa, E. E., and Mustard, J. F.: Response of platelets to tissue injury.
       Biochem. Pharmacol., *17*:171, 1968.
280.   Panner, B.: Nephritis of Schönlein-Henoch syndrome. Arch. Path., *74*:230, 1962.
281.   Patek, A. J., Jr., and Taylor, F. H. L.: Hemophilia. II. Some properties of a substance obtained
       from normal human plasma effective in accelerating the coagulation of hemophilic blood.
       J. Clin. Invest., *16*:113, 1937.
282.   Patterson, J. H., Pierce, R. B., Amerson, J. R., and Watkins, W. L.: Dextran therapy of
       purpura fulminans. New England J. Med., *273*:734, 1965.
283.   Pavlosky, A.: Contribution to the pathogenesis of hemophilia. Blood, *2*:185, 1947.
284.   Pearson, H. A., Shulman, N. R., Marder, V. J., and Cone, T. E., Jr.: Iso-immune neonatal
       thrombocytopenic purpura: clinical and therapeutic considerations. Blood, *23*:154, 1964.
285.   Perkins, H. A.: Brief report: correction of the hemostatic defects in von Willebrand's disease.
       Blood, *30*:375, 1967.
286.   Phillips, L. L.: Homologous serum jaundice following fibrinogen administration. Surg.
       Gynec. Obstet., *121*:551, 1965.
287.   Phillips, L. L., Hyman, G. A., and Rosenthal, R. L.: Prolonged postoperative bleeding in a
       patient with Factor XI (PTA) deficiency. Ann. Surg., *162*:37, 1965.
288.   Philpott, M. G.: The Schönlein-Henoch syndrome in childhood with particular reference to
       the occurrence of nephritis. Arch. Dis. Child., *27*:480, 1952.

289. Pitney, W. R., and Potter, M.: Retention of platelets by glass bead filters. J. Clin. Path., *20*:710, 1967.

290. Pool, J. G.: The effect of several variables on cryoprecipitated Factor VIII (AHG) concentrates. Transfusion, 7:165, 1967.

291. Pool, J. G., Desai, R., and Kropatkin, M.: Severe congenital hypoprothrombinemia in a Negro boy. Thromb. et Diath. Haemorrh., *8*:235, 1962.

292. Pool, J. G., Hershgold, E. J., and Pappenhagen, A. R.: High potency antihemophilic factor concentrate prepared from cryoglobulin precipitate. Nature, *203*:312, 1964.

293. Poole, J. C. F., and French, J. E.: Thrombosis. J. Atheroscler. Res., *1*:251, 1961.

294. Post, R. M., and Desforges, J. F.: Thrombocytopenia and alcoholism. Ann. Int. Med., *68*:1230, 1968.

295. Prentice, C. R. M., Breckenridge, R. T., Forman, W. B., and Ratnoff, O. D.: Treatment of hemophilia (Factor VIII deficiency) with human antihemophilic factor prepared by the cryoprecipitate process. Lancet, *1*:457, 1967.

296. Presley, S. J., Best, W. R., and Limarzi, L. R.: Bone marrow in idiopathic thrombocytopenic purpura. J. Lab. & Clin. Med., *40*:503, 1952.

297. Prichard, R. W., and Vann, R. L.: Congenital afibrinogenemia. Am. J. Dis. Child., *88*:703, 1954.

298. Pritchard, J. A., and Wright, M. R.: Studies to determine the cause of hypofibrinogenemia in placental abruption. Am. J. Med., *27*:321, 1959.

299. Purcell, G., Jr., and Nossel, H. L.: Factor XI (PTA) deficiency: surgical and obstetrical aspects. Obstet. & Gynec., *35*:69, 1970.

300. Quick, A. J.: The prothrombin in hemophilia and in obstructive jaundice. J. Biol. Chem., *109*:73, 1935.

300a. Quick, A. J.: Salicylates and bleeding: aspirin tolerance test. Am. J. Med. Sci., *252*:265, 1966.

301. Quick, A. J.: Clinical Course in Hemophilia. J.A.M.A., *210*:1, 1969.

302. Quick, A. J., and Collentine, G. E.: The role of vitamin K in the synthesis of prothrombin. Am. J. Physiol., *164*:716, 1951.

303. Rabinowitz, Y., and Dameshek, W.: Systemic lupus erythematosus after "idiopathic" thrombocytopenic purpura: a review. Ann. Int. Med., *52*:1, 1960.

304. Rand, M., and Reid, G.: Source of "serotonin" in serum. Nature, *168*:385, 1951.

305. Ratnoff, O. D., Busse, R. J., Jr., and Sheon, R. P.: The demise of John Hageman. New England J. Med., *279*:760, 1968.

306. Ratnoff, O. D., and Colopy, J. E.: Familial hemorrhagic trait associated with deficiency of clot promoting fraction of the plasma. J. Clin. Invest., *34*:602, 1955.

307. Ratnoff, O. D., and Colopy, J. E.: Biology and pathology of initial stages of blood coagulation. Prog. in Hemat., *5*:204, 1966.

308. Ratnoff, O. D., Kass, L., and Lang, P. D.: Studies on the purification of antihemophilic factor, Factor VIII. J. Clin. Invest., *48*:957, 1969.

309. Ratnoff, O. D., and Miles, A. A.: Induction of permeability-increasing activity in human plasma by activated Hageman factor. Brit. J. Exp. Path., *45*:328, 1964.

310. Ratnoff, O. D., and Steinberg, A. G.: Further studies on inheritance of Hageman trait. J. Lab. Clin. Med., *59*:980, 1962.

311. Reid, D. E., Weiner, A. E., and Roby, C. C.: Intravascular clotting and afibrinogenemia: the presumptive lethal factors in the syndrome of amniotic fluid embolism. Am. J. Obstet. & Gynec., *66*:465, 1953.

312. Reid, D. E., Weiner, A. E., Roby, C. C., and Diamond, L. K.: Maternal afibrinogenemia associated with long standing intrauterine fetal death. Am. J. Obstet. & Gynec., *66*:500, 1953.

313. Roberts, H. R., Lechler, E., Webster, W. P., and Penick, G. D.: Survival of transfused Factor X in patients with Stuart disease. Thromb. et Diath. Haemorrh., *13*:305, 1965.

314. Roberts, H. R., Grizzle, J. E., McLester, W. D., and Penick, G. D.: Genetic variants of hemophilia B: detection by means of a specific PTC inhibitor. J. Clin. Invest., *47*:360, 1968.

315. Robinson, A. J., Aggeler, P. M., McNicol, G. P., and Douglas, A. S.: An atypical genetic haemorrhagic disease with increased concentration of a natural inhibitor of prothrombin consumption. Brit. J. Haemat., *13*:510, 1967.

316. Robinson, P. M., Tittley, P., and Smalley, R. K.: Prophylactic therapy in classical hemophilia: a preliminary report. Canad. Med. Assoc. J., *97*:559, 1967.

317. Robson, H. N., and Duthie, J. J. R.: Further observations on capillary resistance and adrenocortical activity. Brit. M. J., *1*:994, 1952.

318. Rodriguez-Erdmann, F.: Treatment of the Shwartzman reaction. New England J. Med., *271*:632, 1964.

319. Rodriguez-Erdmann, F.: Bleeding due to increased intravascular blood coagulation, hemor-

rhagic syndromes caused by consumption of blood-clotting factors (consumption-coagulopathies). New England J. Med., *273*:1370, 1965.

320. Rodriguez-Erdmann, F., and Levitan, R.: Gastrointestinal and roentgenological manifestations of Henoch-Schoenlein purpura. Gastroenterology, *54*:260, 1968.
321. Rodriguez, S. U., Leikin, S. L., and Hiller, M. C.: Neonatal thrombocytopenia associated with anti-partum administration of thiazide drugs. New England J. Med., *270*:881, 1964.
322. Rosenthal, M. C.: Deficiency in plasma thromboplastin component. II. Its incidence in hemophilic population. Critique of methods for identification. Am. J. Clin. Path., *24*:910, 1954.
323. Rosenthal, M. C., and Sanders, M.: Plasma thromboplastin component deficiency. Am. J. Med., *16*:153, 1954.
324. Rosenthal, R. L.: Properties of plasma thromboplastin antecedent (PTA) in relation to blood coagulation. J. Lab. & Clin. Med., *45*:123, 1955.
325. Rosenthal, R. L., Dreskin, O. H., and Rosenthal, N.: New hemophilia-like disease caused by deficiency of a third plasma thromboplastin factor. Proc. Soc. Exper. Biol. & Med., *82*:171, 1953.
326. Rosenthal, R. L., and Sloan, E.: PTA (Factor XI) levels and coagulation studies after plasma infusions in PTA-deficient patients. J. Lab. Clin. Med., *66*:709, 1965.
327. Rosner, F.: Medical history: hemophilia in the Talmud and rabbinic writings. Ann. Int. Med., *70*:833, 1969.
328. Ruffolo, E. H., Pease, G. L., and Cooper, T.: Thrombotic thrombocytopenic purpura. Arch. Int. Med., *110*:78, 1962.
329. Salzman, E. W.: Measurement of platelet adhesiveness: progress report. Thromb. et Diath. Haemorrh., Suppl. *26*:323, 1967.
330. Salzman, E. W., and Britten, A.: In vitro correction of defective platelet adhesiveness in von Willebrand's disease. Fed. Proc., *23*:239, 1964.
331. Saunders, W. H.: Hereditary hemorrhagic telangiectasia. Arch. Otolaryng., *76*:245, 1962.
332. Schaar, F. E.: Familial idiopathic thrombocytopenic purpura. J. Pediat., *62*:546, 1963.
333. Schmid, H. J., Jackson, D. P., and Conley, C. L.: Mechanism of action of thrombin on platelets. J. Clin. Invest., *41*:543, 1962.
334. Schneider, C. L.: Fibrin embolism (disseminated intravascular coagulation) with defibrination as one of the end results during placenta abruptio. Surg. Gynec. & Obstet., *92*:27, 1951.
335. Schneider, C. L.: Rapid estimation of plasma fibrinogen concentration and its use as a guide to therapy of intravascular defibrination. Am. J. Obstet. & Gynec., *64*:141, 1952.
336. Schulman, I., Abildgaard, C. F., Cornet, J., Simone, J. V., and Currimbhoy, Z.: Studies on thrombopoiesis. II. Assay of human plasma thrombopoietic activity. J. Pediat., *66*:604, 1965.
337. Schulman, I., Pierce, M., Lukens, A., and Currimbhoy, Z.: Studies on thrombopoiesis. I. A factor in normal human plasma required for platelet production; chronic thrombocytopenia due to its deficiency. Blood, *16*:943, 1960.
338. Schulman, I., Smith, G. H., Erlandson, M., and Fort, E.: Vascular hemophilia. Am. J. Dis. Child., *90*:526, 1955.
339. Scott, J. S.: Blood coagulation failure in obstetrics, effects of dextran and plasma. Brit. Med. J., *2*:290, 1955.
340. Seip, M.: Hereditary hypoplastic thrombocytopenia. Acta Paediat., *52*:370, 1963.
341. Seligsohn, U., and Ramot, B.: Combined Factor V and Factor VIII deficiency: report of four cases. Brit. J. Haemat., *16*:475, 1969.
342. Serpick, A. A.: Platelet transfusion therapy. J.A.M.A., *192*:625, 1965.
343. Shanbrom, E., and Thelin, G. M.: Experimental prophylaxis of severe hemophilia with a Factor VIII concentrate. J.A.M.A., *208*:1853, 1969.
344. Shapiro, C. M., Texidor, T. A., Robbins, K. C., and Rabiner, S. F.: Clinical remission of purpura hyperglobulinemia. Arch. Int. Med., *124*:81, 1969.
345. Shapiro, S. S., and Carroll, K. S.: Acquired Factor VIII antibodies: further immunologic and electrophoretic studies. Science, *160*:786, 1968.
346. Shapiro, S. S., Martinez, J., and Halburn, R. R.: Congenital dysprothrombinemia: an inherited structural disorder of human prothrombin. J. Clin. Invest., *48*:2251, 1969.
347. Sharp, A. A.: Pathological fibrinolysis. Brit. Med. Bull., *20*:240, 1964.
348. Sharp, A. A.: The significance of fibrinolysis. Proc. Roy. Soc., Series B, Biol. Sci., *173*:311, 1969.
349. Sharp, A. A., Howie, B., Biggs, R., and Methuen, D. T.: Defibrination syndrome in pregnancy. Value of various diagnostic tests. Lancet, *2*:1309, 1958.
350. Sherman, L. A., Goldstein, M. A., and Sise, H. S.: Circulating anticoagulant (antifactor VIII) treated with immunosuppressive drugs. Thromb. et Diath. Haemorrh., *21*:249, 1969.
351. Sherry, S.: Fibrinolysis. Ann. Rev. Med., *19*:247, 1968.
352. Sherry, S.: Thrombolysis by urokinase. J. Atherosclerosis Res., *9*:1, 1969.

353. Shulman, I.: Diagnosis and treatment: management of idiopathic thrombocytopenic purpura. Pediatrics, *33*:979, 1964.
354. Shulman, N. R.: Mechanism of blood cell destruction in individuals sensitized to foreign antigens. Trans. Assoc. Am. Phys., *76*:72, 1963.
355. Shulman, N. R., Aster, R. H., Leitner, A., and Hiller, M. C.: Immunoreactions involving platelets. V. Post-transfusion purpura due to a complement-fixing antibody against a genetically controlled platelet antigen. A proposed mechanism for thrombocytopenia and its relevance in "autoimmunity." J. Clin. Invest., *40*:1597, 1961.
356. Shulman, N. R., Aster, R. H., Pearson, H. A., and Hiller, M. C.: Immunoreactions involving platelets. VI. Reactions of maternal isoantibodies responsible for neonatal purpura. Differentiation of a second platelet antigen system. J. Clin. Invest., *41*:1059, 1962.
356a. Shulman, N. R., and Hirschman, R. J.: Acquired hemophilia. Trans. Assoc. Am. Phys., *82*:388, 1969.
357. Shulman, N. R., Marder, V. J., and Weinrack, R. S.: Similarities between known antiplatelet antibodies and the factor responsible for thrombocytopenia in idiopathic purpura. Physiologic, serologic, and isotopic studies. Ann. N.Y. Acad. Sci., *124*:499, 1965.
358. Simone, J. V., Cornet, J. A., and Abildgaard, C. F.: Acquired von Willebrand's syndrome in systemic lupus erythematosus. Blood, *31*:806, 1968.
359. Smith, H.: Purpura fulminans complicating varicella recovery with low molecular weight dextran and steroids. Med. J. Australia, 2:685, 1967.
360. Soloman, W., Turner, D. S., Block, C., and Posner, A. C.: Thrombotic thrombocytopenic purpura in pregnancy. J.A.M.A., *184*:587, 1963.
361. Soulier, J. P.: Syndromes hémorrhagiques avec atteinte isolée de la résistance capillaire. Le sang, *21*:801, 1950.
362. Soulier, J. P., Josso, F., Steinbuch, M., and Cosson, A.: The therapeutical use of Fraction P.P.S.B. Biblio. Haemat., *29*:1127, 1968.
363. Soulier, J. P., and Larrieu, M. J.: Differentiation of hemophilia into two groups. A study of thirty-three cases. New England J. Med., *249*:547, 1953.
364. Spaet, T. H., and Zucker, M. B.: Mechanism of platelet plug formation and role of adenosine diphosphate. Am. J. Phys. Med., *206*:1267, 1964.
365. Speer, R. J., Ridgway, H., and Hill, J. M.: Activated human Hageman Factor (XII). Thromb. et Diath. Haemorrh., *14*:1, 1965.
366. Staub, H. P.: Postrubella thrombocytopenic purpura. A report of eight cases with discussion of hemorrhagic manifestations of rubella. Clin. Ped., *7*:350, 1968.
367. Stefanini, M.: Management of thrombocytopenic states. Arch. Int. Med., *95*:543, 1955.
368. Stefanini, M.: Basic mechanisms of hemostasis. Bull. N.Y. Acad. Med., *20*:239, 1954.
369. Stefanini, M.: Activity of plasma labile factor in disease. Lancet, *1*:606, 1951.
370. Stefanini, M., and Chatterjea, J. B.: Studies on platelets. IV. A thrombocytopenic factor in normal human blood plasma or serum. Proc. Soc. Exper. Biol. & Med., *79*:623, 1952.
371. Stefanini, M., Chatterjea, J. B., Dameshek, W., Zannos, L., and Santiago, E. P.: The effect of transfusion of platelet-rich polycythemic blood on the platelets and hemostatic function in "idiopathic" and "secondary" thrombocytopenic purpura. Blood, 7:53, 1952.
372. Stefanini, M., and Dameshek, W.: The Hemorrhagic Disorders. Grune and Stratton, New York, 1955.
373. Stefanini, M., and Dameshek, W.: Collection, preservation, and transfusion of platelets. New England J. Med., *248*:797, 1953.
374. Stefanini, M., Roy, C. A., Zannos, L., and Dameshek, W.: Therapeutic effect of pituitary adrenocortotropic hormone (ACTH) in a case of Henoch-Schönlein vascular (anaphylactoid) purpura. J.A.M.A., *144*:1372, 1950.
375. Steinkamp, R., Moore, C. V., and Doubek, W. G.: Thrombocytopenic purpura caused by hypersensitivity to quinine. J. Lab. & Clin. Med., *45*:18, 1955.
375a. Stites, D. P., Hershgold, G. J., Perlman, J. D., and Fudenberg, H. H.: Factor VIII: Detection by hemagglutination inhibition. Hemophilia and von Willenbrand's disease. Science, *171*:196, 1971.
376. Storti, E., Traldi, A., Tosatti, E., and Davoli, P. G.: Synovectomy, a new approach to haemophilic arthropathy. Acta Haemat., *41*:193, 1969.
377. Strauss, H. S.: Acquired circulating anticoagulants in hemophilia A. New England J. Med., *281*:866, 1969.
378. Strauss, H. S., and Bloom, G. E.: Von Willebrand's disease. New England J. Med., *273*:171, 1965.
379. Strauss, H. S., and Merler, E.: Characterization and properties of an inhibitor of Factor VIII in the plasma of patients with hemophilia A following repeated transfusions. Blood, *30*:137, 1967.
380. Sussman, L. N.: Azathioprine in refractory thrombocytopenic purpura. J.A.M.A., *202*:259, 1967.

381. Sutherland, J. M., Glueck, H. I., and Gleser, G.: Hemorrhagic disease of the newborn. Am.
      J. Dis. Child., *113*:524, 1967.
382. Suttie, J. W.: Control of clotting factor biosynthesis by vitamin K. Fed. Proc., *28*:1696, 1969.
383. Szpilmanowa, H., and Stachurska, J.: Hageman factor (Factor XII) activity in synovial fluid
      of rheumatoid arthritis patients and its possible pathogenic significance. Experentia,
      24:784, 1968.
384. Tagnon, H. J., Schulman, P., Whitmore, W. F., and Leone, L. A.: Prostatic fibrinolysin.
      Am. J. Med., *15*:875, 1953.
385. Tagnon, H. J., Whitmore, W. F., and Shulman, N. R.: Fibrinolysis in metastatic cancer of
      the prostate. Cancer, *5*:9, 1952.
386. Talbot, J. H., and Ferrandis, R. M.: Collagen Diseases. Grune and Stratton, New York, 1956.
386a. Taub, R. N., Rodriguez-Erdmann, F., and Dameshek, W.: Intravascular coagulation, the
      Shwartzman reaction and the pathogenesis of T.T.P. Blood, *24*:775, 1964.
387. Thomas, D. P., Ream, V. J., and Stuart, R. K.: Platelet aggregation in Laennec's cirrhosis.
      New England J. Med., *276*:1344, 1967.
388. Tocantins, L. M.: Platelets and the structure and physical properties of blood clots. Am. J.
      Physiol., *114*:709, 1936.
389. Trieger, N., and McGovern, J. J.: Evaluation of corticosteroids in hemophilia. New England
      J. Med., *266*:432, 1962.
390. Tullis, J. L., and Melin, M.: Management of Christmas disease and Stuart-Prower deficiency
      with a prothrombin-complex concentrate (Factors II, VII, IX, and X). Biblio. Haemat.,
      29:1134, 1968.
390a. Umlas, J., and Kaiser, J.: Thrombohemolytic thrombocytopenic purpura (TTP): A disease
      or a syndrome? Am. J. Med., *49*:723, 1970.
391. Van Creveld, S., Ho, L. K., and Veder, H. A.: Thrombopathia. Acta Haemat., *19*:199, 1958.
392. Van Creveld, S., and Paulssen, M. M. P.: Significance of clotting factors in blood-platelets,
      in normal and pathological conditions. Lancet, *2*:242, 1951.
393. Van Creveld, S., Mochtar, I. A., Van Charantevan Der Meulen, C. C. M., Pascha, C. N., and
      Stibbe, J.: Investigation of circulating anticoagulants against AHF (Factor VIII) in three
      patients with hemophilia A. Acta Haemat., *39*:214, 1968.
394. Vandenbroucke, J., and Verstraete, M.: Thrombocytopenia due to platelet agglutinins in
      the newborn. Lancet, *1*:593, 1955.
395. van Itterbeek, H., Vermylen, J., and Verstraete, M.: High obstruction of urine flow as a
      complication of the treatment with fibrinolysis inhibitors of haematuria in haemophiliacs.
      Acta Haemat., *39*:237, 1968.
396. Vernier, R. L., Worthen, H. B., Peterson, R. D., Colle, E., and Good, R. A.: Anaphylactoid
      purpura: pathology of the skin and kidney and frequency of streptococcal infection.
      Pediatrics, *27*:181, 1961.
397. Villalobus, T. J., Adelson, E., and Barila, T. J.: Hematologic changes in hypothermic dogs.
      Proc. Soc. Exper. Biol. & Med., *89*:192, 1955.
397a. Vitsky, B., Suzuki, Y., Strauss, L., and Churg, J.: The hemolytic-uremic syndrome. Am. J.
      Path., *57*:627, 1969.
398. Von Felten, A., Frick, P. G., and Straub, P. W.: Studies on fibrin monomer aggregation in
      congenital dysfibrinogenemia fibrin fraction. Brit. J. Haem., *16*:353, 1969.
399. Waddell, W. W., Jr., Guerry, D., III, Bray, W. E., and Kelley, O. R.: Possible effects of vitamin
      K on prothrombin and clotting time in newly-born infants. Proc. Soc. Exper. Biol. &
      Med., *40*:432, 1939.
400. Waldenström, J.: Incipient myelomatosis or "essential" hyperglobulinemia with fibrino-
      genopenia—a new syndrome? Acta Med. Scandinav., *117*:216, 1944.
401. Wall, R. L., McConnell, J., Moore, D., Macpherson, C. R., and Marson, A.: Christmas disease,
      color blindness and blood group Xg. Am. J. Med., *43*:214, 1967.
402. Wardle, E. N.: Immunoglobulins and immunological reactions in hemophilia. Lancet, *2*:233,
      1967.
403. Ware, A. G., Fahey, J. L., and Seegers, W. N.: Platelet extracts, fibrin formation, and inter-
      action of purified prothrombin and thromboplastin. Am. J. Physiol., *154*:140, 1948.
404. Watson-Williams, E. J., Macpherson, A. I., and Davidson, S.: The treatment of idiopathic
      thrombocytopenic purpura; a review of ninety-three cases. Lancet, *2*:221, 1958.
405. Weber, F. P.: Multiple hereditary developmental angiomata (telangiectases) of the skin and
      mucous membranes associated with recurring hemorrhages. Lancet, *2*:160, 1907.
406. Weiner, A. E., Reid, D. E., and Roby, C. C.: Incoagulable blood in severe premature separa-
      tion of the placenta. A method of management. Am. J. Obstet. & Gynec., *66*:475, 1953.
407. Weiss, H. J.: Analytic review: von Willebrand's disease—diagnostic criteria. Blood, *32*:4, 1968.
408. Weiss, H. J.: Platelet aggregation, adhesion and adenosine diphosphate release in thrombo-
      pathia (platelet Factor 3 deficiency) comparison with Glanzmann's thrombasthenia and
      von Willebrand's disease. Am. J. Med., *43*:570, 1967.

408a. Weiss, H. J., Aledort, L. M., and Kochwa, S.: Effect of salicylates on hemostatic properties of platelets in man. J. Clin. Invest., 47:2169, 1968.

408b. Weiss, H. J., Chervenick, P. A., Zalusky, R., and Factor, A.: A familial defect in platelet function associated with impaired release of adenosine diphosphate. New England J. Med., 281:1264, 1969.

409. Weiss, H. J., and Eichelberger, J. W., Jr.: The detection of platelet defects in patients with mild bleeding disorders. Am. J. Med., 32:872, 1962.

410. Weiss, H. J., and Eichelberger, J. W., Jr.: Secondary thrombocytopathia: platelet Factor 3 in various disease states. Arch. Int. Med., 112:827, 1963.

411. Weiss, H. J., and Kochwa, S.: Studies of platelet function and proteins in 3 patients with Glanzmann's thrombasthenia. J. Lab. & Clin. Med., 71:153, 1968.

412. Whipple, G. H.: Fibrinogen. I. An investigation concerning its origins and destruction in the body. Am. J. Phys. Med., 33:50, 1914.

413. Whissell, D. Y., Hoag, M. S., Aggeler, P. M., Kropatkin, M., and Garner, E.: Hemophilia in a woman. Am. J. Med., 38:119, 1965.

414. Wilde, C., Ellis, D., and Cooper, W. M.: Splenectomy for chronic idiopathic thrombocyopenic purpura. Arch. Surg., 95:344, 1967.

415. Williams, G. A., and Brick, I. B.: Gastrointestinal bleeding in hereditary hemorrhagic telangiectasia. Arch. Int. Med., 95:41, 1955.

416. Winterbauer, R. H.: Multiple telangiectasia, Reynaud's phenomenon, sclerodactyly, and subcutaneous calcinosis: a syndrome mimicking hereditary hemorrhagic telangiectasia. Bull. Johns Hopkins Hosp., 114:361, 1964.

417. Wishart, C., Smith, A. C., Honey, G. E., and Taylor, K. B.: Dental extraction in haemophilia. Lancet, 2:363, 1957.

418. Wolper, J., and Laibson, R. R.: Hereditary hemorrhagic telangiectasis (Rendu-Osler-Weber disease) with filamentary keratitis. Arch. Ophthal., 81:272, 1969.

419. Wright, D. O., Reppert, L. B., and Cuttino, J. T.: Purpuric manifestations of heat-stroke. Arch. Int. Med., 77:27, 1946.

420. Zucker, M. B.: In vitro abnormality of the blood in von Willebrand's disease correctable by normal plasma. Nature, 197:601, 1963.

421. Zucker, M. B., Pert, J. H., and Hilgartner, M. W.: Platelet function in a patient with thrombasthenia. Blood, 28:524, 1966.

XII / Leukocytes

Credit for distinguishing between the red and white corpuscles in the circulating blood has been given to William Hewson.[32] The term "leukocytosis" was introduced by Virchow to indicate a temporary increase in the number of circulating leukocytes; he recognized that increases occurred in a variety of normal and disease states. The association of leukocytosis with infectious processes attracted considerable attention and stimulated numerous investigations. Almost 50 years ago the authors of one book on hematology wrote, "The problem of leukocytosis has been subjected to as much discussion as any question of modern medicine. An exhaustive recital of the work devoted to it, of its methods, and of the results of this work would fill a whole volume and would be out of place in a treatise on blood diseases."[23] Since that time other investigations of the origin, function, and variations in the leukocytes have added to our knowledge but many important details remain to be clarified.

The origin and morphology of the leukocytes are discussed in Chapter I. The present chapter deals with the functions these cells perform, the numbers of the different types of leukocytes that are found in normal circumstances, the variations that occur under different physiologic and pathologic conditions, and the mechanisms that are considered important in producing these changes. Some of the functions of these cells, particularly those concerned in antigen-antibody reactions are discussed in Chapter XV.

Granulocytes

Leukopoiesis

The granulocytes constitute a tissue of considerable size. Only a small part of this tissue is contained in the circulating blood, where the number of granulocytes normally ranges from 2000 to 6000 per cu.mm. Osgood has calculated that the total number of the cells of this series in the hematopoietic organ (marrow) is 18×10^{11}, and in the circulating blood 20×10^9; in the tissue exclusive of the blood and blood-forming organs the calculated total is 12×10^{11}.[50] The quantity and distribution of the cells are better appreciated by considering the total mass of cells rather than the total numbers. It is estimated that the weight of the granulocytic cells in the marrow is 900 gm., in the circulating blood 10 gm., and in other tissues 600 gm. In the normal adult the spleen weighs about 150 gm. and the liver about 1500 gm. Donohue and others, who employed a radioiron technique, calculated that the average total marrow granulocytic forms in man is 11.4×10^9 cells per kg. or 79.8×10^{10} for a 70 kg. man; of this total 61.6×10^{10} are metamyelocytes, bands, and segmented forms, cells that can be released from the marrow quickly. The same authors placed the total of freely circulating granulocytes at 2.1×10^{10} in a 70 kg. man.[21] It has been reported that an equal number of cells, 2.1×10^{10}, is sequestered in the capillaries in the body.[3]

The location and function of the extravascular granulocytes is an intriguing problem. The bone marrow apparently serves as a reservoir of functioning cells as well as an organ of production.[20, 74] Other sites of extravascular accumulation are the lungs, liver, and spleen.[6, 50] Granulocytes may also be found within the vascular compartment arranged along the walls of the capillaries in various tissues, apparently sequestered from the general circulation. The presence of cells in these locations may indicate that they perform some function such as transportation, or it may indicate that the cells accumulate in these areas prior to elimination or destruction. It is also possible that these intravascular aggregates of cells constitute a reserve of motile cells ready to be utilized in the defense of the body. Experimental evidence indicates that leukocytes that have left the intravascular compartment are unable to reenter in significant numbers.[56]

The studies of Craddock and co-workers have provided valuable information about the location and size of the reserve pool of granulocytes.[19, 20, 56] Dogs were subjected to the rapid removal of leukocytes by leukopheresis and the responses were studied under various conditions. From these studies it was concluded that the main source of mature granulocytes that take part in an acute leukocytosis is the marrow reserve. These studies provide information about the mechanism of leukocytosis and emphasize the importance of the large reserve pool of granulocytes in the marrow described by Kindred,[36] Yoffey,[74] and Osgood.[50] More recently, bacterial endotoxin and etiocholanolone have been used to assess bone marrow reserves.[55] A method of measuring the marrow reserve suitable for general clinical use would be of considerable value in managing patients who are being treated with cytotoxic agents.

The factors that control the level of the granulocytes in the circulation in normal and abnormal conditions have not been defined clearly. Infection has been recognized as a stimulus to neutrophilic leukocytosis from the time that leukocytosis was first described. In Ehrlich's and Lazarus' textbook of 50 years ago chemotaxis was accepted as the explanation of the migration of leukocytes into areas of infection, and it was postulated that the marrow cells were stimulated by a chemical that led to increased proliferation and output of these cells.[23] The importance of the reactive ability of the marrow was recognized, for it was known that an injection of oil of turpentine produced leukocytosis in normal individuals but failed to do so in patients with typhoid fever and leukopenia until after the fever and leukopenia had disappeared. More recent studies have provided a better understanding of some of the factors concerned in the leukocytosis of infection. The rate of release of neutrophils from the marrow appears to be influenced by a humoral factor, and the number of such cells circulating through the marrow seem to be regulated by a negative feedback mechanism. Plasma from dogs made neutropenic by vinblastine sulfate, nitrogen mustard, or endotoxin administration induced neutrophilia when infused into normal dogs.[8] Plasma from rats subjected to leukopheresis caused an increase in the rate of leukocyte release from perfused limbs and a decrease in the number of granulocytes in the marrow; the release of cells from the marrow was also influenced by the rate of flow of the perfusion and the number of cells in the perfusate.[29] Other experiments that utilized leukopheresis[19] or the injection of antiserum support this concept, as do the results obtained when mice were irradiated while the marrow of one leg was shielded.[47] The significance of the report of a substance in the urine of normal persons and patients with leukemia that stimulated granulocyte growth in cultures of bone marrow in vitro is uncertain.[59]

At least in special circumstances hormonal factors exert an influence on the circulating leukocytes. It has been shown that ACTH produces an increase in circulating neutrophils and a decrease in circulating eosinophils;[22] the similar response that has been observed in adrenalectomized animals may have been due to contamination of the ACTH material with pituitary growth factors that are known to produce a rise in neutrophils.[28] The administration of cortisone to mice was followed by an increase in the myeloid cells of the marrow associated with an increase in circulating neutrophils.[57] Neutrophilia after steroid administration may be the result not only of increased inflow from the marrow into the blood, but also of decreased outflow from the circulation, possibly as a result of a change in capillary permeability. Although most of the studies indicate that neutrophilic leukocytosis is produced by the rapid release of granulocytes into the circulation followed by the augmented production of these cells in the marrow, an increased life span of the cells in the circulation occurring as a consequence of decreased removal or destruction of the cells could produce the same result.

The life span of the neutrophils has been estimated by different methods and different results have been obtained.[39] Studies that employed transfusion or cross circulation techniques generally indicate a short life span measured in hours; other methods indicate a longer survival. The marrow culture method has indicated that the total life span of the neutrophil is 4.5 days. By the same technique the life span of eosinophils and basophils outside the marrow has been found to be from 8 to 12 days; the time spent within the marrow was found to be the same as that of the neutrophils.[50] Cartwright and associates have utilized radioactive diisopropylfluorophosphate as a label for granulocytes.[4, 9, 14, 15] Their studies have shown that the total blood granulocyte pool (TBGP) consists of two compartments, the circulating granulocyte pool (CGP) and the marginal granulocyte pool (MGP). Cells move freely between these pools which are in equilibrium; the circulating pool constitutes about 44 per cent of the total blood pool, which is about 70×10^7 per kg. of body weight. Calculations in normal subjects indicate that the mean half-time disappearance from the total blood granulocyte pool ($T\frac{1}{2}$) is 6.7 hours. The mean granulocyte turnover rate by this method is 163×10^7 granulocytes per kg. of body weight per day and the turnover time is 10.4 hours. The total granulocyte pool of the marrow was calculated to be 186×10^8 cells per kg. of body weight. The mean generation time of myelocytes is estimated at not more than 2.9 days, and the time necessary for myelocytes to divide, mature, and enter the blood stream is thought to be about 11.4 days. These workers found that the half-time disappearance of labeled granulocytes in chronic myelocytic leukemia was 26 to 89 hours compared to the normal of 6.7 hours; the difference was shown to lie in the cells, not in the subjects, and may be a reflection of the immaturity of the granulocytes in leukemia.

In a review of the question of the life span of the granulocytes Craddock placed the turnover time of the precursor pool at 4 days, the time in the marrow reserve at 5 days, and the duration in the circulation at less than 24 hours.[18] If the neutrophil is not destroyed in the circulation it eventually leaves the blood stream and migrates into the extravascular spaces. The sites most concerned in the removal of leukocytes from the circulation are the lungs, liver, spleen, gastrointestinal tract, bone marrow, striated muscle, and kidney.[6] Studies that employed catheterization of various vessels have revealed that the lungs remove large numbers of leukocytes from the circulation. The removal of cells from the peripheral circulation could be initiated by the administration of histamine, nicotinic acid, and colloidal substances. The fate of the cells trapped in the pulmonary circulation is uncertain, but the following possibilities have been suggested: (1) transient trapping with later entry into the general circulation; (2) migration and excretion through the sputum and gastrointestinal tract; (3) reentry into the general circulation by way of the lymphatics and thoracic duct; (4) disintegration in the lung. A failure of the removal mechanism has been suggested as a cause of leukocytosis in certain diseases, especially leukemia.

Function of the Granulocyte

Although the fact that there are a large number of enzymes and other chemical substances in granulocytes suggests that these cells have multiple functions, their primary function is concerned with the defense of the body against various noxious agents. Studies in patients with cyclic neutropenia and those with agranulocytosis associated with aplastic anemia indicate that the granulocytes play a minor role at most in defense mechanisms other than intracellular killing of phagocytized microorganisms.[53] Such studies indicate no influence on antibody production or the local reactions to endotoxin, or bacterial allergy; the febrile response, however, is mediated by granulocytes and monocytes.[70a] The responses to appropriate stimuli in the form of increased production of C-reactive protein and mucoprotein appear to be unimpaired in the absence of granulocytes.

The importance of phagocytosis as one of the main defense mechanisms of the body was suggested by Metchnikoff in 1882 after he had observed the accumulation of mobile cells about a thorn placed under the skin of the starfish larva.[73] The stimulus responsible for the movement of the leukocyte into the proximity of the offending particle is believed to be chemical in nature and is termed chemotaxis; the actual engulfment of the particle by the leukocyte is termed phagocytosis.

Chemotaxis is termed positive if the leukocyte moves toward the particle, negative if it moves away, and indifferent if it is unaffected by the presence of the particle. Numerous investigators have tried to identify the specific substance or substances responsible for chemotaxis. Crystalline nitrogenous material from inflammatory exudates attracts leukocytes in large numbers when it is placed in the cutaneous tissue of an animal;[44] this substance, called leukotaxine, appears to be a polypeptide. Fractions of complement[1, 46] and cyclic-3'-5'-AMP, produced by bacteria,[39a] influence chemotaxis. The canine eosinophil is attracted by fibrinogen, fibrin, and proteolytic enzymes[58] as well as histamine.[2]

After the granulocyte has been attracted to the site, phagocytosis occurs. The neutrophil is more adept than the eosinophil or basophil at this operation. The younger granulocytes, bands, and metamyelocytes are more avid than the segmented cells in attacking bacteria in the presence of opsonins. Hirsch and Cohn have employed cinemicrophotography to study phagocytosis.[33, 34] They observed that a polymorphonuclear leukocyte moved in a random fashion until the cell came within 10 to 20 microns of a particle or bacillus; at this range chemotaxis became evident and the cell moved in a straight line to the particle. When contact was made the cell and particle became firmly adherent. The cytoplasm of the cell then flowed around the particle and the cell membrane invaginated until it fused to enclose the ingested particle in a ring of cell membrane that had become detached (Fig. 12–1). Phagocytosis was completed within from 30 seconds to 2 minutes.

Various factors influence phagocytosis. It appears to be enhanced in some types of anemia[5] and by an increase in temperature from 0° C to 35° C.[25] It is reduced by high concentration of glucose[37] and by malnutrition.[17] The enhanced phagocytosis of organisms that occurs in the presence of immune sera and complement is known as the opsonic function of the antibody.[75] The manner by which opsonin renders microorganisms more susceptible to destruction is not completely understood. In the absence of opsonin, phagocytes are unable to engulf bacteria floating free in a liquid medium. In such circumstances, cells can phagocytize organisms after they have succeeded in trapping them against a convenient surface, such as the wall of an alveolus or another leukocyte; this process has been termed surface phagocytosis.[71] That the properties of the particle to be engulfed affect the process of phagocytosis was demonstrated by studies that utilized inert solid particles and bacteria.[24, 73] Many bacteria produce antiphagocytic substances which are toxic for the phagocytic cell. Among these are the somatic "0" antigen on the surface of many gram-negative species, exotoxins, and leukocidins. The growing type III pneumococcus resists phagocytosis in a different manner; it produces a polysaccharide "slime" layer composed of long-chained carbohydrate polymers of glucose and glucuronic acid which protects the organism from phagocytosis and contributes to the virulence of this organism.[72]

The vital step of killing ingested microorganisms is accomplished by a fusion of the leukocyte granules (lysosomes) with the phagocytic vacuole followed by the discharge of digestive enzymes into the vacuole. During

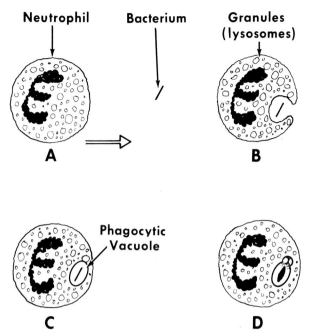

Figure 12-1. Phagocytosis of a bacterium by a neutrophil leukocyte. *A*, Chemotaxis. *B*, Engulfment. *C*, Formation of a phagocytic vacuole. *D*, Fusion of lysosomes and phagocytic vacuole.

phagocytosis, glycolysis is accelerated and acid production is increased; this slight change in pH may suffice to release the bactericidal substances from the granules. The leukocyte granules contain acid and alkaline phosphatase nucleotidase, ribonuclease, deoxyribonuclease, beta glucuronidase, and other substances. It is possible that mere fusion of the granule with the membrane of the phagocytic vacuole may be all that is necessary for the degranulation.

Impaired opsonizing activity associated with diminished phagocytosis and killing of ingested bacteria has been reported in low birth weight infants and in patients with sickle cell disease, both of whom tend be quite susceptible to infections.[26, 68] Failure of these mechanisms, which may be related to the absence or hypofunction of the spleen, probably is an important factor in the frequency and seriousness of pneumococcus and *Salmonella* infections in patients with sickle cell disease.[35] The susceptibility to infections in chronic alcoholics may be related to a depression in the rate of leukocyte mobilization which has been demonstrated to exist for some hours after the ingestion of alcohol; in this circumstance, however, phagocytosis and killing of bacteria were not impaired.[11] Deficiencies in chemotactic ability in enhancement of phagocytosis by serum and in resistance to gram-negative organisms have been reported in association with abnormalities in C-3 and C-5 components of complement.[1, 46]

Lymphocytes

Only a small percentage of the lymphocytes in the body are present in the circulating blood. Osgood has calculated that the total numbers of lymphocytes are as follows: bone marrow, 4×10^{11} (100 gm.); lymphocytic tissue and spleen, 4×10^{11} (100 gm.); peripheral blood, 12×10^9 (3 gm.); total outside the blood and blood-forming organs, 52×10^{11} (1300 gm.).[50] The injection of ACTH has been shown to cause a lymphocytopenia followed by a lymphocytosis,[22] but the factors that control the level of these cells in the circulation under normal circumstances are poorly understood.

The lymphocyte, once considered by many to be a uniform type of cell of doubtful utility, almost a vestigial remnant, is now considered to perform a number of different and important functions, at least some of which are necessary for man's survival. The heterogeneous nature of the lymphocyte line of cells is shown by the wide range of life spans; some survive only a few weeks, some for months, others for years, and a few for decades.[25a] The life span of the lymphocytes in normal individuals and those with chronic lymphocytic leukemia has been calculated to be at least 30 days, one-tenth of which is thought to be spent in lymphatic tissue.[50] Studies that employed the labeling of lymphocytes with radioactive isotopes in man suggest a dual population of lymphocytes, one with a mean age of 2 to 3 days, and a larger number (80 per cent) with a mean age of 100 to 200 days.[52] Similar investigation of two human subjects with chronic lymphocytic leukemia indicated that the lymphocytes had an average life span of 85 days. There was also prolonged retention of isotope in other cells (half-time about 300 days), but whether this indicated a dual population of cells, one of which survived for very long periods, or a specific reutilization of large fragments of nucleic acid or nucleoprotein was uncertain.[31] It has been reported that turnover time of small lymphocytes in the peripheral circulation of the rat, as determined by the continuous H^3-thymidine infusion, is over 100 days.[40]

The function and fate of the lymphocytes that enter the blood stream each day is one of the interesting problems in hematology. The circulation of small lymphocytes, perhaps 80 to 90 per cent of the total, from the blood to lymph nodes and then back to the blood by efferent lymph channels seems well established.[25a] Short-lived lymphocytes constitute a greater portion of this recirculating pool than they do of the peripheral lymphoid tissues. Most of the circulating lymphocytes originate in the thymus, but some may come directly from the marrow; the precursors of the thymus cells arise in the marrow. For the most part, the production of lymphocytes in peripheral lymphoid tissue occurs as the result of antigen stimulation. The recirculation of lymphocytes is probably important in the induction of immune responses.[25a]

Studies of patients with deficiencies in immune reactions, particularly thymic aplasia and the sex-linked recessive form of agammaglobulinemia, as well as experiments with different species of animals and birds, have led to the concept that there are two main types of lymphocytes, one thymus-dependent and one thymus-independent.[45] The source of the thymus-independent lymphocytes in birds is the bursa of Fabricius; collections of small lymphocytes in the wall of the small intestine in man may be the counterpart. Undifferentiated lymphoid cells arise in the marrow. Those that enter the thymus and are modified by the thymus become important in graft rejection, delayed hypersensitivity and graft-host reactions. Cells that by-pass the thymus and enter the bursal tissue (or its equivalent) are thought to develop into cells capable of producing antibodies in the peripheral lymphoid tissues. The lymphocyte is the important specific element in all these reactions, in cell-mediated immunity, in graft rejection, and in immunologic surveillance against microorganisms, and probably against malignant cells as well.

Monocytes

Monocytes or mononuclear macrophages are found normally in the circulating blood, bone marrow, lymph nodes, spleen, and loose connective tissue. They constitute from 3 to 7 per cent of the circulating leukocytes, the total number in the circulation being approximately 0.5×10^{11}. The ratio of those in the tissues to those in the circulating blood has been estimated to be 400:1.[50]

Although numerous origins have been suggested for the monocytes in the peripheral blood, recent work seems to have established that monocytes are formed in the bone marrow.[67] The migration of macrophages of rats and their labeling by tritiated thymidine were suppressed by radiation, but not if the bone marrow was shielded; in addition, labeled cells present in bone marrow suspension that were injected intravenously appeared as labeled macrophages in exudates, but cells from the thoracic duct, lymph nodes, and thymus prepared in the same way and injected intravenously did not produce labeled macrophages.

Cell multiplication occurs in promonocytes in the bone marrow. These are immature cells from 14 to 20 μ in diameter that contain a large nucleus, prominent nucleoli, and a basophilic cytoplasm; the nucleus usually has a single large cleft but may be round. As the monocytes mature, the nucleoli fade, the ratio of nucleus to cytoplasm decreases, and cytoplasmic granules appear. The average generation time of these cells has been computed to be 9.7 hours.[64] The monocytes, which normally are not proliferating cells, rapidly enter the circulating blood. After an average blood transit time of 32 hours (for mice), the monocytes leave the circulation to become macrophages in the lung, peritoneum, and liver (Kupffer's cells) and in areas of inflammation.[65] Under normal conditions, the tissue macrophages originate in the marrow, but under pathologic conditions the tissue macrophages may multiply. Macrophages also form multinucleated cells, giant cells, by fusion of the membranes of various cells.

The endothelial cells, fibroblasts, reticular cells, and dendritic cells are considered by some to belong to a different system because these cells do not have the morphologic characteristics of the mononuclear phagocytes, cannot be shown to be derived from the peripheral blood monocyte, and are not highly phagocytic.[64] Both the fixed and mobile macrophages are considered to be parts of the reticuloendothelial system.[158a]

The macrophage may function in three areas—phagocytosis, delayed hypersensitivity, and antibody formation. One of its main functions is ingestion of extracellular substances, endocytosis; the cell can engulf solid particles (phagocytosis), a function shared by the granulocytes, and, in addition, is able to absorb liquid particles (pinocytosis).

Phagocytosis consists of two stages, the attachment step, or binding of the particle to the surface of the phagocyte, and the ingestion phase. The surface of the mononuclear phagocytic cells has many sites for attachment for various substances; the sites for the attachment of complement can be differentiated from others. The serum components responsible for attachment are called opsonins; opsonic activity requires complement. Specific immune serum is a rich source of opsonins. The active molecules are globulins, possibly immunoglobulins.[49] The attachment of antigen-antibody complexes to specific receptors appears to be an important factor in phagocytosis of certain particles and may be a specific feature of these cells.[49] The physicochemical nature of the particle surface also influences the attachment; certain substances, such as the polysaccharide capsule of pneumococci, interfere with the attachment. The ingestion step is sensitive to temperature changes; glycolysis and respiration are transiently stimulated by phagocytosis, which shows that the process obviously requires metabolic energy.

After the particle is ingested, the lysosomal contents are transferred to the phagocytic vacuoles. This is an essential step in the intracellular digestive process. (The lysosomes have been described in some detail in Chapter I.)

Pinocytosis, the absorption of liquid particles, is a function of macrophages but not of granulocytes, and differs from phagocytosis in several respects.[49] In phagocytosis there is progressive movement of the cytoplasm around the particle, which probably is analogous to the spreading of the macrophages on a glass slide, a concept supported by the observation that spreading on a glass slide is enhanced by the presence of an antigen-antibody combination. Pinocytosis differs in that the vacuole may contain more than one particle, is not accompanied by expenditure of energy, and seems to be the result of invagination of the cell membrane rather than extension of the membrane around the particle.

Chemotaxis apparently requires membrane participation, and a "macrophage-specific" factor that is different from that effective in polymorphonuclear leukocytes has been described; it is present in serum treated with immune complexes but differs from C'5,6,7 complex.[67a] Lymphocytes may release a chemotactic factor for macrophages. In addition, the production of a macrophage migration inhibitory factor by the thymic-dependent lymphocytes has been demonstrated in vitro; this factor correlates with in vivo delayed hypersensitivity.[59a]

The macrophages that are important in cellular immunity are larger and have increased capacity for phagocytosis.[41] Activation, which is an expression of specific immunity recall, can be produced by the transfer of living lymphoid cells but not by the injection of humoral antibody or by passive transfer of specific serum. The macrophage is the main factor in resistance to tuberculin infection.

Cellular immunity and delayed-type hypersensitivity are similar in that committed lymphocytes are necessary for both reactions, in that antilymphocyte globulin blocks both reactions,[41] in that both types of immune reactions are abolished temporarily by x-irradiation, the disappearance being parallel to the loss of circulating monocytes,[66] and in that neither can be induced in recently irradiated subjects. These functions are important in reactions to bacterial infections, in organ transplants, and probably in the rejection of neoplastic cells. The fact that macrophages do react to foreign cells is supported by an increasing body of indirect evidence.

Macrophages also play an important role in viral infections. Some viruses are ingested and destroyed, and others, such as lymphocytic choriomeningitis virus, are ingested by the macrophages but continue to reproduce in them. The latter situation alters reticuloendothelial function and produces hypergamma-globulinemia, which may be important in the pathogenesis of some chronic diseases, such as the "collagen diseases," that at present are poorly understood. The persistence of antigens in the macrophages may be important in the immune response mediated by lymphocytes which come in contact with these cells.

Although the fundamental role in the immune response is played by lymphocytes, macrophages may be important to certain antigens in the antibody formation because the macrophage may process the antigen or act to prevent tolerance. After the macrophage has phagocytized antigen, the antigenic material may be catabolized and the potentially immunogenic molecules eliminated, or some of it may be preserved in the macrophage, part of the immunologic memory process to be available to the lymphocytes at an appropriate time later.[63]

Normal Values

The normal values for the total and differential leukocyte counts in adults according to various authors are shown in Table 12–1. Both the total count and the percentages of the different cells vary with the age of the individual. In the newborn, total counts varying from 3600 to 45,000 per cu.mm. have been reported but the great majority are in the range of 10,000 to 25,000 per cu.mm.;[27, 61] at this time the neutrophils constitute about 60 per cent of the cells. From the second week through the second year, when the total count ranges from 8000 to 13,000 per cu.mm., the lymphocytes predominate and make up from 50 to 69 per cent of the total. During childhood the total count is usually around 8000 per cu.mm. and the range is 4000 to 13,000 per cu.mm.; during the same period the percentage of lymphocytes decreases to a range of 25 to 48 per cent by the twelfth year. At about the fifteenth year the adult values are reached and these are maintained throughout the remainder of the individual's life.

Wintrobe found the following values (mean/cu.mm. and 95 per cent confidence limits) in 105 male medical students: neutrophils, 4300, 1800 to 6700; lymphocytes, 2700; 1500 to 3900; monocytes, 500, 100 to 900; eosinophils, 200, 0 to 600; basophils 40, 0 to 120.[70]

In one report of counts on 663 whites and 123 blacks, the granulocyte

Table 12–1. *Total and Differential Leukocyte Counts in Normal Adults According to Various Authors*

Author	Total (Per) (cu.mm.)	Neutro. (%)	Eosin. (%)	Baso. (%)	Lymph. (%)	Mono. (%)
Osgood et al.[51]	4,000–11,000	33–75	0–6	0–2	15–60	0–9
Sturgis and Bethell[61]	6,000– 7,400	55–67	2–3	0.5–0.7	23–38	4–6
Schilling[60]	5,000– 8,000	51–67	2–4	0–1	21–35	4–8
Wintrobe[69]	5,000–10,000	54–62	1–3	0–0.75	25–33	3–7

counts were lower in blacks (white males, 4463; black males, 3722; white females, 4440; black females, 4098).[12, 13] There were no differences in the levels in hemoglobin, hematocrit, or lymphocytes. A drop in the leukocyte count from 7800 per cu.mm. to 3500 per cu.mm., due mainly to a decrease in neutrophils, has been observed in healthy men in isolation at the South Polar Plateau.[48]

Physiologic Variations

In addition to the variations in leukocytes that are found at different ages, changes occur as a result of other physiologic processes, probably as the result of the shifting of granulocytes from the marginal pool along the vessel walls into the circulating granulocyte pool. These variations, which since the time of Virchow have been recognized to occur independently of disease, have been the subject of several detailed reviews.[27, 61]

Spontaneous fluctuations in the leukocyte count occur during the day. These appear to be inconstant, irregular, and unrelated to the ingestion of food; the changes have been interpreted as indicative of a redistribution of leukocytes within the body rather than an increased production of new cells, because these fluctuations are not associated with an increase in immature cells. An hourly rhythm of the leukocytes and an afternoon increase regardless of food ingestion have been reported but not confirmed.

Strenuous exercise produces a marked leukocytosis. Total counts as high as 27,000 per cu.mm. have been found in marathon runners and football players. Leukocytosis that develops within 11 seconds has also been found after a 100-yard dash. After exercise the count returns to normal within several hours. Although pregnancy is associated with only a slight increase in leukocytes and neutrophils, at the onset of labor there is a marked increase, sometimes with the appearance of myelocytes, that may reach levels of 17,000 to 34,000 per cu.mm.[27, 38, 61]

Other causes of leukocytosis are paroxysmal tachycardia (13,000 to 20,000 per cu.mm.) and convulsions (37,000 to 43,000 per cu.mm.). Emotional states may be associated with changes in the leukocyte counts; the count has been noted to rise from 8000 to 18,000 per cu.mm. with the development of a panic reaction, and to decrease 6000 to 12,000 per cu.mm. in 1 hour when amobarbital administered intravenously induced a change in the emotional status.[45a]

Variations Due to Disease

Changes that occur in the leukocytes in the peripheral blood in disease are often helpful in considering both the diagnosis and prognosis. In general, the changes in the peripheral blood reflect the type of injury, the extent of the process, and the body's reaction to the injury. Significant alterations may occur in the total number of leukocytes, in the proportion of the various cells present, and in the morphologic appearance of the individual cells. After removal of the spleen for any cause there is an increase in the neutrophil count which returns to normal or near normal levels after several weeks or months. At this time the

Table 12–2. Causes of Neutrophilic Leukocytosis

1. Infections: especially with pyogenic bacteria; either localized, as appendiceal abscess, or generalized, as septicemia.
2. Other disorders associated with acute inflammation or cellular necrosis: infarction, collagen disease, acute hemolysis.
3. Neoplasms: leukemia, carcinoma, lymphomas, especially with areas of tissue necrosis and widespread metastases.
4. Intoxications: drugs, chemicals; especially in poisonings with liver damage.
5. Acute hemorrhage.

number of circulating lymphocytes and monocytes rises and apparently remains elevated.

Although no unconditional statements can be made concerning the reaction of the body to infection, certain generalizations can be stated. A leukocytosis is more likely to occur in acute infections than in chronic disorders. A mild infection most often is associated with no change in the leukocytes or with a slight increase to 11,000 or 15,000 per cu.mm. In infectious or destructive processes a marked neutrophilic leukocytosis accompanied by an increase in the younger forms indicates a severe injury and a brisk reaction of the body's defense mechanism. A low or normal total leukocyte count associated with a marked increase in younger forms in the presence of infection indicates either an early stage of the infectious process or a subnormal response to a severe infection. Severe infection and extensive tissue destruction are also manifested by morphologic changes in the granulocytes such as cytoplasmic basophilia, vacuolation of the cytoplasm, and toxic granulation. Bacterial infections, particularly those due to cocci, are apt to be accompanied by an increase in the total leukocyte count and the neutrophilic granulocytes; viral infections are likely to be associated with a low or normal total leukocyte count and a relative or absolute lymphocytosis. Neoplastic disease, leukemia excepted, is usually associated with a normal leukocyte count unless the process is extensive and tissue necrosis has occurred; in this circumstance neutrophilic leukocytosis of marked degree is often present. Neutrophilia has been defined as more than 7500 neutrophils per cu.mm. and neutropenia as less than 1500 per cu.mm. in the venous blood.[51]

The most common causes of increases in neutrophilic granulocytes, lymphocytes, monocytes, and eosinophilic granulocytes are presented in Tables 12–2 to 12–5.

A decrease in the number of circulating leukocytes, which is generally due to a decrease in the granulocytes, is found in a variety of clinical conditions. The

Table 12–3. Causes of Lymphocytosis

1. Infections	(a) Acute: infectious mononucleosis, pertussis; infectious lymphocytosis; other viral and bacillary infections.
	(b) Convalescence: especially viral infections.
	(c) Chronic: tuberculosis, brucellosis, syphilis.
2. Neoplasms	Lymphocytic leukemia, lymphosarcoma.
3. Metabolic disease	Hyperthyroidism.

Table 12-4.   *Causes of Monocytosis*

1. Infections	(a) Bacterial: tuberculosis, subacute bacterial endocarditis, brucellosis, typhoid fever.
	(b) Protozoal: malaria, kala-azar.
	(c) Rickettsial: Rocky Mountain spotted fever.
2. Neoplasms	Monocytic leukemia, Hodgkin's disease, reticuloendotheliosis.
3. During recovery from infections and marrow depression caused by drugs or radiotherapy.	
4. Other causes	p. vera; connective tissue disorders.

most frequent causes of neutropenia are listed in Table 12–6. Although the factors that may produce neutropenia are not as well understood as those that produce anemia, the possible mechanisms can be classified in a similar fashion: (1) diminished production; (2) increased destruction; and (3) the "loss" of leukocytes from the circulation, by sequestration in the various organs or tissues. In the majority of clinical conditions with neutropenia, diminished production appears to be the important mechanism.

Diminished production may be due to a deficiency of essential substances, such as vitamin B_{12} and folic acid, or to the presence of metabolic antagonists, such as aminopterin and 6-mercaptopurine. Diminished granulocytopoiesis may also be the result of damage to the precursor cells in the marrow by irradiation, chemicals, marrow replacement, drug idiosyncrasy, and other, unknown, causes.

The importance of leukocyte antibodies as a mechanism responsible for the production of neutropenia is uncertain. The occurrence of nonspecific transfusion reactions characterized by chills, fever, and leukopenia associated with the presence in the recipient's blood of agglutinins against the donor leukocytes has been reported.[9a] In another study it was found that leukoagglutinins were demonstrable in 38 of 350 patients with hematologic disorders. However, 64 per cent of the patients with leukoagglutinins had no leukopenia and only one of 22 patients with leukopenia had leukoagglutinins. Ninety per cent of the patients with leukoagglutinins had received transfusions, and the likelihood of a positive test was greater after multiple transfusions. Because of this observation and the failure to demonstrate any agglutination of autologous leukocytes, it was concluded that at least the majority of leukoagglutinins are isoagglutinins.[54] A different experience is reported by Tullis, who employed a different technique.[62] He found positive tests for leukocyte antibodies in 59 of 132 sera from patients with leukopenia and in only 11 of 102

Table 12-5.   *Causes of Eosinophilia*

1. Allergic reactions	Bronchial asthma, drug reactions, allergic dermatitis, hay fever, angioneurotic edema.
2. Parasitic infestation	Intestinal (hookworm, tapeworm, ascaris, Taenia echinococcus); especially with muscle invasion by trichina.
3. Skin diseases	Exfoliative dermatitis, pemphigus, dermatitis herpetiformis.
4. Neoplasms	Metastatic carcinoma, myelocytic leukemia, Hodgkin's disease.
5. Other diseases	Periarteritis nodosa, eosinophilic granuloma.

Table 12–6. *Causes of Neutropenia*

1. Infections: acute viral (rubeola, infectious hepatitis); bacterial (brucellosis, typhoid fever); protozoal (malaria, kala-azar); and overwhelming infections (septicemia).
2. Bone marrow damage: aplastic anemia or neutropenia due to unknown cause; irradiation, toxic drugs, and chemicals (benzol, mustard drugs, antimetabolic agents); drug idiosyncrasy (amidopyrine, sulfonamides, and others).
3. Disorders associated with splenomegaly: congestive splenomegaly, diseases of the reticulo-endothelial system (parasitic diseases, chronic infections, neoplasms), Felty's syndrome.
4. Other disorders: disseminated lupus erythematosus, anaphylaxis, "aleukemic" leukemia.
5. Nutritional deficiency: vitamin B_{12}, folic acid.
6. Neutropenia: chronic idiopathic, familial benign, cyclic.

sera from patients with hematologic and hepatic disorders without leukopenia. Antibodies were demonstrated in patients with primary agranulocytosis, primary hypersplenism, secondary hypersplenism, myelophthisic anemia, leukemia, and drug sensitivity. The anti-leukocyte antibody activity, which appeared to be made up of two components, decreased as clinical improvement occurred and the granulocyte counts rose after treatment with steroids or splenectomy.

Splenomegaly from diverse causes, such as portal hypertension, tuberculosis, kala-azar, and involvement by diseases of the lymphoma group, may be associated with a neutropenia that is relieved by splenectomy. Splenectomy may remove an organ of leukocyte destruction, a site of the production of leukocyte antibodies, or a depressive influence on the bone marrow; correction of a large plasma volume may be important in some patients.

The neutropenia that occurs in anaphylactic shock and after the administration of histamine and nicotinic acid is thought to be due to a loss of the leukocytes from the circulation as a result of sequestration in the tissues of the body, particularly the splanchnic circulation, liver, spleen, and lungs.

In some patients with fatal bacterial infections, particularly pneumonia or septicemia, severe leukopenia develops in the absence of medication. The authors have seen several such patients with total leukocyte counts of less than 1000 per cu.mm. and no more than a few hundred granulocytes. Examination of the bone marrow revealed an absence of cells older than myelocytes and an increased number of myelocytes and promyelocytes, nearly all of which stained poorly, contained many vacuoles, and appeared to be degenerating; no evidence of leukemia was found in the autopsies. Whether the severe leukopenia developed acutely or the infections developed in someone with unrecognized chronic neutropenia is uncertain.

Leukemoid Reactions

A leukemoid reaction is defined as a leukocyte response in the peripheral blood that simulates a form of leukemia in its magnitude or in the morphology of the cells involved. High leukocyte counts (up to 100,000 per cu.mm.) involving the neutrophils occur in some patients who have bacterial pneumonia, ulcerative colitis, and other severe infections. The smear usually manifests an orderly increase in the immature cells rather than the "leukemic hiatus;" in the latter conditions young cells such as myeloblasts and promyelocytes or young myelocytes may be increased more than the older myelocytes and meta-myelocytes. A leukocyte count of 15,000 to 25,000 or more occurs in patients with polycythemia vera and may mimic leukemia after hemorrhage which has produced anemia. In myeloid metaplasia, Hodgkin's disease, and advanced carcinoma a very marked leukocytic reaction is sometimes encountered. High eosinophil counts which may exceed 75,000 sometimes occur in Hodgkin's disease, other lymphomas, periarteritis, Loeffler's syndrome, and other disorders. Leukemoid reactions characterized by the presence of blast cells and promyelocytes, often with leukopenia, sometimes occur in patients with disseminated tuberculosis and fungus infection. In such patients the marrow is not usually packed with cells, as is often the case in acute leukemia. (F.S.:III, 136.)

Leukemoid reactions characterized by a great increase in the lymphocytes are seen most often in infectious mononucleosis and whooping cough, but occasionally they occur in tuberculosis and during convalescence from various diseases.

The monocytic type of leukemoid reaction is most likely to occur in tuberculosis, Hodgkin's disease, or reticulum cell sarcoma.

Usually the examination of the bone marrow, special tests of the peripheral blood such as the heterophil agglutination test, and other examinations such as x-rays of the chest and possibly biopsies usually suffice for the recognition of the leukemoid reaction. Nevertheless, in some patients the answer only becomes apparent after the patient has been followed for some weeks or months.

Disorders Associated with Quantitative Defects in Granulocytes

Agranulocytosis (Granulocytopenia)

HISTORICAL INTRODUCTION

Although isolated cases of this disease had been seen prior to that time, it was Schultz's report in 1922 that established agranulocytosis as an entity.[92] This report described five fatal cases that occurred in women whose illness was characterized by necrotic ulceration of the oropharynx accompanied by marked leukopenia and granulocytopenia. After this description additional instances of the same disorder, which was thought to be the result of some infectious agent, were soon recognized. Soon afterward, Roberts and Kracke established that the sepsis which occurred in nearly all patients with the disorder followed the agranulocytosis and was not a causative factor.[91] A further advance in the knowledge of the disease came when Kracke noted that the disease occurred largely in Germany and the United States, particularly in middle-aged women who gave a history of treatment with drugs. He also noted that the coal tar derivatives had come into wide usage in these countries following World War I. The fact that benzene is a leukocyte depressant led him to suspect that benzene or its products should be seriously considered as the cause of the condition, a belief that was strengthened when he was able to produce the hematologic and clinical features of agranulocytosis in rabbits by the subcutaneous injection of benzene and its oxidation products.[81, 82]

Madison and Squier,[84] Plum,[89] and others[83] established that drugs containing amidopyrine were responsible for most cases of agranulocytosis at that time. In 1935 Kracke and Parker noted that of 172 cases that had been reported in the literature, 153 had occurred after the administration of amidopyrine.[83] In the same report they listed 46 American proprietary compounds that contained amidopyrine. Because the number of reported instances of agranulocytosis was small in comparison to the large number of persons who took amidopyrine in one compound or another, an idiosyncrasy was suspected. This was demonstrated conclusively by Madison and Squier in 1934[84] and by Plum in 1935.[89] It was recognized that agranulocytosis could be caused by other drugs and in 1938 Fitz-Hugh listed 14 drugs thought to be responsible.[79] This list was compiled at the beginning of the sulfonamide era and since then the list has lengthened steadily.

MECHANISM OF THE DISEASE

Agranulocytosis was considered to be an infectious disease until it was demonstrated that the primary factor was the reduction of the granulocytes in the peripheral blood, which lowered resistance and led to bacterial invasion.[81, 91] The drugs that were the most common offenders contained a known leukocyte depressant in the form of the benzene ring, and it was known that the marrow of some fatal cases was almost completely devoid of cells of the granulocytic series. Because of these observations it was thought that the responsible drugs or their breakdown products acted by direct suppression of granulocytopoiesis in the marrow.[81, 83, 91] The greater likelihood of a different mechanism was shown by Madison and Squier.[84] They administered small doses of amidopyrine to two patients who had recovered from agranulocytosis caused by amidopyrine; symptoms developed in 2 or 3 hours and the circulating granulocytes diminished greatly or disappeared completely by the twelfth hour; recovery occurred in 4 days. These observations, which were confirmed by others,[77, 89] indicated that some mechanism other than depression of granulocytopoiesis must have acted to produce so profound a change in such a short time.

A possible explanation of the rapid disappearance of the circulating granulocytes in these circumstances was provided by the experiments of Moeschlin and Wagner.[86] Blood was obtained from a Pyramidon sensitive patient 3 hours after the administration of 0.3 gm. Pyramidon. When 300 ml. of this blood was given to two normal recipients, severe granulocytopenia developed in from 20 to 40 minutes and persisted for 3 or 4 hours. The same workers also demonstrated that at the height of the Pyramidon agranulocytosis the plasma and serum contained a substance that caused agglutination of both homologous and heterologous leukocytes. It was suggested that leukocytes agglutinated in this manner were removed from the circulation and destroyed mainly in the lungs. The existence of such a mechanism was demonstrated in guinea pigs which were injected with the anti-leukocyte serum produced by the injection of guinea pig leukocytes into rabbits.[85]

Although the presence of leukocyte antibodies may explain the occurrence of agranulocytosis in certain hypersensitive patients, it appears that this mechanism is not the only one concerned in all instances of agranulocytosis that occur as a result of drug idiosyncrasy. Amidopyrine appears to produce agranulocytosis by means of a true immunologic reaction that may follow the administration of only a very small amount of the drug. However, the agranulocytosis that sometimes follows the administration of sulfonamide compounds probably is the result of another mechanism, because agranulocytosis is rarely seen during therapy with these drugs unless a fairly large amount of the drug has been administered.

The role that the bone marrow plays in the production of agranulocytosis has not been clearly defined. It is probably an important one in the development of the clinical syndrome. The depletion of the granulocytic series of the marrow that is seen at autopsy and the delay in the development of agranulocytosis until 1 or 2 weeks after the last dose of offending drug that is seen in some patients appear to be explained best by the action of the responsible mechanism on all members of granulocytic series in the marrow. The normal and hyperplastic marrows that have been found in some patients with the disorder have been interpreted by some as evidence of partial recovery from previous damage[76, 91] and by others as a maturation arrest.[80] Still another interpretation has been offered, namely that the hyperplasia of the granulocytic elements in the marrow is an effort to compensate for the destruction of leukocytes in the circulation; according to this concept the picture of marrow depletion develops only when the bone marrow has become exhausted.[85, 86] This interpretation appears unlikely in view of the results that have been obtained with leukopheresis experiments.

A recent study of agranulocytosis produced by phenothiazine derivatives, a group of drugs frequently implicated in this disease, showed that the dyscrasia did not occur until after more than 10 days of treatment, usually after more than 20 days, and did not occur if it had not appeared within 90 days.[88] Bone marrow aplasia was demonstrated during the disease and recovery usually occurred within two weeks of discontinuation of the drug. Studies of cultures of human bone marrow cells by means of H^3-thymidine or H^3-uridine suggested that chlorpromazine inhibited cell division in both sensitive and non-sensitive patients. Further investigation disclosed that even in the absence of chlorpromazine, cells from sensitive patients had a lower labeling index than the "normal" group, suggesting an inherent defect, possibly of an enzyme concerned with DNA synthesis. When patients with sensitive marrows, as determined by culture studies, were given varying amounts of chlorpromazine, some developed leukopenia but others adapted to the drug and showed no clinical evidence of toxicity.

The drugs that are most likely to produce a decrease in one or more of the types of cells in the blood because of an idiosyncrasy have been listed and classified by Osgood,[87] and Welch, Lewis, and Kerlan.[93] Osgood's classification is used in Table 12–7 and the additional drugs mentioned by Welch et al. have been included.

Table 12–7. *Drugs That Sometimes Produce Hematologic Abnormalities (Classification and Estimated Risk)*

1. Anticonvulsants	methyl-phenyl-ethyl-hydantoin — high; trimethadione — moderate.
2. Antihistaminics	phenothiazine type — moderate; ethylenediamine type — low.
3. Antimicrobial Agents	arsenobenzol — high; chloramphenicol — high; sulfonamides — moderate; thiosemicarbazone — moderate; streptomycin — low; oxytetracycline, chlortetracycline — low.
4. Antithyroid Agents	thiouracils — high, methimazole — moderate.
5. Sedatives	(2-isopropyl-4-pentenoyl) urea — high; amidopyrine — high; phenacemide — moderate; pyrithyldione — low; chlorpromazine — moderate.
6. Spasmolytics	phenothiazine — moderate; procaine amide — low.
7. Unclassified	gold preparations — high; phenylbutazone — high; nitrophenols — high; mercurial diuretics — low; quinidine — low; quinacrine hydrochloride — low; mercury, amphetamine — low.

CLINICAL MANIFESTATIONS

Agranulocytosis occurs in both sexes and may develop at any age. Prodomal symptoms such as fatigue, headache, weakness, insomnia, and restlessness usually occur. The majority of patients complain of a sore throat. This often progresses rapidly as chills, increasing fever, and dysphagia develop. Unless improvement occurs the temperature rises to 105° F or more, and the patient becomes mentally confused, irrational, prostrated, or stuporous.

Physical examination early in the disease may reveal nothing more than a few small areas of necrosis in the tonsillar areas. Later the areas of necrotic ulceration enlarge as edema and slight reddening of the mucous membranes develop. The cervical lymph nodes become enlarged and slightly tender and in some patients the soft tissue of the neck becomes swollen. At times vaginal and rectal ulcerations occur.

LABORATORY EXAMINATION

The most significant feature is the occurrence in the peripheral blood of severe leukopenia and granulocytopenia unaccompanied by anemia or thrombocytopenia. Many patients develop lymphocytopenia as well as granulocytopenia and the total leukocyte count falls to levels as low as 100 to 2000 per cu.mm. Granulocytes often constitute less than 10 per cent of the total cells, and may be entirely absent. Those that are present often show extreme degrees of toxic granulation. Monocytes often make up an appreciable percentage of the cells, especially during recovery, and a total monocyte count of over 100 per cu.mm. is considered a sign of good prognosis.[90]

The appearance of the bone marrow varies with the stage of the disease. In most of the severe cases at the height of the disease the cells of the granulocytic series are greatly reduced or absent and the percentages of lymphocytes, plasma cells, and reticuloendothelial cells are increased. In other patients, particularly when recovery is taking place, examination of the marrow reveals hyperplasia of the granulocytic series; in such circumstances toxic granulation is evident in many of the younger cells. (F.S.:III, 123–125.)

In severe cases blood cultures often establish the presence of septicemia. Smears made from the ulcerated lesions or sputum often show masses of bacteria accompanied by but few cells.

DIFFERENTIAL DIAGNOSIS

The most important consideration in the differential diagnosis is acute leukemia. The distinction is usually not difficult because leukemia is generally associated with anemia, thrombocytopenia, and hemorrhagic manifestations, which are not a part of agranulocytosis. Examination of the bone marrow and study of smears made from the buffy coat of the peripheral blood nearly always reveal the presence of blasts and other young cells when leukemia is present. A carefully taken history regarding recent exposure to drugs or chemical agents is often helpful.

The presence of agranulocytosis may be suspected in some patients with infectious mononucleosis who have ulcerative pharyngeal lesions and a marked reduction in the granulocytes in the peripheral blood. The degree and distribution of the adenopathy, the presence of pathologic lymphocytes in the blood smear, and the positive heterophil agglutination test usually lead to the recognition of infectious mononucleosis; in doubtful cases a few days of observation generally resolve the difficulty because leukopenia rarely persists for more than a few days in infectious mononucleosis.

Other diseases are less likely to be confused with agranulocytosis. Sepsis is rarely responsible for a leukocyte count of less than 3000 per cu.mm. or a depression of the granulocytes to less than 30 per cent of the total. Other diseases such as those of the lymphoma group, tuberculosis, and subacute bacterial endocarditis are sometimes associated with severe leukopenia. In such patients the underlying disease is usually easily recognized because of splenomegaly or other features that lead to the correct diagnosis.

PROGNOSIS AND TREATMENT

Before antibiotics became available agranulocytosis was a serious disease with a mortality rate in the well developed cases that varied from 50 to 90 per cent. The mortality rate was nearly 100 per cent in patients whose leukocyte counts fell to less than 1000 per cu.mm. and in persons over 60 years of age. The general condition of the patient and the amount of drug that had been administered also appeared to influence the outcome.[76]

In the pre-antibiotic era many forms of treatment were employed in an effort to produce an increase in granulocytes. These included x-ray therapy, blood transfusion, injections of pentose nucleotide, leukocyte concentrates, extracts of liver or bone marrow. The early reports on each method were hopeful but subsequent experience was disappointing. The first real advance in treatment came when Dameshek and Wolfson administered sulfathiazole, a drug known to be capable of producing agranulocytosis, to two moribund patients whose disease was due to some other drug; the therapy appeared to bring the infection under control and the patients recovered.[78]

The most important aspects of treatment are the withdrawal of the offending drug and the administration of an antimicrobial agent to combat infection.

Illustrative Case

This 62 year old white widow was in good health until 6 weeks prior to admission, when she developed hematuria, frequency of urination, dysuria, and suprapubic pain. A diagnosis of urinary tract infection was made and she was treated with a sulfonamide 0.5 gm. three times a day. The urinary symptoms improved and the medication was continued for about 5 weeks. At this time the patient complained of fatigue, lassitude, and chilliness. She was admitted to her community hospital where she was found to have a leukocyte count of 600 per cu.mm. and a temperature of 101° F. She was treated with penicillin, transfusions, and cortisone. Four days later the leukocyte count had risen to 2000 per cu.mm. but granulocytes were still absent from the peripheral blood and she was referred for further treatment.

Physical examination. Temperature 103, pulse 84, respirations 22. There was no ulceration of the nasopharynx or vagina, and the liver, spleen, and lymph nodes were not enlarged. The remainder of the examination was noncontributory.

Laboratory examination. Blood studies on admission: Hct. 55 per cent; W.B.C. 2000 per cu.mm.; differential count (per cent), juveniles 1, bands 6, segmented 9, lymphocytes 70, monocytes 12, basophils, 2; reticulocytes 1.3 per cent; platelet count normal. Bone marrow obtained by aspiration 5 days after the agranulocytosis was recognized was cellular, erythropoiesis was normoblastic in type, and the megakaryocytes were normal. The cells of the granulocytic series were increased. Differential count of the marrow leukocytes (per cent): promyelocytes 0.5, myelocytes 16, juveniles 14, bands 46, segmented cells 18, lymphocytes 5, eosinophils 1. The patient was treated with penicillin, 500,000 units per day. Her temperature returned to normal by the third day and remained normal thereafter. The leukocyte count rose rapidly. On the day after admission it was 3500, the third day 10,000, the sixth day 18,000, the fourteenth day 21,000. One month after discharge from the hospital and about 7 weeks after onset of symptoms of agranulocytosis her hematocrit was 47 per cent, hemoglobin 15 gm. per 100 ml., leukocyte count 5000 per cu.mm., platelets 230,000 per cu.mm. The differential count was normal.

Comment. This elderly patient had agranulocytosis manifested by severe leukopenia associated with normal red cell and platelet counts. The bone marrow specimen which was examined after recovery had begun appeared hyperplastic. That obtained at another hospital a week earlier was either "aplastic or dilute." The extremely low leukocyte count in this patient would have augured a poor prognosis in the days before antibiotics. On treatment with penicillin and supportive measures she made an uneventful recovery. When agranulocytosis is caused by a sulfonamide drug, which was suspected but not proved in this case, the fall in granulocytes usually does not occur until after the patient has been taking the drug for several weeks. The patient was warned against future use of the suspected drug.

Neutropenia

Cyclic Neutropenia

Cyclic neutropenia is a well established but poorly understood entity that was first described by Leale in 1910.[111] Other reviewers have found 30 cases reported in the literature.[102, 114] This rare disorder, which may occur at any age, is characterized by the regular diminution or disappearance of the circulating neutrophilic granulocytes at approximately 21-day intervals. During the neutropenic phase fever, malaise, and oral pharyngeal ulceration usually appear and are often accompanied by arthralgia, headache, sore throat, and lymph node enlargement. Relatively minor intercurrent infections occur commonly but severe infections are unusual.

The careful studies of Page and Good have provided the clearest picture of the disorder.[114] By serial bone marrow studies they showed that the recurrent neutropenia is due to the cyclic arrest of production of the entire neutrophilic series. Neither a neutropenia-producing factor nor leuko-agglutinins could be demonstrated in the blood of the patient. The patient's serum exerted no demonstrable influence on the motility function of normal neutrophils. Although the influence of a hormonal factor could not be excluded, none was demonstrated. The occurrence of neutropenia bore no relationship to menstruation or to the urinary excretion of FSH or 17-ketosteroids. The concentrations of corticotropin and 17-hydroxycorticosteroid in the blood and the response of the adrenal gland to stimulation by corticotropin remained within normal limits without fluctuation throughout the cyclic changes in the neutrophils. In addition, no significant fluctuations were found in the levels of gamma globulin or properdin.

In some patients treatment with corticosteroids and splenectomy appear to modify temporarily the clinical manifestations of the disease without producing a significant alteration in the cyclic neutropenia.[114] Splenectomy appears to produce more lasting benefit in older patients with definite splenomegaly.[102] Antibiotics are important in the treatment of infections during the neutropenic phases but their long-term prophylactic use is not recommended.

Cyclic neutropenia is at times familial.[113] In a study of 20 patients with the familial disorder, the clinical course was similar to that in patients previously reported. It was noted that patients whose minimal neutrophil counts were less than 200 per cu.mm. were most severely affected; none of the "symptom-free" patients had minimal neutrophil counts of less than 500 per cu.mm.

Familial Benign Chronic Neutropenia

This disorder, characterized by constant neutropenia and relatively mild recurring infections, has been reported in several generations of the same family; it is thought to be transmitted as a non-sex-linked dominant.[99] In the reported cases the total leukocyte counts were in the neighborhood of 4000 per cu.mm., but the neutrophil granulocytes were only 300 to 500 per cu.mm. The eosinophils were 300 to 700 per cu.mm.; lymphocytes and monocytes were increased in the peripheral blood and marrow. In the marrow there was a reduction in the number of cells older than myelocytes.

Chronic Idiopathic Neutropenia

Chronic idiopathic neutropenia is a serious disorder.[112, 117] The reported patients have had moderate to severe leukopenia and severe granulocytopenia, and sometimes virtual absence of the granulocytes from the circulating blood. The severity of the disease is reflected in the paucity or lack of granulocytic cells in the areas of infection. In the bone marrow, cells of the granulocytic series are reduced and cells beyond the myelocyte or metamyelocyte stage are absent; nucleated red cells and lymphocytes predominate. Three-fourths of the reported cases have been in women more than 40 years of age. Many have died with pneumonia, septicemia, or abscess formation. Although some patients appeared to respond favorably to corticosteroids, treatment with corticosteroids, immunosuppressive agents, and splenectomy has usually been ineffective.

Other patients who appear to have had the same disease pursue a milder course and are not plagued by infections, even though the circulating granulocyte count may be zero.[98, 109] In one group of 15 patients with chronic idiopathic neutropenia, observed from 1 to 19 years, neutrophil counts varied between 0 and 152 per cu.mm. in the patient with the lowest counts, and between 546 and 823 per cu.mm. in the patient with the highest counts. The frequency of infection was not increased above normal and no serious diseases developed. Bone marrow examinations were made in all the patients, and in each the cellularity was normal or increased; there were normal numbers of band cells and younger forms but segmented cells were virtually absent. Treatment with corticosteroids and splenectomy did not change the blood counts.

Disorders Associated with Qualitative Defects in Granulocytes

The clinical syndromes associated with qualitative leukocyte abnormalities have been classified as (1) a defect in neutrophil leukotaxis; (2) defects in the ingestion phase of phagocytosis; or (3) defects in intracellular killing of organisms.[100a] The latter group, which appears to be more common than the others, has received the most study.

Chronic Granulomatous Disease

Chronic granulomatous disease in childhood which has occurred in at least 60 patients was reported first in 1957.[95, 110] The first six cases reported were in males. Symptoms developed within the first few years of life and the children died within 2 or 3 years. The disease is characterized by suppurative lymphadenitis, particularly in the neck and groin, eczematoid dermatitis about the eyes, nose, and mouth, pulmonary infiltrations, hepatosplenomegaly, lymphadenopathy, recurrent suppurative infections, and granuloma formation. Early observations did not reveal the nature of the disorder, but it was noted that the patients developed leukocytosis in response to infection and had normal or increased gamma globulins. Many of the infections were the result of staphylococci, and others were apparently due to *Klebsiella, Serratia marcescens,* and other organisms that ordinarily do not manifest great virulence. This hereditary disorder is transmitted as a sex-linked recessive and the heterozygous state has been demonstrated in some asymptomatic mothers.[103, 105]

A better understanding of this disorder was provided by the demonstration that, although there was no defect in phagocytosis by the leukocytes, cultures disclosed that organisms phagocytized by cells from patients with the disorder survived much better than they did when exposed to normal cells.[103, 105] They concluded that the defect in killing phagocytized organisms was related to a lack of release of bactericidal factors rather than to their absence, since they found normal quantities of acid phosphatase, glucuronidase, lysozyme, and phagocytin in the lysosomes. A failure of lysozomes to degranulate because of lack of fusion of the lysozome with the phagocytic vacuole was postulated, but normal degranulation has been found subsequently in some patients.[42, 101] Other leukocyte abnormalities in these patients have been demonstrated, including a defect in the hexosemonophosphate shunt, defective hydrogen peroxide production after phagocytosis, and a deficiency in reducing nitroblue tetrazolium; this test has shown that mothers of some patients with chronic granulomatous disease have two populations of granulocytes, one normal and one defective.

Hydrogen peroxide is essential for normal intracellular killing of bacteria and the defect in its production, probably the result of absence of a glucose oxidase enzyme, is the likely explanation of the failure of these cells to kill bacteria which do not themselves produce significant amounts of H_2O_2.[43] Some bacteria, such as streptococci or pneumococci, are killed by the combination of their own H_2O_2 production, peroxidase, and appropriate ions, such as chloride or iodide; other bacteria, such as *S. aureus* and *S. marcescens,* survive and multiply in cells with deficient H_2O_2 production. The importance of hydrogen peroxide was shown by the improved killing of *S. aureus* and *S. marcescens* that followed the in vitro introduction of glucose oxidase absorbed on latex particles into leukocytes of patients with chronic granulomatous disease; phagocytosis of these particles corrected an enzyme defect and promoted peroxide generation.[106]

Job's syndrome, a disorder of young red-headed girls characterized by a life-long history of recurrent colds, abscesses, purulent sinusitis, ear disease, skin lesions, and pulmonary disease, first reported in 1966,[100] may be a variant of chronic granulomatous disease.[101] It appears likely that numerous other enzymatic defects, congenital or acquired, will be found with more careful study of individual patients by the improved methods of investigation becoming available.

Other Disorders

Hereditary myeloperoxidase deficiency in neutrophils and monocytes has been associated with systemic infection with *Candida* and impaired killing of *Candida* and bacteria in vitro.[116]

A familial disorder characterized by susceptibility to infection and deficient phagocytosis has been reported. The defect in phagocytosis was the result of dysfunction of a plasma-mediated factor (opsonin); plasma from normal persons corrected the defect, possibly by adding a labile activator of complement.[112a]

The occurrence of frequent prolonged infections with *Klebsiella* and *E. coli* associated with impaired neutrophil leukotaxis has been reported in a 4 year old child.[117a] The defect was due, at least in part, to an inhibitor in the patient's serum; normal serum largely restored the leukotactic function.

CHEDIAK-HIGASHI SYNDROME

Chediak in 1952 and Higashi in 1954 independently reported instances of the syndrome now known as the "Chediak-Higashi Syndrome."[97, 104] This unusual disorder, apparently inherited as an autosomal recessive, is mainly a disease of childhood, but it also occurs in young adults and a mild form (heterozygote) occurs in middle age. The most characteristic feature is the great enlargement of the granules in the leukocytes, which at times resemble Döhle bodies, and the presence of red-staining bodies in the cytoplasm of the lymphocytes (Fig. 12–2). The abnormalities which are present in nearly all the bands and segmented cells appear in the myelocytes and metamyelocytes in the bone marrow as well; the granules are peroxidase positive. Among the clinical features of this disorder is semi-albinism, which gives a peculiar grayish-brown color to the hair.[118] Upon transillumination of the globe of the eyes, a red light can be readily visualized through the pale blue irides. The optic fundi are pale and nystagmus is usually present. There is an increased incidence of pyogenic infections which may be severe and incapacitating. A tendency to excessive sweating in some patients and hyperpigmentation of the areas of skin exposed to sunlight are common. In some patients, at least terminally, lymphadenopathy, splenomegaly, and hepatomegaly develop and suggest the presence of a lymphoma.

The increased susceptiblity of these patients to infections is not understood completely. The leukocytes react to inflammation and phagocytize particles in a normal fashion. The large granules and inclusions that are characteristic of the cells have been shown to be giant abnormal lysosomes. An abnormality in the limiting membranes of the large lysosomes has been postulated on the basis of histochemical supravital staining.[107] Other abnormalities demonstrated are an increased ability of the leukocytes from these patients both to incorporate radioactive precursors into sphingolipids and to cleave glucosyl ceramide sphingomyelin. Both abnormalities suggests an accelerated turnover of sphin-

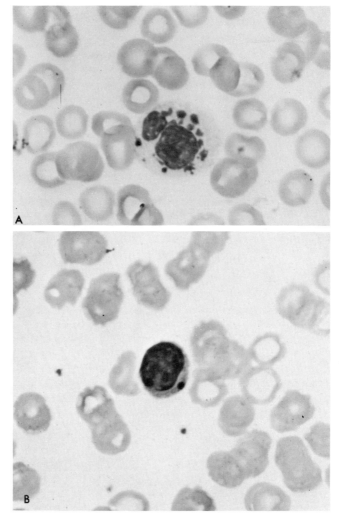

Figure 12-2. Leukocytes in Chediak-Higashi syndrome. *A*, Neutrophil. *B*, Lymphocyte. (F.S.:III, 144.)

golipids. A markedly increased rate of granulocyte turnover reflected by elevation of muramidase is the result of intramedullary cellular destruction.[96]

Infectious Mononucleosis
Synonym: Glandular Fever

Historical Introduction

Credit for the first description of this desease is generally given to Pfeiffer for his report on "Drusenfieber" which appeared in 1889.[154] Pfeiffer described an illness occurring in children 5 to 8 years of age which was characterized by fever of 1 to 10 days' duration, sore throat, adenopathy, splenomegaly, and hepatomegaly. The disorder was considered to be an infectious and epidemic disease. Following this account reports of unusual cases of adenitis that were associated with marked lymphocytosis and resembled lymphocytic leukemia appeared in the literature,[125] but the report of Sprunt and Evans in 1920 provided the first clear description of the disease to which they gave the name "infectious mononucleosis."[166] They studied six young adults whose illness was characterized by fever, enlargement of the cervical, axillary, and inguinal lymph nodes, splenomegaly, and leukocytosis. The differential count was unusual because of an increase in mononuclear elements, chiefly "large lymphocytes;" even more important was the observation that "all types of pathological lymphocytes, some resembling Türk's irritation forms, were to be seen." Study of lymph nodes removed from three patients disclosed definite hyperplasia, distinct from Hodgkin's disease, tuberculosis, and lymphosarcoma, that could not be distinguished from lymphocytic leukemia. It was concluded that the cases constituted a clinical syndrome that had a good prognosis. In the next few years groups of similar cases were reported by Bloedorn and Houghton,[124] Longcope,[149] and Tidy and Morley[172] and it was generally agreed that the disease "glandular fever" and "infectious mononucleosis" were identical.

The abnormal mononuclear cells that had been noted were studied carefully by Downey and McKinlay in 1923.[130] Their observations have been confirmed many times but little has been added to their description. In a study of nine cases they recognized three types of abnormal lymphocytes in the blood and concluded that there was "no danger of confusing the blood picture with leukemia, if well studied."

An important contribution that facilitated the recognition of the disease was made by Paul and Bunnell in 1932.[153] These investigators utilized a sheep cell agglutination test to study the presence of heterophil antibodies in patients with rheumatic fever, and in a group of individuals who served as controls. In their report they stated: "Quite by accident it was discovered that heterophil antibodies were present in a specimen of serum from a patient ill with infectious mononucleosis in much higher concentration than has been described in serum disease or any other clinical condition that we studied." They obtained similar results in three other patients with infectious mononucleosis and, apart from serum sickness and one other exception, failed to find high titers of heterophil antibodies in a large number of other conditions. Since that time the heterophil agglutination test has proved helpful in diagnosing infectious mononucleosis. However, an increasing number of positive tests have since been found in conditions other than infectious mononucleosis and for this reason Davidsohn's differential test has proved valuable.[129]

Comprehensive monographs on infectious mononucleosis have been written by Bernstein[122] and Leibowitz,[146] and Tidy has given an excellent review of the history and clinical features of the disease.[170]

Mechanism of Disease

Ever since infectious mononucleosis was described and epidemics reported, the disease has been considered to be a viral infection, but numerous attempts to isolate an etiologic agent have failed. The degree of infectivity seemed to be low and the incubation period seemed to vary from 1 day[122] to 8 weeks.[137]

In recent years, the studies of Henle and others[133, 135, 135a, 136] on the association of the Epstein-Barr virus (EB virus) and infectious mononucleosis have attracted considerable interest. They have demonstrated the absence of antibodies to EB virus before the development of the disease and their appearance during the acute stage of the disease; in contrast to heterophil antibodies which rise and fall rapidly, those induced by EB virus persist for years. The occurrence of EB virus in culture of cells obtained from patients with Burkitt's lymphoma has stimulated considerable speculation concerning the role of the EB virus in these two diseases and the relationship of the diseases to each other.[130a] Three possibilities have been considered: (1) that EB virus is the etiologic agent of infectious mononucleosis; (2) that it is a superinfection; or (3) that it acts as a latent and poorly immunogenic virus which is activated nonspecifically in subsequent lymphoreticular proliferation. Furthermore, it has been suggested that the different clinical diseases, and even the lack of disease associated with EB virus, may be a reflection of the lymphoreticular response of the patient.

Most of the clinical manifestations of the disease are explained by the pathologic findings. The most complete report is that of Custer and Smith.[128] In a study of nine autopsies they found that the lymph nodes were usually enlarged as a result of an increase in the size of the lymph follicles. Enlargement of the lymph nodes was not invariable and in some cases the architecture of the nodes was blurred and the follicles were inconspicuous. Splenic enlargement occurred in every instance and was associated with lymphocytic infiltration of the trabeculae and capsule. Varying degrees of lymphocytic infiltration were also found in the tissue of the central nervous system, meninges, myocardium, and in the periportal areas of the liver. In this series the bone marrows were normal or hyperplastic. In another study of 23 bone marrow biopsies granulomatous lesions were found in nine.[140]

Clinical Manifestations

Infectious mononucleosis occurs in both sexes and is predominantly a disease of children and young adults. The disease has been reported in a 4 month old infant and in an adult 70 years of age.[170] About 80 per cent of the cases occur between the ages of 15 and 30[122, 138, 145] and the disease is rarely seen in persons over 40. At one time infectious mononucleosis was considered rare in blacks but a more recent report indicates that the incidence in blacks is about the same as that in whites.[175]

Although infectious mononucleosis varies a great deal in its manner of onset, severity, and clinical manifestations, the majority of patients have a similar clinical picture. The patient with infectious mononucleosis usually complains

---

Figure 12–3.   Acute leukemia.
Figure 12–4.   Infectious mononucleosis.

From Heilmeyer, L., and Begemann, H.: Atlas der klinischen Hämatologie und Cytologie. Berlin-Göttingen-Heidelberg, Springer, 1955.

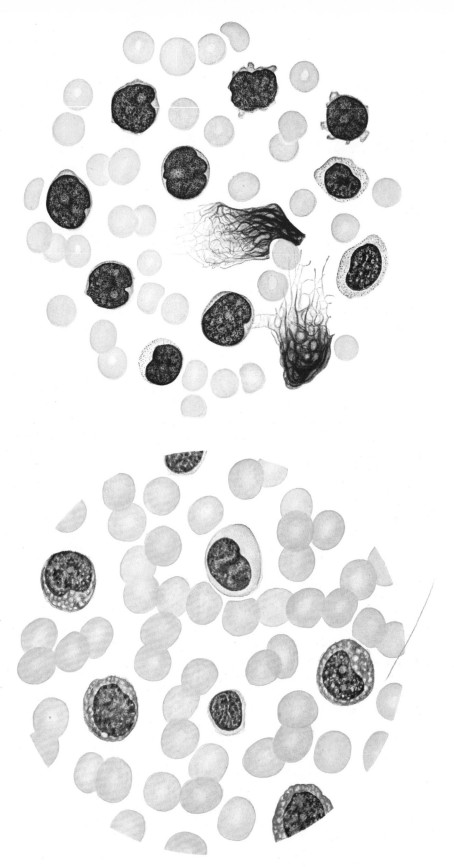

Figures 12-3 and 12-4. *See legends on opposite page.*

of malaise, sore throat, headache, and weakness of several days' duration. Anorexia and cough are not unusual. Fever of less than 102° F is usually present and the pulse is generally normal or slow in proportion to the temperature. Examination of the pharynx usually reveals diffuse infection of the mucous membranes or follicular tonsillitis. Palpable enlargement of the cervical lymph nodes is usually evident when the patient is first seen or develops within a few days. Involvement of the nodes in the cervical region, which is generally bilateral, is soon followed by the appearance of enlargement of the axillary and inguinal nodes. The spleen and liver are often palpable. Usually both the characteristic findings in the blood, a lymphocytosis associated with "pathologic lymphocytes" and the positive heterophil agglutination test, are present when the patient is first seen or develop during the first week or 10 days thereafter. As a rule, the fever subsides by lysis within the first or second week and the symptoms disappear during the second or third week. Convalescence is rapid in most patients. The glandular enlargement often improves within a few days but some residual enlargement may persist for months. In three-fourths of the patients the blood picture returns to normal in 2 months and the heterophil agglutination becomes negative in less than 4 months.

The "usual" clinical picture is not seen in a number of patients with infectious mononucleosis. Some patients are essentially asymptomatic and the presence of the disease is manifested only by painless adenopathy and the characteristic laboratory findings. Other patients become acutely ill with high fever and present the appearance of a severe overwhelming infection. In still other patients the clinical features are dominated by the presence of the disease in a particular organ; in such patients the presenting complaints are abdominal pain, jaundice, hematuria, or disease of the central nervous system.

The essential features of infectious mononucleosis, as emphasized by Tidy, are fever, glandular enlargement, faucial infection, and lymphocytosis.[170] The prominence of these features varies in different patients and various authors have recognized different groups of clinical syndromes. Tidy classified his patients into "glandular," "angiose," and "febrile" types. The "glandular" type occurred most often in children 5 to 11 years of age and was characterized by a temperature of 101° to 103° F, moderate glandular enlargement, and frequent recrudescence. In the "angiose" type the prodromal period lasted from 1 to 3 weeks, following which the patient developed a severe membranous sore throat clinically indistinguishable from diphtheria, peritonsillar edema, and a temperature of 104° F. The "febrile" type was characterized by the sudden onset of malaise, headache, chills, and temperature of 102° to 103° F; a rash was often noted during the first week and glandular enlargement did not appear until from 10 to 21 days had passed.

The incidence of the symptoms and signs in patients with infectious mononucleosis varies in different series.[129, 137, 138, 150, 167, 168, 170, 175] The extremes are shown in Table 12–8.

SKIN LESIONS

Various types of cutaneous eruptions occur and an incidence of 18 per cent was found in one series. The rash usually makes its appearance between the

Table 12–8. *The Incidence of Various Symptoms and Signs in Infectious Mononucleosis as Reported by Different Authors*

SYMPTOMS	PER CENT	PHYSICAL SIGNS	PER CENT
Sore throat	50–80	Fever	70–100
Malaise	25–63	Enlarged nodes	76–100
Headache	35–67	Pharyngitis	68–82
Weakness	13–54	Splenomegaly	26–70
Anorexia	17–41	Hepatomegaly	6–37
Abdominal pain or disease	14–22	Rashes	0–18
Ocular symptoms	6–15	Jaundice	5–8
		Hematuria	1–7

fourth and seventh days, but may appear as late as the twentieth day. The commonest type is a fine macular or maculopapular rash, pink or pinkish-brown in color, that involves mainly the trunk. The rash is often virtually indistinguishable from that seen in rubella. The rash, which may consist of only 8 or 10 lesions, usually appears in a single crop that lasts from 3 to 7 days. Other types of lesions that have been seen less often are erythematous, urticarial, morbilliform, and vesicular. Lesions like those seen in erythema multiforme and erythema nodosum also occur.

Two independent reports that a rash occurred in virtually 100 per cent of patients with infectious mononucleosis who were treated with ampicillin appeared in 1967.[152, 155] Copper-colored macules and papules appeared first on the trunk and quickly spread to involve the entire body; pruritus was almost invariably present. The rash usually appeared from 7 to 10 days after the patient began taking ampicillin and cleared up a week after the drug was stopped; neither antihistaminics nor corticosteroids exerted any effect on the course. These authors noted a rash in less than 15 per cent of patients with infectious mononucleosis who received no antibacterial drugs and in less than 20 per cent of the general population who took ampicillin. The incidence of rash in patients taking tetracycline and penicillin was about the same as that in untreated patients.

LIVER DAMAGE

Although jaundice occurs in only about 6 per cent of patients with infectious mononucleosis, it is probable that some impairment of liver function occurs in a high percentage of patients with the disease. Study of liver tissue obtained by biopsy and at autopsy indicates that the jaundice is due to a form of hepatitis and is not the result of extrahepatic obstruction from enlarged nodes.[128] The lesion consists mainly of periportal infiltration with mononuclear cells; there are minimal changes in the hepatic cells which are not accompanied by necrosis or alteration of the hepatic architecture. A good correlation between the severity of the infiltrative process and the frequency of abnormal liver function tests (BSP, SGPT, and alkaline phosphatase) has been reported.[142] A high incidence of abnormal liver function tests has been found in patients with infectious mononucleosis without jaundice. In one series of 15 patients, the thymol turbidity and BSP tests were found to be positive in all, and the alkaline phosphatase level was elevated in seven of eight patients on whom it was determined. Plasma electrophoresis was performed on six patients and a protein distribution similar to that seen in infectious hepatitis was found; there was a slight decrease in albumin, increase in alpha and beta globulin, and a marked increase in gamma globulin. Other studies have shown a positive thymol turbidity test in 60 to 68 per cent[127, 132, 175] and a positive cephalin flocculation test in 95 per cent.[132] Such studies have led to the conclusion that hepatitis is a feature of nearly all cases of infectious mononucleosis. Although abnormal liver function tests may persist for long periods (up to 22 months in one report),[167] the prognosis for complete recovery is excellent, even in the patients with jaundice. Cirrhosis of the liver has been reported only once and this patient had an alcoholic history.[147]

CENTRAL NERVOUS SYSTEM INVOLVEMENT

Involvement of the central nervous system, first reported in 1931,[131, 141] is a rare complication of infectious mononucleosis. At least 64 cases have been reported.[164] Involvement of the central nervous system has been manifested by headache, nuchal rigidity, drowsiness, stupor, coma, paralysis, convulsions, and changes in the spinal fluid such as pleocytosis, increased protein, and increased pressure. The types of central nervous system involvement were classified by Bernstein and Wolff as follows: (1) serous meningitis; (2) meningitis; (3) encephalitis; (4) meningo-encephalitis; (5) meningitis or meningo-encephalitis with acute polyneuritis; (6) peripheral neuropathy.[123] Meningitis, encephalitis, and meningitis or meningo-encephalitis with polyneuritis, (Guillain-Barré syndrome) make up about three-fourths of the reported cases. Although central nervous system involvement is estimated to occur in less than 1 per cent of the patients with infectious mononucleosis, this complication is responsible for a high percentage of deaths in the disease; when death occurs it is usually the result of respiratory paralysis. Despite a course that is frequently stormy, the prognosis is good in patients with central nervous system involvement; 85 per cent recover within a period that varies from a few days to several months after the onset of the complication.

CARDIAC INVOLVEMENT

The occurrence of cardiac involvement has been reviewed.[139] There is rarely any clinical evidence of cardiac involvement, but pericarditis which was diagnosed by the occurrence of chest pain, pericardial friction rub, electrocardiographic abnormalities, and changes in heart size has been reported nine times.[150, 164] Most of the reported cardiac abnormalities are not obvious and consist of electrocardiographic changes in the T waves, PR interval, or cardiac rhythm. Routine electrocardiograms have revealed abnormalities in from 5 to 50 per cent of patients. Postmortem studies have revealed focal interstitial infiltration of abnormal lymphocytes in the myocardium that appears to offer an explanation for the electrocardiographic findings.[128] Pericarditis has not been present in the autopsied cases. Although the electrocardiographic changes persist for months in some patients, there is little or no evidence that chronic heart disease occurs in patients with infectious mononucleosis.

RUPTURE OF THE SPLEEN

This is a serious complication that has been seen in at least 21 patients with infectious mononucleosis.[164] This complication, which has a mortality rate of about 33 per cent in the reported cases, is one of the most frequent causes of death in infectious mononucleosis.[128] Rupture of the spleen occurs as a consequence of splenic enlargement associated with capsular infiltration and subcapsular hemorrhage. The rupture rarely occurs before the third week of the disease, but has been reported as early as the end of the second week, and as late as 30 days after onset. The presence of this complication is generally manifested by severe pain in the upper abdomen or left upper quadrant followed by circulatory collapse. In some patients the occurrence of this complication has not been recognized because the diagnosis of infectious mononucleosis had not been made prior to the rupture and was not suspected then because of the intraperitoneal hemorrhage was associated with polymorphonuclear leukocytosis.[163] Although rupture of the spleen in infectious mononucleosis is usually termed "spontaneous," the importance of slight trauma associated with a trivial blow or the performance of the physical examination has been emphasized.

HEMATOLOGIC COMPLICATIONS

The most important hematologic complications that occur in infectious mononucleosis are hemolytic anemia and thrombocytopenic purpura. Both complications are rare but each has been reported at least 16 times.[164] In the reported cases the hemoglobin levels have ranged from 4.3 to 9.8 gm. per 100 ml., the reticulocyte count from 7.0 to 37.5 per cent, and the level of indirect reacting bilirubin in the serum from 1.6 to 6.0 mg. per 100 ml.[169] The antiglobulin (Coombs) test has been positive in most of the patients with hemolytic anemia when it has been performed, which suggests that the hyperhemolysis is due to autoimmune antibodies. Both the anemia and the thrombocytopenia disappear spontaneously or with appropriate treatment and no deaths have been reported from these complications. Thrombocytopenia may persist for 6 months or more, but at least partial recovery usually occurs in from 2 to 4 weeks.

HEMATURIA

Hematuria occurs in from 3 to 6 per cent of patients[170, 175] and may be the presenting complaint. Presumably the hematuria results from lymphocytic infiltration in the kidney. Chronic renal disease secondary to infectious mononucleosis has not been reported.

Laboratory Manifestations

The most characteristic abnormalities in the peripheral blood in infectious mononucleosis are leukocytosis, absolute lymphocytosis, and the presence of abnormal lymphocytes. Leukocyte counts of 3000 per cu.mm. or less may occur early in the disease, but the total count is usually elevated by the second week.

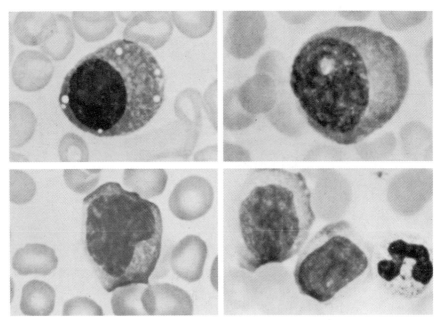

Figure 12-5. Various forms of pathologic lymphocytes seen in patients with infectious mononucleosis.

Counts over 40,000 per cu.mm. are rare. The most constant feature in infectious mononucleosis is the presence of the "pathologic lymphocytes" first described by Sprunt and Evans[166] and classified into three types by Downey and McKinlay.[130] The Type I cell is a highly differentiated mature lymphocyte with a nucleus that has a cloudy appearance due to the presence of a coarse network of chromatin strands or masses that is not sharply separated from the parachromatin. The nucleus is often indented. The cytoplasm is very basophilic and somewhat mottled in appearance. The Type II cell has a nucleus with a coarse chromatin structure somewhat similar to that of the plasma cell. The cytoplasm is less basophilic than the Type I cell and contains fewer vacuoles. The Type III cell, which more closely resembles leukemic cells, has a less differentiated nucleus that contains nucleoli. In Downey and McKinlay's report the Type III cells were uncommon; they were seen in small numbers in only one of nine cases; the Type I and II cells were numerous in all nine cases that were studied.

Other abnormalities, such as nuclear indentation, cytoplasmic vacuolation, and nuclear fenestration, may be seen in lymphocytes of all sizes. In patients who are diagnosed as having infectious mononucleosis, mononuclear cells almost invariably constitute over 50 per cent of the leukocytes at some stage of the disease, and counts as high as 96 per cent have been observed. Abnormal lymphocytes probably occur in all patients with infectious mononucleosis but are not pathognomonic of the disease. Apparently identical cells, for which the name "virocyte" has been suggested, have been observed in the following conditions: infectious hepatitis, virus pneumonia, herpetic infections, rubella, rubeola, roseola infantum, undulant fever, rickettsialpox, and allergic states. In these disorders the percentage of abnormal lymphocytes is generally less than in infectious mononucleosis and elevated total leukocyte counts are unusual. Although absolute lymphocytosis nearly always occurs in infectious mononucleosis it is not a constant finding. An increase in polymorphonuclear cells sometimes occurs in the prodromal phase and early in the disease.

Eosinophilia, which is more likely to develop during convalescence, has been found in 14 per cent of one series,[159] and in 10 per cent of another.[175] The eosinophils are usually less than 15 per cent but counts as high as 21 per cent occur. Except in rare instances complicated by hemolytic anemia and thrombocytopenia, the hemoglobin, red cell count, and platelet counts are normal.

Although the heterophil agglutination (Paul-Bunnell) test is non-specific, it is a very helpful procedure in the diagnosis of infectious mononucleosis.[153] Titers of 1:56,[159] 1:160,[128] and 1:224[129] have been considered confirmatory of infectious mononucleosis if the clinical and hematologic findings are suggestive of the disease. The differential adsorption test of Davidsohn is more specific because agglutinins for sheep cells sometimes occur in normal persons and in patients with serum sickness and other diseases.[129] Davidsohn found that the heterophil antibodies in infectious mononucleosis are not completely removed from the serum by adsorption with guinea pig kidney but are removed completely when adsorbed with beef red cells. The heterophil antibodies found in normal individuals and in patients with serum sickness and other diseases are different in that they are removed from the serum when adsorbed with guinea pig kidney. The test is useful in excluding patients with high titers that are not due to infectious mononucleosis and in establishing the diagnosis of infectious mononucleosis in patients with low titers. The test has been particularly helpful in patients with monocytic leukemia and acute leukemia; titers as high as 1:896 have been seen in these diseases but they could be distinguished from infectious mononucleosis by the guinea pig absorption test.[126, 165] The incidence of positive heterophil agglutination tests in infectious mononucleosis has been reported to be from 50 per cent to 100 per cent. The frequency of positive tests depends on the criteria used for establishing the diagnosis of infectious mononucleosis, the stage of the disease, and the number of the tests performed. The test is usually positive when the patient is first seen but the time of development of a positive test varies from 1 to 89 days.[138] In the vast majority of patients the test will be positive in the first 2 weeks of the disease if it is going to become positive. The heterophil agglutination test may remain positive from 9 days to 63 weeks,[138] but generally it becomes negative in from 2 to 4 months.[122] In one series the test became negative in 75 per cent of the patients within 4 months.[138]

The thymol turbidity, BSP excretion, and cephalin flocculation tests and the serum alkaline phosphatase level have been found to be abnormal in a high percentage of patients with infectious mononucleosis. One review of the literature reports that the various liver function tests were abnormal in from 40 to 100 per cent of 524 cases.[122]

A significant increase in α 2-globulin has been reported in 81 of 85 patients in one series.[158] There was no correlation with the heterophil antibody level, liver function, or lymphocytosis. The elevated level was readily reversed by corticosteroid therapy, and it was inferred that the hypergammaglobulinemia was a manifestation of a response of the reticuloendothelial system, a delayed hypersensitivity reaction, possibly to a virus.

The occurrence of false positive Wassermann and Kahn tests in infectious mononucleosis is well known. Incidences of 2 per cent,[167] 3 per cent,[175] 10 per cent,[137] 18 per cent,[122] and "about half"[170] have been reported. The test usually becomes positive during the second week and reverts to negative by the eighth week, but the duration of positivity varies from a few days to more than 3 months. The finding of a positive routine serologic test for syphilis in a young adult may be the first intimation that the patient may have infectious mononucleosis.

False positive agglutination tests for Br. melitensis, S. typhosa, S. paratyphii A and B, and Proteus X-19 have been reported.[121, 145] In some patients several agglutination tests may be positive at the same time.[121] When repeated titrations have been done, it has been noted that the titers rose abruptly, sometimes to as high as 1:1280, but fell quickly.

Transient urinary abnormalities in the form of red blood cells, white blood cells, albuminuria, and casts have been reported in 3 per cent and 6 per cent of patients.[164]

Diagnosis

The possibility of infectious mononucleosis is suggested by the occurrence of sore throat, fever, enlarged lymph nodes, or lymphocytosis in children and young adults. The presence of more than 50 per cent lymphocytes and more than 10 per cent pathologic lymphocytes is even stronger evidence. Most authors accept a diagnosis of infectious mononucleosis if the clinical and hematologic picture is considered characteristic even if the heterophil agglutination test is negative. However, some consider that patients with a negative heterophil agglutination reaction who have the clinical and hematologic features of infectious mononucleosis really have a different disease that is closely allied to infectious mononucleosis.[138, 162] The actual incidence of positive heterophil agglutination tests is hard to determine because it depends on many factors, including the stage of disease when the test is performed, the number of the tests done, and the criteria that are accepted for the diagnosis of infectious mononucleosis. Titers of over 1:56[159] and over 1:224[129] have been considered diagnostic if the other features of the disease are consistent. It has been recommended that the differential adsorption test be used if the titer is less than 1:224 and the findings suggest infectious mononucleosis, and also in circumstances when the titer is over 1:224 but is associated with no evidence of the disease.[129] If the titer is reduced more than 75 per cent by adsorption with guinea pig kidney, the antibody is probably not of the infectious mononucleosis type.

The diagnosis of infectious mononucleosis may be difficult if the patient is seen before the characteristic hematologic and serologic findings appear, especially when the clinical features are those that are more often associated with other diseases. When jaundice, hematuria, a septic type of fever, adenopathy, or evidence of central nervous system involvement is the presenting complaint the diagnosis may not be considered in sporadic cases when the patient is first seen. When the diagnosis of infectious mononucleosis is considered, repeated examination of the peripheral blood, repeated agglutination tests, and a period of observation may be necessary before the question can be settled.

The "postperfusion syndrome" closely resembles infectious mononucleosis.[156] This syndrome occurs from 1 to 8 weeks (usually 2 to 5 weeks) after openheart surgery and lasts from 1 to 4 weeks. It is characterized by fever (100° to 103° F), splenomegaly, and abnormal lymphocytes in the circulating blood; liver function tests are often abnormal and at times the liver is enlarged. The total leukocyte count is almost invariably normal; lymphocytes constitute 21 to 79 per cent of the cells and atypical cells have ranged from 3 to 60 per cent. In one series of 11 patients who had heterophil tests, three were negative; five had a titer of 1:7 or 1:14, two a titer of 1:28, and one a titer of 1:112. Both Eb virus[134] and cytomegalic virus infection[143] have been incriminated, apparently from exposure to blood containing the live viruses.

The cytomegalic virus may produce a clinical picture resembling that of infectious mononucleosis but without leukocytosis or a positive heterophil test.[157]

The report of a patient with infectious mononucleosis who had a mass in the anterior mediastinum that regressed spontaneously is yet another example of the protean manifestations of this disease and the difficulty one may encounter in making a diagnosis.[174] The rare occurrence of a positive heterophil test in patients with lymphoma is sometimes puzzling but of uncertain significance, especially in view of the recent studies on Burkitt's tumor.

Course and Prognosis

Infectious mononucleosis usually runs an acute course characterized by fever for 10 days or less followed by prompt recovery. A recrudescence of fever and symptoms is not unusual after the temperature has returned to normal for several days. In some patients the manifestations of the disease are so mild that the presence of the disease is recognized only by the laboratory tests. In other patients malaise and weakness may persist for months before complete recovery occurs. Nearly all patients recover completely, but deaths have occurred in some patients with splenic rupture and in some with central nervous system complications.

Treatment

The treatment of infectious mononucleosis is largely symptomatic and supportive. Parenteral fluids may be necessary if the throat is much involved. Prolonged bed rest is not necessary in patients with abnormal liver function tests or abnormal electrocardiograms. Treatment with sulfonamides, penicillin, chlortetracycline, and chloramphenicol has not been found to shorten significantly the duration of symptoms or fever or to reduce the incidence of complications.[120, 159, 161, 173] In certain circumstances corticosteroid drugs appear to be of benefit.[160] A favorable effect with the corticosteroid drugs in the approximately 10 per cent of patients who had the severe form of disease has been reported.[119]

Shortening of the period of fever together with striking improvement in the pharyngeal inflammation, malaise, lethargy, and anorexia was noted; no adverse effect from the treatment was observed.

Illustrative Case

A 17 year old white male student was in excellent health until 2 weeks prior to admission when he first noticed malaise. Ten days prior to admission transient chilly sensations occurred. Five days before admission severe headache appeared and was accompanied by sore throat and enlargement of the cervical lymph nodes. The sore throat became progressively worse and on the day of admission the patient was unable to swallow liquids.

Physical examination. The oral temperature on admission was 100° F. The tonsillar areas were covered with a white, thick, pseudo-membranous type of exudate. There was bilateral enlargement of the cervical and axillary lymph nodes which measured 1 to 3 cm. in diameter. A soft spleen edge was palpable 1 cm. below the left costal margin. The neurologic examination and the remainder of the routine examination were within normal limits.

Laboratory examination. Admission blood studies: Hct. 50 per cent; W.B.C. 14,000 per cu. mm., differential count (per cent), granulocytes 28, lymphocytes 64, monocytes 8. Many of the lymphocytes appeared abnormal: they were large and had an opaque basophilic cytoplasm. The nuclei of many of the smaller cells were indented or fenestrated. Other examinations showed the following: serum bilirubin level 0.7 mg. per 100 ml.; alkaline phosphatase 6.3 (B.U.); thymol turbidity 9.6 units; cephalin flocculation 4 plus in 48 hours; spinal fluid normal. The heterophil agglutination test was positive in dilutions of 1:3564 before adsorption and positive in a dilution of 1:792 after differential adsorption.

A diagnosis of infectious mononucleosis was made. The patient responded well to symptomatic measures and was essentially asymptomatic when discharged from the hospital 8 days later. One month after discharge nodes that measured 1 × 1 cm. were still palpable in the cervical area and in the left axilla. The leukocyte count was 7000 per cu. mm., and the differential count was (per cent): bands 1, segmented 47, lymphocytes 40, monocytes 9, eosinophils 2, basophils 1. A few atypical lymphocytes persisted. The heterophil test was still positive in dilutions of 1:24 after adsorption.

Comment. This patient illustrates most of the typical features of infectious mononucleosis. The majority of patients are young adults who complain of fever, malaise, sore throat, and cervical adenopathy. As often happens, the heterophil agglutination test was positive and the blood smear was typical of infectious mononucleosis when the patient was first seen. The patient is typical of many with the disease in that he had neither clinical jaundice nor elevation of the serum bilirubin but did exhibit evidence of liver dysfunction in the various tests. Because of his severe headache the complication of a meningo-encephalitis was considered but was discarded when the neurologic examination and cerebrospinal fluid proved to be normal.

References

LEUKOCYTES AND LEUKOPOIESIS

1. Alper, C. A., Abramson, N., Johnston, R. B., Jr., Jandl, J. H., and Rosen, F. S.: Increased susceptibility to infection associated with abnormalities of complement-mediated functions and of the third component of complement (C3). New England J. Med., *282*:349, 1970.

2. Archer, R. K.: On the functions of eosinophils in the antigen-antibody reaction. Brit. J. Haem.,*11*:123, 1965.

3. Athens, J. W., Mauer, A. M., Raab, S. O., Haab, O. P., and Cartwright, G. E.: Studies of granulocytic kinetics. J. Clin. Invest., *39*:969, 1960.

4. Athens, J. W., Raab, S. O., Haab, O. P., Boggs, D. R., Ashenbrucker, H., Cartwright, G. E., and Wintrobe, M. M.: Leukokinetic studies. X. Blood granulocyte kinetics in chronic myelocytic leukemia. J. Clin. Invest., *44*:765, 1965.

5. Berry, L. J., Leyendecker, R. M., and Spies, T. D.: Comparative studies on phagocytosis in normal and anemic blood. Blood, Special Issue No. 1, 98, 1947.

6. Bierman, H. R., Kelly, K. H., and Cordes, F. L.: The sequestration and visceral circulation of leukocytes in man. Ann. N.Y. Acad. Sci., *59*:850, 1955.

7. Bloom, B. R., and Bennett, B.: Macrophages and delayed-type hypersensitivity. Seminars Hemat.,*7*:215, 1970.

8. Boggs, D. R.: The kinetics of neutrophilic leukocytes in health and disease. Seminars Hemat., *4*:359, 1967.

9. Boggs, D. R., Athens, J. W., Cartwright, G. E., and Wintrobe, M. M.: Leukokinetic studies. IX. Experimental evaluation of a model of granulopoiesis. J. Clin. Invest., *44*:643, 1965.

9a. Brittingham, T. E., and Chaplin, H., Jr.: Sensitivity to buffy coat a cause of "nonspecific" transfusion reactions. J. Clin. Invest., *36*:877, 1957.

10. Boggs, D. R., Marsh, J. C., and Cartwright, G. E.: Humoral regulation of neutrophil release from bone marrow. J. Clin. Invest., *45*:988, 1966.

11. Brayton, R. G., Stokes, P. E., Schwartz, M. S., and Louria, D. B.: Effect of alcohol and various diseases on leukocyte mobilization, phagocytosis and intracellular bacterial killing. New England J. Med.,*282*:123, 1970.

12. Broun, G. O., Herbig, F. K., and Hamilton, J. R.: Leukopenia in Negroes. New England J. Med.,*275*:1410, 1966.

13. Broun, G. O., Herbig, F. K., and Hamilton, J. R.: Leukopenia in Negroes. New England J. Med.,*277*:899, 1967.

14. Cartwright, G. E., Athens, J. W., Haab, O. P., Raab, S. O., Boggs, D. R., and Wintrobe, M. M.: Blood granulocyte kinetics in conditions associated with granulocytosis. Ann. N.Y. Acad. Sci., *113*:963, 1964.

15. Cartwright, G. E., Athens, J. W., and Wintrobe, M. M.: The kinetics of granulopoiesis in normal man. Blood, *24*:780, 1964.

16. Cohn, Z. A., and Hirsch, J. G.: The isolation and properties of the specific cytoplasmic granules of rabbit polymorphonuclear leukocyte. J. Exper. Med., *112*:983, 1960.

17. Cottingham, E., and Mills, C. A.: Timing of phagocytic changes in malnutrition. J. Lab. Clin. Med., *30*:498, 1945.

18. Craddock, C. G.: The production, utilization and destruction of white blood cells. Progr. in Hemat., *3*:92, 1962.

19. Craddock, C. G., Jr., et al.: Studies of leukopoiesis. The technique of leukopheresis and the response of myeloid tissue in normal and irradiated dogs. J. Lab. & Clin. Med., *45*:881, 1955.

20. Craddock, C. G., Jr., Perry, S., and Lawrence, J. S.: The dynamics of leukopoiesis and leukocytosis, as studied by leukopheresis and isotopic techniques. J. Clin. Invest., *35*:285, 1956.

21. Donohue, D. M., Reiff, R. H., Hanson, M. C., Betson, Y., and Finch, C. A.: Quantitative measurements of erythrocytic and granulocytic cells of the marrow and blood. J. Clin. Invest., *37*:1571, 1958.

22. Dougherty, T. F., and White, A.: Influence of hormones on lymphoid tissue structure and function. The role of the pituitary adrenotrophic hormone in the regulation of the lymphocytes and other cellular elements of the blood. Endocrinology, *35*:1, 1944.

23. Ehrlich, P., and Lazarus, A.: Anemia. Rebman, Ltd., London, 1910.

24. Fenn, W. O.: The phagocytosis of solid particles. III. Carbon and quartz. J. Gen. Physiol., *3*:575, 1920–21.

25. Fenn, W. O.: The temperature coefficient of phagocytosis. J. Gen. Physiol., *4*:331, 1921–22.

25a. Ford, W. L., and Gowans, J. L.: The traffic of lymphocytes. Seminars Hemat.,*6*:67, 1969.

26. Forman, M. L., and Stiehm, E. R.: Impaired opsonic activity but normal phagocytosis in low-birth-weight infants. New England J. Med.,*281*:926, 1969.

27. Garrey, W. E., and Bryan, W. R.: Variations in white blood cell counts. Physiol. Rev., *15*:597, 1935.

28. Gordon, A. S.: Some aspects of hormonal influences upon the leukocytes. Ann. N.Y. Acad. Sci., *59*:907, 1955.

29. Gordon, A. S., Handler, E. S., Siegel, C. D., Dornfest, B. S., and Lo Bue, J.: Plasma factors influencing leukocyte release in rats. Ann. N.Y. Acad. Sci., *113*:766, 1964.

30. Gowans, J. L.: Life-history of lymphocytes. Brit. Med. Bull., *15*:50, 1959.

31. Hamilton, L. D.: Nucleic acid turnover studies in human leukaemic cells and the function of lymphocytes. Nature, *178*:597, 1956.

32. Hewson, W.: The Works of William Hewson. Printed for the Sydenham Society, London, 1846, p. 282.

33. Hirsch, J. G.: Cinemicrophotographic observations on granule lysis in polymorphonuclear leukocyte during phagocytosis. J. Exper. Med., *116*:827, 1962.

34. Hirsch, J. G., and Cohn, Z. A.: Degranulation of polymorphonuclear leukocytes following phagocytosis of microorganisms. J. Exper. Med., *112*:1005, 1960.

35. Kabins, S. A., and Lerner, C.: Fulminant pneumococcemia and sickle cell anemia. J.A.M.A., *211*:467, 1970.

36. Kindred, J. E.: A quantitative study of the hemopoietic organs of young adult albino rats. Am. J. Anat., *71*:207, 1942.

37. Kuna, A., and Chambers, R.: Effect of saccharides on leukocyte movement. J. Clin. Invest., *32*:436, 1953.

38. Kuvin, S. F., and Brecher, G.: Differential neutrophil counts in pregnancy. New England J. Med., *266*:877, 1962.

39. Lawrence, J. S., Ervin, D. M., and Wetrich, R. M.: Life cycle of white blood cells: The rate of disappearance of leukocytes from the peripheral blood of leukopenic cats. Am. J. Physiol., *144*:284, 1945.

39a. Leahy, D. R., McLean, E. R., Jr., and Bonner, J. T.: Evidence for cyclic-3′,5′-adenosine monophosphate as chemotactic agent for polymorphonuclear leukocytes. Blood, *36*:52, 1970.

40. Little, J. R., Brecher, G., Bradley, T. R., and Rose, S.: Determination of lymphocyte turnover by continuous infusion of H³ thymidine. Blood, *19*:236, 1962.

41. Mackaness, G. B.: The monocyte in cellular immunity. Seminars Hemat., *7*:172, 1970.

42. Mandell, G. L., and Hook, E. W.: Leukocyte function in chronic granulomatous disease of childhood. Am. J. Med., *47*:473, 1969.

43. Mandell, G. L., and Hook, E. W.: Leukocyte bactericidal activity in chronic granulomatous disease: correlation of bacterial hydrogen peroxide production and susceptibility to intracellular killing. J. Bacteriology, *100*:531, 1969.

44. Menkin, V.: Factors concerned in the mobilization of leukocytes in inflammation. Ann. N.Y. Acad. Sci., *59*:956, 1955.

45. Meuwissen, H. J., Stutman, O., and Good, R. A.: Functions of the lymphocytes. Seminars Hemat., *6*:28, 1969.

45a. Milhorat, A. T., Small, S. M., and Diethelm, O.: Leukocytosis during various emotional states. Arch. Neurol. & Psychiat., *47*:779, 1942.

46. Miller, M. E., Nilsson, U. R.: A familial deficiency of the phagocytosis-enhancing activity of serum related to a dysfunction of the fifth component of complement (C5). New England J. Med., *282*:354, 1970.

47. Morley, A., and Stohlman, F., Jr.: Studies on the regulation of granulopoiesis. I. The response to neutropenia. Blood, *35*:312, 1970.

48. Muchmore, H. G., Blackburn, A. B., Shurley, J. T., Pierce, C. M., and McKown, B. A.: Neutropenia in healthy men at the South Polar Plateau. Arch. Int. Med., *125*:646, 1970.

49. North, R. J.: Endocytosis. Seminars Hemat., *7*:161, 1970.

50. Osgood, E. E.: Number and distribution of human hemic cells. Blood, *9*:1141, 1954.

51. Osgood, E. E., Brownlee, I. E., Osgood, M. W., Ellis, D. M., and Cohen, W.: Total differential and absolute leukocyte counts and sedimentation rates. Arch. Int. Med., *64*:105, 1939.

52. Ottesen, J.: On the age of human white cells in peripheral blood. Acta physiol. scandinav., *32*:75, 1954.

53. Page, A. R., and Good, R. A.: Studies on cyclic neutropenia. Am. J. Dis. Child., *194*:623, 1957.

54. Payne, Rose: Leukocyte agglutinins in human sera. Arch. Int. Med., *99*:587, 1957.

55. Perry, S., Goodwin, H. A., and Zimmerman, T. S.: Physiology of the granulocyte. J.A.M.A., *203*:937, 1025, 1968.

56. Perry, S., Weinstein, I. M., Craddock, C. G., Jr., and Lawrence, J. S.: The combined use of typhoid vaccine and P³² labeling to assess myelopoiesis. Blood, *12*:549, 1957.

57. Quittner, H. N., Wald, N., Sussman, L. N., and Antopol, W.: The effect of massive doses of cortisone on the peripheral blood and bone marrow of the mouse. Blood, *6*:513, 1951.

58. Riddle, J. M., and Barnhart, M. I.: The eosinophil as a source for profibrinolysin in acute inflammation. Blood, *25*:776, 1965.

59. Robinson, W. A., and Pike, B. L.: Leukopoietic activity in human urine. New England J. Med., *282*:1291, 1970.
59a. Rocklin, R. E., Rosen, F. S., and David, J. R.: In vitro lymphocyte response of patients with immunologic deficiency diseases. New England J. Med., *282*:1340, 1970.
60. Schilling, V.: The Blood Picture. C. V. Mosby Co., St. Louis, 1929.
61. Sturgis, C. C., and Bethell, F. H.: Quantitative and qualitative variations in normal leukocytes. Physiol. Rev., *23*:279, 1943.
62. Tullis, J. L.: Prevalence, nature and identification of leukocyte antibodies. New England J. Med., *258*:569, 1958.
63. Unanue, E. R., and Cerottini, J. C.: The function of macrophages in the immune response. Seminars Hemat., *7*:225, 1970.
63a. Van Furth, R.: The formation of immunoglobulins by circulating lymphocytes. Seminars Hemat., *6*:84, 1969.
64. Van Furth, R.: Origins and kinetics of monocytes and macrophages. Seminars Hemat., *7*:125, 1970.
65. Van Furth, R., and Cohn, Z. A.: The origin and kinetics of mononuclear phagocytes. J. Exp. Med., *128*:415, 1968.
66. Volkman, A., and Collins, F. M.: Recovery of delayed-type hypersensitivity in mice following suppressive doses of x-radiation. J. Immunol., *101*:846, 1968.
67. Volkman, A., and Gowans, J. L.: The origin of macrophages from bone marrow in the rat. Brit. J. Exp. Path., *46*:62, 1965.
67a. Ward, P. A.: Chemotaxis of mononuclear cells. J. Exp. Med., *128*:1201, 1968.
68. Winkelstein, J. A., and Drachman, R. H.: Deficiency of pneumococcal serum opsonizing activity in sickle cell disease. New England J. Med., *279*:459, 1968.
69. Wintrobe, M. M.: Diagnostic significance of changes in leukocytes. Bull. N.Y. Acad. Med., *15*:223, 1939.
70. Wintrobe, M. M.: Clinical Hematology. 6th Ed. Lea & Febiger, Philadelphia, 1967, p. 260.
71. Wood, W. B., Jr., Smith, M. R., and Watson, B.: Studies on the mechanism of recovery in pneumococcal pneumonia. IV. The mechanism of phagocytosis in the absence of antibody. J. Exper. Med., *84*:387, 1946.
72. Wood, W. B., Jr., and Smith, M. R.: The nature and biological significance of the capsular slime layer of pneumococcus Type III. Trans. Assoc. Am. Phys., *62*:90, 1949.
73. Wright, C. S., and Dodd, M. C.: Phagocytosis. Ann. N.Y. Acad. Sci., *59*:945, 1955.
74. Yoffey, J. M.: The quantitative study of the leukocytes. Ann. N.Y. Acad. Sci., *59*:928, 1955.
75. Zarafonetis, C., Harmon, D. R., and Clark, P. F.: The influence of temperature upon opsonization and phagocytosis. J. Bact., *53*:343, 1947.

AGRANULOCYTOSIS AND OTHER DISORDERS OF NEUTROPHILS

76. Dameshek, W.: Leukopenia and Agranulocytosis. Oxford University Press, New York, 1944.
77. Dameshek, W., and Colmes, A.: The effect of drugs in the production of agranulocytosis with particular reference to amidopyrine hypersensitivity. J. Clin. Invest., *15*:85, 1936.
78. Dameshek, W., and Wolfson, L. E.: A preliminary report on the treatment of agranulocytosis with sulfathiazole. Am. J. Med. Sci., *203*:819, 1942.
79. Fitz-Hugh, T., Jr.: Sensitivity reactions of the blood and bone marrow to certain drugs. J.A.M.A., *111*:1643, 1938.
80. Fitz-Hugh, T., Jr., and Krumbhaar, E. B.: Myeloid cell hyperplasia of the bone marrow in agranulocytic angina. Am. J. Med. Sci., *183*:104, 1932.
81. Kracke, R. R.: Recurrent agranulocytosis: Report of an unusual case. Am. J. Clin. Path., *1*:385, 1931.
82. Kracke, R. R.: The experimental production of agranulocytosis. Am. J. Clin. Path., *2*:11, 1932.
83. Kracke, R. R., and Parker, F. P.: The relationship of drug therapy to agranulocytosis. J.A.M.A. *105*:960, 1935.
84. Madison, F. W., and Squier, T. L.: The etiology of primary granulocytopenia (agranulocytic angina). J.A.M.A., *102*:755, 1934.
85. Moeschlin, S., Meyer, H., Israels, L. G., and Tarr-Gloor, E.: Experimental agranulocytosis. Its production through leukocytic agglutination by antileukocytic serum. Acta Haemat., *11*:73, 1954.
86. Moeschlin, S., and Wagner, K.: Agranulocytosis due to the occurrence of leukocyte-agglutinins (Pyramidon and cold agglutinins). Acta Haemat., *8*:29, 1952.
87. Osgood, E. E.: Hypoplastic anemias and related syndromes caused by drug idiosyncrasy. J.A.M.A., *152*:816, 1953.
88. Pisciotta, A. V.: Agranulocytosis induced by certain phenothiazine derivatives. J.A.M.A., *203*:1862, 1969.

89. Plum, P.: Agranulocytosis due to amidopyrine. An experimental and clinical study of seven new cases. Lancet, *1*:14, 1935.
90. Reznikoff, P.: The etiologic importance of fatigue and the prognostic significance of monocytosis in neutropenia (agranulocytosis). Am. J. Med. Sci., *195*:627, 1938.
91. Roberts, S. R., and Kracke, R. R.: Agranulocytosis: Report of a case. J.A.M.A., *95*:780, 1930.
92. Schultz, W.: Ueber eigenartige Halserkrankungen (a) Monozytenangina; (b) Gangränezierende Prozesse und Defekt des Granulozytensystems. Deutsche med. Wchnschr., *48*:1495, 1922.
93. Welch, H., Lewis, C. N., and Kerlan, I.: Blood dyscrasias. A nationwide survey. Antibiotics & Chemother., *4*:607, 1954.

CYCLIC NEUTROPENIA AND OTHER DISORDERS OF NEUTROPHILS

94. Baehner, R. L., and Nathan, D. G.: Quantitative nitroblue tetrazolium test in chronic granulomatous disease. New England J. Med., *278*:971, 1968.
95. Berendes, H., Bridges, R. A., and Good, R. A.: Fatal granulomatous disease in childhood: clinical study of new syndrome. Minn. Med., *40*:309, 1957.
96. Blume, R. S., Bennett, J. M., Yankee, R. A., and Wolff, S. M.: Defective granulocyte regulation in the Chediak-Higashi syndrome. New England J. Med., *279*:1009, 1968.
97. Chediak, M.: Nouvelle anomalie leucocytaire de la charactère constitutionnel et familial. Rev. Hemat., 7:362, 1962.
98. Crosby, W. H.: How many "polys" are enough? Arch. Int. Med., *123*:722, 1969.
99. Cutting, H. O., and Lang, J. E.: Familial benign chronic neutropenia. Ann. Int. Med., *61*:876, 1964.
100. Davis, S. D., Schaller, J., and Wedgwood, R. J.: Job's syndrome. Recurrent "cold" staphylococcal abscesses. Lancet, *1*:1013, 1966.
100a. Douglas, S. D.: Analytic review: disorders of phagocyte function. Blood, *35*:851, 1970.
101. Douglas, S. D., Davis, W. C., and Fudenberg, H. H.: Granulocytopathies: pleomorphism of neutrophil dysfunction. Am. J. Med., *46*:901, 1969.
102. Duane, G. W.: Periodic neutropenia. Arch. Int. Med., *102*:462, 1958.
103. Good, R. A., Quie, P. G., Windhorst, D. B., Page, A. R., Rodey, G. E., White, J., Wolfson, J. J., and Holmes, B. H.: Fatal (chronic) granulomatous disease of childhood: a hereditary defect of leukocyte function. Seminars Hemat., *5*:215, 1968.
104. Higashi, O: Congenital gigantism of peroxidase granules. Tohoku J. Exp. Med., *59*:315, 1954.
105. Holmes, B., Quie, P. G., Windhorst, D. B., and Good, R. A.: A fatal granulomatous disease of childhood: inborn abnormality of phagocytic function. Lancet, *1*:1225, 1966.
106. Johnson, R. B., Jr., and Baehner, R. L.: Improvement of leukocyte bactericidal activity in chronic granulomatous disease. Blood, *35*:350, 1970.
107. Kanfer, J. N., Blume, R. S., Yankee, R. A., and Wolff, S. M.: Alteration of sphingolipid metabolism in leukocytes from patients with the Chediak-Higashi syndrome. New England J. Med., *279*:410, 1968.
108. Klebanoff, S. J., and White, L. R.: Iodination defect in leukocytes of chronic granulomatous disease. New England J. Med., *280*:460, 1969.
109. Kyle, R. A., and Linman, J. W.: Chronic idiopathic neutropenia. New England J. Med., *279*:1015, 1968.
110. Landing, B. H., and Shirkey, H. S.: Syndrome of recurrent infection and infiltration of viscera by pigmented lipid histiocytes. Pediatrics, *20*:431, 1957.
111. Leale, M.: Recurrent furunculosis in an infant showing an unusual blood picture. J.A.M.A., *54*:1854, 1910.
112. Lipton, A.: Chronic idiopathic neutropenia. Arch. Int. Med., *123*:694, 1969.
112a. Miller, M. E., Seals, J., Kaye, R., and Levitsky, L. C.: Familial plasma-associated defect of phagocytosis: new cause of recurrent bacterial infections. Lancet, *2*:60, 1968.
113. Morley, A. A., Carew, J. P., and Baikie, A. G.: Familial cyclical neutropenia. Brit. J. Haemat., *13*:719, 1967.
114. Page, A. R., and Good, R. A.: Studies on cyclic neutropenia. Am. J. Dis. Child., *94*:623, 1957.
115. Quie, P. G., Kaplan, E. L., Page, A. R., Gruskay, F. L., and Malawista, S. E.: Defective polymorphonuclear-leukocyte function and chronic granulomatous disease in two female children. New England J. Med., *278*:976, 1968.
116. Salmon, S. E., Cline, M. J., Schultz, J., and Lehrer, R. I.: Myeloperoxidase deficiency. New England J. Med., *282*:250, 1970.
117. Spaet, T. H., and Dameshek, W.: Chronic hypoplastic neutropenia. Am. J. Med., *13*:35, 1952.

117a. Ward, P. A., and Schlegel, R. J.: Impaired leucotactic responsiviness in a child with recurrent infections. Lancet, 2:344, 1969.

118. Weary, P. E., and Bender, A. S.: Chediak-Higashi syndrome with severe cutaneous involvement. Arch. Int. Med., *119*:381, 1967.

INFECTIOUS MONONUCLEOSIS

119. Bender, C. E.: The value of corticosteroids in the treatment of infectious mononucleosis. J.A.M.A., *199*:529, 1967.

120. Bennike, T.: Penicillin treatment of infectious mononucleosis. Arch. Int. Med., *87*:181, 1951.

121. Bernstein, A.: Antibody responses in infectious mononucleosis. J. Clin. Invest., *13*:419, 1934.

122. Bernstein, A.: Infectious mononucleosis. Medicine, *19*:85, 1940.

123. Bernstein, T. C., and Wolff, H. G.: Involvement of the nervous system in infectious mononucleosis. Ann. Int. Med., *33*:1120, 1950.

124. Bloedorn, W. A., and Houghton, J. E.: The occurrence of abnormal leukocytes in the blood in acute infections. Arch. Int. Med., *27*:315, 1921.

125. Cabot, R. C.: The lymphocytosis of infection. Am. J. Med. Sci., *145*:335, 1913.

126. Carpenter, G., Kahler, J., and Reilly, E. B.: Elevated titers of serum heterophil antibodies in three instances of monocytic leukemia. Am. J. Med. Sci., *220*:195, 1950.

127. Carter, A. B., and MacLagan, N. F.: Some observations on liver function tests in diseases not primarily hepatic. Brit. Med. J., *2*:80, 1946.

128. Custer, R. P., and Smith, E. B.: The pathology of infectious mononucleosis. Blood, *3*:830, 1948.

129. Davidsohn, I., Stern, K., and Kashiwagi, C.: The differential test for infectious mononucleosis. Am. J. Clin. Path., *21*:1101, 1951.

130. Downey, H., and McKinlay, C. A.: Acute lymphadenosis compared with acute lymphatic leukemia. Arch. Int. Med., *32*:82, 1923.

130a. E.B. virus, infectious mononucleosis and Burkitt's lymphoma. Lancet, *2*:887, 1969.

131. Epstein, S. H., and Dameshek, W.: Involvement of the central nervous system in a case of glandular fever. New England J. Med., *205*:1238, 1931.

132. Evans, A. S.: Liver involvement in infectious mononucleosis. J. Clin. Invest., *27*:106, 1948.

133. Gerber, P., Hamre, D., Moy, R. A., Rosenblum, E. N.: Infectious mononucleosis: complement-fixing antibodies to herpes-like virus associated with Burkitt lymphoma. Science, *161*:173, 1968.

134. Gerber, P., Walsh, J. H., Rosenblum, E. N., and Purcell, R. W.: Association of EB-virus infection with the post-perfusion syndrome. Lancet, *1*:593, 1969.

135. Henle, G., Henle, W., and Volker, D.: Relation of Burkitt's tumor-associated type virus in infectious mononucleosis. Proc. Nat. Acad. Sci. U.S.A., *59*:94, 1968.

135a. Henle, G., and Henle, W.: EB virus in the etiology of infectious mononucleosis. Hosp. Pract., *5*:33, 1970.

136. Hirshaut, Y., Glade, P., Moses, H., Manaker, R., and Chessin, L.: Association of herpes-like virus infection with infectious mononucleosis. Am. J. Med., *47*:520, 1969.

137. Hoagland, R. J.: Infectious mononucleosis. Am. J. Med., *13*:158, 1952.

138. Hobson, F. G., Lawson, B., and Wigfield, M.: Glandular fever: A field study. Brit. Med. J., *1*:845, 1958.

139. Houck, G. H.: Involvement of the heart in infectious mononucleosis. Am. J. Med., *14*:261, 1953.

140. Hovde, R. F., and Sundberg, R. D.: Granulomatous lesions in the bone marrow in infectious mononucleosis. Blood, *5*:209, 1950.

141. Johansen, A. H.: Serous meningitis and infectious mononucleosis. Acta Med. Scandinav., *76*:269, 1931.

142. Kilpatrick, Z. M.: Structural and functional abnormalities of liver in infectious mononucleosis. Arch. Int. Med., *117*:47, 1966.

143. Lang, D. J., and Hanshaw, J. B.: Cytomegalovirus infection and the postperfusion syndrome. New England J. Med., *280*:1145, 1960.

145. Leavell, B. S., and McNeel, J. O.: Infectious mononucleosis: Unusual manifestations. Virginia M. Month., *69*:180, 1942.

146. Leibowitz, S.: Infectious Mononucleosis. Modern Medical Monographs. Grune and Stratton, New York, 1953.

147. Leibowitz, S., and Brody, H.: Cirrhosis of the liver following infectious mononucleosis. Am. J. Med., *8*:675, 1950.

148. Litwins, J., and Leibowitz, S.: Abnormal lymphocytes (virocytes) in virus diseases other than infectious mononucleosis. Acta Haemat. *5*:223, 1951.

149. Longcope, W. T.: Infectious mononucleosis (glandular fever) with a report of ten cases. Am. J. Med. Sci., *164*:781, 1922.
150. Lyght, C. E.: Infectious mononucleosis. Journal-Lancet, *58*:91, 1938.
151. Niederman, J. C., McCollum, R. W., Henle, G., and Henle, W.: Infectious mononucleosis. J.A.M.A., *203*:205, 1968.
152. Patel, B. M.: Skin rash with infectious mononucleosis and ampicillin. Pediatrics, *40*:910, 1967.
153. Paul, J. R., and Bunnell, W. W.: The presence of heterophile antibodies in infectious mononucleosis. Am. J. Med. Sci., *183*:90, 1932.
154. Pfeiffer, S.: "Drusenfieber." Jahrb. f. Kinderh., *29*:257, 1889.
155. Pullen, H., Wright, N., Murdoch, J. McC.: Hypersensitivity reactions to antibacterial drugs in infectious mononucleosis. Lancet, *2*:1176, 1967.
156. Reyman, T. A.: Postperfusion syndrome: a review and report of 21 cases. Am. Heart J., *72*:116, 1966.
157. Rifkind, D.: Cytomegalic mononucleosis. Ann. Int. Med., *69*:842, 1968.
158. Rose, K. D.: Serum proteins in infectious mononucleosis. Ann. Int. Med., *64*:826, 1966.
158a. Saba, T. M.: Physiology and physiopathology of the reticuloendothelial system. Arch. Int. Med., *126*:1031, 1970.
159. Schultz, A. L., and Hall, W. H.: Clinical observations in 100 cases of infectious mononucleosis and the results of treatment with penicillin and Aureomycin. Ann. Int. Med., *36*:1498, 1952.
160. Schumacher, H. R., Jacobson, W. A., and Bemiller, C. R.: Treatment of infectious mononucleosis. Ann. Int. Med., *58*:217, 1963.
161. Seifert, M. H., Chandler, V. L., and Van Winkle, W.: Aureomycin in infectious mononucleosis. J.A.M.A., *142*:1133, 1950.
162. Shubert, S., Collee, J. G., and Smith, B. J.: Infectious mononucleosis: A syndrome or a disease? Brit. Med. J., *1*:671, 1954.
163. Smith, E. B., and Custer, R. P.: Rupture of the spleen in infectious mononucleosis. A clinicopathologic report of seven cases. Blood, *1*:317, 1946.
164. Smith, J. N., Jr.: Complications of infectious mononucleosis. Ann. Int. Med., *44*:861, 1956.
165. Southam, C. M., Goldsmith, Y., and Burchenal, J. H.: Heterophile antibodies and antigens in neoplastic diseases. Cancer, *4*:1036, 1951.
166. Sprunt, T. P., and Evans, F. A.: Mononuclear leukocytosis in reaction to acute infections (infectious mononucleosis). Bull. Johns Hopkins Hosp., *31*:410, 1920.
167. Stevens, J. E.: Infectious mononucleosis: a clinical analysis of 210 sporadic cases. Virginia M. Month., *79*:74, 1952.
168. Templeton, H. J., and Sutherland, R. T.: The exanthem of acute mononucleosis. J.A.M.A., *113*:1215, 1939.
169. Thurm, R. H., and Bassen, F.: Infectious mononucleosis and acute hemolytic anemia. Blood, *10*:841, 1955.
170. Tidy, H. L.: Glandular fever and infectious mononucleosis. Lancet, *2*:180, 236, 1934.
171. Tidy, H. L., and Daniel, E. C.: Glandular fever and infectious mononucleosis with an account of an epidemic. Lancet, *2*:9, 1923.
172. Tidy, H. L., and Morley, E. B.: Glandular fever. Brit. Med. J., *1*:452, 1921.
173. Walker, S. H.: The failure of antibiotic therapy in infectious mononucleosis. Am. J. Med. Sci., *226*:65, 1953.
174. Waterhouse, B. E., and Lapidus, P. H.: Infectious mononucleosis associated with a mass in the anterior mediastinum. New England J. Med., *227*:1137, 1967.
175. Wechsler, H. F., Rosenblum, A. H., and Sills, C. T.: Infectious mononucleosis: Report of an epidemic in an army post. Ann. Int. Med., *25*:113, 1946.

XIII / Leukemia

HISTORICAL ASPECTS

In 1845 Bennett,[4] Craigie,[23] and Virchow[141] independently reported patients with undoubted leukemia. Bennett and Craigie attributed the remarkable numbers of white blood cells to the presence of "purulent matter in the blood." In 1846 Virchow, who introduced the term "leukemia," did not agree that the changes in the blood were the result of the invasion of the blood stream by a suppurative process and considered that the hematologic changes were part of a definite pathologic process that involved certain organs in the body. The conflicting claims regarding the priority of discovery of leukemia were reviewed by Osler,[101] who concluded that Virchow deserves priority because he was the first to realize that the increase in white blood cells was an essential feature of the disease to which he gave the name "leukemia." Two forms of leukemia were recognized by Virchow. In one the small forms of white cells predominated and enlargement of the lymph nodes was common; in the second, the large white cells were increased in number and marked splenomegaly occurred. Acute leukemia was first described by Friedrich in 1857,[27, 41] and in 1913 the first case of monocytic leukemia was reported by Reschad and Schilling-Torgau.[111]

CLASSIFICATION

A classification of leukemia and related neoplastic disorders which contains some features of Lukes' classification[81a] and that of Dameshek and Gunz[29] is given in Table 13–1.

Table 13–1. Classification of Leukemia and Related Neoplastic Disorders

Leukemia (Type)	Tumor
1. (a) Granulocytic (myelocytic), acute or chronic	Chloroma (myeloblastoma)
(b) Eosinophilic	
(c) Basophilic	
(d) Myelo-monocytic (Naegeli type)	
2. Lymphocytic, chronic	Lymphosarcoma, well differentiated (small cell)
3. Lymphosarcoma cell	Lymphosarcoma, poorly differentiated
4. Lymphoblastic, acute (stem cell)	Lymphoma, stem cell
5. (a) Monocytic (Schilling type), acute (bone marrow origin?)	Reticulum cell sarcoma? (lymphoma, histiocytic)
(b) Histiocytic (leukemic reticuloendotheliosis) (peripheral origin?)	Reticulum cell sarcoma (lymphoma, histiocytic)
6. Plasma cell	Plasmacytoma, multiple myeloma

THE INCIDENCE OF LEUKEMIA

It is reported that in the last 50 years there has been a threefold to sixfold increase in leukemia, the greatest increase that has occurred in any disease except coronary thrombosis and carcinoma.[72] In England and Wales the incidence of leukemia has increased from 1.7 per 100,000 in 1900 to 5 per 100,000 in 1955;[123] in the United States comparable studies indicate an increase from 1 per 100,000 in 1900 to 6.3 per 100,000 in 1952. Such factors as improved diagnosis, more frequent hospitalization, improved treatment, and the increased number of older persons in the general population do not explain the apparent increase.[21, 58] In the period 1943 to 1952 the incidence of leukemia in males was 7.3 per 100,000 and that for females was 5.77 per 100,000.[47, 82, 114] Gunz has concluded that the leukemia death rate has increased steadily for some years, particularly in the western countries. In the last few decades the rise has been almost entirely in the group over 50 and the only consistent increase in the last 20 years has been in those above 65 years of age; in the last 15 years the rate in children in New Zealand has been declining. In New Zealand the death rate for those 75 years of age and older in the period 1946 to 1950 was 20 per 100,000 and in the period 1961 to 1965 it was 60 per 100,000. In the group over 74 years of age in the United States the mortality rate increased from 15 to 50 per 100,000 between 1940 and 1960; during the same period in those aged 65 to 74 the mortality rate increased from 12 to 25 per 100,000. Little change occurred in persons less than 64 years of age.[54] The disease is more common in Jews than in non-Jews and is less common in blacks than in whites.[83] The incidence in whites and blacks is about the same if the Jewish population is excluded.

Approximately 60 per cent of patients with leukemia have the chronic form of the disease, which occurs more commonly after middle age. Chronic lymphocytic leukemia is slightly more common than chronic granulocytic leukemia.[79] Eosinophilic leukemia is very rare and in some of the reported patients the diagnosis has been questioned;[135] it is probably one type of granulocytic leukemia. Basophilic cell leukemia and mast cell leukemia are even rarer, but have been reported.[29] A recent review of the literature yielded reports of 57 patients considered to have plasma cell leukemia.[106] Acute leukemia occurs most commonly in children and young adults, but an increasing incidence in older persons has been reported.[21, 58]

Etiology and Pathogenesis

In 1894 Osler wrote of leukemia, "Notwithstanding most careful clinical study and thorough histological and bacteriological investigation, the secret of the causative factor of this disease is as profound as it was half a century ago."[101] Although the cause of leukemia is unknown, there is considerable evidence to support the view that leukemia is a neoplasm.[29, 44, 72] The essential alteration is thought to reside in the leukemic cell and be responsible for the failure of the cell to respond to the forces which ordinarily control its reproduction and maturation. The autonomous uncontrolled behavior of these cells appears to be responsible for the clinical manifestations and course of the disease. Whether a single factor or multiple factors are responsible for the essential alteration of the cell is unknown. Because of ignorance on this point the question arises whether or not all of the clinically recognized forms of acute and chronic leukemia are the same disease. Different types of leukemia differ considerably in age distribution, clinical manifestations, survival time, and response to various types of therapy; these differences could be explained by a varied host response as well as by multiple causative factors.

Although our knowledge of many essentials of the leukemic process remains inadequate, a considerable body of information has accumulated relative to the production of leukemia by external agents and the genetic predisposition to leukemia. Much of this evidence has been derived from the study of laboratory animals, but important deductions have also been drawn from consideration of the occurrence of the disease in man.

Miller thinks that the epidemiologic studies have failed to show that leukemia spreads in a manner which suggests infection. He has identified five high risk groups, those in whom the risk of developing leukemia within 10 to 15 years is greater than 1 in 100. These groups are: (1) identical twins of children with leukemia, 1 in 5; (2) patients with radiation-treated polycythemia vera, 1 in 6; (3) those with Bloom's syndrome and Fanconi's aplastic anemia, 1 in 8 up to 26 years old; (4) atomic bomb survivors within 1000 meters of the hypocenter (Hiroshima and Nagasaki), 1 in 6; and (5) children with Down's syndrome, 1 in 95 under 10 years of age.[88]

Ionizing Radiation

Evidence from a number of sources indicates that ionizing radiation can be a leukemogenic agent in man as well as in mice. The incidence of leukemia in physicians is twice that of the general population. In 1950 the incidence in radiologists was reported to be from eight to nine times that in physicians in general; a decade later the incidence was reported as 3.05 per cent in radiologists and 0.51 per cent in physicians who were not radiologists.[85] An increased incidence of chronic myelocytic and acute lymphoblastic leukemia in survivors of atomic bombings in a frequency directly related to the severity of the exposure to radiation appears to be well established.[39, 76, 94] The peak incidence occurred between 4 and 8 years after the irradiation and the first cases were seen as early as 1 to 2 years after exposure.[139] The therapeutic use of x-ray for spondylitis in adults[22] and for thymic enlargement in children[129] has been reported to be responsible for leukemia. In British spondylitic patients the peak occurred 4 to 5 years after radiation, but the incidence remained elevated up to 15 years; in children exposed to radiation before birth, the increased incidence reached its peak between the third and fifth years of life and was not increased after the age of 7. It is suspected that the incidence of leukemia, particularly acute leukemia, is higher in patients with polycythemia vera who have been treated with x-ray or radioactive phosphorus than in those treated by other means.[91, 120] Even the use of diagnostic x-ray during pregnancy has been suspected as a factor in the development of leukemia in childhood.[55, 133] Myelogenous leukemia, acute or chronic, is the type of leukemia usually induced in man by radiation.

DRUGS

The evidence that exposure to benzol (benzene) may produce leukemia is circumstantial, but a number of suspicious instances have been reported.[67, 179a] The individual response to this chemical appears to vary and both the concentration and length of exposure are probably important. The incidence of leukemia in patients with aplastic anemia may be increased, but a leukemogenic action of the drugs involved has not been proved,[20a, 42a] leukemia may develop if an abnormal clone of cells develops in a hypoplastic marrow. The development of acute myelomonocytic leukemia after prolonged treatment with melphalan has been reported.[74a]

INFECTIONS

Severe infections of various types usher in some 50 per cent of the cases of acute leukemia in childhood.[72] Some authors have suspected infection may cause leukemia, but most workers have concluded that such infections occur as a consequence of the preexistent leukemia.[44] Although the chance that bacterial infection may be of etiologic significance seems remote, the possibility that leukemia is caused by a virus becomes increasingly strong.

Studies of the role of viruses in leukemia have been carried out largely in mice and fowl, and the relationship of the leukemia that occurs in these species to that of man is still uncertain.[119] Gross[51] has shown that leukemia may be transmitted to mice by the injection of a suspension of cells or cell-free extracts. He has suggested that a causative virus might be transmitted from parent to offspring and remain dormant for some time. Cell-free extracts of liver, spleen, or lymphatic tumors of AKR* mice have produced leukemia and epitheliomas when injected into newborn mice of the C_3H† strain less than 16 hours old.[52]

---

*AKR strain — mice having a high incidence of spontaneous leukemia.
†C_3H strain — mice having a low incidence of spontaneous leukemia.

This observation suggests a relationship between leukemia and other malignancy in mice, a relationship that is well recognized in man.[92, 140] Other reports have indicated that injections of cell-free extracts of brain from mice or human beings with leukemia cause the development of leukemia in a strain of mice not ordinarily susceptible to the disease.[116, 122] These and other studies demonstrate that leukemia can be produced in both mammals and fowl by the injection of cell-free filtrates.[84] Studies with mice indicate that leukemia and lymphomas can be induced by radiation and chemicals, including methylcholanthrene and urethan. The presence of murine leukemia virus (MuLV) in a majority of those developing active disease supported the concept that a latent leukemogenic virus had been activated, but did not exclude the possibility that it was only a passenger virus.[71]

Although human leukemia has not been proved to be caused by a viral infection, the similarity to animal leukemia and accumulating evidence of various kinds favor the possibility. Virus-like particles have been demonstrated in the plasma of patients with acute or chronic lymphocytic or myelocytic leukemia; these particles, which resemble the murine leukemia virus on electron microscopic examination, were not found in control plasmas,[19] but their morphology is not unique enough to call them a virus on the basis of ultrastructure alone.[27] Particles with the morphology of herpes virus rarely may be seen in the plasma pellets, and it is recognized that forms of virus exist which are difficult to distinguish from mycoplasma. An infectious etiology, probably a virus, is also suggested but not proved by reports of the occurrence of clusters of children with acute leukemia in small communities.[121] The repeated failures to culture a virus from leukemic tissues may be due to the state of the virus in the cells. Replication may be incomplete, the virus consisting of either RNA or DNA without the protein envelope; the cell remains viable and continues to be associated with genetic compound, viral genome.[35] ~~If a virus is the cause of human leukemia it probably remains dormant unless activated by radiation or some unknown factor in the host.~~ Viruses are known to cause leukemia in mice and chickens and probably cause the disease in cats, dogs, and cattle.[34] Studies of the disease in these species suggest that the disease complex is the same in all, and probably similar to that in man.

GENETIC CONSIDERATIONS

In certain highly inbred strains of mice, leukemia develops spontaneously in from 60 to 70 per cent of the animals. This suggests that genetic factors are important under conditions of controlled breeding and that man may be protected by his varied ancestry. Some constitutional susceptibility to leukemia in man was suggested by the studies of Videbaek[140] but later studies have not confirmed his conclusions.[53] Reports of the occurrence of several instances of leukemia in the same family suggest a genetic influence but are not conclusive because some unrecognized factor in the family environment may be responsible for the disease. Observations on the occurrence of leukemia in identical twins do not afford definite evidence of the existence of a hereditary factor in leukemia.[27] In the rare instances of congenital leukemia that have been reported the disease has not been demonstrated in the mother.[109] There has been a report of the occurrence of leukemia in a nine month old child born of a leukemic mother.[24] In all other reported instances of children born of leukemic mothers the offspring have remained free of the disease.[8]

In 1960 Nowell and Hungerford reported a chromosome abnormality in the peripheral blood of two patients with chronic myelocytic leukemia.[99, 100] This abnormality, subsequently termed Philadelphia chromosome, or Ph[1], is an unusually small chromosome thought to be formed from chromosome 21 by deletion or translocation. Subsequent studies have shown that it is present in the majority of the patients with chronic myelocytic leukemia; the relatively few patients without Ph[1] may form subclasses or variants of the disease. The incidence is higher in the marrow preparations than in cultures from the peripheral blood and the abnormality persists in the marrow after treatment. That the abnormality is not produced by the treatment of the leukemia has been shown by its presence in untreated patients. The importance of the Ph[1] chromosome is that it is the first demonstrated consistent chromosome change found in association with a particular neoplasm. The chromosome marker occurs in a majority of marrow cells, including hemoglobin-containing cells, which suggests the involved cell is a progenitor of both cell lines; the abnormality has not been found in cells obtained from lymph nodes.[69] The abnormality has not been found in skin of patients with myelocytic leukemia.[56]

The Philadelphia chromosome, which is found in from 90 to 95 per cent of patients with typical chronic myelocytic leukemia, is an acquired abnormality induced by radiation or some other mutagen; the myeloid progeny of such a stem cell acquire selective growth advantages over adjacent normal cells.[98] Patients with other myeloproliferative disorders and those with the so-called "preleukemic state" rarely have the Philadelphia chromosome. When patients with these disorders progress to a frank leukemic picture, it is often subacute or acute leukemia; although the leukemic cells may then show some abnormality the Philadelphia chromosome is not found. If a "preleukemic" patient has chromosome abnormalities associated with an abnormal cell clone in the marrow when an examination is made, the development of leukemia within a short time is more likely than it is in patients in whom no chromosome abnormality is detectable. Nevertheless, patients who have received radiation may develop abnormal clones of cells that do not progress to leukemia.

In acute leukemia many patients, perhaps 50 per cent, have no demonstrable chromosomal abnormality. In the others chromosomal abnormalities occur, particularly in children with acute lymphoblastic leukemia; the alterations differ from case to case and occur either in a single stem line or in a small number of them. In one instance a Philadelphia chromosome has been found.[105a] The reported association of chronic lymphocytic leukemia with abnormalities in the twenty-first chromosome appears to be a coincidence.[98] Because of the failure to find chromosome changes in some patients with known leukemia, leukemia must be considered in the diagnosis of patients in whom no chromosomal abnormality can be demonstrated.

Chromosomal abnormalities are not consistent in forms of leukemia other than chronic myelogenous. Numerous abnormalities in chromosomal number and structure have been observed in children with acute leukemia. The abnormalities, which have a very high incidence, vary from case to case, but once established in an individual patient they apparently persist.[56] Mongolism is associated with trisomy chromosome number 21 and has an incidence of leukemia 20 times that of the general population.[56]

Gunz and Fitzgerald point out that whatever relationship to the cause of leukemia the changes in the chromosomes are shown to have, the study of the disease by cytogenetic techniques promises to provide a better understanding of both the nature and the treatment of leukemia.[56]

The occurrence of chronic granulocytic leukemia in more than one member of the same family is extremely rare. The great majority of instances of familial leukemia have been of the chronic lymphocytic variety, but not more than 100 of these have been reported.[29] Leukemia has been reported in identical twins 15 times and in non-identical twins three times; in some (but not all) the leukemia appeared to be of the same variety; the development of the leukemia has occurred in the second child within 18 months. The finding of the Philadelphia chromosome in one of identical twins who had leukemia and the failure to find the abnormal chromosome or leukemia in the identical twin, in one instance for as long as 7½ years after the first examination, is further evidence that the chromosomal change is an acquired abnormality.[49]

OTHER FACTORS

It has been suggested that leukemia is the result of an imbalance in the hematopoietic equilibrium. This concept was suggested by the identification of two chemicals, myelokentic acid and lymphokentric acid, in the urine of patients with leukemia or lymphoma.[87] The same materials have been obtained from the sera of patients with these diseases. It is reported that myelokentric acid produces hyperplasia of myeloid elements and lymphokentric acid produces hyperplasia of the lymphoid elements when injected into the guinea pig. It has been suggested that an imbalance in the production of these "humoral hormones" causes leukemia but the evidence is not convincing.

The production of leukemia by the injection of cell-free chromatin particles and microsomal fragments into mice has been reported.[132] It has been suggested that the chromatin particles enter normal cells and alter their function in some undefined manner. The significance of the reported transfer of the neoplastic character of a cell in this manner cannot be determined until further studies that utilize genetic markers are carried out.[77]

The increased cell counts seen in leukemia have been interpreted as a failure of normal elimination of the leukocytes rather than an overproduction of these cells.[9] It has been shown that the lungs, liver, and gastrointestinal tract daily remove large numbers of cells from the circulation. Cross-circulation experiments have demonstrated that the rate of removal of cells from the circulation is decreased in patients with leukemia as compared to the normal. The relationship of this defect to the pathogenesis of leukemia is not established.

There is yet insufficient evidence to support more than speculation about the nature and cause of human leukemia. Nevertheless, the evidence becomes increasingly strong that a virus or virus-like agent may cause altered metabolic activities and behavior in the host cell. Genetically determined host resistance must be of great importance and might well be influenced by ionizing radiation and chemical agents, which would account for the demonstrated role of these factors in leukemia.

Acute Leukemia

All types of acute leukemia, myeloblastic, lymphoblastic, and monoblastic, are much more severe diseases than any of the chronic leukemias. The illness may begin as acute leukemia or the acute form may develop as the terminal event in a patient who has had the chronic form of the disease for months or years. The presence of acute leukemia is characterized by the occurrence of appreciable numbers of young cells, particularly the blast forms, in the circulating blood and bone marrow. The different types of acute leukemia cannot be distinguished from one another with certainty on clinical grounds alone, and, because of the extreme immaturity of the cells, it may be difficult to identify the cell type even after careful hematologic study. Myeloblastic and monoblastic leukemia are rare in children, and lymphoblastic leukemia is uncommon after the age of 30. In one series of 226 patients over 14 years of age with acute leukemia, 11.5 per cent had lymphoblastic leukemia; in those over 30 years of age the incidence was 8.0 per cent.[7] Other authors report that the myeloblastic type is fairly evenly divided among the different age groups; it is generally agreed that the monocytic type occurs most often in the middle and older age groups.[46, 58, 123] All types of acute leukemia are more common in males.

Clinical Manifestations

The clinical characteristics of acute leukemia vary from case to case and depend mainly on the organ systems involved in the disease. The clinical manifestations in patients who have acute leukemia from the onset differ from those that are seen in patients who undergo a transformation from the chronic to the acute form of the disease.

In most children and young adults the disease is acute from the onset but the initial symptoms may give no hint of the seriousness of the underlying disease. In children especially, the onset may be characterized by the development of listlessness, fretfulness, poor appetite, and pallor. In some, aching and pains in the extremities lead to an initial diagnosis of rheumatic fever. In others pain from a pathologic fracture, particularly of a vertebra, may be the initial manifestation. The onset of the disease often resembles that of an acute respiratory infection with fever, malaise, fatigue, and sore throat, or may mimic a severe infection with high fever, headache, sweats, and severe prostration. Such episodes often occur as a result of infections that develop because of the lowered resistance of these patients, but also occur in the absence of demonstrable infection. Abnormal bleeding, such as epistaxis, bleeding gums, ecchymoses, or petechiae, occurs some time in the course of the illness in nearly all patients with acute leukemia and may be present from the onset. A severe hemorrhagic disorder associated with increased intravascular clotting and/or fibrinolytic activity occurs in some patients of acute leukemia, particularly those in whom the promyelocyte is the predominating cell.

The transformation of a chronic leukemia into the acute variety is seen most often in adults with chronic myelocytic leukemia. The change is usually accompanied by increasing weight loss, fever, progressive anemia, and the appearance of a hemorrhagic tendency. A change in type is recognized by a change in the morphology of the peripheral blood and bone marrow that consists of increased numbers of the more immature cells, myeloblasts or promyelocytes. The hematologic changes may be noted in some patients before the changes in the clinical course are apparent.

Hemorrhage or leukocytic infiltrations in the brain and other parts of the central nervous system occur frequently. The incidence of objective signs of neurologic involvement (other than retinal changes) was reported to be 20 per cent in one series of 334 cases.[117] In another series of 163 patients with leukemia of all types the incidence of central nervous system involvement was 35 per cent.[105] Lesions occurred most often in acute myeloblastic leukemia, where intracranial hemorrhage was the commonest manifestation; the frequency of bleeding appeared to be related more to an elevated leukocyte count (over 50,000 per cu.mm.), than to thrombocytopenia (less than 50,000 per cu.mm.). In another series of 117 patients with acute leukemia, intracerebral hemorrhage was not seen in patients whose preterminal leukocyte counts were less than 100,000 per cu.mm., but the occurrence of subarachnoid hemorrhage appeared to be related to thrombocytopenia.[95] Meningeal infiltration was seen oftenest in lymphocytic leukemia, especially in males less than 20 years of age. Meningeal leukemia is often associated with dilatation of the ventricles; significant arachnoid involvement is usually associated with increases in the cerebrospinal fluid pressure, cell count, and protein. Spinal epidural leukemia, which has been reported in only about 43 patients, also occurs most often in young persons with acute leukemia; in two-thirds it was the initial symptom. Involvement of the central nervous system is reported to occur in 26 per cent of children with acute and subacute leukemia of all types.[70] This complication is usually manifested by vomiting, headache, and other signs of increased intracranial pressure, but it may occur associated with a normal cerebrospinal fluid examination; the complication may develop when the disease is apparently under good control. Convulsions, sensory disturbances, papilledema, cranial nerve palsies, and signs of pyramidal tract involvement are not uncommon. Infiltration in other organs such as the bladder and kidney may produce pain and hematuria.

Severe pain may develop about the joints and in the extremities as a result of involvement of the synovial membranes or as a result of subperiosteal infiltration or hemorrhage. Bleeding from the gastrointestinal tract occurs frequently and may be severe.

Physical examination generally reveals marked pallor of the skin and mucous membranes. Petechial hemorrhages and ecchymoses of different sizes occur commonly in all parts of the skin and mucous membranes. Leukemic infiltration of the skin, which has a characteristic purplish color, occurs occasionally but is less common than in chronic leukemia. Not infrequently the gums appear hypertrophic, swollen, and ulcerated, a finding that occurs more often in monocytic leukemia than in the other types. The gums bleed easily when touched and continued spontaneous oozing develops in many patients. Retinal hemorrhages are often present.

A soft spleen edge is usually but not invariably palpable a few centimeters below the left costal margin. Splenomegaly occurs less often in adults than in children with acute leukemia. In adults the observation that the spleen edge is very firm and extends as far down as the umbilicus suggests that the patient has had a chronic leukemia before the onset of the acute phase. In acute leukemia, enlargement of the liver is inconstant, and hepatic tenderness is unusual. Mild or moderate (0.5 to 1.5 cm.) enlargement of the superficial lymph nodes is usually present but the enlargement may be so slight as to escape detection. In children the node enlargement may become massive, particularly in the thorax. Tenderness on light pressure over the bones, particularly the lower portion of the sternum, is commonly demonstrable in acute leukemia.

Chloromas, tumors that consist of masses of myeloblasts, occur most often in children and young adults.[112] They usually involve the bones of the face and cranium, particularly the orbit. The tumors have a characteristic green color that fades rapidly on exposure to air. Hyposulfite and hydrogen peroxide restore the green color.

Laboratory Manifestations

Anemia, which may result from blood loss, decreased blood production, increased hemolysis, or a combination of these factors, occurs in almost every patient with acute leukemia. The anemia is often severe and hemoglobin levels as low as 2 to 3 gm. per 100 ml. are sometimes seen. The erythrocyte count and hematocrit are reduced proportionally and the anemia is generally of the normocytic, normochromic variety.

The most important abnormality in acute leukemia involves the leukocytes. The total leukocyte count varies from subnormal levels of a few hundred to several hundred thousand per cu.mm. Characteristically very immature cells occur in significant numbers. Often in smears prepared with Wright's stain the identity of the young cells can only be surmised by a positive identification of the older cells that are seen. The use of the peroxidase stain is often helpful since the finding of peroxidase positive granules in the young cells indicates a myelogenous or monocytic origin of the cell. The presence of Auer bodies also places the young cells in the myelocytic or monocytic series. On occasions only very immature atypical blast cells are found and the type of leukemia cannot be identified with assurance; such cases are often classified as "stem cell" leukemia. When the total leukocyte count is low the examination of smears made from a concentrate of the leukocytic fraction after centrifugation of the peripheral blood is often useful in demonstrating the presence of immature cells. Study of the peripheral blood in this manner often makes it possible to distinguish between leukemia and aplastic anemia and is also helpful in identifying the type

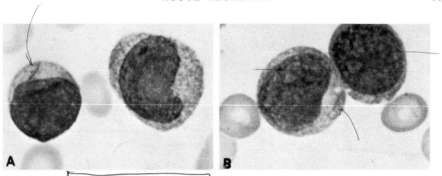

Figure 13–1. Blast cells with Auer bodies. *A*, Monoblasts from patient with acute monocytic leukemia. *B*, Myeloblasts from patient with acute myeloblastic leukemia. (F.S.: II, 59, 64.)

of leukemia. Numerous nucleated red cells are seen commonly in the peripheral blood in all types of acute leukemia.

Thrombocytopenia occurs sooner or later in nearly all types of acute leukemia. Usually the platelets are markedly reduced or absent when the patient is first seen.

Examination of the bone marrow generally reveals infiltration by the immature leukemic cells that are responsible for the disease. In all types of leukemia there is nearly always involvement of the bone marrow, which may be filled with the abnormal cells at a time when there is but little or equivocal evidence of the disease in the peripheral blood.

Diagnosis

The diagnosis of acute leukemia is generally made without difficulty when there is a marked increase in the immature leukocytes in the peripheral blood and bone marrow associated with anemia and thrombocytopenia. On occasion acute leukemia must be distinguished from infectious mononucleosis. The absence of anemia and thrombocytopenia, the absence of blast cells in the peripheral blood, the varied morphologic appearance of the cells in the peripheral blood, the failure to find evidence of significant marrow involvement, and the positive reaction with the heterophil agglutination test usually serve to distinguish infectious mononucleosis without much difficulty (see Fig. 12–5). Aplastic anemia offers more difficulty because anemia, leukopenia, and thrombocytopenia, fever, and abnormal bleeding may occur in both diseases. The presence of lymphadenopathy, splenomegaly, the appearance of the bone marrow, and the study of the smear of the peripheral blood made from a concentrate of the leukocytes nearly always enable one to make the correct diagnosis, but occasionally a period of observation is necessary before this can be done.

Leukemoid reactions in infections usually cause no difficulty because the proportion of very immature cells in leukemia is generally out of all proportion to that seen in severe infections, where there is a more orderly increase in the intermediate and immature forms. Disseminated tuberculosis is an exception; a leukemoid reaction, usually of the myeloblastic type, sometimes develops and so mimics leukemia that the true nature of the primary disease may be discovered only at autopsy.[138] Similar leukemoid reactions have been reported in patients with disseminated histoplasmosis.[11] On occasion, the presence of immature granulocytes and nucleated red cells in the peripheral blood may lead to an initial impression of leukemia in a patient who has metastatic bone marrow involvement; further examinations, including a study of the bone marrow, nearly always reveal the correct diagnosis.

Clinical Course

Acute leukemia probably is a uniformly fatal disease and it usually runs a short course. Before the widespread use of transfusions, antibiotics, and chemotherapeutic agents, the survival time was from 6 days to 6 weeks. The use of corticosteroid hormones, 6-MP, amethopterin, and other drugs has resulted in significant improvement in the outlook for patients with lymphoblastic leukemia, but unfortunately these preparations are relatively ineffective in other types of acute leukemia. The prognosis is worse in children under 1 year of age, and better in those with low or normal leukocyte counts. Other factors, such as the duration of disease before treatment, the condition of the patient, or the initial appearance of the bone marrow, are not related to prognosis. In adults the prognosis has not improved greatly with the newer methods of treatment;[30] patients with the unusual lymphoblastic leukemia often survive more than a year, but those with the other types seldom have a remission that lasts more than 3 or 4 months and rarely live as long as a year. An increasing number of children have survived, some free of evidence of disease, for more than 1 year, some for more than 5 years. Complete bone marrow remission often is accompanied by persistence of the leukemia in the kidney, liver, and other organs.[97]

Treatment

The treatment of acute leukemia involves the use of both supportive measures and specific therapy. Included in the former are the use of blood transfusions for the anemia, fresh blood and platelet concentrates for thrombocytopenia and bleeding, antibiotics for associated infection, and analgesics for pain. Among the most important supportive measures is the attitude of the physician toward the patient and his family. The "human interest" stories in the press have made leukemia a tragic story known to nearly all. The physician's support of members of the family, his sympathetic understanding of their anxieties, and his willingness to take the time to talk with them contribute greatly to their comfort. It is important that the parents of children with leukemia be urged to treat them during periods of remission as they would a normal child. The children should be allowed to return to school and play and normal discipline should be enforced. In this way the overall emotional impact of the disease on the family may be reduced.

In recent years, numerous drugs and combinations of drugs have been used in the treatment of leukemia. Many combinations are under investigation by the various leukemia study groups which have employed a variety of protocols. In such a situation, what is considered the best or even acceptable treatment may vary from one year to the next. Nevertheless, such change and investigation are necessary in a disease such as acute leukemia whose treatment leaves so much to be desired even though definite progress has been made. The progress that has been made is almost entirely confined to children with acute lymphoblastic leukemia. The results of treatment in adults with acute myeloblastic leukemia have been so poor that recently in the American literature there was a short debate about the advisability of treating most adults with acute myeloblastic leukemia with any form of chemotherapy.

Crosby questioned whether all patients with acute myeloblastic treatment (AML) should be treated with the toxic drugs that are employed.[25] He identified six types of AML which he considered to be refractory to treatment: (1) blast crisis, (2) smoldering leukemia, (3) AML with megaloblastosis, (4) myelomonocytic leukemia, (5) promyelocytic leukemia, and (6) AML in the elderly (those over 50). He thought that patients in these groups differ from children and younger adults with the disease, 25 per cent of whom may have a remission with chemotherapy. He suggested that if the physician feels he must treat patients in one of the other groups, milder measures are probably better than aggressive therapy. Boggs and colleagues reported in rebuttal that in their experience in treatment of 146 patients with AML, 33 per cent had remissions which lasted from 2 to 18 months (mean of 8 months) with 6-MP, given in doses of 2.5 mg. per kg. per day for 6 to 8 weeks.[15] They found that the various cell types responded equally well; only in those over 60 was the response poorer than in the group as a whole, and of 24 patients over 60, 18 per cent of those treated 6 weeks or more had a partial or complete remission. Daunorubicine given 1.0 mg. per kg. per day for 5 days has induced complete and partial remission in some adults with acute myeloblastic leukemia.[16] Because of the toxicity of the drug, other agents were used for maintenance therapy.

Although the outlook for adults with acute myeloblastic leukemia remains dismal, prolonged remissions, from 2½ to 9½ years, have been reported. Although the remission rate in patients over 60 years of age is low, the median survival time (5.8 months) and the percentage of patients surviving over 1 year (20 per cent) were little different than those in younger patients.[37]

Prednisone, methotrexate, 6-MP, cyclophosphamide, vincristine and cytosine arabinoside are the drugs used most often in treatment. L-asparaginase and daunorubicin are being tested but have not yet been approved by the F.D.A.

Currently, we are treating most adults with acute myeloblastic leukemia with cytosine arabinoside by the following protocol, which is being evaluated by the Southwest Cancer Chemotherapy Study Group: Intravenous infusions are given at 14-day intervals, either (1) a 48-hour infusion of 400 mg. per M^2 in 24 hours given twice, or (2) a 120-hour infusion of 200 mg. per M^2 in 24 hours, given five times. If the marrow examination prior to the second course is hypocellular and the number of leukemic cells is reduced, the dose of cytosine arabinoside is reduced by 25 per cent. If the marrow cellularity is normal and the leukemic cells reduced, the initial dose is repeated. The dose may be increased if the disease fails to respond. The remission rate may be 25 per cent.

If there is a complete remission (normocellular marrow with less than 10 per cent myeloblasts and promyelocytes, platelets 100,000 per cu.mm. or more, and a circulating granulocyte count of 1500 per cu.mm. or more), maintenance courses (one-half the last induction dose) are given at 14-day intervals three times, then at 21-day intervals three times, and then at 28-day intervals three times. The interval between courses is increased gradually if the patient remains in remission.

The prognosis in children with acute leukemia is not as melancholy as that in adults, but the disease continues to be a most serious one with a grave outlook. Acute leukemia in children treated by induction of remission of prednisone and 6-MP followed by cyclic therapy, alternating 6-MP and methotrexate, produced the following survival rates in "stem cell leukemia": 1 year, 75 per cent; 2 years, 40 per cent; 3 years, 20 per cent; 4 years, 10 per cent; and 5 years, 4 per cent.[145] Zuelzer, who has had considerable experience with cyclic therapy, recommends treatment for induction with a combination of 6-MP and prednisone, followed by oral methotrexate twice a week for maintenance. (F.S.:II, 51.)

Complete remission rates of 96 per cent in newly diagnosed children with acute lymphoblastic leukemia and in 84 per cent of those previously treated have been obtained by the use of vincristine and prednisone.[1] Vincristine was given in a dose of 2 mg. per M^2 per week I.V. and prednisone in a dose of 40 mg. per M^2 per day P.O. A complete remission was defined as 5 per cent or fewer blasts in the bone marrow, 40 per cent or fewer blasts plus lymphocytes in the bone marrow, normal values for all peripheral blood elements, and freedom from all clinical symptoms. Remissions lasted for a mean of 9 to 12 months when maintenance treatment with the methotrexate was given — 30 mg. per M^2 twice a week P.O. or I.M. Reinduction after relapse can often be accomplished with the drugs used initially or a new combination. (F.S.:II, 53.)

Central nervous system leukemia, which is not uncommon in children, is treated either by 1800 r to the skull or by intrathecal methotrexate. In one schedule patients were given methotrexate, 12 mg. per M^2 intrathecally each week for 2 weeks, then each month until evidence of involvement cleared.[1] Another schedule is: 0.2 mg. per kg. of body weight every other day for four doses; a second course to be given if abnormalities persist for more than a week after completion of treatment.[74] (F.S.:II, 56.)

Methotrexate, which is used in treating leukemia, malignant tumors, and some less serious diseases, is a folic acid antagonist. It may produce megaloblastic erythropoiesis and even severe marrow depression; continued therapy may produce severe disturbance in the mucous membrane of the gastrointestinal tract, with ulceration and diarrhea. Pneumonia, thought to be induced by allergy, has been attributed to the drug.[111a]

Combined therapy with daunomycin and prednisone produced a complete remission rate of 65 per cent and a partial remission rate of 15 per cent in 60 children with acute lymphoblastic leukemia who had already had one or more relapses.[131] The protocol which produced remission in 4 weeks was as follows: daunomycin was given 25 mg. per M^2 I.V. "push" q.i.d. for 3 days, then rest 4 days; repeat the weekly course twice, then administer the injection once a week; prednisone was given in a dose 60 mg. M^2 per day throughout. In the group of seven patients with acute myeloblastic leukemia, one had a complete remission and one had a partial remission.

Henderson has given a comprehensive report on the results obtained with various drugs in treating acute leukemia.[64] Prednisone produces a complete remission in approximately 75 per cent of children (median duration, $2\frac{1}{2}$ to 3 months) and 50 per cent of adults with acute lymphoblastic leukemia; in myeloblastic leukemia the remission rate in each group is less than 20 per cent. With vincristine the remission rate in children has been variously reported as from 15 to 57 per cent (median duration, 2 to 10 months) and in adults as from 0 to 40 per cent. The remission rate in children treated with methotrexate is from 20 to 30 per cent (median duration, 2 to 11 months). Purine antagonists, mainly 6-MP, have induced remissions in between 33 and 66 per cent of children with acute lymphoblastic leukemia (median duration, 2 to 5 months). With cyclophosphamide the results are similar. The remission rate in adults with acute myeloblastic leukemia appears to be less than 20 per cent when treated with 6-MP and between 25 and 50 per cent with cytosine arabinoside. When multiple drug combinations are used, the results are better, particularly in children.

Other measures are also important in the treatment of acute leukemia in adults or children. In various circumstances, blood transfusions, platelet concentrates and antibiotics are useful. In addition, allopurinol and a high fluid intake reduce the likelihood of urate nephropathy. For adults the dose is usually 300 to 600 mg. per day, divided into two or three doses; for children over six, the dose is 100 mg. t.i.d., and for those under six, 50 mg./t.i.d.

Illustrative Case

Case 1

This 44 year old surgeon reported that he was in his usual health until about 2 weeks prior to his visit when he first noted malaise and easy fatigue. Two or 3 days before his examination he noticed petechial lesions on the hands while he was scrubbing for an operation and this led him to seek medical advice.

Physical examination revealed no significant abnormality. The patient did not appear pale, had no significant lymphadenopathy, retinal hemorrhage, or hepatomegaly. Roentgenogram of the chest was normal.

Laboratory examination. Hematocrit was 36 per cent, erythrocyte count 3.7 mil. per cu.mm., hemoglobin 12.1 gm. per 100 ml., leukocyte count 67,500 per cu.mm. Study of the peripheral blood revealed that all of the leukocytes were blast cells; most of them gave a positive peroxidase reaction. Some cells were binucleated and others contained unusually large nucleoli. Examination of aspirated bone marrow revealed that the marrow was packed with early progranulocytes and myeloblasts. The platelets were markedly reduced, bleeding time was 8 minutes (normal 1 to 3 minutes), and the prothrombin time was 34 seconds (control of 15 seconds).

Course. The patient was made acquainted with his diagnosis of acute myeloblastic leukemia. He decided to postpone any treatment until he had put his affairs in order and returned home the same day.

On the following day he drew up his will, put his financial affairs in order, and arranged for the care of his patients. Twenty-four hours afterward, he became partially blind because of extensive bilateral retinal hemorrhages. He refused hospitalization and within a few hours massive gastrointestinal and intracranial bleeding occurred. On the following day, 4 days after the diagnosis was made and about 3 weeks after the onset of his first symptoms, the patient died.

Comment. The case illustrates the short fulminating course which acute leukemia sometimes takes with or without therapy in adults. The hematologic abnormalities—anemia, thrombocytopenia, and marked increase in leukocytes that consist nearly entirely of blast cells—are typical. Death in such patients is usually due to hemorrhage or septicemia.

Case 2

This 3 year old white girl was in excellent health until 2 months prior to her first visit in June, 1968, when increasing pallor, bruises, and fatigue were noticed. Two months before admission her family physician found her hemoglobin to be 10.7 gm. per 100 ml. and her leukocyte count 14,500 per cu.mm. with "a normal differential." She was treated with penicillin for tonsillitis, but weakness, pallor, and a tendency to bruise continued until admission.

Physical examination. Temperature, 102° F; pulse 108; height 39½ inches; and weight 34 pounds. Multiple 1 by 1 cm. nodes were palpated in the anterior and posterior cervical areas, both the axillary regions, and the inguinal areas. A systolic murmur was heard over the precordium. On inspiration the liver edge was felt 6 cm. below the right costal margin and the spleen 5 cm. below the left. The remainder of the examination was normal except that she was very pale.

Laboratory examination. Hemoglobin, 5.7 gm. per cent; hematocrit, 16.5 per cent; white count, 15,000 per cu.mm.; and platelets, 5000 per cu.mm. Reticulocytes were 0.2 per cent. Differential count: lymphoblasts, 39 per cent; lymphocytes, 55 per cent (many immature); and segmented cells, 6 per cent. Uric acid was 5.4 mg. per 100 ml.

Course. The patient was treated with platelet concentrates and packed red cells, after which bone marrow aspiration was performed. The cellularity was greatly increased and 95 per cent of the cells were considered to be lymphoblasts; megakaryocytes, myelocytes, erythroid cells, and myeloid cells were significantly diminished.

A diagnosis of acute lymphoblastic leukemia was made and following treatment given: prednisone, 10 mg. every 6 hours; 1.67 mg. of vincristine sulfate intravenously on June 7th and 14th; and allopurinal, 50 mg. three times a day.

On July 3rd the hemoglobin was 8.8 gm. per 100 ml.; hematocrit, 27 per cent; white count, 2400 per cu.mm.; platelets 400,000 per cu.mm.; and reticulocytes, 0.7 per cent; bone marrow examination disclosed remission in the leukemia. She received 1.4 mg. vincristine on July 3rd and July 11th; prednisone was stopped. On August 7th the splenomegaly and hematomegaly had disappeared. The hemoglobin was 11 gm. per 100 ml., hematocrit was 34 per cent, platelets were 470,000 per cu.mm., and white count was 3300 per cu.mm. Differential count showed segmented cells to be 63 per cent, lymphocytes 34 per cent, and monocytes 3 per cent.

The patient continued free of symptoms and with bone marrow remission until February 6, 1969, when slight cervical adenopathy reappeared, blasts became evident in the peripheral blood, and the bone marrow examination disclosed relapse with a large infiltration of lymphoblasts. She was again treated with 35 mg. of prednisone q.i.d. and 1.7 mg. of vincristine intravenously at weekly intervals. One month later she was asymptomatic except for developing alopecia; the peripheral blood was essentially normal except for mild anemia with leukopenia, but the bone marrow examination showed continued relapse with 13 per cent blasts. Vincristine at weekly intervals was continued and on March 30th the patient was asymptomatic and the bone marrow was in remission. Prednisone dosage was tapered, then discontinued, and she was given methotrexate 25 mg. per M^2 (17.5 mg.) twice a week.

The patient continued in clinical and hematological remission until August, when she developed diarrhea accompanied by moderate lymphadenopathy. The hematocrit was 38 per cent, hemoglobin 12.6 gm. per 100 ml., and white count 12,000 per cu.mm.; a bone marrow examination disclosed 35 per cent lymphoblasts. Because of the relapse, the patient was treated with daunomycin, 25 mg. per M^2 per day for 3 days, repeated after a 4-day interval, with vincristine, 1.5 mg. per M^2 per week for four doses, and with prednisone, 10 mg. four times a day for 28 days.

Between September, 1969, and January, 1971, relapses occurred with increasing frequency and became more resistant to all forms of therapy.

Comment. This child was diagnosed as having acute lymphoblastic leukemia 3 years ago. She has had numerous relapses, which have responded to different forms of treatment, but it appears likely that she has entered the terminal refractory stage.

Chronic Lymphocytic Leukemia

In 1924 Minot and Isaacs[90] presented data on 97 patients with chronic lymphocytic leukemia. They noted that the disorder occurred most commonly between 45 and 55 years of age, a decade later than the peak incidence of chronic myelogenous leukemia. The disease occurred in males more than three times as often as in women. Scott[124] in 1957 reviewed a series of 227 patients and found the greatest number of cases occurring between the ages of 60 and 70 years. He noted that there seemed to be a growing number of women with chronic lymphatic leukemia. In 1929[104] a small series revealed a male:female ratio of 4:1; in Scott's series the ratio was more nearly 2:1.

Clinical Manifestations

Chronic lymphocytic leukemia may make its appearance in a variety of ways. The onset is sometimes so insidious that the diagnosis is made before symptoms appear, when an individual undergoes a routine examination or consults his physician for some unrelated complaint. In such circumstances the usual manifestations are previously unrecognized enlargement of the superficial lymph nodes and a moderate increase in the leukocyte count, accompanied by an absolute increase in the small lymphocytes. Probably the most common complaint that leads the patient to seek medical advice is the accidental discovery of enlarged superficial nodes. Any group of nodes may be involved but enlargement of the cervical nodes is most often noted. At times the initial complaint is that of involvement of the lacrimal and salivary glands—Mikulicz's syndrome. Enlargement of the intra-abdominal lymph nodes produces gastrointestinal or abdominal complaints; involvement of the mediastinal nodes may result in cough, hoarseness, or dyspnea.

Abnormalities in the peripheral blood are responsible for the initial symptoms in some patients. If anemia is severe, easy fatigue, exertional dyspnea, and weakness occur. Thrombocytopenia may cause bleeding gums, easy bruising, petechiae, or gastrointestinal bleeding.

A variety of skin lesions occur in about 10 per cent of patients sometime during the course of the disease. Nonspecific lesions such as pruritus, areas of hyperpigmentation, macular and papular eruptions, exfoliative dermatitis, and herpes zoster occur without actual leukemic infiltration of the skin. Specific lesions, the result of actual infiltration of the skin by leukemic cells, are usually discrete and bright red or purple in color. These lesions, which vary greatly in

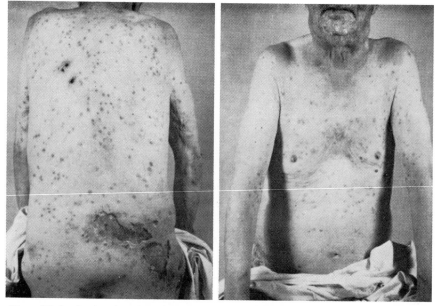

Figure 13–2. Leukemia cutis and herpes zoster in a patient with chronic lymphocytic leukemia.

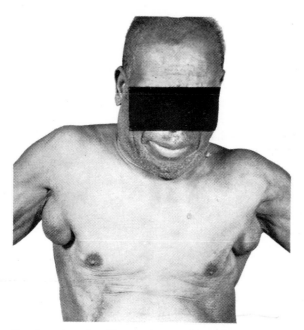

Figure 13–3. Greatly enlarged axillary and cervical lymph nodes in a patient with chronic lymphocytic leukemia.

number, usually measure a few millimeters in diameter. Generalized leukemic involvement of the skin—leukemia cutis universalis—generally produces intense itching. In some patients the disease assumes the form of mycosis fungoides.

Rarer manifestations of chronic lymphocytic leukemia are massive gastrointestinal hemorrhage, visual disturbances, and complaints referable to the skeletal system. Skeletal lesions, such as rarefaction of the bones, pathologic fracture and collapse of vertebrae with cord compression, occur in 5 per cent of the patients with this disease.[128]

On physical examination the most constant abnormality is enlargement of the superficial lymph nodes. In practically every patient some enlargement of at least a few of the superficial lymph nodes occurs. In most patients the individual nodes are moderately enlarged and measure from 2 to 3 cm. in diameter. The nodes are moderately firm, freely movable, and non-tender. Clusters of nodes may measure 10 cm. or more in diameter. Splenomegaly occurs in nearly all patients with chronic lymphocytic leukemia; usually the spleen is moderately firm and extends several centimeters below the left costal margin, but occasionally it fills the entire left side of the abdomen. Hepatomegaly is also an almost constant finding. Retinal hemorrhages may occur without other evidence of abnormal bleeding or in association with ecchymoses, petechiae, and bleeding from the mucous membranes. Leukemic infiltration of the tonsil occurs in a small percentage of the patients and can usually be recognized by its reddish purple color. The leukemic infiltrations of the skin are usually recognized by the reddish purple color and discrete nature of the lesions; if severe pruritus and excoriation are present, the underlying nature of the skin lesions may not be apparent.

Laboratory Manifestations

The most characteristic features of chronic lymphocytic leukemia are increases in the total leukocyte count and the absolute number of small lymphocytes. Severe leukopenia rarely occurs in chronic lymphocytic leukemia. The leukocyte count is nearly always above 15,000 per cu.mm. and often reaches levels of from 200,000 to 400,000 per cu.mm. The majority of the cells in the peripheral blood are small lymphocytes. These constitute 65 to 75 per cent of the cells in the early stage of the disease and usually amount to 95 to 98 per cent of the cells in the more advanced stages. A small number of larger lymphocytes occur at times but the presence of blast forms is unusual.

The amount of bone marrow involved by the leukemic process varies. Nearly always the lymphocytes constitute more than 40 per cent of the cells, and at times the marrow appears packed with them. (F.S.:II, 80–84.)

In some patients anemia is absent when the patient is first seen, but in nearly every patient it develops some time during the course of the disease. The anemia may be the result of leukemic infiltration of the bone marrow, hemorrhage, or hyperhemolysis. In some patients with splenomegaly, apparent anemia with a low hematocrit is in reality hemodilution; the total red cell mass is normal and the plasma volume increased. Unless there has been chronic blood loss the anemia is usually normocytic and normochromic in type. Severe anemia with the hemoglobin as low as 3 or 5 gm. per 100 ml. is sometimes seen, but more often the hemoglobin is above 7.5 gm. per 100 ml. If a hemolytic type of anemia is present it is usually associated with reticulocytosis, polychromatophilia, mild macrocytosis, and the presence of nucleated red cells in the peripheral blood. The degree of hyperhemolysis may be so mild that it is detectable only by cell survival studies, or it may be so severe that it threatens the life of the patient. In the latter situation it is usually of the auto-immune type and the Coombs test is positive. Circulating hemagglutinins are demonstrable in some patients.

Other abnormalities occur less commonly than the changes in the leukocytes and red cells. Among these is an elevation of the basal metabolic rate to plus 20 to 40 per cent, which occurs frequently when the leukemic process is active. A minority of patients with chronic lymphocytic leukemia show disturbances in the plasma protein that resemble those seen in patients with myeloma, an increase in the gamma G globulin fraction or cryoglobulins; others have hypogammaglobulinemia, which may be associated with an increased susceptibility to infection. Although the platelet count is usually normal in patients with chronic lymphocytic leukemia, not infrequently thrombocytopenia develops late in the disease.

Diagnosis

The diagnosis of chronic lymphocytic leukemia is made without difficulty in most patients because generalized lymphadenopathy, leukocytosis, and lymphocytosis are usually present. Not infrequently, chronic lymphocytic leukemia is diagnosed in an asymptomatic stage when the patient has a general examination or enters the hospital for some operation, such as herniorrhaphy. The total leukocyte count is often 10,000 to 12,000 per cu.mm.; from 50 to 70 per cent of the leukocytes in the peripheral blood are small lymphocytes. If a bone marrow is examined, an increased number of lymphocytes is found. At times it may be difficult to distinguish between lymphocytosis due to leukemia and that due to some other cause. Infectious mononucleosis is rare in persons over 40 years of age and lymphocytic leukemia is seen most frequently in older people. Abnormal-appearing lymphocytes of various sizes, particularly large cells, are characteristic of infectious mononucleosis, whereas in chronic lymphocytic leukemia the blood smear contains mainly small lymphocytes or smudge forms. The heterophil agglutination test, which is almost invariably negative in leukemia, is most helpful in younger patients. At times the differential diagnosis between lymphosarcoma and the early stage of chronic lymphocytic leukemia may be difficult. If lymphocytosis in the peripheral blood is inconstant and involvement of the bone marrow is not striking, lymphosarcoma should be suspected. The diseases cannot always be distinguished even after biopsy of a lymph node.

Many patients have clinical pictures that appear to be transitional between leukemia and lymphoma. One group of patients exemplifies the difficulty in distinguishing between the closely related disorders, lymphosarcoma, chronic lymphocytic leukemia, and lymphosarcoma cell leukemia. This problem may or may not be merely a matter of semantics. There are patients with splenomegaly and pancytopenia without lymphocytosis in the peripheral blood. Aspirate of the marrow often produces only a dilute, hypocellular specimen, whereas a biopsy reveals the marrow to be packed with mononuclear cells; most of the cells are small, but some are larger than small lymphocytes. Such patients may improve on corticosteroid treatment or after splenectomy; at operation there may or may not be evidence of disease in the intra-abdominal and retroperitoneal nodes. Whether one should classify the disorder in these patients as an atypical form of chronic lymphocytic leukemia, as lymphosarcoma largely confined to the spleen and bone marrow, or as lymphosarcoma cell leukemia is uncertain.

In lymphosarcoma cell leukemia, the cells are often large and have a reticulated nuclear chromatin, often a single nucleolus, and abundant cytoplasm. In one series of patients in which a distinction was made between chronic lymphocytic leukemia characterized by cells which resemble mature small lymphocytes and chronic lymphosarcoma leukemia characterized by the larger cells, approximately 60 per cent of a series of almost 500 patients were classified as having chronic lymphosarcoma cell leukemia.[143] There was striking similarity in the symptoms, physical abnormalities, and laboratory findings in the patients in the two groups, but the survival rate was higher in patients with chronic lymphocytic leukemia. Of the patients with chronic lymphocytic leukemia, 56 per cent survived 5 years and 31 per cent survived 10 years; of those with chronic lymphosarcoma leukemia, 40 per cent survived 5 years and 14 per cent survived 10 years.

The term "chronic reticulolymphocytic leukemia" has been proposed for the group of patients who have cells in the peripheral blood that are abnormal and that display features of both lymphocyte and reticulum cells on light microscopy.[113] Studies of such cells by special methods indicate that they probably are lymphoid in origin, although transitional forms between lymphocytes and reticulum cells cannot be excluded. The disorder, termed "leukemic reticuloendotheliosis" by some authors, is rare. It is characterized by a chronic course, splenomegaly, anemia, thrombocytopenia, and often leukopenia; its distinguishing feature is the presence in the circulating blood of large mononuclear cells which resemble lymphocytes but have cytoplasmic projections and spongy nuclear chromatin that suggest reticulum cells. Both small and large cells often have folded or indented nuclei. Several nucleoli are visible in some cells. Whether histiocytic leukemia is the same disorder is uncertain.

Clinical Course and Prognosis

The survival time in chronic lymphocytic leukemia as reported by different authors varies considerably. The median (50 per cent survival time) has ranged from 1.5 to 7.7 years as shown in Table 13–2. Although many factors, such as the dating of onset of disease, the selection of patients to be included, and the source of the material, may be partially responsible for the differences, the most favorable results have been obtained by those who used radioactive phosphorus. Five year survivals of 60 per cent and 10 year survivals of over 20 per cent have been reported. About 10 per cent reach the normal life expectancy.

Boggs and colleagues studied the factors influencing survival in 130 patients with chronic lymphocytic leukemia whom they saw between 1945 and 1964.[14] The median survival of the entire group was 6 years. The survival period was 9 years if those who died with other diseases were excluded; a 10

Table 13–2.   Survival in Chronic Lymphocytic Leukemia
(after onset of symptoms)

Author	Date	No. Of Pts.	Avg. Survival Time (Yrs.)	Median (Yrs.)	Treatment
1. Minot et al.[89]	1924	30	3.5		None
		50	3.5		X-ray
2. Leavell[79]	1938	49	3.6	3.0	X-ray
3. Wintrobe and Hasenbush[142]	1939	152	3.3		X-ray
4. Bethell[7]	1942	68	4.9		
5. Tivey[136]*	1954	685		2.8	
6. Osgood et al.[103]	1955	100		4.8	P[32]
7. Reinhard et al.[110]	1959	77†	3.5		P[32]
		25‡	6.5		
8. Feinleib and MacMahon[38]	1960	359		1.5	Various
9. Steinkamp et al.[134]	1963	119†	5.3	5.4	P[32]
		42‡	8.9		
10. Hill et al.[65]	1964	97		7.7	P[32]

*Series collected from literature
†Survival from diagnosis until death
‡Survival since diagnosis (patients living at time of report)

year life span from the time of onset of disease was suggested. Patients who had the poorer prognosis, a survival time of less than 5 years, manifested more clinical or laboratory evidence of disease at the time of diagnosis, were older, and were more likely to have symptoms; these features suggested that the disease probably had been present and asymptomatic for a longer period. Patients treated infrequently survived as long as did those treated regularly; this observation, and the known added hazards of bleeding and infection that follow treatment with radiation, cytotoxic drugs, and corticosteroids, led them to question whether leukemia-directed therapy prolonged survival. This study at least affords strong support for individualizing treatment in each patient.

Many patients with chronic lymphocytic leukemia lead practically normal lives over a course of many years and about one-third die of causes unrelated to leukemia. Generally, however, the disease progresses; the lymph nodes, liver, and spleen increase in size, and other manifestations of the disease, such as weakness, loss of weight, anemia, and bleeding, appear. The appearance of anemia and thrombocytopenia is associated with a relatively poor prognosis. A shortening of the length of remission after treatment, failure of the nodes to regress with therapy, the appearance of skin lesions, and the occurrence of serious bleeding are also signs of more rapid progression of the disease. Death is usually due to uncontrolled leukemia, hemorrhage, or infection, particularly pneumonia. The development of acute blastic transformation is much rarer in lymphocytic leukemia than in granulocytic leukemia, but it occurs occasionally.

The occurrence of auto-immune hemolytic anemia is a serious development. When the anemia is severe, weakness, palpitation, fatigue, and obvious jaundice may be present. Fortunately the hemolytic anemia usually responds to adrenocortical steroid therapy; unfortunately in some patients the auto-agglutination reaction is so strong that cross-matching with donors is extremely difficult or even impossible. This situation is even more hazardous if the patient needs an urgent operation. Whether or not this type of anemia occurs more frequently in patients treated with radiation therapy is uncertain. An incidence of 26 per cent was noted in one series.[102]

Patients with chronic lymphocytic leukemia appear to be more susceptible to bacterial infections, particularly pulmonary infection, than patients with chronic myelocytic leukemia are. The susceptibility to infection in lymphocytic leukemia is thought to be related to the poor response to antigenic stimuli that is manifested by patients with this disease, or it may be the result of hypogammaglobulinemia which favors bacterial infection, especially with *D. pneumoniae*, or of disordered delayed hypersensitivity reaction, which is associated with increased susceptibility to fungal or viral infections.

When patients with known chronic lymphocytic leukemia develop either gastrointestinal bleeding associated with a gastric lesion apparent on a roentgenographic study or a mass in some part of the body, the question arises whether the lesion is a leukemic tumor or some other form of neoplasm. Often only a biopsy will give the answer. We have seen a variety of neoplasms, including carcinoma of the breast, pancreas, colon, prostate, and lung in patients with leukemia. In six reports from the literature, which covered 1261 patients with chronic lymphocytic leukemia, a combined incidence of various sorts of malignancies of 8 per cent was found.[29]

Therapy

As in any serious disease which is incurable, the attitude of the physician is of great importance in the care of the patient. Continuing interest, periodic examinations that are unhurried, a certain amount of optimism regarding the course that the disease will follow in the patient, and a degree of enthusiasm for the treatment that is employed all help the patient to adjust to his disease.

Measures other than the "specific" therapeutic agents have contributed to the improvement in the treatment of leukemia in recent decades. Antibiotics for the treatment of infections and the greater use of transfusions for anemia have saved lives that would have been lost in other years. Adrenocortical steroids are valuable in the treatment of hemorrhagic manifestations or hemolytic anemia when these develop. Splenectomy is occasionally employed in the treatment of the hemolytic anemia and thrombocytopenia but the result is unpredictable and when good is often of short duration.

The most widely used forms of therapy at present are radiation, the alkylating agents, and adrenocortical steroids.

RADIATION THERAPY

Roentgen ray therapy has been used in chronic lymphocytic leukemia for many years. Therapy is most often directed to limited areas such as the spleen or lymph nodes because serious damage to the bone marrow may follow repeated spray irradiation. In chronic lymphocytic leukemia the sensitivity of the nodes to roentgen therapy varies greatly from patient to patient. In some patients the nodes regress promptly but in others they remain refractory despite large doses.

Radioactive phosphorus (P^{32}), which can be administered orally or intravenously, is considered by many to be the best form of radiation therapy.[65, 103, 110] From 20 or 25 per cent of the administered oral dose is lost in the feces and a comparable amount of the intravenous dose is excreted in the urine.[31] The recommended dose of radioactive phosphorus is 0.1 millicurie per kilogram of body weight, given in divided doses of 1 millicurie per day.[102] Excellent results have been reported from therapy of this type administered regularly even when the patient is asymptomatic.

Choice of Therapeutic Agents

In patients with chronic lymphocytic leukemia who are asymptomatic and who have only mild enlargement of the superficial lymph nodes accompanied by a mild leukocytosis and lymphocytosis, it is advisable to defer specific treatment until progression of the disease occurs. Some patients in this category survive 10, 20, or 30 years, or even longer, and lead entirely normal lives without treatment. More often the disease progresses and some form of therapy becomes necessary.

The selection of the treatment depends to some extent on the facilities available to the physician, the amount of contact that can be maintained with the patient, and the manifestations of the disease in each particular patient. Good results have been reported by those who have used radioactive phosphorus either as titrated, regularly spaced radiation aimed at keeping the patient in optimal condition[103] or at irregular intervals determined by a change in the patient's condition.[65] If one is using "irregular" treatment, weight loss, anemia, increasing size of nodes or spleen, fever, and night sweats are more reliable guides than the leukocyte count, which may fluctuate spontaneously or remain elevated for years without any accompanying evidence of progression of the disease. Roentgen ray irradiation is the most effective means available for reducing large localized tumor masses in any location, but in some patients with chronic lymphocytic leukemia, enlargement of the lymph nodes and massive splenomegaly seem to be totally resistant to radiation.

Chlorambucil is perhaps the easier treatment to give and is effective in the majority of patients, but the results obtained appear to be inferior to those obtained with radiation or a combination of chemotherapy and radiation.[63]

Chlorambucil, 2 to 8 mg. a day (usually 6 mg.), or cyclophosphamide, 100 to 200 mg. a day orally, is effective. Patients receiving cyclophosphamide appear to suffer less toxic effects on the platelets and megakaryocytes. Treatment with either chlorambucil or cyclophosphamide is usually given until a satisfactory response occurs; the drug is then discontinued until there is evidence of progression of the disease. Adrenocortical steroids are used only when complications are present or other agents are ineffective.

Relatively large doses of prednisone, from 60 to 100 mg. a day orally, often produce dramatic reduction in the size of the enlarged lymph nodes, a change which often is accompanied by a sharp increase in the leukocyte count of the peripheral blood, which may persist for a month or more. Some patients with chronic lymphocytic leukemia who are febrile and appear to be acutely ill will respond to massive doses of steroids when all other forms of treatment of the leukemia or presumed infection have failed. Because of the undesirable sequelae of steroid treatment, the dosage of the drug is reduced and the drug discontinued as soon as possible. Intermittent therapy, such as administration of the drug two or three days a week, may reduce the incidence of complication. Many patients with auto-immune hemolytic anemia can be maintained in remission with relatively small doses of prednisone, 2.5 to 5 mg. a day, and with this amount the likelihood of complications is much less than with large doses.

Illustrative Case

This 56 year old male real estate broker was in good health until January, 1948, when he consulted his physician because of the sudden onset of left upper quadrant pain which was made worse by inspiration or bending.

Physical examination revealed the patient to be well developed and nourished. Lymph nodes that measured 1 or 2 cm. in size were present in the left supraclavicular region, in both posterior cervical regions, and in both inguinal areas. A firm tender spleen edge extended 6 cm.

below the left costal margin. The liver was not palpable and the remainder of the physical examination was non-contributory.

Laboratory examination. Leukocyte count was 140,000 per
cu.mm.; practically all the cells were small lymphocytes; hemoglobin
13 gm. per 100 ml.; erythrocyte count 3.8 mil. per cu.mm.

Treatment and course. After the acute symptoms of splenic
infarction subsided, the patient was treated by conventional roentgen
ray therapy with 400 r to the splenic area. He improved promptly
and 2 months later the spleen was barely palpable and the leukocyte
count was 12,000 per cu.mm. On several occasions, while the patient
remained asymptomatic, the leukocyte count rose from 20,000 to
130,000 per cu.mm. and then returned to the lower level without treatment. In June, 1956, the spleen again increased in size until it extended to the level of the umbilicus. Following another course of
irradiation to the splenic area the spleen edge receded to the left
costal margin. In the next 3 years the leukocyte count varied between 16,000 and 20,000 per cu.mm. During the next five years the
patient had several exacerbations of his disease, but they responded
to treatment with chlorambucil, 6 mg. per day. He survived an attack
of pneumonia and had little difficulty with a hernia repair. He continued to lead an active life until he died suddenly following a cerebrovascular accident in 1964.

Comment. This case illustrates the commonly observed onset of
chronic lymphocytic leukemia in later years, and the relatively benign
course which the disorder follows in some patients. Over a period of
16 years radiation of the spleen and chlorambucil controlled his disease satisfactorily. Many patients with chronic lymphocytic leukemia
survive for the normal life span and die from causes other than
leukemia.

Chronic Granulocytic Leukemia

Incidence

Chronic granulocytic (myelocytic) leukemia is found in all races and in both
sexes and is primarily a disease of middle age. In 1924 Minot, Buckman, and
Isaacs[89] presented data on 130 patients with chronic myelogenous leukemia. In
this series the commonest age of onset was from 35 to 45 years. Fifty-six per cent
of the patients were males. In 1951 Shimkin, Mettier, and Bierman[127] reviewed
the incidence and distribution of chronic myelogenous leukemia, compared
their data with those of Minot, Buckman, and Isaacs, and noted an increased
incidence of the disease, particularly in women, and an increased age at onset.

Clinical Manifestations

The onset of chronic myelocytic leukemia is usually gradual; occasionally
its presence is discovered during a routine examination. The period between
the appearance of symptoms and the time the patient seeks medical advice is

usually from 8 to 9 months. The most common initial symptoms are the presence of discomfort in the left upper quadrant or the upper abdomen, or the accidental finding of a mass in this area. The patient often complains of a sensation of fullness and gaseous eructations after eating. Not infrequently signs of active disease such as loss of weight, fever, and night sweats are present. Usually the persistence and progression of these relatively mild symptoms lead the patient to seek medical advice.

Less often the disease begins more abruptly. Massive gastrointestinal hemorrhage manifested by either hematemesis or melena may be the first definite indication of disease. Other individuals seek medical advice because of aching in the back and extremities or because of a pleuritic type of pain in the left upper quadrant and lower portion of the left chest which radiates to the left shoulder, evidence of splenic infarction. The occurrence of hemorrhages or infiltrative lesions in the skin may be the first evidence of the disease. Visual disturbance from retinal hemorrhages is at times the initial complaint. In some patients, the initial symptoms are those of anemia—dyspnea on exertion, dizziness, palpitation, easy fatigue, and weakness.

Priapism develops in chronic myelocytic leukemia more often than it does in other types of leukemia, but fortunately it is very rare. In at least one child with this complication, radiation of the penile area was followed by prompt abatement of the priapism before the effect of busulfan was manifest.[50a] Fever from the leukemia per se is a late manifestation of the disease, and when it occurs it often continues until the death of the patient.

The most striking abnormality on physical examination is splenomegaly. Enlargement of the spleen is present in nearly all patients with chronic myelocytic leukemia at the time of the initial examination. In one series of patients the lower border of the spleen extended below the umbilicus at the time of the initial visit in 70 per cent.[125] As the disease progresses the splenomegaly responds less to treatment and sometimes steadily increases in size until it eventually fills the entire left half of the abdomen and occasionally the right lower abdomen as well. The sudden appearance of hernia or uterine prolapse has been noted in some patients with such massive splenomegaly. In most of the patients the splenomegaly is associated with considerable enlargement of the liver, which is usually firm and non-tender. Mild degrees of enlargement of the superficial lymph nodes may be seen in patients with chronic myelocytic leukemia but the enlargement does not reach the degree seen in patients with lymphocytic leukemia; frequently no significant lymphadenopathy is present. Retinal lesions such as engorgement of the veins and white-centered areas of hemorrhage are seen in a high percentage of the patients with chronic myelocytic leukemia. At times leukemic infiltration along the peripheral portion of the distended veins and blurring of the disc margin are present. The skin and mucous membranes are often pale and petechial lesions and ecchymoses are not unusual. Light or moderate pressure on the lower portion of the sternum produces pain in many patients; this tenderness is present during the active phase of the disease and often subsides as the disease responds to treatment.

Roentgenologic examination may reveal osseous lesions in various parts of the skeleton. Subperiosteal new bone formation, osteolytic lesions, and transverse bands of diminished density at the ends of the long bones are the commonest abnormalities.[29, 96, 128] Osteosclerotic lesions are less common. Rarely

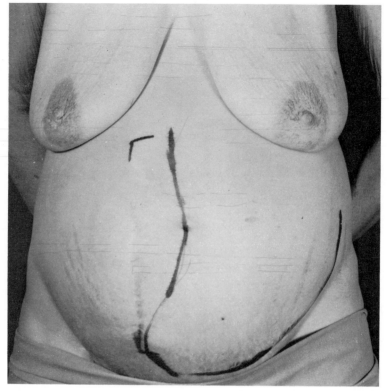

Figure 13–4.   Splenomegaly in a patient with chronic granulocytic leukemia.

the patient may develop acute pain in a joint because of involvement of the synovia by hemorrhage or infiltration with leukemic cells.

Laboratory Manifestations

Anemia occurs at some time in practically all patients with chronic myelocytic leukemia but is not invariably present when the patient is first seen. The anemia tends to increase as the disease progresses and improves as the disease regresses in response to treatment. The anemia is usually normocytic and normochromic. The hemoglobin may be as low as 4 or 5 gm. per 100 ml. but is more often in the range of 7 to 9 gm. per 100 ml. when the patient is first seen. The reticulocyte count is usually normal or slightly elevated. Anemia may be the result of either abnormal bleeding or diminished erythropoiesis secondary to the encroachment on the erythropoietic tissue of the marrow by the leukemic

Figure 13–5.   Chronic lymphocytic leukemia.

Figure 13–6.   Chronic myelocytic leukemia.

From Heilmeyer, L., and Begemann, H., Atlas der klinischen Hämatologie und Cytologie. Berlin-Göttingen-Heidelberg, Springer, 1955.

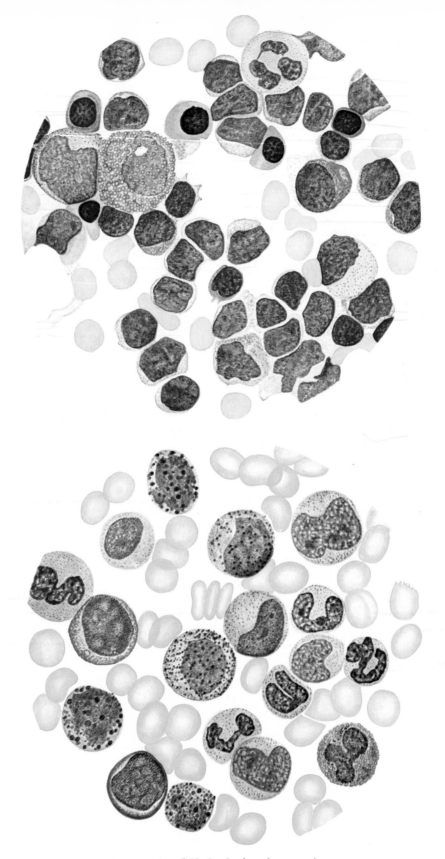

Figures 13–5 and 13–6. *See legends on opposite page.*

cells or hemodilution. Recent studies have shown that in some patients with this disease hyperhemolysis is present.

The most striking abnormality in myelocytic leukemia is found in the leukocytes. The total leukocyte count in different patients ranges from less than 1000 per cu.mm. to more than 1,000,000 per cu.mm. and is commonly between 100,000 and 300,000 per cu.mm. Such high values are the result of an increase in segmented neutrophils, band cells, juveniles, and myelocytes; a few myeloblasts and promyelocytes may be present, but they do not constitute a large percentage of the cells in chronic myelocytic leukemia. The eosinophils and basophils are usually increased.

The platelet count of the patient with chronic myelocytic leukemia is characteristically increased. Platelet counts over 1,000,000 per cu.mm. are sometimes seen. When chronic myelocytic leukemia begins with a picture that resembles aplastic anemia, thrombocytopenia is often present.

Examination of the bone marrow usually reveals a marked increase in cellularity that is due chiefly to an increase in cells of the myeloid series. Often the percentage of the younger cells in this series is increased, but at times the differential count of the marrow falls within normal limits. Even in such circumstances the marked increase in the number of cells of the granulocytic series leaves little doubt about the diagnosis. Erythropoiesis is normoblastic in type and megakaryocytes usually are present in normal or increased numbers.

Search for the Philadelphia (Ph¹) chromosome and determination of the leukocyte alkaline phosphatase value are valuable aids in diagnosis. The Ph¹ chromosome was found in 90 to 95 per cent of one group of patients[98] and in 70 per cent of another group of 61 adult patients.[36] In the latter study, Ph¹-negative patients had lower leukocyte and platelet counts and did not respond as well to therapy. The leukocyte alkaline phosphatase determination was zero or decreased in the overall majority of both groups, but in 9 per cent of the Ph¹-positive group and 20 per cent of the Ph¹-negative group it was elevated. Thus the presence of the Philadelphia chromosome and a low leukocyte alkaline phosphatase value is very strong evidence for a diagnosis of chronic myelocytic leukemia; opposite results are, however, obtained in a minority of patients. Serum muramidase levels, which are most consistently elevated in acute monocytic leukemia,[180a] are also high in some patients with chronic granulocytic leukemia; the elevated level is associated with absence of the Philadelphia chromosome, lower platelet counts and a poorer response to busulfan.[171a] Whether these groups constitute different forms or subclassifications of granulocytic leukemia is uncertain.

Other abnormalities occur in this disease but their significance is not clear. The basal metabolic rate is elevated in relapse but radioactive iodine uptake is normal. The uric acid level of the plasma is often elevated. The serum vitamin B_{12} level is consistently greatly increased, 10 or 12 times the normal, but the level in the circulating leukocytes is less than normal.

Clinical Course and Prognosis

The survival times for chronic myelocytic leukemia that have been reported vary considerably (Table 13–3). With most forms of treatment, the average

Table 13–3. *Survival in Chronic Granulocytic Leukemia*
(after onset of symptoms)

AUTHOR	DATE	NO. OF PTS.	AVG. SURVIVAL TIME (YRS.)	MEDIAN (YRS.)	TREATMENT
1. Minot et al.[89]	1924	52	3.0	2.6	None
		78	3.5		X-ray
2. Hoffman and Craver[66]	1931	82	3.4		X-ray
3. Leavell[79]	1938	87	3.2	2.5	X-ray
4. Tivey[136]*	1954	1090		2.7	
5. Osgood et al.[103]†	1956	100		4.8	P[32]
6. Reinhard et al.[110]	1959	118		2.6	P[32]
7. Feinleib and MacMahon[38]	1960	290		1.0	
8. Haut et al.[60]	1961	30		3.6	Busulfan

*Series collected from literature
†Chronic lymphocytic leukemia and chronic myelocytic leukemia — same survival

survival time from onset of symptoms is probably between 3 and 4 years; the prognosis is better for females than for males by about 6 to 12 months. The 5 year survival rate is probably between 15 and 25 per cent, but a few patients live for 15 or 20 years. The initial course of treatment may be followed by an excellent clinical remission but relapse inevitably occurs. The development of relapse is usually manifested by loss of weight, fever, night sweats, increasing anemia, increasing size of the spleen, and the recurrence of sternal tenderness. The leukocyte count usually rises during relapse but clinical relapse does not invariably follow an increase in the leukocyte count; nevertheless, if the leukocyte count continues to rise over a period of several months a relapse is likely. Subsequent courses of therapy generally bring remissions of shorter duration and the response of the spleen and blood is usually not nearly so satisfactory as in the first remission. As the disease progresses, splenomegaly and anemia become more or less constant features. The course of this disorder is sometimes accompanied by severe attacks of left upper quadrant pain and fever which are the result of splenic infarction or perisplenitis. A transformation into a myeloblastic leukemia is a common cause of death. The terminal stages are usually characterized by cachexia, persistent fever, night sweats, the persistence of anemia, and the occurrence of hemorrhages. The final episode is usually either a bacterial pneumonia or a fungus infection, but in some patients intracranial or gastrointestinal hemorrhage is the terminal event.

Treatment

All forms of treatment available at the present time are palliative. The demonstration of the persistence of the Philadelphia chromosome abnormality in the bone marrows of patients who have been brought into complete clinical and hematologic remission with apparently normal bone marrow indicates the failure to eliminate the disease even temporarily.

Although chronic myelocytic leukemia may be discovered on a routine examination when the patient is asymptomatic, it is rare that more than a few months will elapse before the patient will need some form of treatment. Both supportive and more specific measures are employed in the treatment of chronic myelocytic leukemia.

The most important supportive measures are transfusions and antibiotics. Anemia is treated by transfusion if it is severe or if it fails to respond as the disease improves with specific therapy. Antibiotics are used when infections are present and are not used for prophylaxis because of the possible emergence of a resistant bacterial or fungal infection. Patients with leukemia are prone to infections, and all patients who present with what appears to be a febrile relapse of leukemia should be studied carefully for some superimposed infection, such as pneumonia or pyelitis, that may be treated successfully.

The most effective agents now in use for the treatment of chronic myelocytic leukemia are radiation and chemotherapy with busulfan or 6-mercaptopurine.

RADIATION THERAPY

Roentgen therapy, first used by Pusey in 1902,[107] was for many years the most widely used form of treatment for chronic myelocytic leukemia. Programs of therapy have varied both in the area of the body irradiated and in the amount of radiation given. Radiation is most often directed towards the spleen in single treatments of 100 r. A total of 600 to 1200 r is given over a period of several weeks. Such treatment usually produces a diminution in the size of the spleen, a decrease in the leukocyte count, and improvement in the anemia. The initial remission usually lasts from 6 to 9 months. Subsequent therapy produces shorter remissions and the patient ultimately becomes refractory to further treatment of this type. The major disadvantages of this form of therapy are the necessity of the patient's being near a hospital where the therapy can be administered and the not infrequent occurrence of radiation sickness with anorexia, nausea, and vomiting.

Radiation in the form of P[32] has been used successfully in the treatment of chronic myelocytic leukemia. Radioactive phosphorus, administered orally or intravenously, is selectively concentrated in the rapidly dividing cells of the bone marrow and the leukemic tissue. It has a half-life of 14.3 days and emits soft beta radiation that penetrates only a few millimeters in tissue.[78] The dose must be individually determined and depends on the size of the patient, the amount of marrow involvement, and the extent of the disease elsewhere. The usual initial dose varies from 4 to 8 millicuries. A second, smaller dose, 2 to 4 millicuries, is given if the disease has not been controlled in 6 to 9 weeks. After the disease has been brought under control, the patient returns for periodic visits at intervals of from 3 to 6 months. Osgood advocated that the patient should be treated as soon as the diagnosis is made. An initial dose of 0.5 to 2.5 millicuries of P[32] is given intravenously and an effort is made to keep the disease under control by a plan of "titrated" therapy that consists of small individual doses of P[32] at intervals of from 4 to 12 weeks.[102] Osgood reported that results with this technique are superior to those obtained with other therapeutic regimes in that patients so treated survive longer and spend about 85 per cent of their remaining life span at their usual activities.

CHEMOTHERAPY

Among the earlier treatments used for chronic myelocytic leukemia were the chemotherapeutic agents, arsenic and benzol. These are used rarely if at all at the present time but newer chemotherapeutic agents have assumed an important place in the management of this disease. Among the most important of these are busulfan (1-4-dimethanesulfonyloxybutane), and 6-mercapto-purine (6-MP). Both of these agents can produce serious bone marrow depression, and for this reason blood counts at regular intervals are a necessary part of the routine when these drugs are employed. Busulfan and 6-MP are the preparations that are used most often.

BUSULFAN is considered by many to be the drug of choice in the treatment of chronic myelocytic leukemia at the present time. The use of this drug was initially reported by Galton[45] and the good results that he reported have been amply confirmed.[12, 60b, 68, 115] The initial dose of the drug for the average adult is 4 or 6 mg. a day. The drug is continued until the leukocyte count has fallen to the range of 4000 to 10,000 per cu.mm. This level is reached by over three-fourths of patients in 3 months or less. About half the patients who respond have remissions that last over 6 months, occasionally more than 2 years. The longer remissions are more likely to follow if treatment is continued until the leukocyte count is in the normal range. When relapse occurs, the course of treatment is repeated. Subsequent remissions are usually of shorter duration than the first. We prefer intermittent treatment to continuous treatment with small doses. However, when relapse occurs in 1 to 2 months, maintenance therapy of 2 mg. per day or 2 mg. two or three times a week may be employed. Maintenance therapy is preferred by some authors.[7]

Although adverse effects aside from those on the bone marrow are not common, busulfan in the usual dose (6 to 12 mg. per day initially and a maintenance dose of 2 mg. per day) has produced a variety of toxic reactions. These include generalized skin pigmentation, amenorrhea, gynecomastia, impotence, sterility, alopecia, pulmonary fibrosis, and renal damage with hyperuricemia. Nausea, vomiting, diarrhea, cheilosis, and glossitis are not common but do occur.

6-MERCAPTOPURINE will induce remissions in about one-third of patients with chronic myelocytic leukemia but appears to be inferior to busulfan in this type of disease.[18] However, it is the drug of choice when a myeloblastic transformation occurs in the terminal phase of the disease.[7] This drug is usually given orally in a single daily dose of 2.5 mg. per kg. The usual initial dose of 6-MP of 150 to 250 mg. per day or a maintenance dose of 50 to 100 mg. per day frequently produces bone marrow depression and pancytopenia. Anorexia, nausea, and vomiting occur in about 25 per cent and other toxic effects, such as stomatitis, diarrhea, jaundice, bile stasis, dermatitis, and hyperuricemia, occur less often.

When busulfan is no longer effective, dibromomannitol (DBM) and hydroxyurea sometimes are.[45a] Treatment with DBM, in daily doses of 750 mg. for 7 days repeated after 6 to 8 weeks, seems preferable to daily maintenance therapy with from 100 to 250 mg. because of the difficulty in stabilizing the leukocyte count with maintenance therapy. The reaction to hydroxyurea, either the initial dose of 30 to 40 mg. per kg. daily or maintenance therapy, 20 to 80 mg. per kg. three times a week or 20 to 30 mg. per kg. daily, is difficult to control. Nevertheless, with frequent adjustment of the dosage these drugs are well tolerated. They lower the leukocyte count and often control the adverse hematological features of the disease after control with busulfan has been lost.

The "blast cell crisis," an ominous development, is manifested by an increase in blast cells independent of increases in older cells; increasing enlargement of the spleen and osseous tumors are often present. Prednisone, 6-MP, vincristine, methotrexate, cytosine arabinoside, demecolcine, DBM, and hydroxyurea have been used in treatment in the customary doses. Remissions occur rarely, and usually are of short duration when they do.

Special Therapeutic Problems in the Leukemias

Management of the patient with leukemia who is pregnant requires special consideration. Although there is no evidence that the pregnancy has an adverse effect on the course of any type of leukemia, the hazards of pregnancy and delivery are greatly increased. Another worry is the effect that the antileukemic therapy might have on the unborn child. Because of this possibility an effort is made to avoid any treatment during pregnancy; treatment is given during the first 3 months only if absolutely essential. The treatment of choice in acute leukemia is probably 6-mercaptopurine in the smallest effective dose; sometimes a dose of 50 to 75 mg. a day will suffice. Adrenocortical steroids are useful at times, particularly for the deterioration that sometimes occurs in the mother soon after delivery. Hypofibrinogenemia is another complication in the mother that may require special measures which depend on the mechanism that is responsible. For the patient with chronic leukemia, which is usually granulocytic, busulfan in the smallest effective dose is the preferred treatment.

The question of the advisability of surgical operations arises in some patients with leukemia. In acute leukemia, even in children with remissions, the risk of complications is probably greater; in adults the prognosis is usually so poor that only urgent operations are ever considered. In any patient with any type of leukemia, the decision for or against operation must be an individual one that is made only after an evaluation of all the aspects of the problem.

Not infrequently, patients with chronic leukemia need operations such as prostatic resection, cholecystectomy, hysterectomy, cataract extraction, or pinning of a fractured hip; at times more serious ones such as resection of the colon for carcinoma may be necessary. Although complications of bleeding and infection are not uncommon, the survival rate for patients with chronic lymphocytic leukemia approaches that of other patients of the same age. Patients with chronic myelocytic leukemia have more complications and a more difficult time.[3a] For elective procedures in a patient with uncomplicated chronic lymphocytic leukemia, if the leukocyte count is not over several hundred thousand, it is probably best to operate after his anemia has been corrected. This should be done without treatment with cytotoxic drugs, because of the attendant risk of thrombocytopenia. Mild autoimmune hemolytic anemia is often controlled by corticosteroid drugs, but severe anemia of this type greatly increases the risk and in serious or acute situations may be a fatal factor because the difficulty in cross-matching for transfusion may lead to too great a delay in giving trans-fusions or performing an operation. One patient with early chronic lymphocytic leukemia, an elderly man, survived the insertion of an aortic graft and a hernia repair without difficulty, but died 6 years later when he developed a leaking false aneurysm and a severe auto-immune hemolytic anemia. Death occurred several weeks after onset as a result of a terminal massive hemorrhage at a time when the anemia had been corrected and the antibodies appeared to be becom-ing weaker as a result of treatment with prednisone.

Infections are a recurrent hazard to many patients with leukemia, particu-larly those with chronic lymphocytic leukemia or acute leukemia. With the exception of hepatitis, and vaccinia, patients with lymphocytic leukemia, unless they are on adrenocortical steroid drugs, handle viral infections about as well as normal persons do; bacterial infections are often serious problems. Patients with chronic lymphocytic leukemia are particularly susceptible to pneumonia, and both pneumonia and septicemia are common in acute leukemia. The pro-tection afforded by the granulocytes is probably unimpaired; the total number, the response to infection, and cellular motility are usually normal. The inci-dence of bacterial infections correlates fairly well with the gamma globulin level; from 36 to 64 per cent of patients with chronic lymphocytic leukemia have hypogammaglobulinemia;[86] even in those with normal levels of gamma globulin the antibody production response may be inferior. Maintenance intramuscular injections of gamma globulin (6.6 gm.) every 3 or 4 weeks appears to reduce the incidence and severity of infections in some patients. No significant benefit has been observed when the globulin was used routinely in patients with acute leukemia.[13] Treatment with adrenocortical steroid increases the susceptibility to infections, probably because it reduces the inflammatory response when it de-creases vascular permeability; interference with antibody production may also be important.

Illustrative Case

A 43 year old white housewife enjoyed her usual health until the summer of 1952 when she first noticed increased fatigue, irregular fever, weight loss, and vague abdominal discomfort. In October, 1952, she consulted her physician, who found her to be moderately pale. The spleen was palpable 2 fingerbreadths below the left costal margin. The erythrocyte count was 3 mil. per cu.mm., hemoglobin 9.5 gm. per 100 ml., leukocyte count 57,000 per cu.mm. Differential count (per cent): myelocytes 25, polymorphonuclears 52, lymphocytes 16, eosino-phils 4, basophils 3.

A diagnosis of chronic myelocytic leukemia was made and the patient was treated with roentgen irradiation of the spleen. She responded well and a month later the leukocyte count had fallen to

19,000 per cu.mm. and the hemoglobin had risen to 11.5 gm. per 100 ml. During the next 2 years the patient remained active and was treated with roentgen therapy at intervals.

Late in 1954 her symptoms increased and a hematologic relapse occurred. Because of the decreasing effectiveness of x-ray therapy she was treated with 8.1 millicuries of radioactive phosphorus in January, 1955. Following this therapy the patient was asymptomatic for 8 months.

In October, 1955, she was hospitalized because of a fever of 105° F, roentgenographic evidence of an infiltrate or exudate in the hilar regions of both lungs, hepatomegaly, splenomegaly, and a leukocyte count of 59,000 per cu.mm. The fever and pulmonary abnormalities persisted unchanged for 4 weeks despite numerous antibiotics. Busulfan was then administered orally in a dose of 4 mg. each day. The fever declined gradually and after 3 weeks the patient was afebrile. At this time the leukocyte count was 10,000 per cu.mm., and a roentgenogram revealed clearing of the lung densities. The patient continued active and felt well on a maintenance dose of busulfan, 2 mg. two or three times a week for about 2 years.

In September, 1957, it became necessary to give transfusions every few months because of recurrent anemia. Busulfan was discontinued even though the bone marrow examination at this time revealed greatly increased granulocytic activity associated with hypoplasia of the erythroid series. Several examinations disclosed no reticulocytes in the peripheral blood. In November, 1957, the leukocyte count had risen to 90,000 per cu.mm. and the majority of the cells in the peripheral blood were myeloblasts. Because of the predominance of blast cells, 6-mercaptopurine was administered in a daily dose of 2.5 mg. per kg. The patient again responded well; at the end of 1 month the leukocyte count was 6000 per cu.mm. and the myeloblasts had almost completely disappeared from the smear. Following a remission of several months relapse occurred and the disease was refractory to further treatment. In July, 1958, 6 years after the initial symptoms, the patient died with cachexia, anemia, and pneumonia.

Comment. The onset of the disease in this patient at middle age with vague symptoms of weakness, abdominal discomfort, splenomegaly, anemia, and leukocytosis is the common one. At various times she had clinical remissions with the usual methods of therapy—roentgen ray, radiophosphorus, and busulfan. As is often the case, severe refractory anemia and the blood picture of myeloblastic leukemia developed in the later stages. At this time a brief remission followed the use of 6-mercaptopurine. In the terminal stage the disease was refractory to treatment and a fatal infection occurred.

Eosinophilic Leukemia

Although the existence of eosinophilic leukemia is questioned by some authors and is considered a variant of chronic myelocytic leukemia by others, a number of cases, including 43 with autopsy, have been reported.[5, 6] The following criteria have been proposed for the diagnosis of eosinophilic leukemia: hepatosplenomegaly, lymphadenopathy, and marked persistent eosinophilia, usually accompanied by anemia and thrombocytopenia. Some of the autopsied patients had chloromas; those with evidence of other diseases which might have caused eosinophilia were excluded. The leukocyte counts ranged between 50,000 and 200,000 per cu.mm. Over 60 per cent were eosinophilic granulocytes; blast cells were observed in the peripheral blood of 27 patients and in one constituted 80 per cent of the cells. Features of the disease different from those usually seen in chronic myelocytic leukemia were the high incidence of involvement of the central nervous system (20 per cent) without association of bleeding or thrombocytopenia, and intractable heart failure which occurred in several patients; at autopsy cardiac fibrosis and eosinophilic infiltration of the myocardium were found. The Philadelphia chromosome was not found in the two patients in which it was searched for. Response to treatment was poor.

Monocytic Leukemia

Monocytic leukemia was first described as a distinct clinical entity by Reschad and Schilling-Torgau in 1913.[111] They reported a 33 year old patient who gave a history of exhaustion, inflamed gums, and loss of appetitie of 6 weeks' duration; during the week prior to admission chills and epistaxis occurred. Physical examination disclosed marked pallor, a papular rash, ulcerated bleeding gums, and retinal hemorrhages. The erythrocyte count was 2.2 mil. per cu.mm. and the leukocyte count was 15,000 per cu.mm. Seventy-two per cent of the leukocytes were large mononuclear and transitional cells; many were large, bizarre, lobed cells with basophilic cytoplasm. The patient died in coma 20 days later; on the day prior to death the leukocyte count was 56,000 per cu.mm. and the erythrocyte count was 920,000 per cu.mm. Postmortem examination revealed splenomegaly and infiltration of the marrow, skin, and liver with large mononuclear cells. The bone marrow sections varied in the degree of involvement with leukemic cells from few to many but no tumor masses were found anywhere and apparently it was inferred that the process began in the bone marrow. Erythrophagocytosis was widespread. The authors believed that the case represented acute, large mononuclear and transitional cell leukemia that was distinct from myeloid and lymphatic leukemia.

Although the existence of a third cell type of leukemia was questioned by hematologists who considered the reported cases to be only variants of the other types of leukemia, the occurrence of a monocytic type of leukemia is now accepted generally. Acute monocytic leukemia of the Schilling type is a rare disorder. Much commoner are the acute cases usually classified as "myelo-monocytic leukemia," probably a variety of granulocytic leukemia.

Even rarer is the chronic monocytic leukemia described by Doan and Wiseman.[33] Most cases considered to be chronic monocytic leukemia are the Naegeli type, which in all probability is a variety of granulocytic leukemia; in some patients the number of monocytes and myelocytes in the peripheral blood fluctuates widely from week to week, even from day to day. Almost invariably in these chronic cases the lesions at autopsy are those of chronic granulocytic leukemia.

The patients diagnosed as having histiocytic leukemia or leukemic reticulo-endotheliosis, who may be considered subacute or chronic, usually have marked splenomegaly, histiocytes, or monocytes in the circulating blood, and pancyto-penia.[17] It seems probable that such patients have reticulum cell sarcoma (histiocytic lymphoma) primarily; the leukemic transformation of the blood comes gradually or only in the last few weeks, essentially a terminal development.

Whether these cases are somewhat atypical instances of monocytic leukemia or are a different process altogether is uncertain. The relationship may be similar to that between lymphosarcoma and lymphocytic leukemia, but at times the morphology of the cells from different cases is so different that the possibility of different cellular origins must be considered.

Monocytic leukemia is less common than myelocytic and lymphocytic leukemia. It has been reported to constitute from 2 to 16 per cent of all leu-kemias.[81, 130] Apparently the diagnosis is made more frequently when supra-vitally stained preparations are studied than when fixed smears stained with Wright's stain alone are examined. The chronic form of the disease has been variously defined as that in which the patient survives for 6 months and 12 months after onset of symptoms.

Acute monocytic leukemia affects males more often than females, the proportion of males in one series being 65 per cent.[81] A mean age of 44 years was found in one series[81] but the ages of the reported patients have varied from 11 months[33] to 83 years.[130]

The first clinical manifestation of the disease is usually the gradual onset of weakness and easy fatigue, but in some patients there is an acute onset with high fever, abnormal bleeding, and prostration. Physical examination generally reveals pallor and slight generalized enlargement of the lymph nodes. The spleen is palpable in about three-fourths of the cases; the lower border usually extends from 1 to 4 cm. below the left costal margin, but enlargement of the spleen may not be detected clinically even in the most fulminant cases. Hepato-megaly is usually present. As was first emphasized by Forkner, often the most striking abnormalities on the physical examination are found in the gums and buccal mucosa.[41] Relatively early in the disease the gums are swollen and pale, and later they become ulcerated and necrotic. When such lesions are present they are usually accompanied by moderate enlargement of the cervical lymph nodes. Gingival hyperplasia and other lesions of the oral cavity are seen occa-sionally in other types of acute leukemia but they are much more common in the monocytic type, where the frequency may be about 75 per cent (Fig. 13–7). Anal fissure, sometimes associated with perirectal abscess, is found often enough in patients with this disease to warrant a special search for these lesions. Involvement of the skin in the form of erythematous papular or infiltrative lesions occurs but is not common.

Laboratory examinations generally disclose a severe progressive normo-cytic type of anemia. The leukocyte count is nearly always increased but a low or normal total count is sometimes seen. The initial count is usually in the range of 15,000 to 45,000 per cu.mm., but counts as high as 400,000 per cu.mm. are

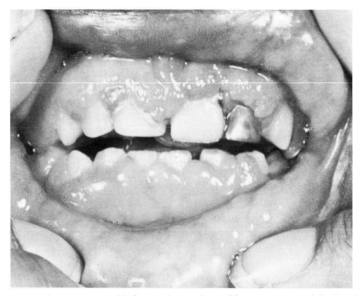

Figure 13–7. Hypertrophied gums in a patient with acute monocytic leukemia.

reported; counts of over 100,000 per cu.mm. are common in the terminal stages. Cells of the monocytic series are increased and constitute from 30 to 90 per cent of the total. Some appear to be normal adult monocytes, but usually blast forms and promonocytes are present; in addition, there are usually large abnormal multilobulated cells that have folded nuclei and pseudopodia or vacuolation in the cytoplasm. Occasionally the predominant cell in the blood resembles the tissue histiocyte more than the circulating monocyte. The peripheral blood often contains nucleated red cells; the platelet count is usually reduced. The bone marrow is hypercellular; blast cells and older cells of the monocytic series predominate. (F.S.:III, 58.)

Acute monocytic leukemia generally runs a rapid course that terminates within 2 or 3 months. Some patients undergo a partial remission when treated with adrenocortical steroids, the alkylating agents, or 6-mercaptopurine; but even in these patients life is rarely prolonged for more than 6 or 8 months. Patients with acute myelomonocytic leukemia respond better than those with the Schilling type when treated with cytosine arabinoside or 6-MP, but even in these patients the remissions are usually measured in months.

Illustrative Case

History. This 41 year old woman was admitted to the obstetrical service of the hospital in the seventh month of pregnancy because of weakness, easy fatigue, and severe ulceration of the mucous membranes of the mouth.

She had had an uneventful gestation until 6 to 8 weeks prior to admission when she noted the onset of mild migratory joint pains.

Four weeks before admission the left elbow became swollen and extremely painful. She was admitted to another hospital where the physical examination revealed only a swollen left elbow with increased heat and the uterus enlarged to a size compatible with a 6 month pregnancy. Laboratory studies at that time revealed: hematocrit 33 per cent, erythrocyte count 3.3 mil. per cu.mm., hemoglobin 9 gm. per 100 ml., platelets 81,000 per cu.mm., and leukocyte count 7200. Differential count (per cent), myelocytes ("monocytoid") 28, juvenile 2, bands 9, segmented 28, lymphocytes 28, monocytes 3, eosinophils 1. Many of the young forms contained Auer rods. Examination of the aspirated bone marrow revealed 12 per cent blast cells and 56 per cent young monocytes of bizarre form.

A diagnosis of acute monocytic leukemia was made. Over the next 10 days the leukocyte count rose to 16,000 per cu.mm. and the patient developed hypertrophy of the gums and severe ulcerative stomatitis. Therapy was then instituted with 6-mercaptopurine, 75 mg. daily by mouth. Over the next 10 days the leukocyte count fell to 3000 per cu.mm., the platelets to 40,000 per cu.mm., and petechiae appeared over the dependent portions of the body. 6-Mercaptopurine was discontinued and the leukocyte count rose to 15,000 per cu.mm. and the petechiae disappeared, though the platelet count persisted at 31,000 per cu.mm. The patient was discharged to her home under the care of her physician.

While at home during the week prior to final admission, she was weak and nauseated and continued to have migratory joint pains. The ulcerative stomatitis worsened and she began to vomit intermittently.

Physical examination. Physical examination on admission revealed an acutely ill woman with fever of 101° and pulse rate of 124. There was marked pallor of skin and mucous membranes. Several ecchymoses were noted over the lower legs. There was a foul ulcerative stomatitis which was associated with marked hypertrophy of the gums. There was moderate anterior and posterior cervical adenopathy. The fundus was 4 fingerbreadths below the xiphoid. Fetal heart rate was 140 per minute.

Laboratory examination. Hematocrit 17 per cent; leukocyte count 3,100 per cu.mm., and differential count (per cent), blast cells 6, promyelocytes 17, myelocytes 5, juvenile 0, bands 5, segmented 17, lymphocytes 46, monocytes 4. Platelets were 15,000 per cu.mm. The patient was treated symptomatically. Transfusions of whole blood and packed cells over the next 8 days brought the hematocrit to 35 per cent. The leukocyte count rose gradually during this period to 12,000 per cu.mm. and the platelet count rose to 38,000 per cu.mm. The differential count remained essentially unchanged.

Treatment and course. Adrenocortical steroid therapy was started on the fourteenth hospital day. The patient went into labor that night and was delivered of a viable premature female infant of 1400 gm. Following delivery her condition deteriorated. She continued to vomit and had several gastrointestinal hemorrhages. Her leukocyte count decreased progressively over the next 6 days to 400 per cu.mm. and no platelets were seen on smear. She died 7 days following delivery, about 3 months after the appearance of the first symptoms of her disease.

Microscopic examination of the placenta and umbilical cord revealed no evidence of leukemic infiltration.

At postmortem examination there was enlargement of the liver, spleen, lymph nodes, and kidneys. The bone marrow was entirely replaced in the axial skeleton and partially in the femur by the leukemic cell, which was a large mononuclear form with a moderate amount of dark cytoplasm and a notched or folded nucleus that contained two or three small nucleoli and a moderately dense chromatin. Microscopic leukemic infiltrates were present in the interstitial tissues of nearly all organs and appeared as gross nodules in the kidneys. The uterine cervix was heavily infiltrated by the leukemic cells as well as by hemorrhage. The uterine cavity contained a necrotic decidual lining in which there were many colonies of bacteria, and bacteria had been disseminated throughout most of the other tissues. The kidneys showed the lesions of lower nephron nephrosis. The axial bone marrow contained broad areas of coagulative necrosis with some foci of acute hypoplasia and regeneration with reticulum cells.

Comment. This patient presents many of the features commonly found in patients with acute monocytic leukemia. The onset of the illness with weakness, easy fatigue, and joint pain is not unusual in any type of acute leukemia but the early development of gingival hyperplasia and ulcerative stomatitis is more common in the monocytic type. Identification of the cell line involved in acute leukemia is often difficult and is particularly so in the monocytic type. Postmortem examination confirmed the clinical diagnosis of monocytic leukemia in this patient. The effect of treatment is difficult to evaluate. At least the patient survived long enough to be delivered of a viable infant.

Erythroleukemia

Synonyms: Di Guglielmo syndrome; erythremic myelosis

Di Guglielmo first described this disorder as one characterized by malignant proliferation of the erythrocytic cells in the bone marrow.[32] He later recognized the occurrence of mixed forms involving both the erythrocytes and the granulocytes, "erythroleukemia." Practically all the patients seen clinically fit into the "mixed" forms of disturbance in both the red cells and the granulocytes and for this reason the syndrome is now considered to be one of the myeloproliferative disorders.[28, 32, 126] Some authors consider that the disorder passes through three stages, namely predominant erythroblastic proliferation, mixed erythroblastic and myeloblastic growth, and preponderant myeloblastic proliferation. Others are unable to recognize these stages and consider the disorder as one with variable proliferation of both the erythroid and myeloid cells, erythroleukemia at all stages.[126] Dameshek considers that some, if not all, instances of refractory normoblastic anemia and acquired sideroblastic anemia are variants of the Di Guglielmo syndrome.[28] The high percentage of patients with "refractory normoblastic anemia" or "acquired sideroblastic anemia" who develop acute myeloblastic leukemia terminally support the concept of a relationship.

The disorder has been reported in patients from 11 to 85 years of age but it occurs most frequently in those 40 years of age or older. Males have outnumbered the females 2:1 in the reported cases. The presenting symptoms are usually weakness, easy fatigue, dyspnea on exertion, and weight loss. Less often bleeding in the skin and mucous membranes or from the gastrointestinal tract occurs. Severe pains of an unusual character occur commonly in the trunk, epigastrium, back, or extremities. Examination of the patient usually discloses pallor and evidence of weight loss. Hemorrhages into the skin, mucous membranes, or fundi are not unusual. Splenomegaly and hepatomegaly have been reported in about one-third of the patients.

Laboratory examinations reveal severe or moderate anemia that is normochromic and normocytic or slightly macrocytic in character. Leukopenia is common, normal counts are not unusual, but leukocytosis is rare. The platelet count is normal or reduced. The reticulocyte count is often 2 to 4 per cent. Study of the peripheral blood usually discloses nucleated red cells and myeloblasts. The erythrocytes on the stained smear may show anisocytosis and poikilocytosis.

Examination of the bone marrow discloses marked hyperplasia, mainly the result of a striking increase in the erythrocyte precursors. Many of the cells are large basophilic multinucleated immature pronormoblasts or stem cells. Some of the cells are megaloblasts or resemble abnormal forms of these cells. Auer bodies are sometimes seen in young cells of the myeloid series.

Studies of the anemia in patients with this disease have disclosed that the serum vitamin B_{12} level is unusually high, the vitamin B_{12} absorption is normal and the anemia fails to respond to either vitamin B_{12} or folic acid. The hemolytic character of the anemia is shown by the increased fecal urobilinogen excretion and the decreased cell survival measured with chromium-tagged cells. Failure of erythropoiesis has been demonstrated by studies with radioactive iron which disclose an increased clearance from the plasma associated with decreased utilization or incorporation into the circulating red cells, the picture of "ineffective" erythropoiesis.[31] Hypertransfusion reduces the bizarre erythroid hyperplasia seen in the disease, but qualitative abnormalities persist.[1a]

The prognosis of the disease is very poor and most patients do not survive for a year after the appearance of the first symptoms. However, a chronic form of the disease does exist and survivals for 10 years or more have been reported. Treatment with steroids, vitamin B_{12}, folic acid and other preparations is ineffective. As the disease pursues its relentless course, the myeloblasts in the marrow increase and nearly always becomes the predominant cell before the patient dies.

Myeloid Metaplasia

Synonyms.   One review lists 25 different names that have been suggested for this syndrome.[158] Those that are used most commonly are: agnogenic myeloid metaplasia, chronic non-leukemic myelosis, aleukemic myelosis, leukanemia, leukoerythroblastic anemia, myelosclerosis, and myelofibrosis.

This syndrome is characterized by splenomegaly, anemia, the presence of nucleated red blood cells and immature granulocytes in the circulating blood, and the occurrence of extramedullary hematopoiesis in the liver and spleen. There is considerable variation in the histologic appearance of the bone marrow in the reported cases. Credit for the first report of a case of this type is usually given to Heuck, who in 1879 reported two cases that were considered to show the chance association of myelogenous leukemia and osteosclerosis.[159] Ever since that time there has been considerable confusion and controversy concerning terminology, classification, and causation of the syndrome. Several comprehensive reviews of the clinical or pathologic aspects of the problem that also contain extensive bibliographies have appeared.[148, 156, 158, 162, 163, 168, 171, 172, 177] Although some authors differ as to what should be classified as "primary" and "secondary" types of this syndrome, some such grouping is desirable for a better understanding of the problem. The clinical manifestations of this syndrome occur in patients known to have some primary disease, such as carcinomatosis, and also in patients in whom no primary disease can be demonstrated. The latter group is usually diagnosed "myelofibrosis" or "agnogenic myeloid metaplasia" or "chronic non-leukemic myelosis."

Secondary or Symptomatic Myeloid Metaplasia

The clinical features of this syndrome, splenomegaly, anemia, young cells in the peripheral blood, and extramedullary hematopoiesis, have been reported in a number of diseases that are sometimes classed as metaplasia, myelophthistic anemia, and space-consuming lesions of the bone marrow. The following diseases have been found to be associated with the syndrome: carcinomatosis, tuberculosis, multiple myeloma, Hodgkin's disease, septicemia, Gaucher's disease, leukemia, neurofibromatosis, and polycythemia vera.[152, 160, 171] The simple occurrence of nucleated red cells in the peripheral blood without other evidence of extramedullary hematopoiesis is not sufficient for the inclusion of a patient in this syndrome. Nucleated red cells have been found in the circulating blood in a number of disorders. They are seen most often in association with hemorrhage, pernicious anemia, hemolytic anemia, leukemia, and carcinoma, but also occur in other disorders such as heart failure, severe infection, and cerebrovascular accidents.[175]

Primary or Agnogenic Myeloid Metaplasia, Non-leukemic Myelosis, Myelofibrosis

Most of the controversy regarding patients in this category has centered around the nature of the underlying process. It has been considered to be: (1) leukemic in nature; (2) a proliferative or neoplastic disorder closely related to but different from myelocytic leukemia and polycythemia; (3) a response of the marrow and reticuloendothelial tissue to injury of some sort.

The evidence for the leukemic nature of the process has been reviewed by Heller, Lewison, and Palin.[158] These authors studied two autopsied cases and one splenectomized patient; the bone marrow of both the autopsied cases showed intense myeloid hyperplasia and only one showed small, widely scattered areas of fibrosis, but the authors emphasized that they considered their comments applicable to cases reported in the literature under the 25 other names as well as the term "aleukemic myelosis" which they used. The authors, who concluded that the syndrome is a form of myelogenous leukemia, considered that the presence of fibrosis in the marrow and osteosclerosis in the bones, the absence of leukemic invasion in the organs, and the appearance of the spleen were not adequate grounds for excluding leukemia.

Wyatt and Sommers[181] studied 30 patients, 20 of whom were autopsied, and concluded that the disorder was non-leukemic in nature. It was thought that the primary lesion was a necrobiosis of the maturing hematopoietic cells, which was followed by overgrowth of the marrow reticulum, ossification, and extramedullary hematopoiesis. The study of the histories and a retrospective analysis for possible causative agents in these cases revealed a list of possible factors similar to those that are considered important in aplastic anemia. This suggested that prolonged marrow exposure to certain substances might be an important factor. A similar conclusion is suggested by another report of six patients with "agnogenic myeloid metaplasia." It was noted that two patients gave histories of heavy exposure to benzol, two had daily exposure to "paint removers," one worked with carbon tetrachloride, and one washed auto parts with "high-test gasoline."[173]

Another hypothesis that has been advanced to explain the disorder is that it is one manifestation of a proliferative disorder that involves the multipotential primitive mesenchymal cells. According to this concept myelofibrosis, myelogenous leukemia, megakaryocytic myelosis, and polycythemia vera are similar and related processes.[151, 163, 180] Cases that show varying degrees of histologic evidence of these different disorders at the same time and others that undergo transition from a typical example of one condition into a typical example of another are interpreted as evidence of the validity of this hypothesis. In the series of patients with myelofibrosis that has been reported, the incidence of preexisting polycythemia vera has varied from 10 to 38 per cent.[168, 172] Myelofibrosis develops in about 10 per cent of patients with polycythemia vera.[180] The increased incidence of myelofibrosis found in survivors of the atomic bomb explosion in Hiroshima, a pattern similar to that found for leukemia, is evidence that ionizing radiation is the causative agent in some patients with the disorder.[147]

The development of aplastic anemia after radiation and certain toxic agents is well recognized. Leukemia develops in some patients who have or have had aplastic anemia, and the development of myeloid metaplasia may be an analogous sequence. It appears evident that the development of massive enlargement of the spleen and liver with myeloid metaplasia seen in many patients is something different from an effort to compensate for a bone marrow rendered functionless by fibrosis. The postmortem examination in some patients discloses lesions that must be closely akin to leukemia; in such patients the evidence of myeloid metaplasia (the proliferation of normoblasts, granulocytes, and megakaryocytes) is so widespread, involving the myocardium, lungs, and other tissues, as well as the liver, spleen, and lymph nodes, that it has every appearance of an invasive process which involves several cell lines rather than one, as is seen characteristically in leukemia.

An unusual type of myeloproliferative disease has been reported in nine children.[172a] The disorder became manifest between 5 months and 4 years of age and was characterized by chronic illness, anemia, and massive splenomegaly in most; there was a leukocytosis of between 2700 and 128,000 per cu.mm. accompanied in nearly all by young cells of the granulocytic series in the peripheral blood. The bone marrow was hyperplastic. The leukocyte alkaline phosphatase was low in the four patients in whom it was measured and the Philadelphia chromosome was not found in four patients who were examined for it. The course of the disease was variable, ranging from early death through improvement after splenectomy to apparent spontaneous complete recovery after 10 or 12 years of illness. The disorder closely resembled chronic granulocytic leukemia, but its familial distribution, the absence of the Philadelphia chromosome, and the apparent recovery in some patients suggests that it is a different disorder.

Although it is probable that the controversy as to the nature and causation of this syndrome will continue, it appears that the concept of this syndrome as a proliferative disorder, which does not exclude a reaction to toxic agents, affords the best working hypothesis at the present time.

Clinical Manifestations

This rather uncommon disorder occurs in either sex. Symptoms generally appear first after the age of 50 but sometimes begin before the age of 40. The onset is usually gradual and the patients complain of weakness and easy fatigue, or of upper abdominal discomfort that is caused by the enlargement of the spleen and liver. Weight loss of 15 to 20 pounds is common. Aching and severe pain in the extremities, leg cramps, and peripheral edema sometimes occur. Cutaneous hemorrhages, either petechiae or ecchymoses, are not unusual and serious gastrointestinal hemorrhage is not rare. Night sweats and fever occur in an appreciable number of patients. Occasionally unexplained ascites develops late in the course of the disease. Attacks of gout or gouty arthritis are a troublesome feature in some of the patients who have high levels of uric acid in the blood.

The most significant feature of the physical examination is the splenomegaly. Palpable enlargement of the spleen is almost invariably present and is sometimes so extreme that the firm spleen fills the entire left side of the abdomen and extends into the right lower quadrant. Hepatomegaly generally occurs but is usually less prominent than the splenomegaly. In some patients, after the spleen is removed, the liver becomes enormous and virtually fills the abdominal cavity. Significant enlargement of the superficial lymph nodes is exceedingly rare. Not infrequently a bleeding tendency is manifested by ecchymoses and petechiae or retinal hemorrhages. Pallor of the skin and mucous membranes is usually evident and jaundice of mild degree is sometimes apparent in the skin and sclerae. The other abnormalities found on the physical examination are those that occur commonly in older persons with a chronic disease associated with anemia, such as evidence of loss of weight, cardiac enlargement, and precordial systolic murmurs.

Laboratory Examination

The most significant hematologic feature of this disorder is an anemia that is characterized by marked anisocytosis and poikilocytosis associated with the occurrence of nucleated red cells and myelocytes or myeloblasts in the peripheral blood. The degree of anemia, the levels of leukocytes and platelets, and the numbers of immature erythrocytes and granulocytes vary within a wide range. Patients with normal or polycythemic blood levels sometimes are also included as examples of this syndrome if immature cells are present in the circulating blood.

In the reported series, which include observations on more than 150 patients, the hemoglobin ranged from 5.0 to 14.0 gm. per 100 ml. and was less than 9.0 gm. per 100 ml. in 21 patients. The mean corpuscular volume varied from 71 to 103 cu. microns, and was normal in 60 per cent of the subjects. The mean corpuscular hemoglobin was normal in 60 per cent and low in the remainder. Examination of the blood smear often suggests the diagnosis because of the presence of a marked degree of poikilocytosis—particularly "teardrop forms" and elongated cells—anisocytosis, and the presence of nucleated red cells. The changes in the peripheral blood are not diagnostic. The nucleated red cells are usually few in number, less than 5 per 100 leukocytes, but occasionally they outnumber the leukocytes. Most often these cells are late normoblasts but basophilic and polychromatophilic normoblasts and cells that resemble megaloblasts are sometimes seen. The reticulocyte count is often normal but mild or moderate reticulocytosis of 3 to 5 per cent is common.

The leukocyte count is usually elevated but the range in the reported cases is from 1200 to 92,000 per cu.mm. Myeloblasts, progranulocytes, and myelocytes are usually found in the peripheral blood. It has been noted that the number and identity of the immature granulocytes in the peripheral blood represent a "shift to the left" rather than a "leukemic hiatus." The authors have seen marked diminution and even the disappearance of the immature leukocytes follow a series of transfusions in several patients with this disorder but such a change has not been found in patients with leukemia who have been treated similarly. Eosinophilia, monocytosis, and basophilia sometimes occur in myelofibrosis. The alkaline phosphatase stain in patients with myelofibrosis gives variable results; low, normal, and high values have been found. Although a differentiation between leukemia and myelofibrosis cannot be made by this reaction a high value favors myelofibrosis. The Philadelphia chromosome, which occurs in a high percentage of patients with chronic myelocytic leukemia, is rarely found in patients with myelofibrosis. (F.S.:II, 73.)

The platelets are often large and the total count varies widely in different patients. Neither a marked reduction to less than 100,000 per cu.mm. nor a marked increase to over a million per cu.mm. is uncommon, but a normal or slightly increased count is usual.

*Polychromato-
philie*

Tear drop

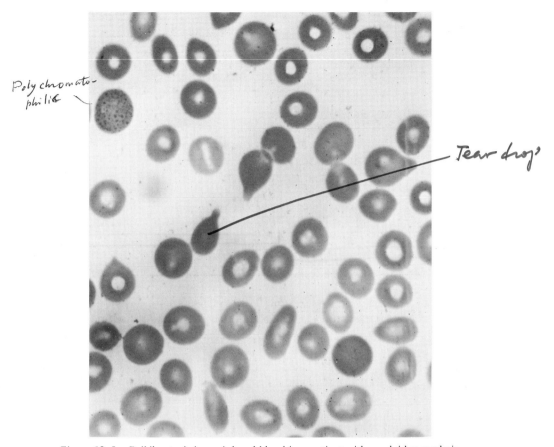

Figure 13–8. Poikilocytosis in peripheral blood in a patient with myeloid metaplasia.

Specimens of bone marrow obtained by aspiration are usually very hypocellular, but normal cellularity or even hyperplasia of some or all elements is found in some patients. Biopsy specimens obtained by operation or the Vim-Silverman needle and postmortem marrows show increased fibrosis as well as hypocellularity although some marrows contain areas of hyperplasia. Hickling has studied the bone marrow histology in 68 patients with the disorder.[162] He concluded that the marrow undergoes a transition ranging from general hyperplasia involving all of the normal hematopoietic cells, followed by megakaryocytic hyperplasia, to varying degrees of fibrosis and eventual bony replacement of nearly all the marrow. Between these extremes he recognized seven categories. Splenic aspiration and hepatic puncture usually reveal extramedullary hematopoiesis in the form of nucleated red cells, young granulocytes, and megakaryocytes. (F.S.:II, 74–79.)

Other laboratory tests are frequently abnormal in patients with this disorder. Uric acid levels in the blood are elevated in more than half the patients and in many of these the levels are twice the normal value. The liver function tests are often mildly abnormal. Serum bilirubin and fecal urobilinogen excretion are usually increased in patients who have significant hyperhemolysis. The

Coombs test is occasionally positive. Abnormalities of coagulation in the form of defective platelet function or an abnormality in a plasma coagulation factor have been found in some patients.

Roentgenograms of the bones, particularly of the long bones, may show a decreased density of the inner surface of the central area of bone and patchy irregular densities in the spongiosa.[179] The changes may be indistinguishable from those sometimes found in leukemia. Increased bone density was demonstrated on roentgenograms in one-fourth of the patients in one series.[168]

Differential Diagnosis

1. Leukemia
2. CGL
3. II to ca., T.B.,

When a patient presents with splenomegaly and anemia associated with nucleated red cells and immature granulocytes in the peripheral blood, the important differential diagnosis is between chronic myelocytic leukemia and the myeloid metaplasia syndrome. The appearance of marked poikilocytosis in the smear is suggestive but not diagnostic of myeloid metaplasia. Failure to obtain a specimen that is consistent with leukemia by marrow aspiration strongly suggests that leukemia is not present; however, the diagnosis of leukemia cannot be discarded in this circumstance because hypocellular samples and "dry taps" are sometimes obtained in patients with leukemia even when the marrow is packed with cells. The distinction between the leukemia and myeloid metaplasia sometimes cannot be made until after a surgical biopsy of the bone marrow or a needle aspiration of the liver. A splenic aspiration biopsy which reveals young granulocytes, normoblasts, and megakaryocytes is strong evidence of myeloid metaplasia, but the risks of the procedure have restricted its use in most institutions. Although a diagnosis of myelofibrosis with myeloid metaplasia is not justified without a biopsy of the bone marrow that demonstrates fibrosis, it must be remembered that fibrosis in the bone marrow occurs in other conditions, particularly in leukemia. Sometimes even after these studies the evidence is inconclusive and the distinction between these two disorders cannot be made with assurance until after a longer period of observation.

A search for the Philadelphia chromosome and determination of the leukocyte alkaline phosphatase help distinguish chronic myelocytic leukemia from myeloid metaplasia. The Philadelphia chromosome is present in from 90 to 95 per cent of patients with chronic myelocytic leukemia and is present rarely, if at all, in patients with myeloid metaplasia. Nowell indicates that it is not found in myeloid metaplasia,[98] but positive results have been reported by others.[157] This is not too surprising, since the Philadelphia chromosome is present in megakaryocytes and red cell precursors as well as granulocytes in chronic myelocytic leukemia. Nearly all patients with myeloid metaplasia have a normal or increased score with the leukocyte alkaline phosphatase determination while patients with chronic myelocytic leukemia have subnormal values; a subnormal value is not diagnostic of chronic granulocytic leukemia but an elevated value is strong evidence against the diagnosis.

If leukemia appears to be excluded, further study for possible causes of the secondary type of extramedullary hematopoiesis, such as carcinomatosis, tuberculosis, and other disorders, is indicated. If these appear to be excluded and the appearance of the bone marrow biopsy is consistent, a diagnosis of myelofibrosis, non-leukemic myelosis, or agnogenic myeloid metaplasia is made. A history of previous exposure to toxic substances or of preceding polycythemia vera favors this diagnosis. Although the age of the patient, the history of exposure to chemicals, pancytopenia, and hemorrhagic tendency may be similar to the findings in patients with the aplastic anemia syndrome, the presence of the splenomegaly and the character of the cells in the peripheral blood suffice to distinguish between the two conditions.

Treatment and Course

There is no specific treatment for this disorder, which is usually a chronic one that continues over a period of 1 to 20 years or more.[158, 161, 165] An average survival of 2 or 3 years after diagnosis and an 8 per cent survival for more than 5 years are reported in one series.[149] In this series, 20 per cent of the patients had terminal leukemia. Weakness, recurrent anemia, and complaints referable to the enlarged spleen are the most common symptoms but severe gastrointestinal hemorrhages occur occasionally. Bone pain, phlebothrombosis, and pulmonary embolism with infarction are troublesome at times. Blood transfusions, which constitute the main form of therapy, are usually given as often as indicated by the patient's symptoms. Neither iron nor vitamin B_{12} is of any value in the uncomplicated case. Splenic irradiation has been recommended as a form of therapy for patients with discomfort from enlarged spleens accompanied by leukocytosis because of the results seen in seven patients.[161] Such therapy has also been considered contraindicated because of potential damage to an area of extramedullary hematopoiesis.[150] The effectiveness of this type of therapy could not be evaluated in one group of 14 patients.[168]

For many years splenectomy was considered contraindicated because of the high operative mortality rate and because it appeared that the operation removed a needed area of hematopoiesis. A different opinion was expressed by Green, Conley, Ashburn, and Peters,[156] who reported that in a series of 24 patients splenectomy was rarely harmful and sometimes produced beneficial effects. In the authors' experience, most patients have not improved significantly after splenectomy. Others, however, have reported favorable results.[149, 153, 165] In one study, of 35 patients who were treated with splenectomy, 14 responded well and survived up to 8 years.

Splenectomy is most likely to be helpful in the patients with hemolytic anemia who require large numbers of transfusions and in those with associated thrombocytopenia. Pronounced discomfort in the splenic area and severe hypermetabolism manifested by sweats and weight loss have also been considered indications for splenectomy. The dangers and ineffectiveness of the operation in some patients are apparent from published reports. Of 28 patients who had splenectomy, 12 died at operation or in the immediate, postoperative period and 7 others died within 1 year.[155, 167, 172] Excellent results were obtained in a small number of patients. Since there is appreciable risk associated with the operation in patients with this disorder, splenectomy is not indicated in the patients who can be managed adequately by other forms of treatment. In elderly patients and those with very high platelet counts splenectomy is contraindicated because of the risk of operation and the chance of postoperative complications such as thrombosis and hemorrhage secondary to thrombocytosis.

The anemia in this disorder is often the result of multiple factors, such as hypocellularity of the marrow, ineffective erythropoiesis, increased hemolysis, bleeding, hemodilution, and the effectiveness of extramedullary hematopoiesis; even folic acid deficiency is sometimes a factor. Studies with radioactive iron and chromium have shown that in only about a quarter of the patients does the spleen play an important role in hyperhemolysis. Evidence provided by studies of this type also indicate that the extramedullary hematopoiesis is very slight or ineffective. Paroxysmal nocturnal hemoglobinuria develops in some patients.[60a]

Androgen, prednisone, and busulfan are usually employed in treatment. Androgens, first seriously studied by Gardner and Pringle, have proved to be very effective in many patients: from one-half to three-quarters experience either complete remission or distinct improvement.[154, 166] Results appear to be better in women, in patients who have had polycythemia vera, in those who have had splenectomy, or in those in whom the spleen is not massively enlarged. Testosterone enanthate, 6 mg. per kg. of body weight intramuscularly once a week, dianabol, 5 mg. four times a day, or oxymetholone, 40 to 100 mg. per day, is effective. Unfortunately, virilizing effects may be troublesome, particularly in women. Corticosteroids produce benefit in some patients, especially those with hyperhemolysis or thrombocytopenia and bleeding. Busulfan, 6 mg. a day, benefits some patients, probably by reducing hyperhemolysis, but a variety of effects have occurred; hematologic improvement unaccompanied by a diminution in the size of the spleen occurs in some patients and in others splenomegaly diminishes without any improvement in the peripheral blood. Busulfan may produce an adverse effect on the remaining marrow elements and the use should be discontinued if thrombocytopenia develops. The authors have seen severe pulmonary fibrosis and bone marrow aplasia in a patient treated continuously for over 2 years. Intermittent therapy should be used if possible. Busulfan is a useful agent, however, in treating thrombocytosis that is sometimes present and apparently a factor in both phlebothrombosis and bleeding.

The prognosis for patients with myeloid metaplasia is only slightly better than for those with chronic leukemia. Although the survival time varies from a few weeks to more than 20 years, the median survival time in one group of 143 patients was about 4.0 years.[168] The mortality rate was greatest during the first year. The 3 year survival rate in the disease is about 30 per cent, the 5 year survival about 20 per cent, and the 10 year survival about 10 per cent. Death is most often the result of thrombosis or hemorrhage. Other patients die with heart failure and a few develop chronic myelocytic leukemia or acute myeloblastic leukemia as a terminal event.

Illustrative Case

A 40 year old white librarian was largely asymptomatic when an "abdominal tumor" was found on routine physical examination in October 1945. At that time the erythrocyte count was 6.6 mil. per cu.mm. and the hematocrit 62 per cent. A diagnosis of polycythemia vera was made and during the next 4 years she received a total of 3250 r of x-radiation to the spleen and a total of 460 r over the long bones. Phlebotomies were performed at frequent intervals. Following treatment with radiophosphorus in 1950 she had a good symptomatic remission and in 1953 the blood values were: Hct. 49 per cent, Hb. 12.7 gm. per 100 ml., R.B.C. 6 mil. per cu.mm., W.B.C. 13,000 per cu.mm., platelets 516,000 per cu.mm. During the late spring and summer of 1954 the patient noticed progressive weakness, easy fatigue, slight dyspnea on exertion, easy bruisability, and recurrent left upper quadrant pain. Because of these symptoms she was admitted to the hospital on August 2, 1954.

Physical examination. Loud systolic murmurs were heard in the aortic area and in the mitral region. The liver was palpable three fingerbreadths below the right costal margin; the spleen filled the entire left side of the abdomen. The remainder of the physical examination was non-contributory.

Laboratory examination. Admission blood studies disclosed: Hct. 28 per cent, R.B.C. 2.8 mil. per cu.mm., Hb. 8.4 gm. per 100 ml., retics. 0.7 per cent, W.B.C. 7400 per cu.mm.; differential count (per cent), myelocytes 2, juveniles 2, bands 7, segs. 68, lymphs. 18, monocytes 1, eosinophils 1, basophils 1. There were 5 nucleated red cells per 100 white cells. The serum bilirubin was 0.54 mg. per 100 ml. Bone marrow obtained by aspiration and also by surgical biopsy of the iliac crest revealed marked hypoplasia.

Treatment and course. The patient responded moderately well to steroid therapy but in the fall of 1955 her symptoms and anemia increased. A hemolytic factor was demonstrated by finding an average daily fecal urobilinogen excretion of 245 mg. per day over a 4-day period at a time when the hemoglobin was 8.8 gm. per 100 ml. Eight months later the anemia was more severe and the fecal urobilinogen excretion was measured at 380 mg. per day. Because of the hemolytic element splenectomy was performed in September 1956. The spleen weighed 1975 grams. Microscopic study of the spleen revealed the presence of many islands of myeloid tissue associated with evidence of erythropoiesis and an increased number of megakaryocytes. The findings were considered to be characteristic of myeloid metaplasia. The patient did well symptomatically following splenectomy and 6 months later, in April 1957, hemoglobin was 9.4 gm. per 100 ml., red count 3 mil. per cu.mm., hematocrit 31 per cent, platelets 500,000 per cu.mm., and reticulocyte count 5.1 per cent. Immature cells of the myelocytic series and eosinophilia were present in the peripheral blood. Daily fecal urobilinogen excretion (average of a 4-day period) was found to be 125 mg.

In the fall of 1957 the patient's symptoms changed and from then on heart failure was a problem. In addition to the systolic murmurs at the base and apex, which had been noted throughout her course, a low pitched rumbling presystolic murmur was heard in the mitral area. She became increasingly refractory to treatment and in April 1958 she died after an episode of abdominal pain.

At autopsy the usual manifestations of congestive heart failure were present. In addition there was marked coronary arteriosclerosis as well as calcific aortic valvulitis and calcification of the annulus fibrosus of the mitral valve. Of particular interest was the presence of generalized fibrosis of the bone marrow associated with areas of hypercellularity and evidence of extramedullary hematopoiesis in the liver.

Comment. This patient's course is similar to that seen in many patients with myelofibrosis. At one time she had well developed polycythemia vera which was treated with phlebotomies, x-radiation, and radiophosphorus. About 8 years after the polycythemia was first recognized she developed anemia. This was associated with fibrosis in the bone marrow, marked splenomegaly, the presence of immature leukocytes and red cells in the peripheral blood, and evidence of hematopoiesis in the spleen. Splenectomy produced only moderate temporary benefit and the patient succumbed to recurrence of the anemia and heart failure several years later. The relationship of the myelofibrosis to the preceding polycythemia vera and to the radiation therapy is interesting but difficult to interpret. The occurrence of both syndromes in the same patient has led some to consider that both these disorders are examples of myeloproliferative syndromes. At the present time, androgen probably would be used in treating a patient of this type.

Hemorrhagic Thrombocythemia

The clinical features of hemorrhagic thrombocythemia are splenomegaly, anemia, abnormal bleeding, usually from the nose or gastrointestinal tract, and thrombocytosis; an abnormal tendency to thrombosis is sometimes manifest. The platelet counts are from 1.0 mil. to 5.0 mil. per cu.mm., or even more, and megakaryocytes in the bone marrow are often strikingly increased. Whether or not this syndrome constitutes a separate clinical entity is debatable. Unquestionably some patients with myelofibrosis, polycythemia vera, and chronic myelocytic leukemia develop all the features of the syndrome during the course of their illness; others have the fully developed syndrome when they first consult their physician. Abnormal bleeding is the result of the excessive number of platelets and their poor function; both bleeding and thrombocytosis are often controlled by treatment with busulfan, radioactive phosphorus or melphalan.[4a] (F.S.:II, 77–79.)

References

LEUKEMIA

1.   Acute Leukemia Group B: acute lymphocytic leukemia in children. J.A.M.A., *207*:923, 1969.
1a. Adamson, J. W., and Finch, C. A.: Erythropoietin and regulation of erythropoiesis in Di Guglielmo's syndrome. Blood, *36*:590, 1970.
2.   Anderson, R. C.: Familial leukemia: A report of leukemia in five siblings, with a brief review of the genetic aspects of this disease. Am. J. Dis. Child., *81*:313, 1951.

3. Baldini, M., Fudenberg, H. H., Fukutake, K., and Dameshek, W.: The anemia of the Di Guglielmo syndrome. Blood, 14:334, 1959.

3a. Bender, A., and Leavell, B. S.: Surgical procedures in patients with chronic leukemia. Virginia M. Month., 94:753, 1967.

4. Bennett, J. H.: Case of hypertrophy of the spleen and liver in which death took place from suppuration of the blood. Edinburgh Med. & Surg. J., 64:413, 1845.

4a. Bensinger, T. A., Logue, G. L., and Rundles, R. W.: Hemorrhagic thrombocythemia; control of postsplenectomy thrombocytosis with melphalan. Blood, 36:61, 1970.

5. Bentley, H. P., Jr., Reardon, A. E., Knoedler, J. P., and Krivit, W. K.: Eosinophilic leukemia. Am. J. Med., 30:310, 1961.

6. Benvenisti, D. S., and Ultmann, J. E.: Eosinophilic leukemia (report of five cases and review of literature). Ann. Int. Med., 71:731, 1969.

7. Bethell, F. H.: The relative frequency of the several types of chronic leukemia and their management. J. Chron. Dis., 6:403, 1957.

8. Bierman, H. R., Aggeler, P. M., Thelander, H., Kelly, K. H., and Cordes, F. L.: Leukemia and pregnancy. J.A.M.A., 161:220, 1956.

9. Bierman, H. R., Byron, R. L., Kelly, K. H., and Cordes, F.: The behavior of leukemic cells during continuous cross-transfusions between patients with leukemia and other neoplastic diseases. Cancer Res., 11:236, 1951.

10. Binger, C. M., Ablin, A. R., Feuerstein, R. C., Kushner, J. H., Zoger, S., and Mikkelsen, C.: Childhood leukemia. New England J. Med., 280:414, 1969.

11. Bird, R. M., and Marshall, R. A.: Unusual hematological manifestations in disseminated histoplasmosis. Trans. Am. Clinical & Climatological Assoc., 79:177, 1967.

12. Blackburn, E. K., King, G. M., and Swan, H. T.: Myleran in treatment of chronic myeloid leukemia. Brit. Med. J., 1:835, 1956.

13. Bodey, G. P., Nies, B. A., Mohberg, N. R., and Freireich, E. J.: Use of gamma globulin in infection in acute leukemia patients. J.A.M.A., 190:1099, 1964.

14. Boggs, D. R., Sofferman, S. A., Wintrobe, M. M., and Cartwright, G. E.: Factors influencing the duration of survival of patients with chronic lymphocytic leukemia. Am. J. Med., 40:243, 1966.

15. Boggs, D. R., Wintrobe, M. M., and Cartwright, G. E.: To treat or not to treat acute granulocytic leukemia. Arch. Int. Med., 123:568, 1969.

16. Bornstein, R. A., Theologides, A., and Kennedy, B. I.: Daunorubicine in acute myelogenous leukemia in adults. J.A.M.A., 207:1301, 1969.

17. Bouroncle, B. A., Wiseman, B. K., and Doan, C. A.: Leukemic reticuloendotheliosis. Blood, 13:609, 1968.

18. Burchenal, J. H., et al.: Clinical evaluation of a new antimetabolite 6-mercaptopurine in the treatment of leukemia and allied diseases. Blood, 8:965, 1953.

19. Burger, C. L., Harris, W. W., Anderson, N. G., Bartlett, T. W., and Kniseley, R. M.: Virus-like particles in human leukemic plasma. Proc. Soc. Exper. Biol. & Med., 115:151, 1964.

20. Carbone, P. P., Tjio, J. H., Whang, J., Block, J. B., Kremer, W. B., and Frei, E.: The effect of treatment in patients with chronic myelogenous leukemia: hematologic cytogenetic studies. Ann. Int. Med., 59:622, 1963.

20a. Cohen, T., and Creger, W. P.: Acute myeloid leukemia following seven years of aplastic anemia induced by chloramphenicol. Amer. J. Med., 43:762, 1967.

21. Cooke, J. V.: The occurrence of leukemia. Blood, 9:340, 1954.

22. Court-Brown, W. M., and Abatt, J. D.: The incidence of leukemia in ankylosing spondylitis treated with x-rays. A preliminary report. Lancet, 1:1283, 1955.

23. Craigie, D.: Case of disease of the spleen in which death took place in consequence of the presence of purulent matter in the blood. Edinburgh Med. & Surg. J., 64:400, 1845.

24. Cramblett, H. G., Friedman, J. L., and Najjar, S.: Leukemia in an infant born of a mother with leukemia. New England J. Med., 259:727, 1958.

25. Crosby, W. H.: To treat or not to treat acute granulocytic leukemia. Arch. Int. Med., 122:79, 1968.

26. Dalton, A. J., Rowe, W. P., Mitchell, E. Z., and Pugh, W. W.: Detection of virus particles in leukemia-lymphoma by electron microscopy. Proc. International Conference on Leukemia-Lymphoma. J. D. Zarafonetis, Ed. Lea & Febiger, Philadelphia, 1968, p. 87.

27. Dameshek, W.: The outlook for eventual control of leukemia. New England J. Med., 250:131, 1954.

28. Dameshek, W., and Baldini, M.: The Di Guglielmo syndrome. Blood, 13:192, 1958.

29. Dameshek, W., and Gunz, F.: Leukemia. Grune & Stratton, New York and London, 1964.

30. Dameshek, W., Necheles, T. F., Finkel, H. E., and Allen, D. M.: Therapy of acute leukemia, 1965. (Edit.) Blood, 26:220, 1965.

31. Diamond, H. D., Craver, L. F., Woodard, H. Q., and Parks, G. H.: Radioactive phosphorus. I. In the treatment of lymphatic leukemia. Cancer, *3*:779, 1950.
32. Di Guglielmo, G.: Acute erythremic disease. In Proceedings of the Sixth Congress of the International Society of Hematology. Grune & Stratton, New York, 1958, p. 33.
33. Doan, C., and Wiseman, B.: The monocyte, monocytosis and monocytic leukosis. Ann. Int. Med.,*8*:383, 1934.
34. Dutcher, R. M.: Viruses as etiologic factors in leukemia. In Dameshek, W., and Dutcher, R. M. (Eds.): Perspectives in Leukemia. Grune & Stratton, N.Y., 1968, p. 13.
35. Enders, J. F.: Thoughts on future contributions of virology to medicine. New England J. Med., *271*:969, 1964.
36. Ezdinli, E. Z., Sokal, J. E., Crosswhite, L., and Sandberg, A. A.: Philadelphia chromosome–positive and negative chronic myelocytic leukemia. Ann. Int. Med., *72*:175, 1970.
37. Fairbanks, V. F., Shanbrom, E., Steinfeld, J. L., and Beutler, E.: Prolonged remissions in acute myelocytic leukemia in adults. J.A.M.A., *204*:574, 1968.
38. Feinleib, M., and MacMahon, B.: Variation in the duration of survival of patients with chronic leukemias. Blood, *15*:332, 1960.
39. Folley, J. H., Borges, W., and Yamawaki, T.: Incidence of leukemia in survivors of the atomic bomb in Hiroshima and Nagasaki, Japan. Am. J. Med., *13*:311, 1952.
40. Forkner, C. E.: Clinical and pathological differentiation of acute leukemias with special reference to acute monocytic leukemia. Arch. Int. Med., *53*:1, 1934.
41. Forkner, C. E.: Leukemia and Allied Disorders. The Macmillan Co., New York, 1938.
42. Fraumeni, J. F., Vogel, C. L., and DeVita, V. T.: Familial chronic lymphocytic leukemia. Ann. Int. Med., *71*:279, 1969.
42a. Fraumeni, J. F., Jr.: Bone marrow depression induced by chloramphenicol or phenylbutazone; leukemia and other sequellae. J.A.M.A., *201*:828, 1967.
43. Freymann, J. G., Vander, J. B., Marler, E. A., and Meyer, D. G.: Prolonged corticosteroid therapy of chronic lymphocytic leukaemia and the closely allied malignant lymphomas. Brit. J. Haem., *6*:303, 1960.
44. Furth, J.: Recent studies on the etiology and nature of leukemia. Blood, *6*:964, 1951.
45. Galton, D. A. G.: Myleran in chronic myeloid leukemia. Lancet, *1*:208, 1953.
45a. Galton, D. A. G.: Chemotherapy in chronic myelocytic leukemia. Seminars in Hematol., *6*:323, 1969.
46. Gauld, W. R., Innes, J., and Robson, H. N.: A survey of 647 cases of leukemia 1938–1951. Brit. Med. J., *1*:585, 1953.
47. Gilliam, A. G.: Age, sex, and race selection at death from leukemia and the lymphomas. Blood, *8*:693, 1953.
48. Goh, K., and Swisher, S. N.: Specificity of Philadelphia chromosome: cytogenetic studies in cases of chronic myelocytic leukemia and myeloid metaplasia. Ann. Int. Med., *61*:609, 1964.
49. Goh, K., Swisher, S. N., and Herman, E. C., Jr.: Chronic myelocytic leukemia and identical twins. Arch. Int. Med., *120*:214, 1967.
50. Goh, K., Swisher, S. N., and Rosenberg, C. A.: Cytogenetic studies in eosinophilic leukemia. Ann. Int. Med.,*62*:80, 1965.
50a. Graw, R. G., Skeel, R. T., and Carbone, P. P.: Priapism in a child with chronic granulocytic leukemia. J. Pediat., *74*:788, 1969.
51. Gross, L.: Mouse Leukemia. Ann. N.Y. Acad. Sci., *54*:1184, 1952.
52. Gross, L.: A filterable agent, recovered from Ak leukemic extracts, causing salivary gland carcinomas in C3H mice. Proc. Soc. Exper. Biol. & Med., *83*:414, 1953.
53. Guasch, J.: Hérédité des Leucémies. Le sang, *25*:384, 1954.
54. Gunz, F. W.: The leukemia-lymphoma problem. Proc. International Conference on Leukemia-Lymphoma. C. J. D. Zarafonetis, Ed. Lea & Febiger, Philadelphia, 1968, p. 13.
55. Gunz, F. W., Borthwick, R. A., and Rolleston, G. L.: Acute leukemia in an infant following excessive intrauterine irradiation. Lancet, *2*:190, 1958.
56. Gunz, F. W., and Fitzgerald, P. H.: Chromosomes and leukemia. (Edit.) Blood, *23*:394, 1964.
57. Gunz, F. W., Fitzgerald, P. H., and Adams, A.: An abnormal chromosome in chronic lymphocytic leukemia. Brit. M. J., *2*:1097, 1962.
58. Gunz, F. W., and Hough, R. F.: Acute leukemia over the age of fifty. Blood, *11*:882, 1956.
59. Haddow, A., and Timmis, G. M.: Myleran in chronic myeloid leukemia. Lancet, *1*:207, 1953.
60. Hampton, J. W.: Leukocyte anticoagulant with myelogenous leukemia. Am. J. Med., *48*:408, 1970.
60a. Hansen, N. E., and Killmann, S.: Paroxysmal nocturnal hemoglobinuria in myelofibrosis. Blood, *36*:428, 1970.
60b. Haut, A., Abbott, W. S., Wintrobe, M. M., and Cartwright, G. E.: Busulfan in the treatment of chronic myelocytic leukemia. The effect of long-term intermittent therapy. Blood, *17*:1, 1961.

61. Heath, C. W., Jr., and Hasterlik, R. J.: Leukemia among children in a suburban community. Am. J. Med., *34*:796, 1963.

62. Heath, C. W., Jr., and Moloney, W. C.: The Philadelphia chromosome in an unusual case of myeloproliferative disease. Blood, *26*:471, 1965.

63. Heilmeyer, L., Mossner, G., and Hess, K.: Lymphocytic leukemia: Symptomatology and results of therapy in 160 cases. Klin. Wchnschr., *37*:790, 1959.

64. Henderson, E. S.: Treatment of acute leukemia. Seminars Hemat., *6*:271, 1969.

65. Hill, J. M., Loeb, E., and Speer, R. J.: Colloidal zirconyl phosphate P^{32} in chronic leukemia and lymphomas. J.A.M.A., *187*:106, 1964.

66. Hoffman, W. J., and Craver, L. F.: Chronic myelogenous leukemia. J.A.M.A., *97*:836, 1931.

67. Hueper, W. C.: Occupational Tumors and Allied Diseases. Charles C Thomas, Springfield, Ill., 1942, pp. 594–599.

68. Huguley, C. M., Jr., et al. (The Southeastern Cancer Chemotherapy Cooperative Study Group): Comparison of 6-mercaptopurine and busulfan in chronic granulocytic leukemia. Blood, *21*:89, 1963.

69. Hungerford, D. A.: The Philadelphia chromosome and some others. (Edit.) Ann. Int. Med., *61*:789, 1964.

70. Hyman, C. B., Bogle, J. M., Brubaker, C. A., Williams, K., and Hammond, D.: Central nervous system involvement by leukemia in children. Blood, *25*:1, 1965.

71. Igel, H. J., Huebner, R. J., Turner, H. C., Katin, P., and Falk, H. L.: Mouse leukemia virus activation by chemical carcinogens. Science, *166*:1624, 1969.

72. Kaplan, H. S.: On the etiology and pathogenesis of the leukemias: A review. Cancer Res., *14*:535, 1954.

73. Kidd, H. M., and Thomas, J. W.: Level of vitamin B_{12} in circulating leukaemic leucocytes. Brit. J. Haem., *8*:64, 1962.

74. Koler, R. D., Seaman, A. J., and Osgood, E. E.: Continuous therapy of acute leukemias— comparison of therapeutic agents. In Proceedings of the Sixth Congress of the International Society of Hematology. New York, Grune & Stratton, 1958, p. 149.

74a. Kyle, R. A., Pierre, R. V., and Bayrd, E. D.: Multiple myeloma and acute myelomonocytic leukemia. New England J. Med., *283*:1121, 1970.

75. Kyle, R. A., McParland, C. E., and Dameshek, W.: Large doses of prednisone and prednisolone in the treatment of malignant lymphoproliferative disorders. Ann. Int. Med., *57*:717, 1962.

76. Lange, R. D., Moloney, W. C., and Yamawaki, T.: Leukemia in atomic bomb survivors. Blood, *9*:574, 1954.

77. Law, L. W.: Recent advances in experimental leukemia research. Cancer Res., *14*:695, 1954.

78. Lawrence, J. H., Dobson, R. L., Low-Beer, B. V. A., and Brown, B. R.: Chronic myelogenous leukemia: A study of 129 cases in which treatment was with radioactive phosphorus. J.A.M.A., *136*:672, 1948.

79. Leavell, B. S.: Chronic leukemia. A study of the incidence and factors influencing the duration of life. Am. J. Med. Sci., *196*:329, 1938.

80. Leavell, B. S., and Twomey, J.: Possible leukemoid reaction in disseminated tuberculosis: Report of a case with Auer rods. Trans. Am. Clin. & Climatol. Assoc., *75*:166, 1964.

81. Lynch, M. J.: Monocytic leukemia. Canad. Med. Assoc. J., *70*:670, 1954.

81a. Lukes, R. I.: Pathological picture of the malignant lymphomas. Proc. International Conference on Leukemia—Lymphoma. C. J. D. Zarafonetis, Ed. Lea & Febiger, Philadelphia, 1968, p. 333.

82. MacMahon, B., and Clark, D.: Incidence of the common forms of human leukemia. Blood, *11*:871, 1956.

83. MacMahon, B., and Koller, E. K.: Ethnic differences in the incidence of leukemia. Blood, *12*:1, 1957.

84. Maduros, B. P., and Schwartz, S. O.: Viral etiology of leukemia. Advances Int. Med., *11*:107, 1962.

85. March, H. C.: Leukemia in radiologists 10 years later; with review of pertinent evidence for radiation leukemia. Am. J. M. Sc., *242*:137, 1961.

86. Miller, D. G.: Patterns of immunological deficiency in lymphomas. Ann. Int. Med., *57*:703, 1962.

87. Miller, F. R., and Turner, D. L.: The action of specific stimulators on the hematopoietic system. Am. J. M. Sc., *206*:146, 1943.

88. Miller, R. W.: The viral etiology of leukemia: an epidemiologic evaluation. Proc. International Conference on Leukemia-Lymphoma. C. J. D. Zarafonetis, Ed. Lea & Febiger, Philadelphia, 1968, p. 23.

89. Minot, G. R., Buckman, T. E., and Isaacs, R.: Chronic myelogenous leukemia. J.A.M.A., *82*:1489, 1924.

90. Minot, G. R., and Isaacs, R.: Lymphatic leukemia: Age, incidence, duration and benefit derived from irradiation. Boston Med. & Surg. J., *191*:1, 1924.

91. Modan, B., and Lilienfeld, A. M.: Polycythemia vera and leukemia. The role of radiation treatment. Medicine, *44*:305, 1965.

92. Moertel, C. G., and Hagedorn, A. B.: Leukemia or lymphoma and coexistent primary malignant lesions: A review of the literature and a study of 120 cases. Blood, *12*:788, 1957.

93. Mollin, D. L., and Ross, G. I. M.: Serum vitamin B_{12} concentrations in leukemia and in some other haematological conditions. Brit. J. Haem., *1*:155, 1955.

94. Moloney, W. C., and Kastenbaum, M. A.: Leukemogenic effects of ionizing radiation on atomic bomb survivors in Hiroshima City. Science, *121*:308, 1955.

95. Moore, E. W., Thomas, L. B., Shaw, R. K., and Freireich, E. J.: The central nervous system in acute leukemia. Arch. Int. Med., *105*:451, 1960.

96. Nesbitt, J., III, and Roth, R. E.: Solitary lytic bone lesion in an adult with chronic myelogenous leukemia. Radiology, *64*:724, 1955.

97. Nies, B. A., Bodey, G. P., Thomas, L. B., Brecher, G., and Freireich, E. J.: The persistence of extramedullary leukemia infiltrates during bone marrow remission of acute leukemia. Blood, *26*:133, 1965.

98. Nowell, P. C.: Chromosome abnormalities in human leukemia and lymphoma. Proc. International Conference on Leukemia-Lymphoma. C. J. D. Zarafonetis, Ed. Lea & Febiger, Philadelphia, 1968, p. 47.

99. Nowell, P. C., and Hungerford, D. A.: Chromosome studies on normal and leukemic human leukocytes. J. Nat. Cancer Inst., *25*:85, 1960.

100. Nowell, P. C., and Hungerford, D. A.: Chromosome studies in human leukemia. II. Chronic granulocytic leukemia. J. Nat. Cancer Inst., *27*:1013, 1961.

101. Osler, W.: In Pepper, W. A. (Ed.): System of Practical Medicine by American Authors. Vol. 11. Philadelphia, 1894, p. 215.

102. Osgood, E. E., and Seaman, A. J.: Treatment of chronic leukemias. Results of therapy by titrated regularly spaced total body radioactive phosphorus or roentgen irradiation. J.A.M.A., *150*:1372, 1952.

103. Osgood, E. E., Seaman, A. J., and Koler, R. D.: Results of a 15 year program of treatment of chronic leukemia with titrated regularly spaced total body irradiation with P^{32} or x-ray. In Proceedings of the Sixth Congress of the International Society of Hematology. New York, Grune & Stratton, 1956, p. 44.

104. Panton, P. N., and Valentine, F. C. O.: Chronic lymphoid leukemia. Lancet, *216*:914, 1929.

105. Phair, J. P., Anderson, R. E., and Namiki, H.: The central nervous system in leukemia. Ann. Int. Med., *61*:863, 1964.

105a. Propp, S., and Lizzi, F. A.: Philadelphia chromosome in acute lymphocytic leukemia. Blood, *36*:353, 1970.

106. Pruzanski, W., Platts, M. E., and Ogryzlo, M. A.: Leukemic form of immunocytic dyscrasia (plasma cell leukemia). Am. J. Med., *47*:60, 1969.

107. Pusey, W. A.: Report of cases treated with roentgen rays. J.A.M.A., *38*:911, 1902.

108. Rand, J. J., Moloney, N. C., and Sise, H. S.: Coagulation defects in acute promyelocytic leukemia. Arch. Int. Med., *123*:39, 1969.

109. Reimann, D. L., Clemmens, R. L., and Pillsbury, W. A.: Congenital acute leukemia. J. Pediat., *46*:415, 1955.

110. Reinhard, E. H., Neely, C. L., Samples, D. M.: Radioactive phosphorus in the treatment of chronic leukemias: Long-term results over a period of 15 years. Ann. Int. Med., *50*:942, 1959.

111. Reschad, H., and Schilling-Torgau, V.: Ueber ein neue Leukämie durch echte Uebergansformen (Splenozytenleukämie) und ihre Bedeutung für die Selbständigkeit dieser Zellen. München med. Wchnschr., *60*:1981, 1913.

111a. Robertson, J. H.: Pneumonia and methotrexate. Brit. Med. J., *2*:156, 1970.

112. Ross, R. R.: Chloroma and chloroleukemia. Am. J. Med., *18*:671, 1955.

113. Rubin, A. D., Douglas, S. D., Chessin, L. N., Glade, P. R., and Dameshek, W.: Chronic reticulolymphocytic leukemia. Am. J. Med., *47*:149, 1969.

114. Sacks, M. S., and Seeman, I.: A statistical study of mortality from leukemia. Blood, *2*:1, 1947.

115. Schilling, R. F., and Meyer, O. O.: Treatment of chronic granulocytic leukemia with 1,4-dimethane-sulfonyloxybutane (Myleran). New England J. Med., *254*:986, 1956.

116. Schoolman, H. M., Spurrier, W., Schwartz, S. O., and Szanto, P. B.: The induction of leukemia in Swiss mice by means of cell free filtrates of leukemic mouse brain. Blood, *12*:694, 1957.

117. Schwab, R. S., and Weiss, S.: Neurologic aspects of leukemia. Am. J. Med. Sci., *189*:766, 1935.

118. Schwartz, D. L., Pierre, R. V., Scheerer, P. S., Reed, E. C., Jr., and Linman, J. W.: Lymphosarcoma cell leukemia. Am. J. Med., *38*:778, 1965.

119. Schwartz, S. O.: Etiology of leukemia: a case for the virus theory. Blood, *11*:1045, 1956.
120. Schwartz, S. O., and Ehrlich, L.: The relationship of polycythemia vera to leukemia: a critical review. Acta Haemat., *4*:129, 1950.
121. Schwartz, S. O., Greenspan, I., and Brown, E. R.: Leukemia cluster in Niles, Illinois: immunologic data on families of leukemic patients and others. J.A.M.A., *186*:106, 1963.
122. Schwartz, S. O., Schoolman, H. M., and Szanto, P. B.: The acceleration of the development of AKR lymphoma by means of cell-free filtrates. Cancer Res., *16*:559, 1956.
123. Scott, R. B.: Leukaemia. Lancet, *1*:1053, 1957.
124. Scott, R. B.: Leukaemia. Lancet, *1*:1162, 1957.
125. Scott, R. B.: Leukaemia. Lancet, *1*:1099, 1957.
126. Sheets, R. F., Drevets, C. C., and Hamilton, H. E.: Erythroleukemia (Di Guglielmo Syndrome). Arch. Int. Med., *111*:295, 1963.
127. Shimkin, M. B., Mettier, S. R., and Bierman, H. R.: Myelocytic leukemia: an analysis of incidence, distribution, and fatality. Ann. Int. Med., *35*:194, 1951.
128. Silverman, F. N.: The skeletal lesions in leukemia. Am. J. Roentgenol., *59*:819, 1948.
129. Simpson, C. L., Hempelmann, L. H., and Fuller, L. M.: Neoplasia in children treated with x-rays in infancy for thymic enlargement. Radiology, *64*:840, 1955.
130. Sinn, C. M., and Dick, F. W.: Monocytic leukemia. Am. J. Med., *20*:588, 1956.
131. Southwest Cancer Chemotherapy Study Group: Clinical study of daunomycin and prednisone for induction of remission in children with advanced leukemia. New England J. Med., *280*:171, 1969.
132. Stasney, J., Cantarow, A., and Paschkis, K. E.: Production of neoplasms by injection of fractions of mammalian neoplasms. Cancer Res., *10*:775, 1950.
133. Stewart, A., Webb, J., Giles, D., and Hewitt, D.: Malignant disease in childhood and diagnostic irradiation in utero. Lancet, *2*:447, 1956.
134. Steinkamp, R. C., Lawrence, J. H., and Born, J. L.: Long-term experience with the use of P^{32} in the treatment of chronic lymphocytic leukemia. J. Nucl. Med., *4*:92, 1963.
135. Thomas, J. R.: Eosinophilic leukemia presenting with erythrocytosis. Blood, *22*:639, 1963.
136. Tivey, H.: Prognosis for survival in chronic granulocytic and lymphocytic leukemia. Am. J. Roentgenol., *72*:68, 1954.
137. Tobin, M. S., Kyung-Suk-Kim, and Kossowshy, W. A.: Adrenocorticotrophic-hormone deficiency in chronic myelogenous leukemia after treatment. New England J. Med., *282*:187, 1970.
138. Twomey, J. J., and Leavell, B. S.: Leukemoid reactions to tuberculosis. Arch. Int. Med., *116*:21, 1965.
139. Upton, A. C.: The role of radiation in the etiology of leukemia. Proc. International Conference on Leukemia-Lymphoma. C. J. D. Zarafonetis, Ed. Lea & Febiger, Philadelphia, 1968, p. 55.
140. Videbaek, A.: Heredity in Human Leukemia. H. K. Lewis & Co., London, 1947.
141. Virchow, R.: Weisses Blut und Milztumoren. Med. Ztg., *15*:157, 163, 1846.
142. Wintrobe, M. M., and Hasenbush, L. L.: Chronic leukemia. Arch. Int. Med., *64*:701, 1939.
143. Zacharski, L. R., and Linman, J. W.: Chronic lymphocytic leukemia versus chronic lymphosarcoma cell leukemia. Am. J. Med., *47*:75, 1969.
144. Zuelzer, W. W.: Implications of long-term survival in acute stem cell leukemia of childhood treated with composite cyclic therapy. Blood, *24*:477, 1964.
145. Zuelzer, W. W.: Therapy of acute leukemia in childhood. Proc. International Conference on Leukemia-Lymphoma. C. J. D. Zarafonetis, Ed. Lea & Febiger, Philadelphia, 1968, p. 451.
146. Zuelzer, W. W., and Flatz, G.: Acute childhood leukemia: A ten-year study. Am. J. Dis. Child., *100*:886, 1960.

MYELOID METAPLASIA

147. Anderson, R. E., Hoshino, T., and Yamamoto, T.: Myelofibrosis with myeloid metaplasia in survivors of atomic bomb in Hiroshima. Ann. Int. Med., *60*:1, 1964.
148. Block, M., and Jacobson, L. O.: Myeloid metaplasia. J.A.M.A., *143*:1390, 1950.
149. Bouroncle, B. A., and Doan, C. A.: Myelofibrosis: clinical, hematologic and pathologic study of 110 patients. Am. J. Med. Sci., *243*:697, 1962.
150. Cook, J. E., Franklin, J. W., Hamilton, H. E., and Fowler, W. M.: Syndrome of myelofibrosis. Arch. Int. Med., *91*:704, 1953.
151. Dameshek, W.: Some speculations on the myeloproliferative syndromes. Blood, *6*:372, 1951.
152. Erf, L. A., and Herbut, P. A.: Primary and secondary myelofibrosis (a clinical and pathological study of thirteen cases of fibrosis of the bone marrow). Ann. Int. Med., *21*:863, 1944.
153. Fishman, N., and Ballinger, W. F.: Splenectomy for agnogenic myeloid metaplasia and myelofibrosis. Arch. Surg., *90*:240, 1965.

154. Gardner, F. H., and Pringle, J. C., Jr.: Androgens and erythropoiesis. II. Treatment of myeloid metaplasia. New England J. Med., *264*:103, 1961.
155. Gilbert, H. S., and Wasserman, L. R.: Hemorrhage in surgery in myelofibrosis, multiple myeloma, leukemia and lymphomas. Ann. N.Y. Acad. Sci., *115* (art. 1):169, 1964.
156. Green, T. W., Conley, C. L., Ashburn, L. L., and Peters, H. R.: Splenectomy for myeloid metaplasia of the spleen. New England J. Med., *248*:211, 1953.
157. Heath, C. W., Jr., and Moloney, W. C.: The Philadelphia chromosome in an unsual case of myeloproliferative disease. Blood, *16*:471, 1965.
158. Heller, E. L., Lewisohn, M. G., and Palin, W. E.: Aleukemic myelosis. Chronic non-leukemic myelosis, agnogenic myeloid metaplasia, osteosclerosis, leukoerythroblastic anemia and synonymous designations. Am. J. Path., *23*:327, 1947.
159. Heuck, G.: Zwei Fälle von Leukämie mit eigenthümlichen Blut-resp. Knochenmarksbefund. Virchows Arch. f. Path. Anat., *78*:475, 1879.
160. Hickling, R. A.: Chronic non-leukemic myelosis. Quart. J. Med., *6*:253, 1937.
161. Hickling, R. A.: Treatment of patients with myelosclerosis. Brit. Med. J., *2*:411, 1953.
162. Hickling, R. A.: The natural history of chronic non-leukemic myeloses. Quart. J. Med., *37*:267, 1968.
163. Hutt, M. S. R., Pinninger, J. L., and Wetherley-Mein, G.: The myeloproliferative disorders. With special reference to myelofibrosis. Blood, *8*:295, 1953.
164. Jackson, H., Jr., Parker, F., Jr., and Lemon, H. M.: Agnogenic myeloid metaplasia of the spleen. A syndrome simulating other more definite hematologic disorders. New England J. Med., *222*:985, 1940.
165. Jensen, M. K.: Splenectomy in myelofibrosis. Acta. Med. Scandinav., *175*:533, 1964.
166. Kennedy, B. J.: Effect of androgenic hormone in myelofibrosis. J.A.M.A., *182*:116, 1962.
167. Koler, R. D.: Prognosis in the myelofibrosis–myeloid metaplasia syndrome. Clin. Res. Proc., *5*:57, 1957.
168. Linman, J. W., and Bethell, F. H.: Agnogenic myeloid metaplasia. Its natural history and present day management. Am. J. Med., *22*:107, 1957.
169. Lynch, E. C.: Uric acid metabolism in proliferative diseases of the marrow. Arch. Int. Med., *109*:639, 1962.
170. Mitus, W. J., Coleman, N., and Kissoglou, K. A.: Abnormal (marker) chromosomes in two patients with acute myelofibrosis. Arch. Int. Med., *123*:192, 1969.
171. Nakai, G. S., Craddock, C. G., and Figueroa, W. C.: Agnogenic myeloid metaplasia. Ann. Int. Med., *57*:419, 1962.
171a. Perillie, P. E., and Finch, S. C.: Muramidase studies in Philadelphia chromosome-positive and chromosome-negative chronic granulocytic leukemia. New England J. Med., *283*:456, 1970.
172. Pitcock, J. A., Reinhard, E. H., Justus, B. W., and Mendelsohn, R. S.: A clinical and pathological study of seventy cases of myelofibrosis. Ann. Int. Med., *57*:73, 1962.
172a. Randall, D. L., Reiquam, C. W., Githens, J. H., and Robinson, A.: Familial myeloproliferative disease: new syndrome closely simulating myelogenous leukemia in childhood. Am. J. Dis. Child., *110*:479, 1965.
173. Rawson, R., Parker, F., Jr., and Jackson, H., Jr.: Industrial solvents as possible etiologic agents in myeloid metaplasia. Science, *93*:541, 1941.
174. Roberts, B. E., Miles, D. W., and Woods, C. G.: Polycythemia vera and myelosclerosis: a bone marrow study. Brit. J. Haemat., *16*:75, 1969.
175. Schwartz, S. O., and Stansbury, F.: Significance of nucleated red blood cells in peripheral blood. J.A.M.A., *154*:1339, 1954.
176. Silver, R. T., Jenkins, D. E., Jr., and Engle, R. L., Jr.: Use of testosterone and busulfan in the treatment of myelofibrosis with myeloid metaplasia. Blood, *23*:341, 1964.
177. Silverstein, M. N., Gomes, M. R., Re-Mine, W. H., and Elveback, L. R.: Agnogenic myeloid metaplasia, natural history and treatment. Arch. Int. Med., *120*:546, 1967.
178. Szur, L., and Smith, M. D.: Red-cell production and destruction in myelosclerosis. Brit. J. Haem., *7*:147, 1960.
179. Vaughan, J. M., and Harrison, C. V.: Leuco-erythroblastic anaemia and myelosclerosis. J. Path. & Bact., *48*:339, 1939.
179a. Vigliani, E. C., and Saita, G.: Benzene and leukemia New England J. Med., *271*:872, 1964.
180. Wasserman, L. R.: Polycythemia vera—its course and treatment: Relation to myeloid metaplasia and leukemia. Bull. N.Y. Acad. Med., *30*:343, 1954.
180a. Wiernik, P. H., and Serpick, A. A.: Clinical significance of serum and urinary muramidase activity in leukemia and other hematologic malignancies. Amer. J. Med., *46*:330, 1969.
181. Wyatt, J. P., and Sommers, S. C.: Chronic marrow failure, myelosclerosis and extramedullary hematopoiesis. Blood, *5*:329, 1950.

XIV / Malignant Lymphomas (Lymphoma, Lymphoblastoma)

The Diagnosis of the Patient with Enlarged Lymph Nodes

The most accurate clinical diagnoses are made either by histologic study of diseased tissue or by the demonstration of the presence of the agent responsible for the disease. In clinical practice the physician usually begins his diagnostic examination with the history and physical examination. With the recognition of some particular sign or symptom complex, such as lymphadenopathy, the physician proceeds with the differential diagnosis by an orderly consideration of the different diseases that are known to produce the manifestations that have been observed. The probability of the presence of one or more of the diseases under consideration increases as other evidence is found that supports those particular possibilities. This evidence is obtained by a systematic study of the patient that includes various laboratory tests and special procedures, such as a biopsy. The investigation is directed toward the "probable" diseases first and specific tests for "possible" but "improbable" disorders are deferred.

Enlarged lymph nodes, which provide the focal point of the diagnostic study in certain patients, occur in a number of different diseases. Probably the commonest causes are regional infections, such as infected wounds, dermatitis, pharyngitis, sinusitis, and abscessed teeth. Lymphadenopathy also occurs with relatively benign systemic infections, such as rubella, infectious mononucleosis, and viral hepatitis, and with more serious infections, such as tuberculosis, brucellosis, syphilis, fungal diseases, and tularemia. Enlargement of lymph nodes may be due to the presence of neoplastic disease, such as metastatic carcinoma, leukemia, lymphosarcoma, Hodgkin's disease, reticulum cell sarcoma, and giant follicular lymphosarcoma. Mild degrees of enlargement occur in serum sickness and hyperthyroidism. Moderate enlargement occurs in disseminated lupus erythematosus and Boeck's sarcoid.

HISTORY

As is true with nearly all diagnostic problems, an accurate history is almost essential. Even the age of the patient is helpful information because the more benign systemic infections, such as rubella and infectious mononucleosis, are common in children and young adults but are rare in middle-aged and older persons. Both the duration of the adenopathy and the presence or absence of various symptoms help in deciding which of the possible diagnoses are more probable. The recent development of adenopathy does not exclude a neoplasm from consideration, but the persistence of enlargement for some months makes an acute infection unlikely. Localizing symptoms, such as pain and tenderness in the gland, and evidence of associated inflammation, such as pharyngitis, favor infection. A history of weight loss, recurrent fever, night sweats, and pruritus suggests the presence of systemic disease, most often one of the lymphoma group.

PHYSICAL EXAMINATION

The physical examination, particularly the characteristics of the superficial nodes, generally gives helpful information. The distribution, size, consistency, and mobility of the nodes are important, as is the presence or absence of tenderness. Probably the most important observation is whether the adenopathy is generalized or localized. If the involvement is generalized, some systemic disease becomes the primary consideration and regional adenitis can be excluded. If the involvement appears to be localized, the presence of systemic disease is not excluded but the first consideration is given to a careful search for some associated disease, either infection or neoplasm, in the area drained by the enlarged lymph nodes. In any patient with enlarged nodes, the size is estimated carefully and is best recorded in centimeters rather than in less accurate terms, such as "pea-sized" and "egg-sized." An estimate of the size of the nodes gives some indication of the probability of the presence of certain diseases. The nodes in hyperthyroidism and serum sickness are rarely more than 0.5 or 1.0 cm. in diameter; and in disseminated lupus they seldom measure more than 1.0 to 3.0 cm. In the diseases of the lymphoma group the nodes are sometimes greatly enlarged. Careful estimations of the size of the nodes, and the constancy of the size, are helpful in following the progress of the disease while the patient is under observation. The presence of tenderness in a node usually indicates that infection is present but marked tenderness also occurs in the nodes of some patients with other diseases, particularly Hodgkin's disease. Fixation of a node to the skin or deeper tissues indicates that the infection or neoplasm has involved the surrounding area. Sinus tracts or scars over an area of adenopathy suggest tuberculosis or fungal disease. A relatively small node that is stony hard in

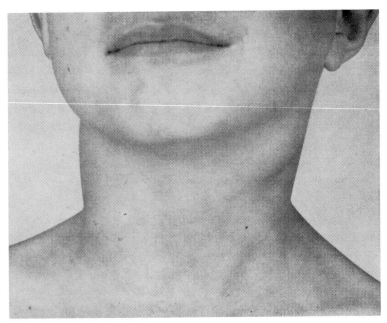

Figure 14–1. Enlargement of cervical lymph node in a patient with Hodgkin's disease.

consistency suggests metastatic carcinoma, but extremely hard nodes that measure several centimeters in diameter also occur with calcification, in sarcoma, and in tuberculosis. In diseases of the lymphoma group characteristically the nodes are moderately firm, rubbery, and somewhat resilient, but many exceptions occur. The normal bean-shaped contour of the node is more apt to be maintained with infection than with neoplasm.

Other details of the physical examination are also important. The detection of a focus of infection in an area related anatomically to the adenopathy usually warrants a diagnosis of regional adenitis. The presence of splenomegaly and hepatomegaly suggests some generalized infectious process or a disease of the lymphoma group. If the spleen is firm and extends halfway to the level of the umbilicus or below, it is probable that the patient has some chronic disorder such as a disease of the lymphoma group rather than an acute infection, such as infectious mononucleosis or viral hepatitis.

LABORATORY EXAMINATION

Laboratory examinations sometimes establish the diagnosis in patients with large lymph nodes and at other times permit the exclusion of certain diseases from further consideration. The routine studies of the blood, such as the hematocrit, leukocyte count, and differential count, are indicated. By such means leukemia usually can be detected if present and the diagnosis of other diseases, such as infectious mononucleosis, can be provisionally established or excluded. An increase in the granulocytes favors bacterial infection or Hodgkin's disease and an increase in "pathologic" lymphocytes favors infectious mononucleosis or a viral infection. Monocytosis suggests Hodgkin's disease, tuberculosis, or brucellosis. The presence of anemia indicates that the patient probably has more than a localized acute infection. More definitive information is provided by specific examinations such as the heterophil agglutination test and agglutination tests for brucellosis and tularemia. Skin tests for tuberculosis and fungal diseases are sometimes helpful. Repeated attempts may be necessary to demonstrate the presence of "lupus erythematosus cells." In certain patients other studies, such as the electrophoretic study of the serum proteins and aspiration of bone marrow to obtain material for culture and cytologic study, are important.

ROENTGENOGRAPHIC EXAMINATION

Roentgenographic examinations often give valuable information about the nature of the process that is manifested by enlargement of the superficial nodes. A roentgenogram of the chest is usually necessary in order to detect disease in the lungs and determine the presence of involvement of the nodes in the hilar areas or mediastinum. The location, number, and appearance of the lesions in the lung may indicate the probability of tuberculosis, fungal disease, primary or metastatic carcinoma, or other disease. Details of the appearance and location of the involved nodes in the hilar areas and mediastinum may help to distinguish between Boeck's sarcoid and one of the lymphoma group. Examination of the gastrointestinal tract may reveal the presence of a primary carcinoma that was first suggested by the presence of Virchow's node behind the origin of the left sternocleidomastoid muscle. Radiologic evidence of diffuse infiltration of the stomach and hypertrophied rugal folds favors lymphosarcoma over Hodgkin's disease and other disorders that may present with superficial adenopathy. Evidence of skeletal involvement indicates that the adenopathy is part of a serious disorder even though the roentgenographic appearance of the osseous lesion may not permit the differentiation between the several possibilities.

LYMPH NODE BIOPSY

If the diagnosis is not made by other means, biopsy of a lymph node is often necessary. The decision as to the need for a biopsy is reached after an evaluation of each patient individually. In one situation it may be apparent at the initial examination that a biopsy should be done promptly; in another circumstance it may be decided that biopsy can be deferred for further observation and the performance of other tests. If an undiagnosed enlargement of the lymph node in an adult does not subside significantly within a few weeks, biopsy is nearly always indicated.

Although no fast rules can be made for the performance of the biopsy, the observance of some simple guides is helpful to both the pathologist and the clinician. Although the pathologist bases his diagnosis on the histologic appearance of the specimen, it is helpful if pertinent clinical data are submitted along with the biopsy specimen. It is important that the pathologist receive representative tissue that is suitable for study. If more than one node is enlarged, the selection of the one to be biopsied is important. In general, cervical or supraclavicular nodes are preferable to axillary nodes; nodes from all of these sites are preferable to nodes from the femoral area because the latter often have undergone alteration as a result of previous infection in the lower extremities. When the patient has a disease that involves the lymph nodes without significant enlargement of the superficial lymph nodes, frequently the diagnosis can be established by a supraclavicular biopsy, or percutaneous liver biopsy; on occasion thoracotomy or laparotomy may be necessary to establish a diagnosis. Whenever possible the biopsy is performed and the diagnosis established before the patient receives any specific therapy, because both irradiation and chemotherapy can so change the appearance of the node that histologic diagnosis is difficult or impossible. Careful handling of the node at the time of operation is important because trauma can distort the histologic appearance of the lesion. Even when the diagnosis seems certain and infectious processes seem to be excluded, it is advisable to send part of the node for histologic examination and part for bacteriologic study. Unless this is done, even tuberculosis or a fungal infection may pass unrecognized. If the biopsy of a node does not provide a definite diagnosis, a second biopsy may be indicated; if no suitable node is available at the time, periodic examination for the appearance of such a node is advisable.

FURTHER STUDY

If the biopsy establishes a diagnosis of Hodgkin's disease or some other lymphoma, further examinations to disclose the extent of the disease are necessary to determine the stage of the disease. These examinations include x-ray of the chest, inferior vena cavogram, lymphangiograms, liver function tests, and liver biopsy; on occasion laparotomy may be necessary.

Classification

Malignant lymphoma is a term used to designate a group of diseases — Hodgkin's disease, lymphosarcoma, reticulum cell sarcoma, giant follicle lymphoma, and more uncommon related disorders — that have certain features in common. These diseases, which involve mainly the lymphoid structures of the body, cannot be distinguished from each other by their clinical manifestations. An accurate diagnosis is made only by microscopic study of a specimen of involved tissue, usually a lymph node. Although of unknown etiology, the diseases are generally considered to be neoplastic in nature.

The term "malignant lymphoma" is a convenient one for various reasons. In clinical practice it provides a designation for a provisional diagnosis until a more accurate one can be made. In addition, the histologic study of biopsy material sometimes makes it possible to place a disorder in this group of diseases even though a more precise diagnosis cannot be made with certainty. In this circumstance the patient often can be treated properly without benefit of an accurate diagnosis because the same principles of therapy and the same therapeutic agents are used in the management of the different diseases. It is convenient to group these diseases for the purpose of a clinical discussion because of the similarities in clinical manifestations, methods of diagnosis, treatment, and prognosis.

Hodgkin's disease is named after Thomas Hodgkin who first described the disorder in 1832.[32] In 1893 Kundrat recognized lymphosarcoma as a disease entity different from leukemia.[43] Giant follicular lymphoma, sometimes called "Brill-Symmers disease," was described by Brill, Baehr, and Rosenthal in 1925[9] and by Symmers in 1927.[77] Roulet has been given credit for first clearly identifying reticulum cell sarcoma as a distinct type of tumor.[71]

Numerous classifications have been proposed for this group of diseases that involve the lymphoid tissue primarily. The classification shown here, which divides the lymphomas into four main groups, is a useful one for clinical purposes.

Classification of Malignant Lymphomas

1. Hodgkin's disease.
2. Lymphosarcoma.
3. Reticulum cell sarcoma.
4. Giant follicular lymphoma (Brill-Symmers disease, nodular lymphoblastoma).

Some idea of the relative frequency of these diseases is given by the diagnoses made in one series of 618 cases of "lymphoma." When classified according to the aforementioned system, the various forms of Hodgkin's disease constituted 37 per cent, lymphosarcoma 35 per cent, reticulum cell sarcoma 20 per cent, and giant follicle lymphoma 8 per cent.[27] Lukes, who advocates discarding the term "reticulum cell sarcoma" and questions whether Hodgkin's disease should be included in the lymphoma group, has proposed the classification of the malignant lymphomas and their relationship to the various kinds of leukemia that is shown in Table 14–1.[53]

Although a specific diagnosis can usually be made by the histologic study of involved tissue, at times the pathologist may have difficulty in identifying the disease from the study of material obtained by biopsy. Different nodes from the same patient have been diagnosed as different diseases and changes considered to be characteristic of Hodgkin's disease, sarcoma, and giant follicle lymphoma have been reported in the same lymph node.[78] The apparent transition of giant follicle lymphoma into the other diseases in the group is well known.[15, 78] In one series of 84 patients with malignant lymphoma, biopsies were repeated after intervals that varied from 1 month to 15 years (average 2.3 years) and a histologic

Table 14–1. *Classification of Malignant Lymphomas and Leukemia*

MALIGNANT LYMPHOMA	LEUKEMIA
Diffuse or nodular	
1. Lymphocytic (well differentiated)	1. Chronic lymphocytic leukemia
2. Lymphocytic (poorly differentiated)	2. Lymphosarcoma cell leukemia
3. Stem cell	3. "Stem cell" or acute lymphocytic leukemia
4. Histiocytic	4. Histiocytic leukemia; monocytic leukemia (Schilling type)
5. Hodgkin's disease	

diagnosis different from the initial one was made in 23 per cent; in most instances the lesion had become less differentiated in appearance.[27] In another series a transition from the biopsy material was found in 39 per cent of the autopsied cases; in over one-half of the autopsies lesions of more than one of the lymphoma group occurred.[15] Although many pathologists consider that the histologic features of these diseases, with the exception of giant follicle lymphoma, remain relatively constant, the inconstancy that has been noted in some cases has led to the suggestion that the whole lymphoma group is but a single neoplastic entity that has a number of variants.[15]

Hodgkin's Disease

The extensive literature on Hodgkin's disease that appeared prior to 1948 has been the subject of several excellent reviews.[34, 36] The clinical manifestations, histologic appearance, methods of diagnosis, and variable natural history of the disease are well established. Despite the numerous attempts that have been made to solve the problem, the cause (or causes) of Hodgkin's disease has not been established. A recent review indicates that the data suggestive of a viral etiology are increasing. Although the occurrence of Hodgkin's disease in association with other diseases, notably tuberculosis and fungal infections, has suggested more than a chance association, all efforts to establish tuberculosis, the avian tubercle bacillus, diphtheroids, and other bacilli and fungi as causes of Hodgkin's disease have proved unsuccessful.[8, 34, 41]

The varied clinical manifestations of Hodgkin's disease may appear at any age and in either sex. The disease occurred most frequently in the third decade in one series[74] but in another study an even distribution was found in the first seven decades.[36] Males are affected more commonly than females, the ratio being about two to one.[27, 74]

The clinical manifestations of Hodgkin's disease are varied because virtually any organ in the body may be involved by the disease process. The incidence of lesions in various locations noted, either during life or at autopsy, in two series that totaled 485 patients[30, 35] are as follows: lungs, 33 per cent; mediastinum, 33 per cent; liver and spleen, 50 per cent and 70 per cent; skin, "common," and 38 per cent; bones, 20 per cent and 7 per cent. Involvement of the nervous system occurred in 12 per cent of another series.[75] Actual renal involvement occurs in only 13 per cent of patients with Hodgkin's disease; ureteral obstruction, at times bilateral, caused by disease in the pelvis is much more common. Retroperitoneal fibrosis has produced the same picture.[42] The disease is rarely found in the tonsils, but the salivary glands are involved in some patients.

Although nearly any sign or symptom may be the presenting one, the commonest initial symptom is painless enlargement of one or more lymph nodes. An initial manifestation of this sort, usually in the cervical nodes, occurs in about 85 per cent of patients with Hodgkin's disease.[35] The initial sites of involvement in one series were as follows: superficial lymph nodes in the cervical region, 60 to 80 per cent; axillary lymph nodes, 6 to 20 per cent; inguinal lymph nodes, 6 to 12 per cent; mediastinal lymph nodes, 6 to 11 per cent. Enlargement of the retroperitoneal lymph nodes, liver, and spleen were seen less commonly in the early stages.[79] The next most frequent symptoms are pain in the back, abdomen, or chest, weakness, loss of weight, and fever. Cough, dyspnea, and pruritus occur less often but are not rare. Severe pain in the abdomen, back, or chest after the ingestion of alcohol is a rare but striking symptom in some patients; the mechanism of the pain, which also occurs in other malignancies, is unknown.

Pruritus is an unusual early symptom in patients with Hodgkin's disease but develops in many during the course of the illness. This symptom, which is considered to be a sign of activity of underlying disease, may be extremely disagreeable and difficult to control unless the disease undergoes a remission.

Fever occurs sometime during the course of the disease in nearly every patient with Hodgkin's disease. The fever may be continuous, intermittent, or cyclic. An irregular type of fever that rises to 100° to 103° F at night occurs frequently and generally signifies that the disease is not confined to the superficial lymph nodes. The well known "Murchison" or "Pel-Ebstein" type of fever occurs in only a minority of patients. In this syndrome the temperature curve shows successive daily rises over a period of about a week until it reaches a peak of 103° to 105°, then subsides gradually to normal. After an interval of 10 days to 2 months, another febrile episode appears. The periods of remission gradually shorten unless the course of the disease is changed by therapy. When this type of fever occurs it generally signifies mediastinal or intra-abdominal disease. A remittent type of fever similar to that seen in septicemia occurs in some patients with the acute fulminating type of Hodgkin's disease, even in the absence of demonstrable infection.

The immunologic status of many patients with Hodgkin's disease is abnormal.[60] Characteristically, there is impairment of the delayed hypersensitivity reaction, as measured by the response to tuberculin and other antigens, particularly those of fungal origin, and impairment of homograft rejection. Patients with localized disease may react normally to these tests; reactivity diminishes in those with more advanced stages of the disease. In advanced Hodgkin's disease, a state of "lymphocytic paralysis" develops; immunologic impairment has been correlated with the degree of lymphocyte reduction, either in the peripheral blood or in the lymph nodes. The impaired reactivity seen in patients with the active disease may improve, and even return to normal, when treatment induces a remission. Associated with the immunologic defect in Hodgkin's disease is an increased incidence of tuberculosis, cryptococcosis, histoplasmosis, nocardial infections, and various viral and bacterial infections, particularly in the late stages of the disease.

The presence of disease in the nervous system most often becomes evident because of pressure on the spinal cord or the fifth, sixth, seventh, eighth, or ninth cranial nerve.[75] Involvement of the brain is generally associated with disease of the cranial bones and the epidural tumor that causes cord compression is nearly always an extension from a lesion in a vertebra or from the adjacent mediastinal or retroperitoneal lymph nodes. Peripheral neuritis in the lower extremities is a troublesome symptom in some patients; non-invasive peripheral neuropathy is unusual but it is sometimes severe. Acute paraplegia and massive necroses affecting both the gray and the white matter in the cord associated with a pathologic picture different from "progressive multifocal leukoencephalopathy" have been reported in patients with Hodgkin's sarcoma and nodular lymphoblastoma who had no invasion of the spinal cord by tumor.[65] It appears likely that the attacks of herpes zoster, which are fairly common, are caused by involvement of the ganglia by the herpes virus rather than by Hodgkin's disease because the herpetic lesions disappear spontaneously without treatment (Fig. 14–2).

Hodgkin's disease involving the gastrointestinal tract is found in 20 to 50 per cent of autopsied patients, but primary involvement is rare, occurring in approximately 3 per cent.[23, 38] Approximately 50 patients with primary involvement of the small bowel have been reported.[21] In one series of 123 autopsied patients with Hodgkin's disease, 22 had lesions in the gastrointestinal tract, 16 in the stomach, 2 in the small intestines, and 4 in the colon. Nontumorous involvement of the gastrointestinal tract produced symptoms such as bleeding or obstruction more often than actual involvement by tumor did. Involvement of the gastrointestinal tract is a sign of poor prognosis. The survival time of the patients who have pain or a mass in the abdomen, vomiting, or bleeding is no more than half that of those without these manifestations; 75 per cent have been considered unsuitable for surgery or have died shortly after surgical operation, and only a small number have survived for more than 6 months.

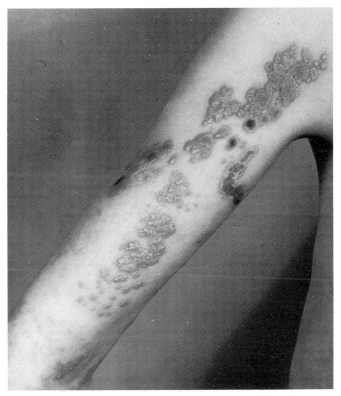

Figure 14–2. Herpes zoster in a patient with Hodgkin's disease.

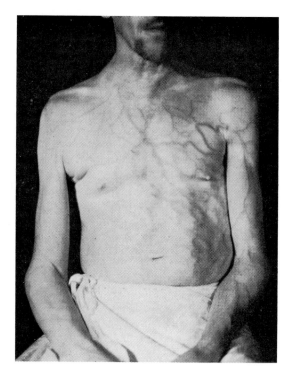

Figure 14-3. Infrared photograph demonstrating collateral circulation in a patient with Hodgkin's disease and superior vena caval obstruction.

Jaundice occurs in from 3 to 8 per cent of patients with Hodgkin's disease.[49] Antemortem diagnosis of the cause of jaundice may be difficult. In autopsies on 57 jaundiced patients, the causes of jaundice were: liver involvement with Hodgkin's disease, 70.2 per cent; no satisfactory explanation, 14.0 per cent; hemolytic anemia, 5.2 per cent; extrahepatic obstruction due to tumor, 3.5 per cent; hepatitis, 3.5 per cent; choledocholithiasis, 1.8 per cent; cirrhosis, 1.8 per cent. Although the jaundice may last from a few days to a year, in more than 90 per cent of the cases its appearance is a preterminal event. Treatment is largely ineffective when the icterus is caused by intrahepatic involvement.

The variety of clinical manifestations that Hodgkin's disease may produce has been emphasized.[35, 56] Pruritus or exfoliative dermatitis may be the first manifestation of the disease. Disease in the intrathoracic region may present as an asymptomatic mediastinal tumor found on the roentgenogram or with evidence of the superior mediastinal syndrome (see Fig. 14-2). Intrathoracic disease may also be responsible for an unproductive cough, dyspnea, or pleural effusion. The first evidence of the disease sometimes appears in the abdominal region in the form of a retroperitoneal tumor, splenomegaly, or hepatomegaly. Skeletal involvement, which is most likely to occur in the vertebrae, is usually associated with pain that may be present for weeks before an osseous lesion is demonstrable in the roentgenograms. Hodgkin's disease is often found to be the cause of a persistent "fever of undetermined origin." In still other patients splenomegaly, anemia, and other abnormalities in the peripheral blood are the principal manifestations of the disease.

Abnormalities that are demonstrable by physical examination depend on

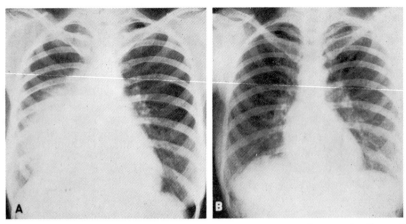

Figure 14–4. Chest roentgenograms of a patient with Hodgkin's disease. The diagnosis of the intrathoracic tumor (*A*) was established by biopsy. The patient responded unusually well to radiation and had no evidence of recurrence 12 years later (*B*). Although treated for recurrence of disease in the neck and elsewhere, she has no clinical evidence of disease 28 years after diagnosis. A review of her biopsy disclosed Hodgkin's disease, nodular sclerotic type.

the presence of the disease in various organs or systems in different parts of the body. Most commonly the lymph nodes, spleen, and liver are involved. The degree of lymphadenopathy, which is usually greatest in the cervical region, varies from slight to marked. The nodes are usually firm and rubbery in consistency, but may be either soft or stony hard. They are rarely tender and usually are not fixed to the skin or underlying structures. Occasionally the size of the nodes, especially in the cervical and submandibular areas, varies spontaneously from day to day. Palpable splenomegaly occurs in about from 50 to 70 per cent of patients at some stage of the disease. The degree of enlargement found in different patients varies from a barely palpable spleen to one that nearly fills the entire left half of the abdominal cavity; usually the lower edge of the spleen is above the level of the umbilicus. Less commonly the examination reveals evidence of ascites, pleural effusion, pericardial effusion, superior vena caval obstruction, and neurologic involvement.

Laboratory examinations often disclose abnormalities, particularly in the peripheral blood. Normocytic anemia of some degree occurs in nearly all patients at some time during the course of the disease. Very rarely pancytopenia is present when the patient is first seen. The anemia is usually the result of diminished erythropoiesis but in some patients increased hemolysis is important. The total and differential leukocyte counts are often normal early in the disease but a transitory increase in lymphocytes sometimes occurs. An increase in blood platelets and an absolute increase in monocytes have been reported to be constant throughout the disease.[10] In the more advanced stages of the disease leukocyte counts often rise to levels of 15,000 to 20,000 per cu.mm. or more. The leukocytosis is associated with an increase in cells of the granulocytic series and a decrease in lymphocytes.[1, 10] Often, in the late stages, when lymphocytic paralysis develops very few lymphocytes, 1000 cu.mm. or less, are found in the circulating blood. Eosinophilia of considerable degree occurs in some patients. Toxic granulation is often prominent and large bizarre platelets are often present. The erythrocyte sedimentation rate is usually elevated and the leukocyte alkaline phosphatase reaction increased when the disease is active. The electrophoretic pattern of the serum proteins may reveal a reduction in albumin associated with an increase in globulin in the moderately advanced cases. Abnormalities in the proteins similar to those found commonly in multiple myeloma sometimes occur in Hodgkin's disease when there is an increase in plasma cells.[3, 45] Reed-Sternberg cells can be found in bone marrow smears only rarely, but the diagnosis has been made in 25 per cent of patients when aspirated bone marrow was studied in paraffin sections;[64] such a result probably indicates a sample which includes a large percentage of Stage IV patients. Massive proteinuria is seen in some patients with Hodgkin's disease who develop amyloidosis.[13a] (F.S.: II, 89, 90, 91)

Lymphosarcoma and Reticulum Cell Sarcoma

Lymphosarcoma and reticulum cell sarcoma occur at any age but the highest incidence is found in the fifth and sixth decades. The incidence in males is approximately twice that in females.[27, 76]

The first evidence of disease is usually visible and palpable enlargement of superficial lymph nodes. In one series of 1269 patients the disease made its appearance in this way in 65 per cent.[68] The cervical nodes were involved in 35 per cent and the axillary, inguinal, and abdominal nodes were each involved in about 12 per cent; mediastinal involvement was much less common. Intra-abdominal and mediastinal lymphosarcoma are causes of initial symptoms much more often in children than in adults. The involved nodes, which are generally moderately firm and resilient, are movable unless local invasion has occurred.

Although lymphosarcoma, reticulum cell sarcoma, and Hodgkin's disease cannot be distinguished from each other by the clinical manifestations in the individual patient, the diseases follow somewhat different patterns. Splenomegaly is less common and auto-immune hemolytic anemia is more common in lymphosarcoma than in Hodgkin's disease (20 per cent compared to 50 to 70 per cent),[35, 76] fever occurs less often,[27] and anemia develops later.[76] The "Murchison-Pel-Ebstein" type of fever curve, which was observed during the course of the disease in 16 per cent of one group of patients with Hodgkin's disease, is rare in other members of the lymphoma group.[27] Nearly any organ in the body can be involved by either of these diseases. Intrathoracic disease is the presenting symptom in only 5 per cent of patients with lymphosarcoma but about one-half of them develop clinical evidence of such involvement during the course of the disease; in 35 per cent it is mediastinal, 30 per cent pleural, and 20 per cent lungs. No part of the body is immune to involvement.

Lesions of the gastrointestinal tract occur more commonly than in Hodgkin's disease;[27, 35, 76] in lymphosarcoma and reticulum cell sarcoma, the clinical incidence is reported to be 10 per cent and the frequency at autopsy 50 per cent.[68] The stomach, small intestine, or colon may be involved.

In an autopsy series of 125 patients with reticulum cell sarcoma, 50 per cent had the disease in the gastrointestinal tract. The small intestine was involved most often, but lesions occurred frequently in the stomach and colon.[23] The report also included 75 patients with lymphosarcoma; 27 per cent had involvement of the gastrointestinal tract, most often in the stomach or colon. As in patients with Hodgkin's disease, involvement of the gastrointestinal tract with these diseases, except as the initial manifestation, was a sign of poor prognosis. Clinical symptoms such as bleeding, obstruction, and perforation occurred as often in patients without actual involvement of the gastrointestinal tract as in those with invasion; in the former group ulceration, sometimes associated with prednisone and other therapy, was a frequent problem. The gastric lesion most often consists of a diffuse infiltration that may be recognized on the roent-genologic examination of the stomach because of the presence of exaggerated, stiffened rugae and diminished peristalsis. The most frequent site of disease in the small bowel is the terminal ileum, where the lesion may produce bleeding or intestinal obstruction.

Renal involvement, which is often not recognized clinically, occurs in about half of the patients with lymphosarcoma and reticulum cell sarcoma. In one group of patients, actual renal involvement occurred in 39 per cent of those with lymphosarcoma and in 46 per cent of those with reticulum cell sarcoma. Various types of involvement occur.[42] The most common lesions are multiple

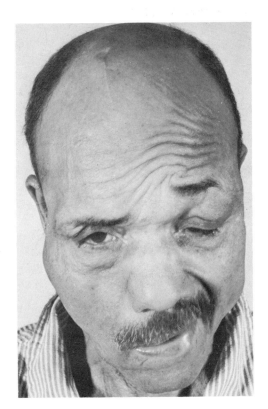

Figure 14–5. Lymphosarcoma involving the parotid gland with facial paralysis.

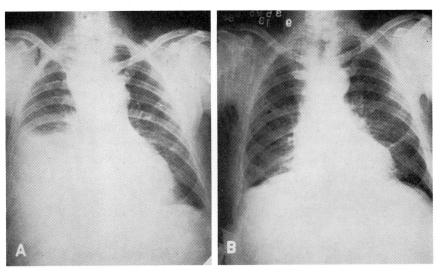

Figure 14–6. Chest roentgenograms in a patient with lymphosarcoma, showing mediastinal adenopathy and hydrothorax before therapy (*A*); appearance after irradiation (*B*).

nodules, cortical infiltration, possible evidence of the leukemic transformation, and invasion from a retroperitoneal tumor. More than half the patients have some impairment of the renal function, most often from disease outside the genitourinary tract, obstruction from tumors, or retroperitoneal fibrosis before the disease has run its course. The typical picture of the nephrotic syndrome occurs in some patients. At times renal vein thrombosis may be the responsible mechanism, but in other patients neither involvement by tumor nor vascular complications can be found; in these patients an abnormality in immunologic mechanism has been postulated. Other forms of renal disease that occur are amyloidosis and post-radiation nephritis.

Involvement of the nasopharynx and tonsillar areas, rare in Hodgkin's disease, occurs oftener in lymphosarcoma. Lesions of the nervous system and skeleton occur more frequently in reticulum cell sarcoma than in lymphosarcoma.[27] When reticulum cell sarcoma involves the skeleton, the disease is usually widespread; in some patients, however, the disease appears to be primary in bone, and in these 50 per cent have been reported to have 5 years of survival after radiotherapy.[80]

Abnormalities occur in both the peripheral blood and bone marrow of many patients with lymphosarcoma and reticulum cell sarcoma. Lymphocytosis of the peripheral blood, which is sometimes due partly to an increase in the large lymphocytes, is seen more often in these disorders than in Hodgkin's disease. Some patients who are diagnosed as having lymphosarcoma later develop the peripheral blood picture of lymphocytic leukemia; this occurred in 7.3 per cent of adults and 13 per cent of children in one series.[67] Acute leukemia was extremely rare except in children. Eosinophilia and polymorphonuclear leukocytosis sometimes occur but are less frequent than in Hodgkin's disease. At times patients with lymphosarcoma present with splenomegaly with or without evidence of hypersplenism. In some the disease progresses slowly to involve the intra-abdominal lymph nodes and then the bone marrow. In this stage, when the total leukocyte count and the differential count are normal or nearly so and the bone marrow is infiltrated with small lymphocytes, either as nodules or as diffuse involvement, it is difficult to know whether to make a diagnosis of "aleukemic lymphocytic leukemia" or "lymphosarcoma with involvement of the bone marrow." In some patients the disease progresses to a more characteristic picture of chronic lymphocytic leukemia with predominance of small lympho- cytes in the peripheral blood. Other patients with lymphosarcoma, possibly those whose tumors contain the larger cell types, develop a picture of "leukosar- coma" characterized by the presence of cells resembling immature large lympho- cytes; some cells have nucleoli and others have indented or folded nuclei. The "leukemoid" picture in these patients may persist or may be transient. Similar changes occur in some patients with reticulum cell sarcoma; these are not as frequent but sometimes develop late in the disease, most often in the last few months. (F.S.: II, 86, 88)

Hemolytic anemia of the auto-immune type occurs in some patients and at times is accompanied by thrombocytopenia. The antiglobulin (Coombs) test is positive in at least half of the patients with malignant lymphoma who develop severe hemolytic anemia;[44] in some reports on the association of auto-immune hemolytic disease and lymphoma, only patients with positive tests are included.[70] Abnormalities in the serum protein, such as moderate decreases in albumin and gamma globulin and moderate increases in the alpha-1 and alpha-2 fractions, occur commonly; the occurrence of "myeloma-type" proteins is not rare.[3] An increased percentage of lymphocytes and an increase in the number of large mononuclear or reticulum cells in the bone marrow suggest the diagnosis of lymphosarcoma or reticulum cell sarcoma. When material obtained by aspira- tion of the marrow is studied by the paraffin section method, a positive diagnosis may be made in some of the patients with reticulum cell sarcoma. In lympho- sarcoma and giant follicle lymphoma a positive diagnosis can be made less often in this way.[64]

Giant Follicular Lymphoma

Giant follicular lymphoma (nodular lymphoblastoma, Brill-Symmers dis- ease) is about two and a half times as common in males as in females and occurs most often in the fifth or sixth decade.[27, 28] Less than 5 per cent of the cases occur in individuals under 20 years of age. This disorder has a more benign course than the other members of the lymphoma group but its tendency to undergo transition to lymphosarcoma, reticulum cell sarcoma, Hodgkin's disease, and lymphocytic leukemia is recognized.[4, 15, 24, 27, 28, 78] (F.S.: II, 85)

Transformation into another type of lymphoma usually occurs after the disease has been present for 5 years. The most frequent transformation in one group of 64 patients was to lymphosarcoma;[26] other patients developed reticulum cell sarcoma, chronic lymphocytic leukemia, and acute leukemia; in this series transformation into Hodgkin's disease did not occur. The 5-year survival was

72 per cent; 10 years, 60 per cent; and 15 years, 40 per cent. All of the patients who died had lymphosarcoma or leukemia.

The most common initial manifestation is enlargement of the superficial lymph nodes or spleen. The involvement of the nodes is usually more or less generalized but localized disease also occurs. In one report the disease appeared to be localized at onset in one-half and generalized in one-third.[26] Twenty per cent developed lesions in the vertebrae or other parts of the skeleton; none had neurological involvement. Enlargement of the mediastinal nodes may produce marked impairment of respiration. Enlargement of the retroperitoneal, mesenteric, and mediastinal nodes is common. The presence of the disease in these locations is often associated with ascites or hydrothorax and the frequent occurrence of chylous ascites has been reported. The incidence of splenomegaly in giant follicular lymphoma is reported to be 33 per cent.[28] Fever, cachexia, and other constitutional manifestations are rare. Although anemia is unusual until late in the disease,[4, 28] the frequent development of hemolytic anemia, thrombocytopenic purpura, and leukopenia in patients with splenomegaly has been reported.[24] Involvement of the skin, nervous system, and skeleton is rare.

Although radiotherapy has been reported to produce the best results in patients with this disease even when the disorder is not localized,[26] some patients respond well to small doses of chemotherapeutic agents for a number of years.

Other Disorders

Mycosis Fungoides

Mycosis fungoides is usually considered to be a form of malignant lymphoma of the skin.[7] The most common initial manifestation is some benign or nonspecific dermatitis, such as psoriasiform or neurodermatitis. After an interval that varies from months to decades, but which is usually several years, cutaneous tumors appear in all cases; in some patients the tumors are apparent at the onset. Infection, especially staphylococcal septicemia or pneumonia (or some other disease), may lead to the death at this stage of disease; in this circumstance autopsy discloses no evidence of lymph node or visceral involvement by malignant lymphoma. Most often adenopathy appears, accompanied by visceral involvement; histologic study of the nodes or the visceral lesions shows either a transition phase between normal and lymphoma or a definite malignant lymphoma which often is difficult to classify precisely. Although nearly all patients with mycosis fungoides are dead within 3 years after the diagnosis is established, an occasional patient lives more than 10 years after adenopathy appears. Patients with a localized cutaneous form of the disease sometimes remain well for decades and die from some other cause.

The disease is usually treated by radiation or the alkylating agents combined with topical measures. Topical nitrogen mustard is the treatment of choice for treating skin plaques.[31a] The regime used at the University of Virginia utilizes a solution of 10 mg. of HN_2 in 20 ml. of distilled water. A physician or nurse wearing rubber gloves applies sterile 4 × 4 gauze flats soaked in the solution to the lesions for 5 minutes; in intertriginous areas the soaks are applied for only 1 minute. The treatment usually is given three times a week for 1 week. Advanced disease is treated by radiotherapy, intravenous nitrogen mustard, chlorambucil, or methotrexate.[31a] In the advanced stage, severe pruritus and widespread ulcerating infected lesions may present a distressing problem, one that taxes the ingenuity of the physician and the fortitude of the patient.

Burkitt's Tumor

This disorder, now considered to be a lymphoma, was described first in 1958 by Burkitt, who observed the disease in 38 Ugandan children between the ages of 2 and 14.[11] Its most characteristic feature is rapidly growing osteolytic tumors that involve one or more quadrants of the jaw; tumors also occur in the salivary glands, kidneys, adrenals, liver, heart, retroperitoneum, and other sites. Central nervous system involvement, manifested by cranial nerve palsies and paraplegia from compression, is common but usually responds well to treatment. The disease differs from the other types of lymphoma in that involvement of the superficial lymph nodes and the spleen is uncommon or minimal. This lymphoma is a disease of childhood, and in parts of Africa it comprises half of the tumors in children under 14 years of age. The distribution of the disease across Equatorial Africa has led to the suggestion that it is caused by an arthropod-borne virus.

The tumor is a malignant neoplasm of predominantly undifferentiated lymphoreticular cells which have a uniform and characteristic appearance in tissue sections and imprints.[13] The recommended classification is "malignant lymphoma, undifferentiated Burkitt's type." The disease is not confined to the continent of Africa; a number of patients have been reported from the United States and other parts of the world. In American patients, the jaw is involved less often than it is in the African cases, but the ovary, the intra-abdominal organs, and the bone marrow are involved more often. Patients with the African form of the disease rarely have a terminal leukemic blood picture, but this has developed in about 30 per cent of the American series. (F.S.: II, 92)

Untreated Burkitt's lymphoma follows a rapidly fatal course (death usually occurs in less than 6 months), but the disease apparently responds well to treatment with cyclophosphamide, 40 mg. per kg. intravenously. About two-thirds of the patients, even some of those with Stage III and IV disease, obtain complete remission on such treatment. In 9 patients treated with x-ray and a variety of chemotherapeutic agents, the mean survival time was only 2.5 months; in a group of 12 patients who received six or more injections of cyclophosphamide intravenously at intervals of 3 or 4 weeks, six patients survived from 52 to 112 weeks. Neurological involvement which occurred in some patients responded well to intrathecal methotrexate, 10 mg. weekly for a minimum of four courses.[13]

The serologic aspects of Burkitt's tumor have created considerable interest. Although these have not been completely clarified, in every clinically confirmed case of African Burkitt's tumor the patient has had high levels of antibodies against a herpes-like virus; only 50 to 60 per cent of other Africans have similar titers. The herpes-like virus appears to be widely distributed in man. In young adults it is associated with infectious mononucleosis. The exact relationship of this virus to Burkitt's tumor and other diseases has not been defined.

Study of patients with Burkitt's lymphoma in Uganda has shown that many have delayed hypersensitivity responses to autologous tumor antigens; sustained remission was correlated with a positive reaction.[24a]

Histiocytic Medullary Reticulosis

Histiocytic medullary reticulosis, first described by Scott and Robb-Smith in 1939,[72] is a rare disorder; 63 cases from virtually all parts of the world had been reported by 1968, the largest series being a group of 14 patients from Uganda.[73] Most of the reported patients have been middle-aged or older, but some have been less than 20 years of age. The clinical manifestations of the disease are fever, wasting, lymphadenopathy, and hepatosplenomegaly; late in the disease abdominal pain, jaundice, hemolytic anemia, leukopenia, thrombocytopenia, and bleeding occur in a majority of patients. The disease is rapidly fatal; most patients have died within 10 weeks of onset and only an occasional patient has survived from 6 to 15 months. Treatment with corticosteroids, 6-MP, alkylating agents, and vincristine and splenectomy have produced no more than short remissions.

The characteristic feature of the disease is a diffuse proliferation of the histiocytes and their precursors throughout the reticuloendothelial system. Erythrophagocytosis occurs frequently but is not specific for this disorder, since it also occurs in other lymphomas and various infections. The criteria suggested for a diagnosis are as follows: (1) sections that disclose proliferation of abnormal cells of the histiocytic series, not classified as Sternberg-Reed giant cells, with a tendency to erythrophagocytosis, must be found in at least two of the following organs: liver, lymph nodes, spleen, or bone marrow; and (2) there should be no evidence of local tumor formation in the liver, spleen, and marrow.[73] Sections of the liver and lymph nodes usually are better than those of the bone marrow for diagnosis.

Diagnosis

The presence of one of these diseases is suggested by the clinical manifestations but the antemortem diagnosis can be made only by biopsy. A suitable superficial node is usually available. Preference is given to cervical, supraclavicular, and axillary nodes; femoral and inguinal nodes are used only if no other is suitable. When none of the superficial lymph nodes is significantly enlarged, the diagnosis can sometimes be made by a supraclavicular biopsy, particularly if disease is present in the lung or mediastinum. At times the diagnosis can be made by the biopsy of a local tumor mass or by needle aspiration of an enlarged liver. Study of stained smears made from material obtained by needle aspiration of a lymph node is also a helpful procedure in experienced hands. The diagnosis can be made only rarely by a study of stained smears made from aspirations of the bone marrow, but examination of either a surgical biopsy of the marrow or paraffin sections made from aspirated material is more likely to yield the diagnosis. This type of examination of the bone marrow may be a very helpful procedure when the diagnosis is obscure.[64] Cell blocks made from pleural or ascitic fluid rarely provide a positive diagnosis in diseases of the lymphoma group.

A "negative" report of a biopsy does not mean that the presence of one of these diseases has been excluded. If the pathologist can make no diagnosis on the specimen other than "lymphoid hyperplasia" or "hyperplastic lymphadenitis" another biopsy should be performed. If no suitable nodes are available the patient should be examined periodically in the expectation that a lesion suitable for biopsy will develop later.

Hodgkin's disease, lymphosarcoma, reticulum cell sarcoma, and giant follicle lymphoma must be distinguished from other diseases that may produce similar clinical manifestations. The possibility of one of the lymphoma group is suggested by enlargement of superficial lymph nodes, splenomegaly, prolonged fever, mediastinal tumors, hemolytic anemia, exfoliative dermatitis, and spinal cord compression. Infectious mononucleosis, tuberculosis, brucellosis, sarcoidosis, disseminated lupus erythematosus, and carcinomatosis often present problems in differential diagnosis. The difficulty can be resolved only by demonstrating the presence of one of the lymphoma group histologically or by satisfying the diagnostic criteria for the other disease under consideration. Whether or not the patient has lymphoma may remain uncertain even after biopsy if he has been taking anticonvulsant drugs.[34a, 74a]

In the majority of patients the distinction between lymphosarcoma and chronic lymphocytic leukemia is made without difficulty because of the increases in total leukocyte count and percentage of lymphocytes that are found in most patients with leukemia. However, in the occasional patient this differential diagnosis is not easy because there seems to be a close relationship or overlapping between the two diseases. It is known that some patients who are diagnosed as having lymphosarcoma from a node biopsy at a time when the blood and bone marrow appear entirely normal later develop the hematologic features of lymphocytic leukemia. The term "leukosarcoma" has been used to designate these transitional cases. In some such patients the classic features of leukemia develop later but in others the abnormalities in the peripheral blood prove to be transient, and at necropsy months or years later there is no evidence of widespread invasion of the various organs that usually occurs in leukemia. In still others the abnormalities in the blood, such as a mild absolute lymphocytosis, persist but a frankly leukemic picture does not develop. A leukocyte count of 30,000 per cu.mm. has been taken as the criterion of leukemia in some series when lymphocytes constitute more than half the cells.[67]

Management of the Patient with Malignant Lymphoma

It is important to establish a histological diagnosis before treatment is started; unless the biopsy suffices to place the diagnosis, at least in this group of diseases, treatment is best deferred except in unusual circumstances. The decision regarding the type and amount of treatment must be based on a careful evaluation of the individual patient and must take into consideration the condition of the patient as well as the type, extent, and location of disease. An evaluation of this sort is important because any treatment can prove deleterious or even fatal to the patient if given injudiciously. Close collaboration between an internist and radiotherapist and at times the surgeon is essential in deciding on the initial plan for staging and treatment of the patient and continues to be important throughout the course of the disease. Regular follow-up examinations constitute an important part of the program. Not only do these visits allow the physician to follow the course of the disease, but they also constitute an important part of the supportive treatment. The psychological aspect of the management becomes even more important when the disease is relapsing or progressing despite treatment; a moderately aggressive and hopeful attitude toward therapy is most likely to produce the best results at any stage of the disease and is usually best for the patient's morale.

The same therapeutic agents are employed in the treatment of patients with the different diseases of the lymphoma group and the same general plan of therapy can be followed in each disease. In the treatment of diseases that have such varied clinical manifestations, it is important to have a basic plan of therapy that can be followed through the variety of different symptoms and situations that may develop.

In formulating or following a plan for a patient with any disease of the lymphoma group, the patient is classified according to the severity or extent of the disease, as Peters first recommended for Hodgkin's disease.[61] Her studies first clearly showed that the prognosis in Hodgkin's disease was related to (1) the extent of the disease, for which she established three stages; (2) the type of treatment given (those with local treatment did not survive nearly as well as those receiving regional treatment); and (3) the presence or absence of symptoms (patients with symptoms had a much poorer prognosis than those who were asymptomatic). These observations have had a great influence on the management of patients with Hodgkin's disease.

Stages of Lymphoma

A Committee on the Staging of Hodgkin's Disease that was appointed at a 1965 symposium sponsored by the American Cancer Society and the National Cancer Institute has recommended the following categories:[66]

STAGE I. Disease limited to one anatomic region or to two contiguous anatomic regions on the same side of the diaphragm.

STAGE II. Disease in more than two anatomic regions or in two non-contiguous regions on the same side of the diaphragm.

STAGE III. Disease on both sides of the diaphragm, but not extending beyond the involvement of lymph nodes, spleen, and/or Waldeyer's ring.

STAGE IV. Involvement of the bone marrow, lungs, parenchyma, pleura, liver, skin, bone, kidneys, gastrointestinal tract, or a tissue or organ in addition to lymph nodes, spleen, or Waldeyer's ring.

All stages should be subclassified as "A" or "B" to indicate the absence or presence, respectively, of systemic symptoms. The following documented symptoms, otherwise unexplained, are significant: fever, night sweats, and pruritis.

Other symptoms of Hodgkin's disease are important to document, but are not considered sufficient, in themselves, to place a patient in the "B" subgroup. These include weight loss, weakness, fatigue, anemia, leukocytosis, leukopenia, lymphadenopathy, elevated sedimentation rate, cutaneous anergy, or pain induced by alcohol.

If a more detailed classification is desired, it is recommended that patients with the disease limited to one anatomical region be designated "Stage I_1," and those with disease limited to two contiguous regions on the same side of the diaphragm as "Stage I_2."

Rosenberg and Kaplan, in order to better correlate staging with prognosis, proposed that patients with Hodgkin's and other forms of lymphoma be more precisely categorized according to the extent of extranodal involvement:[69a] Stage I_E, involvement of a single extralymphatic organ or site; Stage II_E, one or more node regions, same side of diaphragm and Stage III_E, both sides of diaphragm with single areas of non-node involvement; and Stage III_S, splenic involvement. Stage IV would be reserved for patients with multiple extra-lymphatic foci.

In order to properly classify a patient according to these stages of disease, the Committee recommended that the following studies be performed:

1. Careful clinical history with special attention to the systemic symptoms described above.

2. Complete physical examination.

3. Complete blood count, including white cell count, differential, hematocrit or hemoglobin, platelet count, and erythrocyte sedimentation rate.

4. Posteroanterior and lateral chest films; whole lung scan in the presence of hilar adenopathy.

5. Skeletal survey, or if this is not feasible, x-ray examination of the thoracolumbar spine and pelvis.

6. Retroperitoneal studies to include lower extremity lymphangiography, if possible, and an excretory urogram.

7. Bone marrow examination with a histologic section of marrow clot or, if possible, a needle (or open marrow) biopsy.

8. Liver function tests, including a serum alkaline phosphatase.

9. Renal function tests, including a urinalysis.

10. Documentation of cutaneous anergy.

Intravenous pyelograms, inferior vena cavograms, and lymphangiograms are made in patients who appear to have Stage I disease or Stage II disease above or below the diaphragm. These studies usually are not indicated in patients with generalized disease or in those with recognized disease below the diaphragm not confined to the groin areas unless such studies are considered to be of special value in defining the field to be used in radiation treatment of a particular patient. Roentgenographic study of the gastrointestinal tract is made in patients who have symptoms suggesting involvement, but these examinations are not done routinely; x-rays of areas of the skeleton are taken when involvement is suspected.

In one report of 100 patients with Hodgkin's disease, 27 were found to be in Stage I, 30 in Stage II, 33 in Stage III, and 10 in Stage IV.[40] Symptoms which

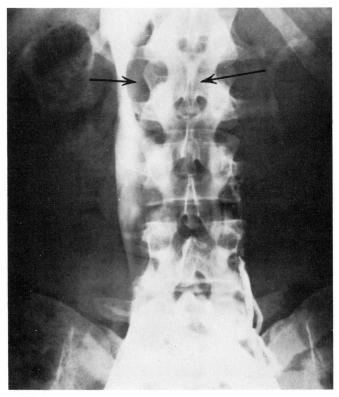

Figure 14–7. Inferior vena cavogram showing enlarged intra-abdominal nodes in a patient with Hodgkin's disease.

placed them in the "B" category (fever, sweats, or pruritis) were found in three patients in Stage I, 12 in Stage II, 16 in Stage III, and 8 in Stage IV. The examinations made to classify the stage of the disease are valuable. Many patients who would be considered to be in Stage I or II on the basis of the information provided by the usual clinical examinations are in reality in Stage III or IV, which makes a difference in the planning of treatment and also the estimation of prognosis.

In another group of 100 patients with Hodgkin's disease, abnormal lymphangiograms were found in 35 per cent of those thought to be Stage I, 51 per cent of those thought to be Stage II, and 89 per cent of those known already to be Stage III.[59] Similar results have been reported by others.[16] In a large series of 192 patients with Hodgkin's disease, investigation disclosed that only two of 20 patients with cervical Stage I disease had abnormal lymphangiograms, whereas the same examination was abnormal in all six of those with Stage I disease in the groin. In the same study, lymphangiograms were abnormal in 90 per cent of those with Stage IIB and Stage III disease. Lymphangiograms were abnormal in from 60 to 75 per cent of patients with lymphosarcoma and reticulum cell sarcoma who were thought to be in Stage I; the examination disclosed disease in over 80 per cent of those classed as Stage II and over 90 per cent in Stage III.[59]

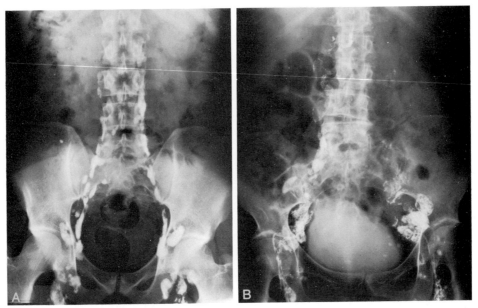

Figure 14–8. Lymphangiograms. *A*, Normal. *B*, Abnormal; Hodgkin's disease, Stage III A. (Courtesy of Dr. Anne Brower.)

Although the determination of the stage of disease is a significant advance in the management of the patients with Hodgkin's disease and other lymphomas, interpretation of the lymphangiograms is often difficult. The level of error is probably at least 10 per cent, usually but not always due to a false negative reading, which may occur when a node does not fill because it is replaced by tumor, or for some other reason. Some patients have more extensive disease, particularly below the diaphragm, than is disclosed by any of the studies.

Because of the imperfections in these staging procedures we, and others, have adopted a more aggressive approach to classifying certain types of patients.[28a, 51b, 69a] Preliminary results suggest its value. We hope that more accurate staging will lead to more precise radiotherapy and a better prognosis for some patients and to avoiding unnecessary radiation, with its potential damage to different organs. The procedures include the following: (1) abdominal operation; (2) splenectomy; (3) removal of obviously enlarged nodes for histological study; (4) removal of apparently normal nodes if none appears diseased; and (5) two wedge and two needle biopsies of the liver. Splenectomy is performed because there seems to be little correlation between spleen size and histologic evidence of Hodgkin's disease and also because large doses of radiation to the splenic region may damage the left kidney. Currently the procedure is usually recommended for the following types of patients: (1) Stage IB and IIB with demonstrated disease above the diaphragm; (2) Stage IA and IIA disease involving the mediastinum; (3) Stage IA or IIA disease above the diaphragm with equivocal lymphangiograms or vena cavograms; (4) Stage IIIA; and (5) Stage IA or IIA below the diaphragm.

The results of laparotomy in 100 consecutive untreated patients have proved valuable and interesting.[69a] Half the patients with splenomegaly did not have disease in the spleen (on the usual pathologic examination); one-third of the normal sized spleens were diseased. Liver involvement was not found in the absence of splenic involvement; in addition, the larger the spleen, the greater the likelihood of hepatic involvement. In 57 patients with "negative" lymph-angiograms, only two patients were found to have para-aortic node involvement. Nodes were found in 17 of 23 patients with "positive" lymphangiograms; nodes were also found in three of 20 patients with "equivocal" lymphangiograms.

Lymphangiography and vena cavography are not without risk. The complications of lymphangiography include oil embolism to the lung, kidney, brain, or liver, cellulitis at the site of the cutdown, and allergy to the injected dye. Transient pain, fever, hematoma, and pulmonary embolism also occur in some patients after vena cavography. Fatal reactions have been reported.[29, 58] Because of these complications, the following conditions are generally contraindications to lymphangiography: (1) pulmonary disease, symptomatic or asymptomatic: (2) history of allergy to iodine: and (3) known generalized Stage III disease, particularly with palpable involvement below the diaphragm.[48]

The value of the bone marrow biopsy in staging patients with Hodgkin's disease is shown in one report of 28 patients with Stage III or IV disease; in 11 the biopsy was positive; 6 patients previously considered to be in Stage III were found to be in Stage IV.[81] In our experience, positive biopsies are much less common.

If a patient with Hodgkin's disease has abnormal liver function tests, a liver scan or percutaneous needle biopsy may be employed to more accurately determine the presence of liver involvement and assess its extent. Unfortunately, the results of these procedures often have been negative or equivocal when the presence of disease has been demonstrated later by operation or postmortem examination.

Histologic Classification of Hodgkin's Disease

Lukes and Butler have proposed a histological classification of Hodgkin's disease that offers certain advantages over that proposed by Jackson and Parker.[35] The modification of the Lukes and Butler classification, which was adopted at the 1965 Conference on Hodgkin's Disease,[54] distinguishes four histological types: (1) lymphocytic predominance; (2) nodular sclerosis; (3) mixed cellularity; and (4) lymphocytic depletion. The presence of Reed-Sternberg cells is a "sine qua non" for the diagnosis of Hodgkin's disease of any type.

A comparison of the two classifications of Hodgkin's disease based on Luke's review of 377 patients[54] is given in Table 14-2. In their original study of 301 patients, Jackson and Parker found the following distribution: paragranuloma, 12 per cent; granuloma, 80 per cent; and sarcoma, 8 per cent. Some difference in age distribution in the two series may be responsible for the discrepancies and the frequency of patients classed as sarcoma.

The Lukes classification has the advantage of providing a more definitive diagnosis for the type of disease which correlates better with prognosis and may

Table 14–2. *Histologic Classification of Hodgkin's Disease*

JACKSON & PARKER		LUKES & BUTLER	
Type	*Incidence (%)*	*Type*	*Incidence (%)*
Paragranuloma	8	Lymphocytic predominance	15
Granuloma	91	Mixed	39
Sarcoma	1	Nodular sclerosis	40
		Lymphocytic depletion	6

reflect the status of the body's resistance to the disease. The nodular sclerosis picture occurs most often in the mediastinum, and many patients with this disease have a good prognosis, even if pulmonary tissue is involved.

Treatment and Prognosis

HODGKIN'S DISEASE

Studies by Rosenberg and Kaplan, which included detailed clinical, laboratory, and radiologic evaluation as well as biopsy of equivocal areas, in 100 consecutive untreated patients with Hodgkin's disease, indicated that Hodgkin's disease probably arises in a single focus and usually spreads along adjacent lymphoid channels. "Skipped" areas appeared in less than 25 per cent, and these were usually in the mediastinum. The good effects noted by Peters with "prophylactic" or "complementary" treatment of adjacent areas in patients with Hodgkin's disease point to the same conclusion, although she considers that there may be two types of Hodgkin's disease, one unifocal and the other multifocal in origin.[62] The latter is seen mainly in patients with Stage III disease. Both of these observations indicate that the radiation treatment of the patient with Hodgkin's disease should be directed toward areas of probable involvement and not limited to those actually demonstrated.

In a careful consideration of the controversial issues in the treatment of patients with Hodgkin's disease, Rubin concluded that no study to date has clearly demonstrated the value of prophylactic extended field irradiation.[71a] Likewise, the possible value of chemotherapy as an adjunctive or prophylactic treatment following radiotherapy has not been assessed. Thus it may be some years before the methods of treatment now commonly used and often strongly advocated can be fully evaluated. Both radiotherapy and chemotherapy are used in treatment, the details depending largely on the stage of the disease.[14a, 69a]

Most authorities now agree that high voltage dosage radiation which aims at cure is the treatment of choice for patients with localized Hodgkin's disease. Even in patients with advanced disease, the more aggressive radiation therapy brings a higher rate of remission and better palliation. In our institution patients with Stage I, II, and IIIA disease are treated with high voltage radiation in large doses, 3500 to 4000 rads given in several weeks; with such treatment the 5-year survival is approximately double that of patients treated with 2000 rads or less.[39]

On the assumption that Hodgkin's disease spreads to contiguous areas via the lymphatics, treatment is directed both at the involved areas and toward the adjacent drainage areas. The pattern of the area above the diaphragm to be radiated is "T" shaped, a "mantle" that includes the cervical and supraclavicular areas on both sides, both axillary regions, and the mediastinum, front and back. Therapy below the diaphragm is directed in an inverted "Y" pattern with radiation to the para-aortic areas, the inguinal and femoral areas on both sides, and the splenic area. Radiation is directed away from normal tissue as much as possible.

The reports of Peters[62] and Kaplan[39] indicate that in patients with Hodgkin's disease treated with 2500 to 4000 rads, the 5-year survival in those who have Stage I or IIa disease is between 75 and 90 per cent and is between 10 and 50 per cent in those with Stage III disease. In all categories there are patients who survive from 10 to 20 years; if the patient survives 5 or 10 years, the chances are excellent that he will survive for 15 or 20 years. Patients who have Stage IV disease, especially those with a IVB classification, have a poor prognosis (usually measured in months), but newer methods of chemotherapy and combined chemotherapy and radiation often provide a better outlook for these patients.

The hazards of radiation to the skin and bone marrow elements have been known for many years. Radiation also usually produces transient but uncomfortable laryngitis and esophagitis, and gastrointestinal symptoms of anorexia, nausea, and diarrhea appear in some patients receiving radiation to the abdominal region. The use of high voltage therapy has meant a lessening of damage to the skin and administration of larger doses to the interior organs.

As a consequence of these higher doses, other sequelae, including pulmonary fibrosis, radiation damage to the spinal cord, and cardiac embarrassment from fibrosis of the pericardium, have been reported following such therapy.[22] These complications are serious and may be fatal. It may be the high voltage radiation rather than the recurrence of the lymphoma that is responsible for pericardial effusion, apparent cardiac enlargement, and constrictive pericarditis. Cardiac damage does not occur frequently enough to deter the physician from using this form of therapy when it is indicated, but such therapy should not be used unless there is a good chance of more than a palliative effect. In one report,[38] the most significant complication of high voltage large dose therapy was radiation pericarditis. This was noted in six out of 114 patients with clinical evidence of recurrence of Hodgkin's disease. Two were treated by aspiration and chemotherapy and eventually died of constrictive pericarditis. In the other four patients pericardectomy was performed; Hodgkin's disease was found in one, but the other three have done well.

Long-term survival after radiation therapy may be followed in months or years by retroperitoneal fibrosis, interstitial fibrosis of the kidney, dilated lymphatics, telangiectasia, fibrosis, or stricture of the bowel which may be associated with malabsorption and perhaps chronic pancreatitis. As a result of the effect of radiation on the bone marrow, months may be required for hematological recovery sufficient to permit the effective use of chemotherapy.[38] When it is necessary to give chemotherapy after a shorter interval, the development of cytopenia of one sort or another often causes modification of the treatment regime and limits its effectiveness.

If the patient with Hodgkin's disease relapses after his initial treatment, or if the disease presents as Stage IIIB, IVA, or IVB, palliative doses of radiation may be given to selected areas; usually the treatment of choice in patients in the later stages utilizes chemotherapeutic agents. The number of agents now available is so large and the variety of protocols or plans of management so great that a physician in family practice or a general internist is often bewildered by the possible choices. Numerous drugs and combinations of drugs are being evaluated.

Nitrogen mustard was one of the first agents to be used in the treatment of Hodgkin's disease, and the dose of 0.4 mg. per kg. of body weight given intravenously is very effective in many patients. Preinjection medication with a barbiturate and a drug such as chlorpromazine appreciably reduces the frequency of nausea and vomiting. Most often the full amount of nitrogen mustard is given in a single injection. Leukopenia and thrombocytopenia usually develop in 1 to 2 weeks, and in ordinary circumstances administration of the drug is not repeated for 6 or 8 weeks. Other alkylating agents, such as chlorambucil in a dose from 2 to 6 mg. a day or cyclophosphamide, are also effective; cyclophosphamide may be given intravenously in a dose of 500 mg., to be followed by oral preparation in doses of 50 to 150 mg. a day. Thrombocytopenia, which may be prolonged, occurs more often during treatment with chlorambucil than with cyclophosphamide. Vinblastine, a periwinkle derivative given in a dose of 0.1 mg. per kg. intravenously at intervals of 1 week, often produces gratifying remission in patients with Hodgkin's disease. One must check the leukocyte count before administering this drug; it is usually withheld if the count is less than 3500 per cu.mm.

Adrenal corticosteroids have a place in the treatment of patients with Hodgkin's disease. They sometimes produce regression in the size of the involved nodes and organs;[31] more often they are effective in reducing fever and increasing appetite to help the patient gain weight and strength; they may also be useful if an auto-immune hemolytic anemia (which is unusual in Hodgkin's disease) or thrombocytopenia and bleeding develop. The usual initial dose is 40 to 60 mg. of prednisone a day, followed by the smallest effective maintenance dose, which may be 150 mg. 2 or 3 days a week or 5 to 10 mg. a day. Patients taking prednisone should also take an antacid; in those with a positive tuberculin test, and probably in all patients who take the drug for more than a few weeks, 300 mg. of isoniazide a day is advisable as a protective measure. The dangers of long-term treatment with prednisone include the development of gastrointestinal bleeding, osteoporosis, diabetes mellitus, occasional psychotic reactions, and the Cushingoid syndrome; probably more important is the occurrence of pneumonia or a perforation of a viscus which goes unrecognized because the prednisone has suppressed the clinical evidences of these complications. The frequency of disseminated fungus infections is also increased. Many of the complications of the therapy can be avoided if the drug is given on alternate days rather than every day.[55, 79a]

Evidence is accumulating that appears to show that treatment with several agents simultaneously is more effective than therapy with a single agent. The programs usually combine several different agents, which have different modes of action and different types of toxic reactions. One program of this type utilizes 50 to 100 mg. of cyclophosphamide a day orally, and 0.1 mg. per kg. of vinblastine intravenously once a week. Another combines vinblastine intravenously, 0.1 mg. per kg. a week, with chlorambucil, 4 mg. a day by mouth. Other protocols employ three or four agents. Probably the one with the most promise is quadruple therapy ("MOPP") with prednisone, vincristine, nitrogen mustard, and procarbazine, four compounds with different actions, each of proven value.[18]

One protocol for quadruple therapy, or the MOPP regime, is the following:

1. Nitrogen mustard	6 mg. per M^2 I.V.	day 1 and day 8 of each 28-day period for
2. Vincristine	1.4 mg. per M^2 I.V.	6 cycles
3. Procarbazine	50 mg. per M^2 per os on day 1, 100 mg. on day 2, and 100 mg. on days 3 through 10	
4. Prednisone	40 mg. per M^2 on days 1 through 10, first and fourth courses only	

The dose of nitrogen mustard is reduced to one-half if the bone marrow is moderately impaired; if severe leukopenia or thrombocytopenia develops, the scheduled treatment is omitted. Patients with significant urea retention are not recommended for treatment in this manner.

In one group of 43 patients, stage IVA or B, the MOPP regime produced complete remission in 81 per cent within 6 months.[18] Approximately three years after the study was initiated, the median duration of remission could not be determined but was between 29 and 42 months; relapses occurred as early as two months and as late as 42 months. Median survival time for the 35 patients achieving a complete remission was over 42 months; for the others it was 20 months. A complete remission rate of 70 per cent was obtained in 27 patients who received prior treatment, although previous treatment with both radiotherapy and chemotherapy seemed to limit the response.[51a] These results can be compared with stage IVA or B patients treated with single agents, in whom the remission rate appeared to be between 10 and 30 per cent, and the survival time two years or less. The major toxic effects of the MOPP regime are transient nausea and vomiting; leukopenia, which may be dose-limiting; alopecia in 30 per cent, nearly always transient; and neurotoxicity, usually mild and temporary. When relapse occurs in patients who obtained remission on the MOPP regime, we usually employ single agents for further therapy—nitrogen mustard, procarbazine, cyclophosphamide, chlorambucil, vinblastine, or vincristine.

LYMPHOSARCOMA AND RETICULUM CELL SARCOMA

In treating patients with lymphosarcoma, reticulum cell sarcoma, and nodular lymphoma, the same principles for staging and treatment utilized in Hodgkin's disease are followed. In a group of patients with localized lymphoreticular sarcoma treated with radiation reported by Easson,[19] the 5-year survival was 50 per cent and the 10 and 15 year survival 45 per cent, figures comparable to those obtained in patients with Hodgkin's disease who received the same type of treatment. If the disease is considered to be localized Stage I, an attempt at cure is made with high voltage radiation and the patient is given a dose of 4000 rads; if the disease is Stage II or III, radiation may still be the treatment of choice, or it may be combined with chemotherapy.

Surgical removal of localized areas of disease in the stomach or small bowel has, in our experience, given better results than other types of treatment, but surgery is not used in an effort to cure patients with Stage I disease. Splenectomy may be necessary even in patients with widespread disease if severe hemolytic anemia that is not controlled by prednisone develops, especially when radioisotopic studies show active destruction of the red cells by the spleen. Splenectomy also may be indicated when thrombocytopenia or leukopenia seems to be causing bleeding or infections or to avoid intensive radiation of the left upper quadrant. Operation is also necessary when perforation of a viscus or intestinal obstruction occurs.

In patients in Stage IIIB or Stage IV, and in some with Stage IIIA disease, chemotherapy is usually employed. Although individual patients with lymphosarcoma or reticulum cell sarcoma have remained in remission for many years on continued or periodic treatment with one of the alkylating agents, usually chlorambucil for lymphosarcoma and cyclophosphamide for reticulum cell sarcoma, a higher incidence of remission is reported in patients treated with a combination of agents.

Vincristine is more effective in lymphosarcoma and reticulum cell sarcoma and less effective in Hodgkin's disease than vinblastine. The usual dose of vincristine is 0.01 mg. per kg. I.V. initially, increasing at weekly intervals to a dose of 1.0 to 3.0 mg. (usually 1.0 or 1.5 mg.) a week in adults.

One schedule, a "high dose" regime reported to produce remissions in 100 per cent of patients with lymphosarcoma and 85 per cent of those with reticulum cell sarcoma (compared to remissions in about 50 per cent by cyclophosphamide alone), is as follows:[33]

1. Cyclophosphamide, 15 mg. per kg., I.V. } each week for 6 weeks
   Vincristine, 25 micrograms per kg., I.V.

2. Prednisone, 1 mg. per kg. per day.

At the end of the 6-week period, the patient receives methotrexate, 0.5 mg. per kg. either orally or intramuscularly twice a week. The low dose regime, which was less effective, particularly in reticulum cell sarcoma, is similar but uses different doses of the drugs: cyclophosphamide, 10 mg. per kg.; vincristine, 17 micrograms per kg.; and prednisone, 0.6 mg. per kg. If the patient has leukocyte counts of less than 5000 and platelet count of less than 100,000, only 75 per cent of the scheduled dose should be administered; it should be 50 per cent of the dose if the leukocyte count is between 3000 and 4000 and the platelet count is over 75,000. With leukocytes less than 3000 and platelets over 75,000, 25 per cent of the scheduled dose is given, and with a leukocyte count less than 2000 and platelets less than 75,000, the scheduled dose is omitted.

Prednisone alone in large dosage, 60 to 100 mg. per day, often produces prompt and striking diminution in the size of the tumor masses of lymphosarcoma. Suppression of the disease may continue for many months on a maintenance dose of prednisone, either a small daily dose or a dose of 100 to 150 mg.

three times a week. Prednisone given on alternate days in a dose as high as 80 mg. is effective in many diseases and produces few side effects; in addition the cellular immune mechanism, as measured by delayed-type skin reactions, is not inhibited.[55]

GIANT FOLLICULAR LYMPHOMA

Patients with giant follicular lymphoma (Brill-Symmers disease) probably respond best to radiotherapy directed toward the involved areas. When this is impractical, as is sometimes the case, they often respond well to therapy with nitrogen mustard, cyclophosphamide, or chlorambucil for long periods.

Special Problems in Therapy

When chemotherapeutic agents are used in treating patients with lymphomas, possible toxic effects must be watched for; many are uncommon but some are serious.[12] Nitrogen mustard may produce thrombophlebitis or necrosis of tissue if the drug escapes from the vein; marrow depression is a regular effect of the drug and for this reason the course should not be repeated in less than 4 weeks, preferably in not less than 8 weeks. Chlorambucil, which is usually prescribed in a dose of 0.1 to 0.2 mg. per kg. per day, or 6 to 12 mg. per day, occasionally produces gastrointestinal upset and exfoliative dermatitis. The marrow depression caused by this drug is moderate in degree and is gradual in onset; recovery after discontinuance of chlorambucil is usually prompt, but on occasions the platelet count remains depressed for many months. Cyclophosphamide, which may be administered orally, intravenously, intramuscularly, intrapleurally, or intraperitoneally in a dose of 2 to 3 mg. per kg., may produce a wide variety of toxic effects. Leukopenia is not uncommon, but thrombocytopenia occurs less often than it does with nitrogen mustard or chlorambucil. Alopecia which is reversible, nausea and vomiting, non-bacterial cystitis, transient hepatic toxicity, and mucosal ulceration have been reported. Triethylamine (TEM) is rarely used at the present time because of its unpredictable and inconstant absorption; chlorambucil and cyclophosphamide are at least as effective and much easier to regulate. Vinblastine in therapeutic amounts regularly produces leukopenia, which usually remits in from 7 to 14 days; in addition, transient alopecia and peripheral neuritis may occur. Vincristine is much less likely to produce leukopenia, but produces alopecia, which is transient but sometimes extensive in 20 per cent or less of patients. Vincristine does, however, often produce neurologic toxicity which at times is severe. The manifestations include loss of deep tendon reflexes, neuritic pain, weakness, foot drop, hoarseness, diplopia, ptosis and constipation; even postural hypotension has been suspected. The neurologic defects usually disappear slowly when the drug is discontinued. Allopurinol, 300 to 600 mg. per day, is often given with a large fluid intake to prevent urate deposition in patients with lymphomas treated with chemotherapeutic agents when appreciable cellular destruction is anticipated.

Certain clinical situations require special consideration in treatment. Patients with masses in the superior mediastinum, compression of the spinal cord, or involvement of the central nervous system are treated cautiously and kept under close supervision because serious consequences may follow any increase in pressure. When a lesion of this type is irradiated, only a small dose is employed. A steroid drug is often given in this situation in an effort to reduce the size of the tumor mass quickly or minimize the possibility of swelling secondary to radiation. The use of nitrogen mustard or TEM has been recommended in these situations because of the belief that the effects of these chemicals are different from those of x-rays and induce regression of the lesion without producing active congestion or edema.[83] We have seen one patient with Hodgkin's disease with signs and symptoms of spinal cord compression who developed temporary paraplegia twice after courses of nitrogen mustard. A mediastinal mass often responds well to treatment and a long remission ensues. Unfortunately, intracranial and intraspinal lesions rarely respond for more than short remissions with any form of treatment. Close collaboration with a neurologist is often helpful in localizing the lesion to be treated and in the general management of the patient. Not infrequently considerable damage to the spinal cord has occurred before the lesion is recognized and varying degrees of paralysis outlast the regression of the tumor masses. Laminectomy rarely produces significant or lasting benefit but is probably advisable in an acute compression.

Recurrent hydrothorax is a difficult problem to manage if it is not relieved by treatment of the intrathoracic disease. Intrapleural nitrogen mustard or the instillation of a radioactive isotope, such as gold, is sometimes effective. After preliminary sedation, nitrogen mustard, 0.4 mg. per kg., is instilled in a single injection into the pleural cavity after about half of the fluid has been removed and a free flow of fluid is still present; after instillation, the position of the patient is changed every 5 to 10 minutes over a period of 1 hour to insure more uniform distribution through the cavity.[82] Nitrogen mustard instillation has also been employed to treat recurrent ascites; chylous ascites often responds to corticosteroids. Herpes zoster in patients with lymphoma is treated by analgesic drugs, usually aspirin, supplemented by sedation, usually phenobarbital, and care of the local lesion if required; special treatment of the lymphoma is not necessary unless there is other evidence of relapse.

Patients with Hodgkin's disease are prone to infection with *Cryptococcus neoformans* (Torula histolytica). Disseminated disease including meningitis formerly was considered uniformly fatal. When this complication is treated with amphotericin B, remission or even a cure of this complication is sometimes obtained. Pneumocystis carinii pneumonia which has been diagnosed antemortem by needle biopsy of the lungs, and successfully treated with pentamidine isethionate occurs in some patients with long-standing Hodgkin's disease.[5] In one report, both tuberculosis and pyogenic infection were commoner than disseminated fungus disease in 137 patients with Hodgkin's disease.[50] Fever from Hodgkin's disease per se occurs twice as often as fever from infection; the latter was rarely seen except in advanced stages of the disease.

Pregnancy may present a problem in patients with a lymphoma. There is no evidence that pregnancy causes any aggravation or acceleration of lymphoma. Because of danger to the fetus, either form of treatment, chemotherapy or radiation, is given before or after pregnancy rather than during pregnancy if possible. No area below the diaphragm is irradiated during the first 3 months of pregnancy, the most dangerous time for the fetus, if it can be avoided. Should it be necessary later, the fetus is protected as well as possible. In some circumstances local irradiation and prednisone or an akylating agent have been used successfully during the latter part of the pregnancy. Vinblastine sulfate has been administered orally, 5 mg. per day 5 days a week, throughout pregnancy which ended with the birth of a normal thriving infant.[2]

Splenectomy is sometimes performed on selected patients with these diseases when severe leukopenia, thrombocytopenia, or hemolytic anemia occurs and fails to respond to other measures. The procedure appears to be particularly effective in patients with giant follicle lymphoma.[24] The response to splenectomy in patients with lymphoma who have auto-immune hemolytic anemia is unpredictable; probably less than half of such patients respond to this procedure, but in some the results are excellent.[44]

Prognosis

The statistics regarding prognosis of patients with Hodgkin's disease and the other lymphomas which have been recorded in the literature in the past are of little value at present. Improved histological classification of the tumors, the classification of patients by clinical stages, and improved methods of treatment with radiation and drugs have changed the picture. The knowledge that in former years patients with Hodgkin's disease survived for 2 or 3 years on the average is of little relevance, and the same is probably true in lymphosarcoma and reticulum cell sarcoma.

OTHER FACTORS IN PROGNOSIS

Despite advances in diagnosis and staging, it is virtually impossible to give an accurate prognosis in an individual patient with lymphoma; some with what appears to be localized disease have a rapid downhill course, probably because of undetected disease elsewhere, while others who appear to have generalized disease from the outset may respond well to treatment and survive for decades.[14, 46] Perhaps the most important factor in survival in patients with Hodgkin's disease, as in those with other malignancies, is the resistance on part of the patient to the tumor, the host-tumor relationship; at present there is no satisfactory way to evaluate this factor. Nevertheless, certain considerations aid the physician in estimating prognosis. (1) Patients with localized Stage I disease do better than those with more widespread disease; the outlook is particularly poor when organ involvement and systemic symptoms such as fever, weight loss, and weakness are present. (2) Women with Hodgkin's disease have a better outlook than men. (3) Patients with Hodgkin's sarcoma (lymphocytic depletion of Lukes) have a worse prognosis than other patients with Hodgkin's disease. (4) Patients with nodular lymphosarcoma usually have a better prognosis than those in the other groups.

Easson has reported that the long-term survival in patients with localized lymphosarcoma and with reticulum cell sarcoma is as good as that in patients with Hodgkin's disease. In general, however, patients with reticulum cell sarcoma do not fare as well as those with Hodgkin's disease or lymphosarcoma with a comparable degree of involvement. Patients who have primary localized involvement in the stomach or small intestine with reticulum cell sarcoma or lymphosarcoma often survive for many years after treatment.

The clinical stage of the disease is usually the best guide to prognosis, particularly in patients with Hodgkin's disease. The histologic picture also gives considerable aid in estimating the prognosis in Hodgkin's disease. Lukes reviewed patients with Hodgkin's disease who had been in the Army and found that the nodular sclerosis type occurred in 40 per cent and was the most common type.[52] The majority of patients with lymphocytic (or histocytic) predominance had Stage I disease, whereas the diffuse fibrosis and reticular types (lymphocytic depletion) occurred in over 80 per cent of cases with Stage II and III. Nodular sclerosis was seen most often in disease of the superior mediastinum and cervical region. The prognosis was most favorable in the lymphocytic predominance and nodular sclerosing types, which comprised 79 per cent (44 cases) of patients who survived 15 years. Patients with Stage I disease of the nodular and diffuse types had median survivals of 16 and 9.5 years; in patients with Stage III disease and the picture of lymphocytic depletion, the median survival was approximately 0.5 year. Patients in Stage I disease and nodular sclerosis had a median survival of 11 years.

The encouraging results of treatment in patients with these diseases, together with the realization that the long-term survivors with these diseases who were free of clinical disease 8 or 10 years after onset had as good a life expectancy as the general population of the same age group, led Russell and Easson to introduce the concept of a cure in these diseases.[19] Their definition of a cure was, "... of when in time — probably a decade or so after treatment — there remains a group of disease-free survivors whose progressive death rate from all causes is similar to that of a normal population of the same sex and age constitution." Such a definition, even though it may provoke some semantic difficulties, provides a stimulating and refreshing outlook for both the patient and the physician.

Illustrative Cases

HODGKIN'S DISEASE

CASE 1

This patient was 21 years old in 1946 when it was noted that her abdomen did not return to normal size following delivery of a normal child. One month later she was found to have enlargement of the inguinal nodes, cervical nodes, and right axillary nodes. Biopsy of a lymph node at this time was interpreted as "hyperplastic lymph node." Two months later the patient developed night sweats, pleural effusion, and ascites. A repeat biopsy of a cervical node at this time was interpreted as "Hodgkin's disease."

During the next 12 years the patient received therapy at intervals that varied from 6 months to 3 years. She was usually treated with high voltage radiation but at various times was treated with nitrogen mustard, TEM, and chlorambucil. On nine occasions, courses of x-ray therapy were given to the mediastinum, spleen, and various superficial nodes. During all this time she was managed on an ambulatory basis and led on active life.

In the spring of 1958 the patient developed anemia (hematocrit of 27 per cent), thrombocytopenia (platelet count 20,000 to 40,000 per cu.mm.), and leukopenia (white cells 1000 to 1500 per cu.mm.). It was thought that the pancytopenia was the result of splenomegaly associated with Hodgkin's disease or a combination of this factor and the effect of treatment on her bone marrow. She was treated with prednisone, frequent transfusions, and small doses of chlorambucil and was only slightly incapacitated until October, 1958. At this time she was admitted to the hospital with a history of severe frontal and occipital headache of 8 days' duration. Six days prior to admission she noticed ecchymoses around the eyes and complained of diplopia. She also reported transient weakness and numbness of the left hand and wrist. The hematocrit was 21 per cent, white count 1400 per cu.mm., and platelets 3000 per cu.mm. Marked weight loss was apparent. It was thought that the patient had advanced Hodgkin's disease and that she had suffered an intracranial hemorrhage because of the thrombocytopenia. When lumbar puncture was performed the opening pressure was found to be 600 mm. The fluid contained 250 red cells and 80 neutrophils per cu.mm. The spinal fluid protein was 10 and the sugar was 48. Examination of the cerebrospinal fluid revealed numerous Cryptococcus organisms. Despite treatment with prednisone, amphotericin B, and other measures, the patient's condition deteriorated rapidly, generalized convulsions developed, and she died a few days later, 12 years and 2 months after the onset of the first symptoms.

Postmortem examination revealed splenomegaly and enlargement of the lymph nodes. The presence of Hodgkin's disease was identified in the lymph nodes. However, the striking finding was the severe generalized systemic infection with Cryptococcus organisms which were present throughout the lungs, kidneys, brain, and meninges.

Comment.   This patient is somewhat unusual in that she survived for over 12 years with Hodgkin's disease. She responded well to different forms of treatment on numerous occasions even though the disease was generalized when first diagnosed. She illustrates the fact that generalized disease at onset does not necessarily mean a poor prognosis. As sometimes happens in diseases of the lymphoma group, the initial node biopsy did not reveal the diagnosis. The final episode was generalized Cryptococcosis with meningitis; death appeared to be due to this infection rather than the progression of the Hodgkin's disease. Cryptococcosis, which is not an uncommon development in patients with lymphoma, was apparently present in this patient for some months without being recognized.

CASE 2

A 14 year old white male high school student and athlete was in good health until 6 weeks before admission. At this time he noticed painless enlargement of a lymph node in the left side of this neck. He gave no history of sore throat, fever, pain, sweating, weight loss, pruritus, or rash. He consulted his physician, who prescribed antibiotics without improvement and then referred him to the hospital.

Physical examination was entirely normal except for a moderately firm, freely moveable node measuring 1 by 3 cm. in the left anterior cervical region. The laboratory examinations, which included blood counts, urinalysis, heterophil agglutination test, liver function tests, and bone marrow biopsy, were normal.

The lymph node was removed and Hodgkin's disease was diagnosed. Subsequent examinations were aimed at staging the disease. X-ray of the chest, intravenous pyelogram, inferior vena cavogram, and lymphangiograms were considered to be normal. The patient was classified as Hodgkin's disease, Stage I.

He received cobalt radiation, 3500 r, to the "T" pattern above the diaphragm; except for mild pharyngitis he had no difficulty with the treatment. Periodic follow-up examinations during the past 5 years have shown no evidence of recurrence.

Comment. This young man had Hodgkin's disease, clinically Stage I, and was treated with a large dose of high voltage radiation. He responded well; over 75 per cent of such patients treated in this way survive 5 years or more.

LYMPHOSARCOMA

This 65 year old white saleslady was well until December, 1955, when she noticed small purpuric lesions on the palms of the hands. During the next month the cutaneous lesions increased and became generalized. These lesions persisted and during the following 6 weeks the patient noticed cramping pains and edema in the legs, mild anorexia, and weight loss of 10 pounds. She was admitted to the hospital on March 17, 1956.

Physical examination. Signs of hydrothorax were present bilaterally. The spleen was palpable 3 fingerbreadths below the left costal margin and multiple orange-sized masses were palpable throughout the abdomen. Pitting edema was present in both legs. The trunk, back, and upper arms were covered with maculopapular hemorrhagic rash. The remainder of the examination was essentially normal.

Laboratory examination. Hematocrit, white count, differential count, urinalysis, blood urea, stool examination, and prothrombin times were normal. Roentgenogram of the chest revealed small bilateral pleural effusions. Bone marrow examination disclosed the normoblastic type of erythropoiesis associated with a moderate increase in lymphocytes, a pattern that was thought to be consistent with lymphosarcoma or lymphocytic leukemia. Biopsy of an axillary lymph node was diagnosed as "lymphosarcoma."

Course. She was treated with a total of 12.5 mg. of TEM in three doses and was discharged from the hospital. She was readmitted 3 weeks after the last dose of TEM and 4 weeks after the first dose with a 4 day history of fever, unproductive cough, pain in the left chest, and dyspnea. The intra-abdominal masses had become much smaller and the skin lesions had cleared almost completely. On admission the hematocrit was 35 per cent, white count 250 per cu.mm., and the platelet count 136,000 per cu.mm. Thoracentesis was performed on several occasions, and penicillin was administered because of the granulocytopenia and pneumonia. She improved promptly, and 10 days after admission the white count had risen to 2200 per cu.mm. One month later, 2 months after the last dose of TEM, the hematocrit was 40 per cent, the white count was 4000 per cu.mm., and the differential count was normal.

The patient was largely asymptomatic and received no treatment for a year, when enlargement of the supraclavicular lymph nodes and intra-abdominal nodes recurred. The patient was given 5 mg. of TEM and developed nausea, vomiting, and diarrhea despite the fact that she had taken chlorpromazine before the TEM. The patient's abdominal nodes decreased in size remarkably. The patient felt well for 5 months, at which time the superficial and intra-abdominal lymph nodes again increased in size. At this time a prolonged course of TEM consisting of a total of 57.5 mg. was administered over a 6-month period. At the end of this time the axillary and supraclavicular nodes measured about 2 cm. in diameter, the intra-abdominal masses remained, but the patient was largely asymptomatic and continued to work.

Five months after her last dose of TEM (18 months after her first admission), swelling of the legs and marked enlargement of the superficial and intra-abdominal nodes recurred. Treatment with chlorambucil 6 mg. a day was started when the leukocyte count was 3000 per cu.mm. One month later there was less swelling in the abdomen, the superficial nodes were no longer enlarged, the intra-abdominal masses appeared smaller, and the dose of chlorambucil was reduced to 4 mg. per day. Two months after beginning chlorambucil, no enlargement of the superficial lymph nodes could be detected and the intra-abdominal masses were just palpable. Four and a half months after chlorambucil was started the patient reported that she was entirely asymptomatic. Examination at this time revealed no enlargement of the superficial lymph nodes, liver, spleen, or any detectable intra-abdominal masses. This excellent remission lasted for 8 years during which time only three courses of chlorambucil have been necessary.

Interval note. In September, 1965 the patient lost 8 pounds in weight, had abdominal discomfort, and developed palpable intra-abdominal nodes. She was again treated with chlorambucil, 6 mg. a day for 4 months, at the end of which time she had regained her weight, her abdominal symptoms had subsided, and no intra-abdominal masses could be felt. The patient continued in complete remission from February, 1966 until June, 1969, at which time she was admitted with left lower quadrant mass and two "coin" lesions in the lower portion of the left lung, which were thought to be tumor nodules. She was again treated with chlorambucil. Abdominal symptoms and the mass in her abdomen disappeared, and 6 weeks later x-ray of the chest showed complete resolution of the lesions, which were thought to be lymphosarcoma. Treatment was continued until October 1, 1969. Since then the patient has again been in complete remission; now, in 1971, 15 years after the onset of her disease, she has no clinical evidence of her disease.

Comment. The course of the lymphosarcoma in this patient illustrates many instructive features: (1) the onset with skin lesions and generalized involvement of the lymph nodes; (2) the decision to treat the patient with an alkylating agent rather than radiation because of the widespread distribution of the disease; (3) the occurrence of severe granulocytopenia 3 to 4 weeks after the administration of TEM; (4) the excellent remissions obtained with small amounts of TEM early in the course of the disease; (5) the variable incidence of toxic manifestations after administration of different amounts of this drug; (6) the increasing resistance of the lymphosarcoma to TEM; (7) the excellent remission obtained with chlorambucil after the patient had become resistant to TEM; (8) the time required to obtain the remission with chlorambucil (4½ months); (9) the relatively good prognosis of some patients with lymphosarcoma that is already widespread when the patient is first seen.

References

1. Aisenberg, A. C.: Lymphocytopenia in Hodgkin's disease. Blood, *25*:1037, 1965.
2. Armstrong, J. G., Dyke, R. W., Fouts, P. J., and Jansen, C. J.: Delivery of a normal infant during the course of oral vinblastine sulfate therapy for Hodgkin's disease. Ann. Int. Med., *61*:106, 1964.
3. Azar, H. A., Hill, W. T., and Osserman, E. F.: Malignant lymphoma and lymphatic leukemia associated with myeloma-type serum proteins. Am. J. Med., *23*:239, 1957.
4. Baehr, G.: The clinical and pathological picture of follicular lymphoblastoma. Trans. Assoc. Am. Physicians, *47*:330, 1932.
5. Baker, W. H., and Castleman, B.: Cough and pulmonary infiltrates in a man with Hodgkin's disease of over four years' duration New England J. Med., *277*:39, 1967.
6. Blanchard, B. B.: Peripheral neuropathy (non-invasive) associated with lymphoma. Ann. Int. Med *56*:774, 1962.
7. Block, J. B., Edgcomb, J., Eisen, A., and VanScott, E. J.: Mycosis fungoides. Medicine, *34*:228, 1963.
8. Bostick, W. L.: Evidence for the virus etiology of Hodgkin's disease. Ann. N.Y. Acad. Sci., *73*:307, 1958.
9. Brill, N. E., Baehr, G., and Rosenthal, N.: Generalized giant lymph follicle hyperplasia of lymph nodes and spleen. J.A.M.A., *84*:668, 1925.
10. Bunting, C. H.: Blood platelets and megalokaryocytes in Hodgkin's disease. Johns Hopkins Hospital Bull., *22*:114, 1911.
11. Burkitt, D.: Sarcoma involving jaws in African children. Brit. J. Surg., *46*:218, 1958–59.
12. Calabresi, P., and Welch, A. D.: Chemotherapy of neoplastic diseases. Ann. Rev. Med., *13*:147, 1962.
13. Carbone, P. P., Bernard, C. W., Bennett, J. M., Ziegler, J. L., Cohen, M. H., and Gerber, P.: NIH Clinical Staff Conference. Burkitt's tumor. Ann. Int. Med., *70*:817, 1969.
13a. Case Records, Mass. Gen. Hosp.: Massive proteinuria in a patient with Hodgkin's disease. New England J. Med., *284*:95, 1971.
14. Chawla, P. L., Stutzman, L., DuBois, R. E., Kim, U., and Sokal, J. E.: Long survival in Hodgkin's disease. Am. J. Med., *48*:85, 1970.
14a. Constable, W., and Leavell, B. S.: The management of Hodgkin's disease. Vir. Med. Month., *97*:381, 1970.
15. Custer, R. P., and Bernhard, W. G.: The interrelationship of Hodgkin's disease and other lymphatic tumors. Am. J. Med. Sci., *216*:625, 1948.
16. Davidson, J. W., and Clarke, E. A.: Influence of modern radiological techniques on clinical staging of malignant lymphomas. Canad. Med. Assoc. J., *99*:1196, 1968.
17. DeVita, V. T., Emmer, M., Levine, A., Jacobs, B., and Berard, C.: Pneumocystis Carinii Pneumonia. New England J. Med. *280*:287, 1969.
18. DeVita, V. T., Jr., Serpick, A. A., and Carbone, P. P.: Combination chemotherapy in the treatment of advanced Hodgkin's disease. Ann. Int. Med., *73*:881, 1970.
19. Easson, E. C.: Long-term results of radical radiotherapy in Hodgkin's disease. Cancer Research, *26*:1244, 1966.
20. Easson, E. C., and Russell, M. H.: The cure of Hodgkin's Disease. Brit. Med. J., *1*:1704, 1963.

21. Edwards, R. T.: Hodgkin's sarcoma of the small bowel. Virginia M. Monthly, *96*:521, 1969.
22. Editorial. J.A.M.A., *206*:2309, 1968.
23. Ehrlich, A. N., Stalder, G., Geller, W., and Sherlock, P.: Gastrointestinal manifestations of malignant lymphoma. Gastroenterology, *54*:1115, 1968.
24. Evans, T. S., and Doan, C. A.: Giant follicle hyperplasia: a study of its incidence, histopathologic variability, and the frequency of sarcoma and secondary hypersplenic complications. Ann. Int. Med., *40*:851, 1954.
24a. Fass, L., Herberman, R. B., and Ziegler, J.: Delayed cutaneous hypersensitivity reactions to autologous extracts of Burkitt-lymphoma cells. New England J. Med., *282*:776, 1970.
25. Finkbeiner, J. A., Craver, L. F., and Diamond, H. D.: Prognostic signs in Hodgkin's disease. J.A.M.A., *156*:472, 1954.
26. Firat, D., Stutzman, L., Studenski, E. R., and Pickren, J.: Giant follicular lymph node disease clinical and pathological review of sixty-four cases. Am. J. Med., *39*:252, 1965.
27. Gall, E. A., and Mallory, T. B.: Malignant lymphoma: a clinico-pathologic survey of 618 cases. Am. J. Path., *18*:381, 1942.
28. Gall, E. A., Morrison, H. R., and Scott, A. T.: The follicular type of malignant lymphoma. A survey of 63 cases. Ann. Int. Med., *14*:2073, 1941.
28a. Glatstein, E., Guernsey, J. M., Rosenberg, S. A., et al.: The value of laparotomy and splenectomy in the staging of Hodgkin's disease. Cancer, *24*:709, 1969.
29. Gold, W. M., Youker, J., Anderson, S., and Nadel, J. A.: Pulmonary-function abnormalities after lymphangiography. New England J. Med., *273*:519, 1965.
30. Goldman, L. B.: Hodgkin's disease: an analysis of 212 cases. J.A.M.A., *114*:1611, 1940.
31. Hall, T. C., Choi, O. S., Abadil, A., and Krant, M. J.: High-dose corticoid therapy in Hodgkin's disease and other lymphomas. Ann. Intern. Med., *66*:1144, 1967.
31a. Hayness H. A., and VanScott, E. J.: Therapy of mycosis fungoides. Prog. Derm., *3*:1, 1968.
32. Hodgkin, T.: On some morbid appearances of the absorbent glands and spleen. Medico-Chirurg. Tr. London, *17*:68, 1832. Quoted from Major, R. H.: Classic Descriptions of Disease. Charles C Thomas, Springfield, Ill., 1955.
33. Hoogstraten, B., Owens, A. H., Lenhard, R. E., Gildewell, O. J., Leone, L. A., Olson, K. B., Harley, J. B., Townsend, S. R., Miller, S. P., and Spurr, C. L.: Combination chemotherapy in lymphosarcoma and reticulum cell sarcoma. Blood, *33*:370, 1969.
34. Hoster, H. A., and Dratman, M. B.: Hodgkin's disease—Part I. 1832–1947. Cancer Res., *8*:1, 1948.
34a. Hyman, G. A., and Sommers, S. C.: The development of Hodgkin's disease and lymphoma during anticonvulsant therapy. Blood, *28*:416, 1966.
35. Jackson, H., Jr., and Parker, F., Jr.: Hodgkin's disease. New England J. Med. I. General considerations, *230*:1, 1944; II. Pathology, *231*:35, 1944; III. Symptoms and course, *231*:639, 1944; IV. Involvement of certain organs, *232*:547, 1945; *233*:369, 1945.
36. Jackson, H., Jr., and Parker, F., Jr.: Hodgkin's Disease and Allied Disorders. Oxford University Press, New York, 1947.
37. Jacobson, L. O., et al.: Nitrogen mustard therapy. J.A.M.A., *132*:263, 1946.
38. Johnson, R. E., Kagan, A. R., Hafermann, M. D., and Keyes, J. W.: Patient tolerance to extended irradiation in Hodgkin's disease. Ann. Int. Med., *70*:1, 1969.
39. Kaplan, H. S.: Long-term results of palliative and radical radiotherapy of Hodgkin's disease. Cancer Res., *26*:1250, 1966.
40. Kaplan, H. S.: Clinical Evaluation and Radiotherapeutic Management of Hodgkin's Disease and the Malignant Lymphomas New England J. Med., *278*:892, 1968.
41. Kassel, R.: Etiological considerations in Hodgkin's disease. Ann. N.Y. Acad. Sci., *73*:335, 1958.
42. Kiely, J. M., Wagoner, R. D., and Holley, K. E.: Renal complications of lymphoma. Ann. Int. Med., *71*:1159, 1969.
43. Kundrat: Ueber Lympho-Sarkomatosis. Wien. klin. Wchnschr., *6*:211, 1893; *6*:234, 1893.
44. Kyle, R. A., Kiely, J. M., and Stickney, J. M.: Acquired hemolytic anemia in chronic lymphocytic leukemia and the lymphomas. Arch. Int. Med., *104*:61, 1959.
45. Leavell, B. S., and Thorup, O. A.: Personal observations.
46. Lacher, M. J.: Long survival in Hodgkin's disease. Ann. Int. Med., *70*:7, 1969.
47. Lacher, M. J., and Durant, J. R.: Combined vinblastine and chlorambucil therapy of Hodgkin's disease. Ann. Intern. Med., *62*:468, 1965.
48. Lee, B. J.: Lymphangiography in Hodgkin's disease: indications and contraindications Cancer Res., *26*:1084, 1966.
49. Levitan, R., Diamond, H. D., and Craver, L. F.: Jaundice in Hodgkin's disease. Am. J. Med., *30*:99, 1961.
50. Lobell, M., Boggs, D. R., and Wintrobe, M. M.: The clinical significance of fever in Hodgkin's disease. Arch. Intern. Med., *117*:335, 1966.

51. Lockwood, I. H.: Lymphosarcoma of the gastro-intestinal tract. J.A.M.A., *150*:435, 1952.

51a. Lowenbraun, S., DeVita, V. T., and Serpick, A. A.: Combination chemotherapy with nitrogen mustard, vincristine, procarbazine and prednisone in previously treated patients with Hodgkin's disease. Blood, *36*:704, 1970.

51b. Lowenbraun, S., Ramsey, H., Sutherland, J., and Serpick, A. A.: Diagnostic laparotomy and splenectomy for staging Hodgkin's disease. Ann. Int. Med., *72*:655, 1970.

52. Lukes, R. J.: Prognosis and relationship of histologic features to clinical stage. J.A.M.A., *190*:914, 1964.

53. Lukes, R. J.: The pathologic picture of the malignant lymphomas. Proc. Internat. Conference on Leukemia. Zarafonetis, C. J. D., Ed. Lea & Febiger, Philadelphia, 1968, p. 333.

54. Lukes, R. J., and Butler, J. I.: Pathology and nomenclature of Hodgkin's disease. Cancer Res., *26*:1063, 1966.

55. MacGregor, R. R., Sheagren, J. N., Lipsett, M. B., and Wolff, S. M.: Alternate-day prednisone therapy. New England J. Med., *280*:1427, 1969.

56. Middleton, W. S.: Some clinical caprices of Hodgkin's disease. Ann. Int. Med., *11*:448, 1937.

57. Minot, G. R., and Isaacs, R.: Lymphoblastoma (malignant lymphoma): age and sex incidence, duration of disease, and the effect of roentgen-ray and radium irradiation and surgery. J.A.M.A., *86*:1185, 1926.

58. Nelson, B., Rush, E. A., Takasugi, M., Wittenberg, J.: Lipid embolism to the brain after lymphography. New England J. Med., *273*:1132, 1965.

59. Owens, A. H., Jr., and Blazek, J. V.: Lymphography in the management of neoplastic disease. Johns Hopkins Med. J., *122*:55, 1968.

60. Perry, S., Thomas, L. B., Johnson, R. E., Carbone, P. P., and Haynes, H. A.: Hodgkin's disease (clinical staff conference). Ann. Int. Med., *67*:424, 1967.

61. Peters, M. V.: A study of survivals in Hodgkin's disease treated radiologically. Am. J. Roentgenol., *63*:299, 1950.

62. Peters, M. V.: Prophylactic treatment of adjacent areas in Hodgkin's disease. Cancer Res., *26*:1223, 1966.

63. Peters, M. V., and Middlemiss, K. C. H.: A study of Hodgkin's disease treated by irradiation. Am. J. Roentgenol., *79*:114, 1958.

64. Pettet, J. P., Pease, G. L., and Cooper, T.: An evaluation of paraffin sections of aspirated bone marrow in malignant lymphomas. Blood, *10*:820, 1955.

65. Richter, R. V., and Moore, R. Y.: Non-invasive central nervous system disease associated with lymphoid tumors. Johns Hopkins Hosp. Bull., *122*:271, 1968.

66. Rosenberg, S. A.: Report of the Committee on Staging of Hodgkin's Disease Cancer Res., *26*:1310, 1966.

67. Rosenberg, S. A., Diamond, H. D., and Craver, L. F.: Lymphosarcoma: the effects of therapy and survival in 1269 patients in a review of 30 years' experience. Ann. Int. Med., *53*:877, 1960.

68. Rosenberg, S. A., Diamond, H. D., Jaslowitz, B., and Craver, L. F.: Lymphosarcoma: a review of 1269 cases. Medicine, *40*:31, 1961.

69. Rosenberg, S. A., and Kaplan, H. S.: Evidence for an orderly progression in the spread of Hodgkin's disease. Cancer Res., *26*:1225, 1966.

69a. Rosenberg, S. A., and Kaplan, H. S.: Hodgkin's disease and other malignant lymphomas. Calif. Med., *113*:23, 1970.

70. Rosenthal, M. C., Pisciotta, A. V., Komninos, Z. D., Goldenberg, H., and Dameshek, W.: The auto-immune hemolytic anemia of malignant lymphocytic disease. Blood, *10*:197, 1955.

71. Roulet, F.: Das primäre Retothelsarkim der Lymphknoten. Virchows Arch. f. Path. Anat., *277*:15, 1930.

71a. Rubin, P.: Controversial issues in the treatment of Hodgkin's disease. In Moore, C. V., and Brown, E. B. (eds.): Progress in Hematology, Vol. 5. Grune & Stratton, New York, 1966, p. 180.

72. Scott, R. B., and Robb-Smith, A. H. T.: Histiocytic medullary reticulosis. Lancet, *237*:194, 1939.

73. Serck-Hanssen, A., and Purohit, G. P.: Histiocytic medullary reticulosis (report of 14 cases from Uganda). Brit. J. Cancer, *22*:506, 1968.

74. Shimkin, M. B., Oppermann, K. C., Bostick, W. L., and Low-Beer, B. V. A.: Hodgkin's disease: an analysis of frequency, distribution, and mortality at the University of California Hospital, 1914–1951. Ann. Int. Med., *42*:136, 1955.

74a. Sparberg, M.: Diagnostically confusing complications of diphenylhydantoin therapy. Ann. Int. Med., *59*:914, 1963.

75. Sparling, H. J., Jr., Adams, R. D., and Parker, F., Jr.: Involvement of the nervous system by malignant lymphoma. Medicine, *26*:285, 1947.

76. Sugarbaker, E. D., and Craver, L. F.: Lymphosarcoma: a study of 196 cases with biopsy. J.A.M.A., *115*:17, 1940.

77. Symmers, D.: Follicular lymphadenopathy with splenomegaly. Arch. Path., *3*:816, 1927.
78. Symmers, D.: Giant follicular lymphadenopathy with or without splenomegaly. Its transformation into polymorphous cell sarcoma of the lymph follicles and its association with Hodgkin's disease, lymphatic leukemia and an apparently unique disease of the lymph nodes and spleen. A disease entity believed heretofore undescribed. Arch. Path., *26*:603, 1938.
79. Ultmann, J. E., Cunningham, J. K., and Gellhorn, A.: The clinical picture of Hodgkin's disease. Cancer Res., *26*:1047, 1966.
79a. Walton, J., Watson, B. S., and Ney, R. L.: Alternate-day vs. shorter-interval steroid administration. Arch. Int. Med., *126*:601, 1970.
80. Wang, C. C.: Treatment of primary reticulum-cell sarcoma of bone by irradiation. New England J. Med., *278*:1331, 1968.
81. Webb, D. I., and Silver, R. T.: Hodgkin's disease: value of bone-marrow biopsy. New England J. Med., *279*:46, 1968.
82. Weisberger, A. S., Levine, B., and Storaasli, J. P.: Use of nitrogen mustard in treatment of serous effusions of neoplastic origin. J.A.M.A., *159*:1704, 1955.
83. Wintrobe, M. M., Cartwright, G. E., Fessas, P., Haut, A., and Altman, S. J.: Chemotherapy of leukemia, Hodgkin's disease and related disorders. Ann. Int. Med., *41*:447, 1954.

XV / Proliferative Disorders of the Lymphoreticular System Associated with Plasma Protein Abnormalities

The lymphoreticular system, with its lymphocytes, plasma cells, macrophages, and reticular cells, has the unique function of selectively attacking effete cells of the body and substances in the body which are "foreign" or "not self." This system is able to recognize the presence of a foreign substance and then mount an immune response to rid the organism of the offending material. It serves to protect the body from the effects of exogenous and endogenous agents, such as microorganisms or toxins, is responsible for the rejection of allografts and xenografts, and may be an important determinant of the level of host resistance to endogenous tumors.[32] Absence of any one of the components of this cellular system is almost always associated with infection or malignant tumor.

The injection of immunologically competent cells of the lymphoreticular system into an allogenic animal incapable of rejecting them may cause a syndrome referred to as the graft-versus-host reaction. In laboratory animals, this syndrome includes splenomegaly, hepatomegaly, anemia, lymphopenia, defective growth and weight loss (runting), and, usually, death. Similar syndromes have been noted in humans following the inadvertent introduction of immunologically competent cells by transplantation or transfusion into a recipient whose immunologic system is incompetent and unable to reject them.

Cells of the Lymphoreticular System

LYMPHOCYTES

Lymphocytes are produced in the bone marrow and lymphoid tissue throughout the body.[65, 106, 120, 164] Histochemical studies have shown that these cells contain a number of enzymes and other substances, including acid phosphatase,[186] glycogen,[153] dipetidase, and tripeptidase.[75] Changes in the cytochemistry have been reported in cells thought to be lymphocytes changing into macrophages.[153]

The function of the lymphocyte in the circulation and in other tissues throughout the body continues to be the subject of considerable controversy. It has been considered by many to be an adult cell, perhaps more vestigial than functional because it was thought to possess neither nucleoli nor power of movement. Others have always considered it to be a young cell, capable of forming other cells normally or in times of stress. The observation that enormous numbers of lymphocytes enter the circulation each day via the thoracic duct, the visualization of nucleoli by means of supravital stains, and the newer types of microscopy, the recognition of a characteristic type of motility, and the demonstration that these cells contain a large amount of deoxyribonucleic acid have all combined to produce a reawakening of interest in lymphocytes.[202] At the present time, most of the interest and controversy related to the lymphocyte is concerned with its possible function as a hematopoietic cell or as a vital part of the defense mechanism of the body.[194]

The ability of even small lymphocytes to form other lymphocytes homoplastically is considered established by some because of the demonstration of mitoses in material from lymph nodes, bone marrow, and spleen.[153] Nevertheless, mitoses are seen much more often in large and medium-sized lymphocytes than in small lymphocytes in the germinal centers of lymph nodes. The discrepancy between the large number of lymphocytes present in the body and the infrequent occurrence of mitosis in lymphoid tissue may be explained by a heteroplastic origin from reticulum cells or by a long life span of at least 21 days, as measured by studies with DNA labeled with radioactive phosphorus.[153] Yoffey has calculated that, for every lymphocyte normally present in the circulation, three lymphocytes enter the circulation each day from the thoracic duct and 23 are present in the bone marrow.[202] The function of the large number of lymphocytes contained in the marrow but not organized into lymphoid tissue remains an unsettled problem. According to one concept, these are resting primitive cells, able to be transformed into blast cells of various types, including erythrocyte precursors, and the main function of the small lymphocyte is cellular production.[28, 57, 106, 202] It has also been suggested that the large number of lymphocytes in the tissues and their reaction to adrenocortical steroids indicate that these cells have a role in protein metabolism.[195]

Views of the lymphocyte that are contrary to those just presented have been expressed by Gowans.[86] Gowans states that the small lymphocyte has a long life span, measured in months, and that its transformation into another cell type, either in the bone marrow or in areas of inflammation, has not been demonstrated unequivocally. From his own studies, he concluded that the large number of small lymphocytes that enter the venous system from the thoracic duct each day are cells that have recirculated from the blood.

The lymphocyte is concerned with antibody formation. Results obtained with the fluorescent antibody technique are consistent with the hypothesis that a small amount of antibody is formed in lymphocytes.[54] These studies show, however, that the major portion of the antibody formation takes place in plasma cells, and it is possible that the most important function of the lymphocyte in this connection is in the production of the plasma cells.[153] The lymphocyte is assigned to still another role in antibody production in the "reutilization hypothesis."[88] Antibodies are not self-replicating, and it has been suggested that the transfer of immune reactions by the lymphoid tissue occurs because the nucleic acids of the lymphocytes, which provide templates for the proteins concerned in antibody synthesis, act as mediators when large fragments of the nucleic acids of small lymphocytes are phagocytized by reticulum cells, which later become transformed into new lymphocytes or plasma cells.[53, 88, 195]

The use of tissue culture for the study of lymphocytes has provided much information about these cells. Studies of this type have shown that the small lymphocytes of human peripheral blood can undergo transformation into a large "blast-like" cell capable of mitosis.[26] They have demonstrated that these cells synthesize both deoxyribonucleic and ribonucleic acids. This transformation, termed "blastogenesis," has been reviewed.[156] When small lymphocytes from normal human blood are cultured with phytohemagglutinin, blastogenesis occurs; similar changes have been observed in cells exposed to tuberculin-purified protein derivative, homologous leukocytes, and antiserum to leukocytes. Of great interest is the observation that blastogenesis does not occur in lymphocytes of patients with chronic lymphocytic leukemia on exposure to phytohemagglutinin.[133] Blastogenesis is also absent in mixed cultures containing bloods from pairs of monozygotic twins, although it occurs in mixed cultures of blood from unrelated individuals.[7] The significance of blastogenesis in normal cell development or in various diseases has not been determined. It has not been demonstrated that the blast-like cells can phagocytize debris or produce soluble antibodies; there is no convincing evidence that the cells found in normal peripheral blood are derived from these cells in vivo and it is uncertain whether small lymphocytes may be derived from them.[158]

Many of the important and controversial aspects of the lymphocyte problem have been the subject of recent reviews.[62−64, 76a, 107, 122b, 158, 201]

PLASMA CELLS

Since the discovery of antibodies by von Behring in 1890, a great body of data has accumulated as the result of attempts to find the site of antibody production.[124] The lively discussions which have resulted[71] may be due in part to the confusion arising from the morphologic similarities of the young lymphocyte and plasma cell and to the variations in experimental methods used by various investigators. Recently, the evidence that the plasma cell is the major site of antibody production has become almost indisputable.[53, 54, 109] It has been demonstrated that a marked increase in plasma cells occurs in the spleens of animals receiving repeated injections of antigen; tissue explants from the spleen of these animals continue to produce antibody in vitro. These tissue explants contain plasma cells. By means of the fluorescein-labeled antibody technique, it has been shown that the antibody develops in the plasma cells in response to the second injection of antigen; the production of antibody is associated with a marked increase in the number of plasma cells.

The plasma cell is only rarely phagocytic,[35] and the various inclusion bodies that sometimes occur in the cytoplasm are probably formed intracellularly.

THE MACROPHAGE

The macrophage is important in the immune response even though it does not produce antibodies.[66, 73] In special circumstances, macrophages may arise from tissue histiocytes and some investigators have concluded that the main source of macrophages at sites of inflammation is the circulating lymphocytes.[152] More recent work, however, indicates that in animals and man the macrophages derive from the circulating monocytes, which in turn come from a primitive cell in the bone marrow. The number of macrophages that arise from lymphocytes is small at best.[10, 185, 188, 200]

Most studies of the biochemistry of the macrophage have been performed on relatively pure suspensions of cells obtained from the lungs or peritoneal cavity of laboratory animals. These have shown that most of the biochemical activity of the cell appears to be directed to the formation of lysosomes. Hydrolytic enzymes are synthesized in the endoplasmic reticulum and transferred to the Golgi apparatus, where they are packaged into small vesicles. These primary lysosomes then join small pinosomes, discharge their hydrolases, and form the secondary lysosomes or digestive granules.[49] In vitro studies of mouse,[50] chicken,[178] and horse[19] monocytes have revealed sequential transformation into macrophages with an increase in cell size, number of mitochondria, and lysosomes. Macrophages synthesize other cellular constituents and some proteins important in resistance to infection.[141] The macrophage does not appear to make antibody, but does produce interferon and one component of complement.[84]

The mechanism that recognizes an antigen that gains access to the body as "foreign" or "not self" and brings it into contact with the immunological system is not completely understood. Chemotaxis of macrophages has been difficult to demonstrate, possibly because of their slow movement.[108a] Recently sensitized lymphocytes have been demonstrated to elaborate a chemotactic factor for mononuclear cells[194] as well as a migration inhibitory factor (MIF) which inhibits random migration of normal macrophages in vitro.[27] These factors may play a major role in the accumulation of macrophages at sites of infection or allergic reactions. The specificity of the immunologic activity of the macrophage seems to be increased by globulin components of the serum known as cytophilic antibodies.[132] The cytophilic antibodies bind to the macrophage in such a way that the cell is subsequently able to adsorb antigen. There is evidence that the cytophilic antibodies may occur "naturally" without known prior immunization.[131a]

Structural units which consist of macrophages surrounded by lymphocytic cells have been observed in lymph nodes of immunized animals. Such clones suggest a physical means of transfer between cells, and actual physical joining between the cytoplasm of macrophages and lymphocytes has been reported.[166]

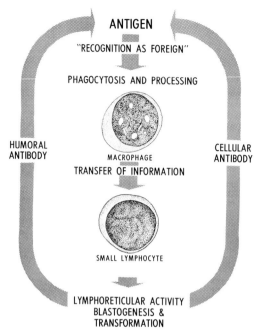

Figure 15–1. Antigen processing. Schematic representation of the response of the body to an invasion by a foreign substance. The means by which the substance is "recognized as foreign" is not clearly understood, but thymic lymphocytes are believed to be involved.

In addition, it has been demonstrated that labeled RNA, which had been produced in macrophages incubated with tritiated cytidine and then extracted, was incorporated into lymph node cells after incubation.[74]

Antigen appears to be unable to stimulate antibody production by antibody-producing cells directly on first exposure or possibly even on subsequent exposures, but the evidence is not conclusive.[59] Apparently the antigen must first be engulfed and processed by the macrophage before the message can be transferred to the antibody-producing cells. Antigen is initially localized in macrophages and later in the reticulum cells in lymphoid follicles. Once in the macrophage, antigen becomes associated with large granules, probably lysosomes. Later macrophage RNA, with or without antigen fragments, is passed to the lymphocytes which cluster about the macrophage.[80] Soon thereafter, new antibody-forming cells appear in the spleen and lymph nodes. Significant titers of antibody do not appear for 3 to 4 days after stimulation, although minute quantities may be detected in the first 24 hours. Stimulation or depression of macrophage activity in vivo is accompanied by stimulation or depression of antibody production.

RETICULAR CELLS

The term "reticular cell" has not been used with accuracy in the past, because of the inability of investigators using the light microscope to clearly differentiate the reticular cells of the lymphoid tissue from macrophages.[153a, 194a] Electron microscopy reveals that reticular cells resemble fibroblasts and are intimately related to the fibrillar material of the lymphoid tissue. They contain no obvious phagocytosed particles.[27b] These findings have prompted recent investigators to suggest that the term be reserved for those cells involved in the formation of fibrillar stroma.[131a]

The reticular cells of the lymphoid follicle have dendritic processes which are in close contact with lymphocytes and blood vessels.[127a, 194b] Antigen has been seen to be retained on the surface of these processes.[127a]

Immunoglobulins: Nomenclature, Structure, and Function

Knowledge of the plasma proteins has increased as the direct result of improved methodology. As is usual in times of rapid technical advances, some overlapping in definition and confusion in terminology has resulted. The various techniques employed in the study of plasma proteins allow different views of the various fractions and the technique employed in any given circumstance will therefore depend on the immediate aim of the investigator.

Ammonium sulfate has been used for many years to precipitate proteins from solution. The 50 per cent saturation of plasma will result in the precipitation of the globulins. The major protein which remains in solution is albumin and it in turn is precipitated when the concentration of ammonium sulfate is increased to 100 per cent. The two main classes of plasma protein, globulin and albumin, may be separated by this simple treatment.

A major advance occurred when Tiselius published the results of his investigations of the behavior of plasma proteins in an electrical field. He was able to identify three globulin fractions which he termed alpha (α), beta (β), and gamma (γ). The apparatus used was too expensive and cumbersome for most laboratories, and widespread interest in electrophoresis did not develop until the method was simplified.

In addition to the study of plasma proteins in an electrical field, investigators characterized their behavior in high centrifugal fields. These experiments were carried out in the ultracentrifuge, where the movement of the protein molecules as a function of their net mass is defined in terms of Svedberg units (S). One S unit is equivalent to a distance of 10^{-13} cm. in 1 second in a force field of 1 dyne; routinely, however, the fields are $> 10^8$ dynes.

When the plasma proteins were studied in this manner, three major fractions were defined:

A = 4S – molecular weight, 70,000
G = 7S – molecular weight, 160,000
M = 19S – molecular weight, 1,000,000

These studies are generally carried out at various concentrations and extrapolated to infinite dilution at 20° C so that the sedimentation rates are not complicated by interactions between the macromolecules.

The smallest protein is present in the largest amount and is mostly albumin (A). That of intermediate size is almost all gamma globulin (G). The proteins of greatest molecular weight are present in the smallest quantity and referred to as macroglobulins (M).

Electrophoresis, using a variety of quasisolid supporting mediums, is now employed clinically to characterize the plasma proteins. When filter paper is used as a supporting medium, the plasma proteins may be separated into six components: albumin, α_1, α_2, β, and γ globulin, and fibrinogen (Fig. 15–1). If serum rather than plasma is used, the fibrinogen is not present. This technique has found widespread clinical application and with careful control gives good reproducibility (Fig. 15–2). Among supporting mediums other than those derived from cellulose, starch and agar gel have been most useful. Each allows further definition of the plasma proteins.

Starch gel electrophoresis allows separation on the basis of the size and shape of the molecule as well as that based on electrical charge. This results in many subdivisions of the major plasma proteins.

Electrophoresis of plasma proteins in agar achieves a separation similar to that of paper (Fig. 15–3). This supporting medium has the advantage that electrophoresis and immunodiffusion may be carried out together in one process known as immunoelectrophoresis. This technique afforded a new approach and new insights. Of particular interest was the finding that gamma globulin is composed of three major fractions,[11] γG, γA, γM, and two minor fractions γD and γE. These fractions are closely related chemically, immunologically, and functionally, and the term *immunoglobulins* has been applied to them.[93]

Extensive studies of the subunits which result from enzymatic digestion[77, 125, 148] or chemical cleavage[47, 68, 99] of the immunoglobulins have contributed much to our knowledge of their structure. The fragments resulting

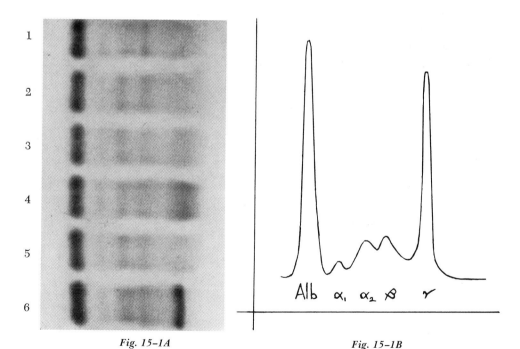

Fig. 15–1A   *Fig. 15–1B*

Figure 15–1A. Electrophoresis on cellulose acetate sheet. Note the heavy broad gamma fraction typical of a polyclonal gammopathy in no. 4 and compare to the heavy sharp gamma fraction in no. 6 which is typical of a monoclonal gammopathy.

Figure 15–1B. Quantitative analysis of the various fractions separated by electrophoresis may be obtained by the use of a densitometer, the main components of which are a photoelectric cell and galvanometer. This is the densitometer record of the electrophoretic pattern of serum no. 6 in *A*. The areas under the curves may be determined by planimetry, by weighing, or by an automatic integrator attached to the densitometer.

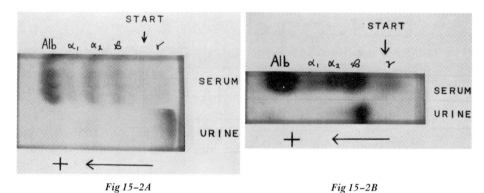

Fig 15–2A   Fig 15–2B

Figure 15–2A. Paper electrophoresis of serum and concentrated urine from patient with multiple myeloma. The abnormal protein is found in the urine but is not apparent in the serum.

Figure 15–2B. Paper electrophoresis of serum and urine from patient with multiple myeloma. The abnormal protein is found in both the urine and the serum.

from papain digestion have been termed S (slow) or F (fast) on the basis of their relative electrophoretic mobilities. Those resulting from chemical cleavage of disulfide bonds are termed L (light) or H (heavy) chains on the basis of their respective molecular weights. Although they are not identical, the S chains are similar to the L fragments and the F chains resemble the H fragments.[47] The products of chemical cleavage unlike those obtained by enzymatic degradation, probably resemble the intact substituent polypeptide chains of the protein molecule.

The H chains are the portion of the molecule which characterize the class and are responsible for the antigenic specificity of the five known immunoglobulins.[68] The molecular weights of these fragments range from 53,000 (γG) to 75,000 (γE); they contain the carbohydrate moiety, carry the Gm (a) specificity, and are unrelated to Bence Jones protein.[68, 142]

The L chains have a molecular weight of approximately 25,000 and contain no carbohydrate; they are the site of InV genotype specificity.[174] Two antigenic types of L chains have been identified and designated as kappa (I,B) and lambda (II,A); others may be found. The L chains have solubility and thermal characteristics similar to the Bence Jones proteins and the normal microglobulins.[67, 68, 151] In each divalent antibody molecule there appear to be two chains, both of which contain antigen combining sites.[119, 142] Since a pair of one of the two known types of L chains comprises part of each immunoglobulin molecule, they are probably responsible for the antigenic cross reactions among the five classes of immunoglobulins and with their abnormal counterparts in disease.

The immunoglobulin molecule is presently thought to be composed of two like H chains, which will determine the class of immunoglobulin, and two like L chains, all connected by disulfide bridges (Fig. 15–4).

γG (γ, γ_2, 7Sγ, 6.6Sγ, γ_{ss} IgG)

γG globulins comprise nearly 70 per cent of the total serum gamma globulin. The majority of acquired antibodies are in this fraction which crosses the

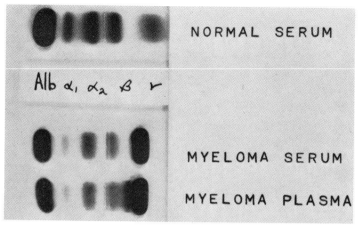

NORMAL SERUM

Alb α₁ α₂ β γ

MYELOMA SERUM

MYELOMA PLASMA

Figure 15–3. Agar gel electrophoresis. Note the fibrinogen band just in front of the abnormal gamma fraction in the myeloma plasma.

placental membrane and is responsible for the early passive immunity of the newborn. The γG fraction has a molecular weight of approximately 168,000 and is thought to originate in the plasma cell.

γG globulin has been divided into four heavy chain subclasses on the basis of antigenic differences. The subclasses have been variously termed γG₁ (We, 2b), γG₂ (Ne, 2a), γG₃ (Vi, 2c), and γG₄ (Ge, 2d). Production of the four different subclasses is believed to be controlled by four separate, closely linked genetic loci.[87]

γA (γ₁A, β₂A, IgA)

γA has a molecular weight of approximately 170,000 and constitutes about 12 per cent of the serum immunoglobulins. In the serum, greater than 90 per

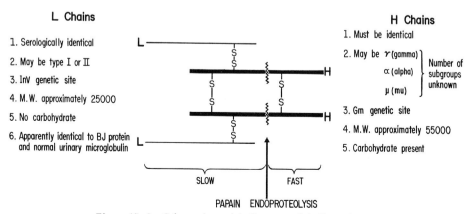

L Chains

1. Serologically identical
2. May be type I or II
3. InV genetic site
4. M.W. approximately 25000
5. No carbohydrate
6. Apparently identical to BJ protein and normal urinary microglobulin

H Chains

1. Must be identical
2. May be γ (gamma)
   α (alpha) } Number of subgroups unknown
   μ (mu)
3. Gm genetic site
4. M.W. approximately 55000
5. Carbohydrate present

SLOW   FAST

PAPAIN ENDOPROTEOLYSIS

Figure 15–4. Schematic model of gamma globulin molecule.

cent of the γA is present as 7S monomers with small amounts of 9S, 11S, and higher polymers. The carbohydrate content of γA measures about 5 to 10 per cent. Two subclasses of γA, γA₁, and γA₂ (Le and He) have been identified on the basis of antigenic differences in the H chains.[187]

γA is the predominant immunoglobulin found in external secretions (saliva, tears, colostrum, and gastrointestinal and respiratory fluids), where it is present as an 11S molecule which consists of a dimer of 7SγA complexed to a glycoprotein called the T (transport) component or secretory piece.[154a, 182, 183] This 11S complex is known as secretory γA. The 7SγA portion of secretory γA is thought to be synthesized by plasma cells located beneath the epithelial cells of the mucosal surfaces, whereas the T component is thought to be made in the epithelial cells.[184] This antibody system has been referred to as the secretory IgA system.[181]

γM (γ₁M, 19Sγ, β₂M, γ-Macroglobulin, IgM)

γM globulins have a molecular weight of approximately 850,000 and represent about 5 per cent of the total serum gamma globulins. Like the γA fraction, these globulins contain a carbohydrate fraction which comprises 10 to 12 per cent of their weight. Certain isohemagglutinins, Rh antibodies, cold hemagglutinins, and heterophile antibodies have been identified in this group. They do not cross the placental membrane and are not found in newborn serum. (The Rh antibodies that cross the placenta are believed to be 7SγG antibodies.) These large units may be dissociated into five subunits of 170,000 molecular weight, which, although they have some similarity to the other gamma globulins, are not identical. They may polymerize into 24S and 32S fractions.[142]

γD (1gD)

Immunoglobulin D (γD) is a 7S globulin with a pair of distinctive heavy chains designated delta (δ) and a normal complement of either kappa (κ) or lambda (λ) chains.[84, 94, 160, 162] The median value of γD in the serum is 3 mg. per cent, and its half-life is 2.8 days. It is primarily intravascular in location (73 per cent), and no unique role has as yet been discovered for it.

γE (1gE, 1gND)

The reaginic antibodies belong to the recently identified immunoglobulin class γE (1gE) and not to γA (1gA), as was believed in the past.[20, 101, 105] γE, which has a molecular weight of approximately 200,000, is present in normal serum in very small amounts. The heavy chains, which have been designated epsilon (ε), and both kappa (κ) and lambda (λ) chains have been identified.[21] γE (1gE) is a γ1 glycoprotein with a sedimentation coefficient of 8.5 and has a carbohydrate content of 10.7 per cent. It is probably divalent, but does not have complement-fixing activity.[101] γE (1gE) from selected sera reacts with a

Table 15–1. *Nomenclature for the Human Immunoglobulins*

I. Major Classes of Immunoglobulin Molecules

PROPOSED BY WHO REPORT*	SYNONYMS
γG or IgG	γ_2, 7Sγ, 6.6Sγ, γ
γA or IgA	γ_1A, β_2A
γM or IgM	γ_1M, 19Sγ, γ-Macroglobulin, β_2M
γE or IgE	IgND
γD or IgD	

II. Constituent Polypeptide Chains

Heavy (Fast) Chains

PROPOSED BY WHO REPORT*	SYNONYMS
γ (gamma)	γ_2-H
α (alpha)	γ_1A-H, β_2A-H
μ (mu)	γ_1M-H, β_2M-H
ϵ (epsilon)	
δ (delta)	

Light (Slow) Chains

PROPOSED BY WHO REPORT*	SYNONYMS
κ (kappa)	Type I, B
λ (lambda)	Type II, A

*Bull. World Health Organ., *30*:447, 1964.

number of antigens. It is capable of sensitizing human skin for Prausnitz-Kustner (P-K) reactions and human leukocytes for histamine release.[102] Recently, investigators have implicated γE immunoglobulin in the release of the slow-reacting substance of anaphylaxis (SRS-A) from monkey lung in vitro.[103]

Low Molecular Weight Antibodies (γM, Microglobulins, γL Globulins)

The original reports in 1958 of low molecular weight antibodies in the urine have been confirmed and extended.[16, 23] These proteins have the electrophoretic mobility of γ globulins, a molecular weight range of approximately 10,000 to 40,000, and sedimentation constants from 1.6 to 5.7S.[78, 154] Two types of low molecular weight γ globulins have been identified in normal urine and related antigenically to the S fragment of papain-digested γG. They appear to have the thermal and solubility characteristics of Bence Jones proteins[176, 180] and normal L chains.[23] The source of these proteins is not known, but they appear to arise from de novo synthesis rather than as the result of asynchronous chain production in the synthesis of normal multichained immunoglobulins and may represent the normal counterparts of Bence Jones proteins.[23,151]

Synthesis of Immunoglobulins

The germinal (reticular) centers and plasma cells of human lymphoid tissue appear to be the site of origin of human immunoglobulins.[122] The small lymphocytes do not appear to participate in this activity. The cells may produce both L and H chains, but rarely, if ever, both types of L chains. The ratio of cells producing kappa L chains to those producing lambda L chains is approximately two to one.[27]

Recent evidence indicates a qualitative difference between primary and secondary antibody responses.[14] The initial response appears to be the rapid rise in the serum concentration of γM immunoglobulins,[118] followed by a slow rise in the γG fraction. The γM fraction has a rather short half-life of 5.1 days compared to the 23 days half-life of γG.[12] It appears that the γM immunoglobulin is the body's initial antibody defense.

The immunoglobulins are increased in chronic infections, collagen diseases, and cirrhosis. One or more of the immunoglobulins is decreased in diseases with immune paralysis, such as primary or secondary hypogammaglobulinemia.

Uncontrolled proliferation of cells of the reticuloendothelial system may result in the production of a homogeneous protein closely related to one or more of the immunoglobulins. Waldenström[191] has used the word "gammopathy" to indicate a primary "essential" disturbance of γ-forming templates in conditions characterized by disturbed gamma globulin formation. Burnet[33] proposed that multiple myeloma be considered the result of unlimited proliferation of a single clone of plasma cells producing excessive amounts of a homogenous protein. This concept has been extended[191] to include all instances of homogeneous hypergammaglobulinemia in the term "monoclonal gammopathies" and those in which heterogeneous hypergammaglobulinemia occurs as "polyclonal gammopathies."

Immunologic Mechanisms

Understanding of the relationship between the structure and the function of the cells of the lymphoreticular system is incomplete. Recent progress has resulted from studies in comparative immunobiology,[42, 127, 129, 144] the use of laboratory techniques to create animal models of immunologic deficiency states,[55, 135] and the study of individuals with congenital or acquired immunologic abnormalities.[60, 61, 100, 130]

COMPARATIVE IMMUNOBIOLOGY

Our environment contains many substances capable of stimulating an immunologic response when introduced into the body through the skin, the respiratory system, or the gastrointestinal tract. The progressive development of the capacity of the human to elaborate an immune response to these substances has now been traced through the phylogenetic scale.

Invertebrates produce agglutinins, and bacteriocidins and have the capacity to wall off offending substances with fibrous tissue. Lower vertebrates have a primitive thymus and spleen, circulating lymphocytes, and the beginnings of adaptive immunity; plasma cells appear in later species. Amphibians and reptiles have lymph nodes and a true lamina propria plasma cell system. They are able to produce multiple immunoglobulin types. The egg-laying mammals are the first to have Peyer's patches and tonsils.

All major components of the evolving lymphoreticular system have persisted in mammals with the exception of the avian bursa, and even this structure may be represented in mammals by the Peyer's patch system.

EXPERIMENTAL STUDIES

Laboratory experiments have established the role of the avian bursa of Fabricius and the thymus in immune development.[50, 130, 147] These studies have led to a concept that two cell populations exist in the lymphoid system. The cell-mediated immune responses appear to be related to a thymus-dependent population of small lymphocytes, whereas immune globulin and antibodies are dependent upon the cell line of the bursa-dependent lymphocytes. The Peyer's patch type of lymphoid tissue in mammals may be equivalent to the avian bursa of Fabricius. Good has suggested that the stem cell population of the bone marrow provides cells to both the thymus and the avian bursa or the mammalian bursa-equivalent.[85]

Thymus-dependent lymphocytes localize in the paracortical areas of the lymph node, where they are capable of undergoing blast transformation and proliferation and are responsible for those immune responses termed cellular immunity: homograft rejection, delayed-type hypersensitivity, and graft-versus-host reactions. The population of thymus-independent or bursa-equivalent lymphocytes is localized in the cortical region of the lymph nodes where they can undergo blast transformation and differentiation into lymphocytes and plasma cells capable of synthesizing immunoglobulins with antigen specificity (Fig. 15–5).

CLINICAL STUDIES

In 1952, Bruton reported the first studies of a patient with an immunologic deficiency state associated with agammaglobulinemia. Some 20 immunologic deficiency states have been identified and studied since that initial report.[85] These studies have provided further support for the concept that two compartments of lymphoid cells differentiate under separate influences in man and have separate functional roles in the immunologic process.

Both congenital and acquired immunologic deficiency states have been described.

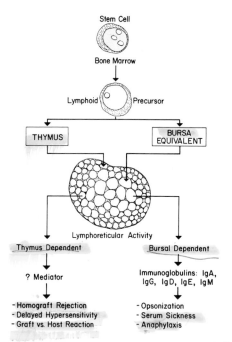

Stem Cell

Bone Marrow

Lymphoid   Precursor

THYMUS   BURSA
                        EQUIVALENT

Figure 15–5. The two-population concept of the immunologic system.

Lymphoreticular Activity

Thymus Dependent   Bursal Dependent

? Mediator   Immunoglobulins: IgA,
                    IgG, IgD, IgE, IgM

- Homograft Rejection   - Opsonization
- Delayed Hypersensitivity   - Serum Sickness
- Graft vs. Host Reaction   - Anaphylaxis

Congenital Immunologic Deficiency States

Sex-linked recessive form of agammaglobulinemia. Patients with this disorder regularly demonstrate a marked decrease in IgG, a decrease or absence of IgM, and an absence of IgA. They either fail to form antibody or form antibody poorly against a variety of antigens. Plasma cells are absent or markedly reduced and germinal centers in lymphoid tissue are absent; in addition, there is absence of follicular structure in the poorly developed Peyer's patches. The plasma cell system in the lamina propria of the intestinal tract and in the secretory glands is lacking and there is no plasma cell response to potent antigens. Thymic structure is normal, as is the number of circulating lymphocytes, bone marrow lymphocytes, and lymphocytes in thymus-dependent areas of the lymph nodes and spleen.

Patients with the sex-linked recessive form of agammaglobulinemia are able to develop delayed-type hypersensitivity and reject primary allografts as well as develop second-set responses, which demonstrates cellular immunologic memory.[85] Skin allograft rejection is delayed in some cases.

There appears to be an isolated deficiency of thymus-independent lymphocytes in this condition. The thymus-dependent lymphocytes seem to be intact. The disorder resembles that which results from bursectomy and irradiation in the chicken.[55]

Congenital aplasia of the thymus gland (DiGeorge's Syndrome). The opposite picture is found in children with the syndrome described by DiGeorge in 1965.[61] These children have neither thymus nor parathyroid glands as the result of a failure of the derivatives of the third and fourth pharyngeal pouches to develop. Normal or slightly reduced numbers of lymphocytes circulate in the blood, but there is an absence of lymphocytes in the thymus-dependent areas of lymphoid tissue. Germinal centers, plasma cells, and immunoglobulins develop normally.

These two examples of immunologic deficiency states in man demonstrate clearly the differences between the loss of thymus-dependent lymphocytes on the one hand and the loss of thymus-independent lymphocytes and plasma cells on the other, and add support to the concept of a two-population lymphoid system.[83]

Swiss type (autosomal recessive) agammaglobulinemia. A third important disorder of immunologic function is found in the Swiss type of agammaglobulinemia. Patients with this disorder lack the ability to produce humoral antibody and have a marked decrease or absence of all immunoglobulins. They do not develop delayed-type hypersensitivity or cell-mediated immunity and they do not reject allografts. There may be a marked reduction of lymphocytes in their peripheral blood at varying times in the course of their illness. Examination of the bone marrow reveals a decrease in lymphocytes and an absence of plasma cells. Germinal centers are not found in the lymph nodes. Tonsils, adenoids, Peyer's patches, and the plasma cell system of the lamina propria system are absent, and the thymus is virtually absent.

Swiss type agammaglobulinemia is a genetic disorder transmitted as a simple autosomal recessive trait. It would appear to be a defect in the stem cell differentiation as both systems are involved.

Other Immunologic Deficiency States

A large variety of congenital immunological deficiency states have now been reported and classification of these disorders has proved difficult.[89, 172] The role of the multipotential stem cell, various sites of differentiation, and factors that may expand the cell population must be taken into account in any system of classification that is based on pathophysiology. The possibility of inadvertant transfer of material with immunologic potential which can not be rejected by these patients must also be considered.[168]

Acquired Immunologic Deficiency States

The acquired immunologic deficiency states are a heterogenous group characterized by altered function of lymphocytes, plasma cells, or both which result in failure to mount an adequate immunologic response. They are characterized by lowered immunoglobulin concentrations and/or alteration in number and function of lymphocytes or plasma cells. They occur in either sex. The onset is usually later than that of the congenital variety and may follow a specific infectious disease, such as measles. The disorder may be temporary or may persist.

Immunologic disorders accompany certain malignancies of the hematopoietic system with relative regularity. Malignant disease of the hematopoietic system is known to alter specific cell lines and study of the function of these cells in relation to their disordered structure has allowed further insight into the function of the immunologic system.

Hodgkin's disease.   Hodgkin's disease is a disease of the lymphoreticular system. Patients with this disorder have long been recognized to have a disordered immunologic potential. They have diminished ability to develop delayed-type hypersensitivity and reject skin grafts, yet maintain normal or elevated levels of immunoglobulins and their capacity to mount a humoral antibody response. They have more difficulty mounting an immunologic response to infections with tuberculosis, cryptococcus and low-grade pyogenic organisms than to the more virulent organisms, such as pneumococcus or streptococcus. These patients have a selective deficiency of thymus-dependent lymphocytes. A pronounced peripheral lymphopenia often develops as the disease progresses.[2, 3, 113]

Multiple myeloma.   Multiple myeloma contrasts sharply with Hodgkin's disease in the manner in which it affects immunologic responsiveness. The plasma cell system is involved and the antibody response to virulent pyogenic infections is suboptimal. The amount of normal circulating immunoglobulin may be deficient, although there usually is a large amount of globulin synthesized by the myeloma cell. The immunologic deficiency of these patients appears to result from the defect in the thymus-independent lymphoid and plasma cell system.[52] They retain the capacity to develop delayed-type hypersensitivity, to reject homografts, and to exhibit second-set reactions.

Chronic lymphocytic leukemia.   Patients with chronic lymphocytic leukemia are often unable to develop or to express delayed-type hypersensitivity; they may also fail to develop humoral antibodies in response to antigenic challenge. Available evidence indicates that both functional components of the lymphoreticular system are deficient, perhaps as a result of a defect at the stem cell level, an abnormality which would affect thymus-dependent and thymus-independent lymphocytes.[52]

Disorders of Plasma Cells and Lymphocytes Associated with Immunoglobulin Abnormalities

Multiple Myeloma

Multiple myeloma is an unusual and interesting disease in many respects. The symptomatology is extremely varied, and striking abnormalities are often apparent on the physical and roentgenologic examinations. The introduction of the needle aspiration of the bone marrow has made the tumor cells easily available for histologic study and a number of different cellular abnormalities have been observed. The disease has been of wide interest to investigators because it is characterized by a number of metabolic disturbances, particularly in protein metabolism. Recent advances in diagnostic techniques have served to broaden the spectrum of this disorder. Intensive study has contributed not only to a better understanding of the disease process, but extensively to the understanding of the synthesis, structure, and genetics of normal gamma globulins.

HISTORICAL ASPECTS

Multiple myeloma was first reported in 1847 in a tradesman who presented with "mollities ossium" (soft bones) and urine containing large quantities of "animal matter." The patient was studied by Drs. MacIntyre and Watson and a urine specimen was sent to Dr. Henry Bence Jones with the following note:[18]

Saturday, Nov. 1st, 1845

Dear Dr. Jones: The tube contains urine of very high specific gravity. When boiled it becomes slightly opaque. On the addition of nitric acid, it effervesces, assumes a reddish hue, and becomes quite clear; but as it cools, assumes the consistence and appearance which you see. Heat reliquefies it. What is it? . . .

Dr. Bence Jones described the peculiar properties of the unusual urinary protein which bears his name.[18] The name multiple myeloma was given to the disorder by von Rustizky in 1873.[16] Prior to 1900 it was thought that different cellular types were responsible for the tumor in different individuals. In 1900 Dr. James H. Wright established that the myeloma cell is related to the plasma cell and concluded that the neoplasm arises from an abnormal proliferation of these cells.[199] These conclusions have been confirmed many times, particularly since the introduction of marrow aspiration by Arinkïn in 1929.[6]

PATHOGENESIS AND PATHOLOGIC PHYSIOLOGY

Multiple myeloma is considered to be a malignant neoplasm that arises in the bone marrow and involves the skeleton primarily. The clinical features of the disease are attributable to the location of the tumor and to abnormalities in protein metabolism. Although multiple myeloma appears to be primarily a widespread disorder of the bone marrow, solitary osseous tumors and extraskeletal nests of myeloma cells are found occasionally. Whether these lesions are metastatic from some skeletal site or arise from precursors in situ in response to some stimulus is unknown.[115]

A tumor which has many of the characteristics of multiple myeloma has been established in mice.[149] It has been demonstrated that it is the tumor and not the host that determines the characteristics of the myeloma protein. The cells comprising any single tumor appear to have but one protein pattern and continue to produce the same protein after serial transplants. Multiple myeloma has also been studied in tissue culture.[123] These studies provide evidence that both Bence Jones protein and gamma globulin are produced by myeloma cells grown in vitro.

Myeloma cells are apparently responsible for the production of the abnormal proteins that are found in the serum and urine of patients with the disease. Recent evidence indicates that the abnormal urinary and serum proteins that occur in any one patient with multiple myeloma are closely related to but distinct from the plasma proteins of other patients with multiple myeloma as well as from the normal serum proteins.[90, 150, 170] As in the other diseases with disordered synthesis of serum proteins, excessive production of L and H chains occurs. There may be synchronous production of excessive amounts of one type of L chain and one class of H chain resulting in the appearance of homogeneous myeloma protein in the serum and no proteinuria. On the other hand, the rate of synthesis of L chains may exceed the rate of synthesis of H chains and the excess of L chains may appear in the serum in addition to the myeloma protein. The L chains are of low molecular weight and are rapidly excreted by the kidney. As a consequence, they are found in very low concentration in the serum but may appear in large amounts in the urine. The L chains have the thermal and solubility characteristics of Bence Jones protein.

Of particular interest is the recent discovery of γD and γE myeloma. The discovery of these disorders brought to light two new classes of immunoglobulin. γD myeloma has been shown to represent about 1 per cent of all myelomas. Only two patients with γE myeloma have been described to date.[17, 20, 21, 72, 96, 134, 203]

As much as 20 or 30 gm. of Bence Jones protein may be excreted in the urine each day. When it is recalled that from 70 to 90 gm. of protein is available in the daily diet of the adult, it is apparent that the amount excreted as Bence Jones protein constitutes a considerable diversion of protein from the usual metabolic needs. This remarkable excretion of protein continues independently of any exogenous source of protein.[150] The prolonged excretion of Bence Jones protein in the urine may produce renal insufficiency. Apparently the protein is not specifically toxic to the renal tissue but is precipitated in the tubular lumen, and results in the eventual loss of the proximal nephron unit.[76]

Table 15–2. *The Relationship of Structural Subunits of Normal Gamma Globulin to the Abnormal Proteins Found in Proliferative Disorders of Plasma Cells and Lymphocytes*

DISEASE	L CHAIN	H CHAIN	URINE PROTEIN	SERUM PROTEIN
Multiple myeloma	Type κ or λ	γ (gamma)	BJP	γ G myeloma
	Type κ or λ	α (alpha)	BJP	γ A myeloma
	Type κ or λ	δ (delta)	BJP	γ D myeloma
	Type κ or λ	ϵ (epsilon)	BJP	γ E myeloma
	Type κ or λ	———	BJP	Light chain
	Type κ or λ	μ (mu)	BJP	γ M myeloma
Macroglobulinemia	Type κ or λ	μ (mu)	BJP	Macroglobulin
Heavy chain disease		γ (gamma)	γ (gamma)	γ (gamma)
		μ (mu)	μ (mu)	μ (mu)
		α (alpha)	α (alpha)	α (alpha)
		δ (delta)*	δ (delta)*	δ (delta)*
		ϵ (epsilon)*	ϵ (epsilon)*	ϵ (epsilon)*

*Expected but not found.

Vacuolation and precipitation of protein have been observed within the tubular epithelium,[171] and it has been suggested that these tubular lesions may be the cause of renal tubular reabsorption defects like those of the adult Fanconi syndrome.[70] Recent investigators suggested that renal insufficiency in multiple myeloma is secondary to intratubular localization of light chains with consequent tubular atrophy.[114] For some obscure reason nitrogen retention which results from renal lesions in multiple myeloma is rarely accompanied by the hypertension usually seen in other forms of renal disease severe enough to produce azotemia.

Sixty per cent of the patients with multiple myeloma will have either Type I or Type II Bence Jones proteinuria. The designation Type I or Type II includes a spectrum of proteins—perhaps varying only by a single amino acid in its primary structure. Thus, Type I Bence Jones protein obtained from the urine of one patient with myeloma would share many antigenic characteristics with a Type I Bence Jones protein from a second patient with myeloma but would have one or more points of difference. The same is true of the serum globulins. The serum and urinary proteins are unique for each patient.

As many as 20 per cent of patients with multiple myeloma may have a reduction in serum immunoglobulins and have no detectable serum M components. The disorder is called light chain disease or Bence Jones myeloma.[48, 94, 196] Patients show a marked increase in free light chains, usually of one type, in the serum, and marked Bence Jones proteinuria. Renal insufficiency is common, as are anemia and widespread osteolytic lesions. The prognosis in this disorder is poorer than that in γG or γA myeloma.

As a result of the increased production of protein the level of the serum protein, particularly the globulin fraction, is usually increased in multiple myeloma. The increase usually involves the gamma globulin but in some instances the alpha and beta fractions are most affected. Despite the large amount of gamma globulin that is often present in the circulating blood these patients are usually able to respond with only a poor antibody response to antigenic challenge.[171] It is not known whether this deficiency is the result of the diversion of protein needed for antibody formation into other channels or of a disorganization of antibody formation in the plasma cells. The increased susceptibility of patients with multiple myeloma to pulmonary infection may be a consequence of the increase in serum protein, which causes an increase in the blood viscosity and leads to thrombosis of the small pulmonary vessels. Pulmonary infection is also favored by the subnormal antibody response and the decreased pulmonary ventilation that is secondary to painful fractures of the ribs or vertebrae.[171]

Another example of the profound alteration in protein metabolism in this disease is the occasional occurrence in the serum of a cold precipitable globulin. This protein, known as cryoglobulin, is found in multiple myeloma but may occur in other diseases.[122a] When it is present in large quantities the cryoglobulin may precipitate in the blood in areas of lower temperature such as the ears, nose, fingers, or toes, and in this way produce thrombosis, ulceration, or gangrene. Raynaud's phenomenon may occur in these circumstances.[56] As the amount of cryoglobulin increases, the critical temperature rises, with the result that precipitation sometimes occurs in deeper structures in the body.

The cryoglobulins may be IgG, IgM, or mixed IgG-IgM proteins. Some have been reported to have rheumatoid factor activity and others to bind complement.[88a, 122a] The physicochemical properties of these proteins responsible for their cryoprecipitation are not known.[122a]

An unusual abnormality of protein metabolism, a form of amyloidosis, is found in approximately 5 or 10 per cent of the patients with multiple myeloma.[37, 44, 115, 171] The distribution of amyloid material is similar to that seen in primary amyloidosis. It has been found in the bones, voluntary muscles, skin, liver, spleen, gastrointestinal tract, adrenal glands, kidneys, tongue, heart, and synovial tissues. In the latter circumstance clinical features that resemble rheumatoid arthritis may occur. It has been suggested that primary amyloid may result from a metabolic defect in the reticuloendothelial cell. Recent studies have not supported the suggested relationship between immunoglobulins, Bence Jones proteins, and amyloid.[13, 44, 144] (F.S.: II, 97)

Hypercalcemia is not unusual in multiple myeloma.[16, 37, 108, 115, 171] It may occur as the result of hyperproteinemia which affords the plasma a greater calcium binding capacity or as the result of bone destruction with a release of more calcium into the blood than can be excreted by the kidneys. The decreased renal function often found in multiple myeloma may also contribute to the hypercalcemia.[1] Serum calcium levels as high as 16 or 18 mg. per 100 ml. occur without any significant disturbance in the levels of the serum phosphorus or alkaline phosphatase. Gastrointestinal dysfunction, weakness, apathy, polydipsia, and polyuria are found in association with moderate increases of serum calcium; very high levels of serum calcium may lead to vascular collapse and death.[1]

The anemia in multiple myeloma was previously considered to be the result of a decrease in red cell production.[43] Recently another factor, dilution of the red cell mass, has been shown to be important.[27a, 93a, 93b, 110a] The colloid osmotic effect produced by the hyperglobulinemia appears to be the most likely cause of the increase in plasma volume and dilution of the red cell mass. Plasmapheresis produces a decrease in the M protein concentration with a resultant decrease in plasma volume, accompanied by an increase in the peripheral hematocrit.[93b]

CLINICAL MANIFESTATIONS

Multiple myeloma occurs in all races and is about twice as common in males as in females.[171] Prior to the introduction of sternal biopsy it was reported to constitute 0.03 per cent of all malignancies.[81] It is characteristically a disease of older persons. The disease has been reported in patients less than 20 years of age,[26] but 95 per cent of the patients in one series were over the age of 40 years.[171] In a group of 50 patients reviewed by the authors all were past 40 years of age and 80 per cent were over 50 years of age.[115]

The commonest presenting symptom is pain, which occurs sometime during the course of the disease in nearly all patients; unfortunately it is often disabling and difficult to control. The pain is due to involvement of the bones and to pressure on the adjacent nerves. Compression fractures of vertebrae, which occur in about one-half of the patients, are most likely to be found in the upper lumbar and lower dorsal vertebrae.[16, 81, 171] Pathologic fractures of the ribs are common and fractures of the femur, sternum, ilium, humerus, clavicle, and pubic bones are not rare. In some patients the discomfort is mild and poorly localized but in others the occurrence of a fracture is accompanied by the sudden onset of severe girdle-like pain in the chest or abdomen. Pain with and without fracture occurs commonly in the hips, legs, shoulders, and arms, but is rare in the neck and head. At times pain is not a prominent feature and the history is mainly that of recurring attacks of fever or pneumonia. The diagnosis of such episodes may be puzzling if other manifestations of multiple myeloma are not evident. Attacks of this nature, which were seen in 50 per cent of one series, are most likely to occur in patients with greatly elevated serum globulin levels.[81, 171] Whether these transient pulmonary manifestations are episodes of pulmonary infarction or pneumonia is uncertain. The clinical picture is usually that of fever, cough, mucopurulent sputum, and roentgenologic evidence of patchy infiltration in the lungs.

The frequent occurrence of radicular pain and evidence of cord compression in multiple myeloma is well known but the occurrence of peripheral neuritis without compression is not so widely recognized. The frequency of all types of neurologic involvement in multiple myeloma has been placed at 10 per cent,[37] 14 per cent,[16] 18 per cent,[108] and 40 per cent.[81, 171] In the last series cord compression, with or without paraplegia, was seen in about 14 per cent of the patients, all of whom had roentgenologic evidence of compression fracture of the spine. Thirty per cent of those with neurologic manifestations evidenced involvement of the spinal roots or peripheral nerves in the absence of vertebral collapse. Involvement of a nerve was manifested by radicular pain or other evidence of peripheral neuritis such as foot drop, hypesthesia, paresthesia, weakness, or muscular atrophy. Cranial nerve involvement appears to be unusual.

Renal insufficiency occurs not infrequently in multiple myeloma and may dominate the clinical picture.[16, 37, 108, 171] There have been reports of death due to acute renal failure following intravenous pyelography in patients with multiple myeloma.[30, 110, 136] The factors responsible are unknown but may be related to dehydration and to stasis of urine flow produced by the abdominal compression resulting in precipitation of Bence Jones protein in the renal tubules. It is noteworthy that spontaneous anuria unassociated with pyelography has also been reported in patients with multiple myeloma.[11] Renal failure, which is secondary to involvement of the kidney by the disease, is unusual in the absence of Bence Jones proteinuria.[171] Hypertension is usually absent in these cases even when severe azotemia is present. The occurrence of azotemia without hypertension should arouse the suspicion of multiple myeloma.

Other less common manifestations of multiple myeloma are psychotic episodes that are often associated with marked elevation of the serum calcium, arthritis associated with deposits of amyloid in synovial membranes, and the presence of palpable tumors overlying the involved bones.

Significant loss of weight during the course of the disease was observed in 63 per cent of one series.[108]

Physical examination may disclose nothing more than is usually found in patients of the same age group. Probably the most frequent finding is tenderness on pressure over the areas of osseous involvement. Palpation should be gentle in these patients. One of the authors once had the experience of producing a fracture of the sternum while testing for sternal tenderness, and then produced another in the humerus when he helped the patient change position. Among the commonest signs on physical examination are those associated with compression of the spinal cord and involvement of the peripheral nerves.

Rarely, extra-osseous lesions may be responsible for the patient's presenting complaint. Moderate enlargement of the superficial lymph nodes is seen frequently. Palpable enlargement of the liver occurs in from 11 to 40 per cent of the patients, and in from 2 to 25 per cent the spleen is moderately enlarged.[171] Palpable tumor masses are seen in a minority of patients and then usually only in the later stages of the disease.[16, 171] Multiple myeloma should be considered in the differential diagnosis of skin and subcutaneous masses, lymphadenopathy, hepatosplenomegally, and pulmonary, pleural, mediastinal, and abdominal masses.[69]

Abnormalities of the skeleton that are demonstrable by x-ray constitute one of the most characteristic features of multiple myeloma. The most typical changes are the presence of multiple, clearly defined, punched-out lesions that involve several different bones (Fig. 15–6). The size of the lesions varies from a diameter of 1 or 2 mm. to areas as large as 10 to 12 cm.; the lesions are charac-

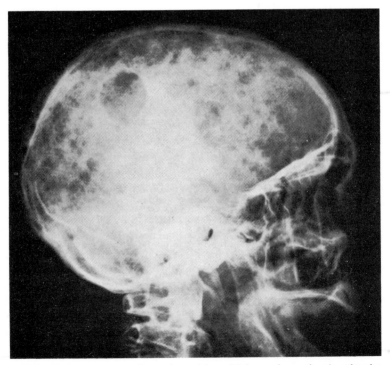

Figure 15–6. Roentgenogram of a patient with multiple myeloma showing the characteristic "punched-out" lesions.

terized by the absence of any osteoblastic reaction.[92, 171] In some patients such definite lesions are absent and roentgenograms show only generalized demineralization similar to that seen in senile or postmenopausal osteoporosis. In both types of lesions pathologic fractures, particularly compression fractures of the vertebral bodies, are common. Since the advent of sternal puncture and more detailed study of the plasma proteins as diagnostic measures it has become evident that some patients, perhaps 5 to 12 per cent, with undoubted myeloma have no demonstrable abnormalities in the roentgenograms at the time the diagnosis is made.[16, 92, 115, 171, 193] Demonstrable lesions occur most commonly in the spine, ribs, sternum, and clavicle; lesions of the skull, extremities, pelvic girdle, and shoulder girdle occur about half as often.[81] Lesions of the mandible occur less often.

LABORATORY EXAMINATION

Many abnormalities occur in the peripheral blood in patients with multiple myeloma. Anemia is one of the commonest features and is rarely absent throughout the course of the disease. In one series the hemoglobin ranged from 6 to 10 gm. per 100 ml. and the erythrocyte count ranged from 2 to 4 mil. per cu.mm.[171] The anemia is usually normocytic but when severe it may be macrocytic. The leukocyte count is usually normal but in one large series 20 per cent of the patients had leukocytosis and 40 per cent had leukopenia.[171] Examination of a smear of the peripheral blood may suggest the diagnosis because of the presence of rouleaux formation or plasma cells, or other abnormal mononuclear cells that resemble the abnormal cells found in the bone marrow. These cells may become so numerous in the peripheral blood that a diagnosis of "plasma cell leukemia" is made. Normoblasts and myelocytes appear in the peripheral blood not infrequently but are most likely to be seen in the advanced stage of the disease. The platelet count is normal in most patients but thrombocytopenia has been reported to occur in about 25 per cent.[171] (F.S.: II, 93)

Examination of bone marrow obtained by aspiration reveals a diagnostic or suspicious cell pattern in approximately 80 per cent of the cases of multiple myeloma.[115] The most characteristic finding is the presence of "myeloma" cells, which may constitute from 4 to 98 per cent of the cells present.[37, 115] These cells, which vary from 15 to 40 microns in diameter, usually have a single eccentrically placed nucleus. The chromatin pattern of the nucleus is finely divided and often contains several small nucleoli or a single large nucleolus. Various types of inclusions are sometimes seen in the cytoplasma of myeloma cells. Some cells appear vacuolated (Mott cell) and others contain protein particles that are thought to originate in the cell. One such protein forms the Russell bodies, which appear eosinophilc with Wright's stain and sometimes resemble whole erythrocytes or fragments of erythrocytes. Other cells contain protein particles, and have a bluish color when stained with Wright's stain, and still others contain definite protein crystals (Fig. 15–7). In many patients the typical "myeloma" cells are not seen but instead there is a large increase in cells that appear to be mature plasma cells. It is extremely rare for such cells to constitute more than 30 or 40 per cent of the total cells in the marrow in any disease other than multiple myeloma. (F.S.: II, 94–96)

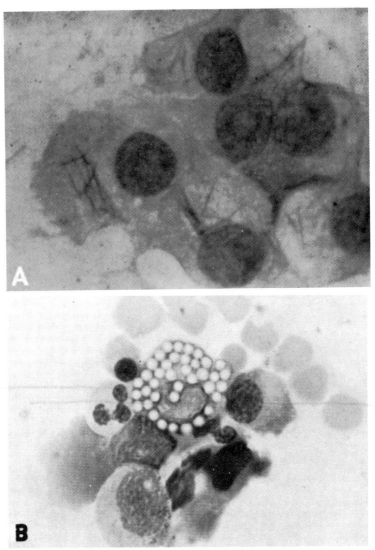

Figure 15-7. *A,* Myeloma cells with thin needle-shaped inclusion bodies which stained bright red with Wright's stain. *B,* Plasma cells containing Mott bodies; bone marrow aspiration, multiple myeloma.

Less pronounced increases in the marrow plasma cells occur in a number of disorders such as hypersensitivity states, collagen diseases, disseminated carcinomatosis, chronic infection (particularly the granulomatous types), and cirrhosis of the liver.[38, 41, 104, 159, 198] Multinucleated plasma cells are seen commonly both in myeloma and in other disorders.

A serum protein abnormality that is demonstrable by electrophoresis occurs in about 75 per cent of patients with myeloma.[138] An additional 18 per cent of patients, who fail to show characteristic changes on serum electrophoresis, have Bence Jones protein in the urine. If electrophoresis of the urinary protein is performed in addition to the serum electrophoresis, diagnostic abnormalities are found in over 93 per cent of patients with multiple myeloma.[138] In the majority of patients the abnormality consists of a sharp peak in the gamma fraction of the serum protein, but occasionally the increase is found only in the alpha or beta fraction.[1] Although a pattern of this type indicates the presence of a protein abnormality that is most likely associated with multiple myeloma, such changes are not diagnostic of multiple myeloma because they have been described in patients with lymphoma, leukemia, and amyloid disease. An "M" spike may occur in the absence of any clinical disease and is referred to as "benign monoclonal gammopathy." Myeloma cannot be excluded by the occurrence of a normal electrophoretic pattern because as many as 20 per cent of patients with multiple myeloma may have a normal serum protein pattern.[37, 94, 108, 138, 150] The total protein is found to be over 8.0 gm. per 100 ml. in about 72 per cent of patients.[16, 171] The increase occurs in the globulin fraction, and may amount to 10 or 11 gm. per 100 ml. Cryoglobulinemia, the presence in the circulating blood of a globulin that precipitates at temperatures lower than 37° C, occurs in only a small percentage of patients with multiple myeloma. Such globulins are not diagnostic of multiple myeloma, for they occur in other diseases, particularly those of the lymphoma group, as well (see Fig. 15–8).

The protein originally described by Bence Jones is found in the urine of 40 or 50 per cent of the patients with multiple myeloma when the urine is examined in the usual fashion by differential heating and acidification. When precipitin tests and electrophoresis are employed the abnormal protein can be demonstrated in virtually every case.[51, 138] The kidney plays a major role in the catabolism of Bence Jones protein.[197] The fragments of Bence Jones protein found in the urine of some patients with multiple myeloma are most likely formed during excretion of these proteins by the kidney.[40]

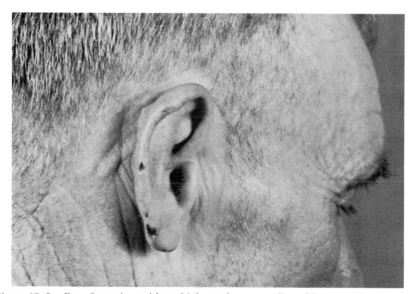

Figure 15–8. Ear of a patient with multiple myeloma complicated by cryoglobulinemia, showing ulceration and scarring.

Other abnormalities are often found in the peripheral blood. The commonest of these is a greatly elevated sedimentation rate, which occurs in the vast majority of patients with multiple myeloma, particularly if the serum protein is increased. When rouleaux formation is prominent on the blood smear the sedimentation rate is usually greatly increased. Hypercalcemia with values of 12 to 18 mg. per 100 ml. has been reported in from 20 to 39 per cent of patients.[16, 37] Even when the calcium is markedly elevated the levels of the serum phosphorus and the alkaline phosphatase are normal or slightly elevated. Hypercalcemia and negative calcium balance are believed to be due to an increased bone resorption rate, since urinary and fecal loss of calcium, bone acretion rate, and the miscible pool of calcium are normal or increased.[91] As is usually true in patients with any type of chronic renal disease, marked elevation of the urea nitrogen and other changes occur when renal failure develops in patients with multiple myeloma.

DIAGNOSIS

The classic case of multiple myeloma is usually recognized without difficulty. In the middle-aged or elderly individual the occurrence of pain, particularly radicular pain associated with compression fractures of the spine, and anemia suggests the diagnosis. If increases in the level of serum globulin and Bence Jones proteinuria are demonstrated, multiple myeloma is very probable. The diagnosis is established by finding "myeloma" cells or greatly increased numbers of plasma cells in the bone marrow; the presence of a sharp gamma peak on plasma electrophoresis usually has the same significance.

When many of the commoner features of the disease are absent or when some particular manifestation dwarfs the other features, the diagnosis may be more difficult. In older persons multiple myeloma must be considered in the differential diagnosis of any unexplained anemia, particularly if proteinuria is present. The diagnosis also should be considered in patients whose roentgenograms show osteoporosis or lytic lesions of the skeleton; the absence of osteoblastic changes, involvement of multiple vertebral bodies, involvement of the skull, and particularly the mandible, are all points that favor the diagnosis of multiple myeloma. Some patients with multiple myeloma come under observation first because of renal insufficiency, uremia, anemia, and proteinuria, and for this reason the diagnosis should be considered in all patients with these manifestations who are middle-aged or older, especially if hypertension is absent. Not infrequently the patient consults a physician because of radicular pain, paraplegia, or some other neurologic difficulty and attention may first be focused on the nervous system. Perhaps the diagnosis of multiple myeloma is most likely to be missed in patients who present with fever and roentgenologic evidence of pneumonia and in those whose complaints are particularly suggestive of peripheral neuritis or arthritis. In such patients difficulties usually arise because of the failure to consider multiple myeloma in the differential diagnosis. If multiple myeloma is present the diagnosis can nearly always be established by careful study of the bone marrow and the electrophoretic pattern of the protein in the serum and urine. All three of these examinations are usually abnormal if multiple myeloma is present; failure to find evidence of multiple myeloma in any of the three practically excludes the disease from further consideration.

COURSE AND PROGNOSIS

Multiple myeloma is a fatal disease with an average survival time of less than 2 years from the onset of symptoms.[16, 37, 81, 108, 121, 146, 171] The median survival time in one series was 13 months[42] and in another 15 months.[16] Although some patients succumb to the disease within a few weeks after onset of symptoms, others occasionally survive for 8, 11, or more years.[37, 51, 108] The 3 years survival rate appears to be only from 5 to 15 per cent.[16, 37] The prognosis is better if the disease appears to be localized;[16, 37] in one group of 18 such patients, 10 survived for more than 2 years and 3 survived from 3.8 to 9.8 years.[37] The status of the "solitary" myeloma is uncertain. At best it seems to be exceedingly rare because prolonged observation of patients suspected of belonging in this category almost invariably reveals widespread disease sooner or later, sometimes after 6 to 10 years have elapsed. The prognosis in an individual case bears little relationship to the apparent degree of maturity of the tumor cells in the marrow.[16, 25, 108]

A recent study compared the clinical and biochemical features of the difficent immunologic types of multiple myeloma.[94] In a group of 212 patients, 53 per cent were found to have γG myeloma, 22 per cent had γA myeloma, and 20 per cent had Bence Jones proteinuria without a demonstrable abnormality in the serum. The rest of the patients had γD, γM, or γE myeloma. Six patients had typical myelomatosis without detectable paraprotein in their urine or serum.

The patients with γG myeloma had the most severe depression of the normal immunoglobulins and the highest incidence of infection. The growth rate of the tumor, based on paraprotein doubling time, was the slowest and there was less hypercalcemia. Bence Jones proteinuria occurred in 62 per cent of these patients.

The course of patients with γA myeloma was more likely to be complicated by hypercalcemia and amyloidosis than was that of the patients with γG myeloma. Seventy per cent had Bence Jones proteinuria.

Patients with Bence Jones myeloma (light chain disease) appeared to have the fastest tumor growth, more osteolytic lesions, hypercalcemia, and amyloidosis. Renal failure was relatively common and this group of patients had a worse prognosis than did the first two groups.

Patients with γD myeloma protein represent 1.5 per cent of those with myelomatosis. All of these patients had a heavy excretion of Bence Jones protein, 90 per cent of which was λ-type light chains.[72] Renal failure, hypercalcemia, extraosseous lesions, and amyloidosis were common.

In approximately 0.5 per cent of the patients in this series, γM paraprotein was present in the serum. Such patients have been differentiated from those with Waldenstrom's macroglobulinemia by the morphology of the bone marrow cells and the absence of the hyperviscosity syndrome.[94]

A small percentage of patients with multiple myeloma lead active lives relatively free from symptoms for a period of years. Unfortunately the vast majority have a very distressing course characterized by pain, fractures, disability, progressive weakness, and cachexia. Remissions sometimes occur but these are usually short and the disease soon resumes it relentless, painful, and crippling course.

TREATMENT

Treatment of multiple myeloma is unsatisfactory for the majority of patients. Non-specific measures such as immobilization of fractures, body braces for vertebral involvement, and analgesics for pain add greatly to the comfort of patients. If anemia is present the use of androgens may be effective[43] but blood transfusions are usually required. Laminectomy is often necessary in patients who develop paraplegia; other operations may be performed if indicated and if the patient's general condition is satisfactory.

A variety of chemical agents have been used in the treatment of multiple myeloma in the past. Nitrogen mustard, TEM, radioactive phosphorous, and stilbamidine have all proved to be ineffective[37] and the vinca alkaloids and antimetabolites have been tried without significant success.[117] Urethan (ethylcarbomate) has been widely used with but limited success. Symptomatic improvement, usually of short duration, occurred in 20 to 30 per cent of patients, and a smaller percentage of patients demonstrated objective improvement, increased hematocrit, decrease in the serum globulin, and improvement in the radiologic appearance of the bone lesions.[37, 108, 163] Little if any improvement occurred, however, when the drug was administered in doses that could be tolerated by most patients.[177] Nausea and vomiting occurred frequently and there was the occasional development of severe leukopenia or hepatic damage.[108]

Therapy of multiple myeloma has improved somewhat in recent years. Reports from several cooperative group studies indicate that response rates of 25 to 50 per cent may be achieved with the alkylating agents melphalan (l-phenylalanine mustard) and Cytoxan (cyclophosphamide). In those patients who were responsive to therapy, the median survival was 40 months from the start of therapy, whereas non-responders lived only 9 months.[117, 177]

Melphalan (l-phenylalanine mustard) has been highly effective in the treatment of some patients with multiple myeloma, but those with severe renal involvement or Bence Jones myeloma do not respond as well.[4] Hematologic toxicity has been a common complication and has caused a reduction in most of the dosage schedules employed when the drug was first introduced.[24, 137] Various therapeutic regimens have been employed. The drug has been given continuously or intermittently. One report recommends the use of 0.05 mg. per kg. daily until toxicity occurs. When the hematologic values return to base line levels, the drug is reinstituted at 0.02 to 0.03 mg. per kg. per day and decreased further if toxicity recurs.[29] Others [4, 98] have employed intermittent therapy. They give the drug in a dose of 0.15 mg. per kg. per day for 7 days and repeat the course every fifth week, or they give 0.25 mg. per kg. per day for 4 days and repeat the course every 6 weeks. We employ intermittent therapy which appears to be less toxic and at least as effective as continuous therapy.

Cytoxan (cyclophosphamide) has been reported to be as effective as melphalan.[117, 157] One group used a dosage regimen of 2.0 mg. per kg. per day by mouth with adjustment in the schedule to allow administration of the maximum dose short of serious cytopenia; the mean dosage in their series was 1.47

mg. per kg. per day.[111] Others have used different drug regimens.[39, 157] Side effects have included hemorrhagic cystitis, which occurred in 9 to 10 per cent of patients, alopecia, which occurred in 3.5 per cent, and hematologic toxicity.

Prednisone has not proved to be particularly effective when used alone, but when used in addition to an alkylating agent it may provide objective and subjective improvement.[4, 116]

Roentgen radiation has an important place in the treatment of some patients with multiple myeloma. When therapy is directed toward specific lesions, pain is often relieved promptly and spontaneous fractures may heal more rapidly. It has also been observed in some patients with relatively localized disease that therapy directed toward specific lesions may eradicate the evidence of disease in those locations.[37]

Should hypercalcemia occur, a low calcium diet and a high fluid intake will promote urinary excretion of calcium and prevent nephrocalcinosis.[8] Adrenocortical steroids often reduce the high calcium levels but their mechanism of action is unknown.[1] Sodium ethylene diamine tetracetic acid (EDTA), a chelating agent, has not been successful in the treatment of hypercalcemia; the results are transient and the drug may produce serious nephrotoxic effects and further renal impairment.[8, 97]

The effect of sodium fluoride on calcium metabolism in multiple myeloma has been under study recently to determine if it might have a place in the treatment of bone lesions. Following the administration of this salt, a coarsening of bone trabeculae has been noted by histologic and radiographic studies.[36] Calcium balance has become progressively more positive and the bone crystal appears to be more stable.[46, 131] Patients with severe bone pain are often relieved.[45] The reported effects of sodium fluoride are of great interest, but the value of the drug is uncertain and it must be pointed out that at the dosage recommended for treatment of demineralizing bone disease it remains an experimental drug and requires an investigative license from the Food and Drug Administration for its use.[46]

A recent study failed to show any reduction in the frequency of major infections in patients with multiple myeloma who were treated prophylactically with γ globulin. The use of appropriate antibiotics when necessary is recommended.[165]

Efforts to treat other aspects of myeloma have been more successful. Acute renal failure resulting from the disease has been successfully treated with dialysis while awaiting the effect of chemotherapy; apparently the renal dysfunction is reversible in some patients.[31] When the plasma volume is expanded and the hematocrit is low, congestive heart failure may develop. Plasmapheresis is particularly effective when transfusion may further compromise the circulation; the blood volume is reduced and the hematocrit is raised.

Illustrative Case

When this 59 year old black female was first seen in the medical outpatient clinic of the University of Virginia Hospital, she was found to have essential hypertension and marked obesity. Symptoms of low back and joint pains were attributed to osteoarthritis and a body weight of 295 pounds. After 8 years of good health she was seen again with severe low back pain of 6 months' duration and anemia thought to be secondary to "dietary iron deficiency." She was treated by physiotherapy and given ferrous sulfate. Three months later she was admitted to the hospital with a respiratory infection manifested by chest pain, purulent sputum, and fever.

Physical examination. T—102°, P—80, R—18, BP 130/90, weight 215 pounds. There was marked splinting of the chest on respiration and breath sounds were difficult to hear. Inspiratory rales were heard at the right base posteriorly. Tenderness on pressure over the sternum and right lower anterior ribs was noted. The lower border of the liver was palpated 8 cm. below the costal margin and was nontender. There was no splenomegaly.

Laboratory studies. Hematocrit, 18 per cent; hemoglobin, 6.8 gm. per cent; W.B.C., 5800 per cu.mm. Differential count (per cent): bands 2, segmented forms 30, lymphocytes 56, plasma cells 10, monocytes 2. Urine: negative. (No Bence Jones protein was demonstrated.) Urea 56 mg. per cent. Total protein 14.6 gm. per cent. Electrophoretic pattern: 34 per cent albumin, 3 per cent alpha-1 globulin, 7 per cent alpha-2 globulin, 9 per cent beta globulin and 47 per cent gamma globulin. The gamma globulin fraction contained a large sharp spike. Marrow aspiration revealed 60 per cent immature plasma cells. Staphylococci were cultured from the sputum. X-rays of the chest revealed elevation of the right diaphragm but no parenchymal infiltration. Multiple radiolucent defects were noted in the clavicles, ribs, and skull. X-rays of the cervical and thoracic spine revealed marked hypertrophic degenerative change with loss of interspaces.

Course. A diagnosis of multiple myeloma and acute bronchitis was made. The patient was treated with penicillin and Prostaphlin and was given two units of whole blood. In 24 hours her chest pain was relieved, her sputum was clear, and she was afebrile.

Initially she was treated with melphalan, 6 mg. daily by mouth for 2 weeks. She developed the expected leukopenia but noted little if any improvement. Laboratory studies: W.B.C. 3200 per cu.mm.; differential count (per cent) segmented forms 56, lymphocytes 39, monocytes 3, eosinophil 1, basophil 1; hematocrit, 24 per cent. The medication was stopped to await a rise in leukocyte count.

One month later the leukocyte count was 4200 per cu.mm. with a normal differential and the hematocrit 26 per cent. The platelet count was 135,000 per cu.mm. Total protein had fallen to 10.0 gm. per cent. Electrophoresis revealed 31 per cent albumin, 2 per cent alpha-1 globulin, 5 per cent alpha-2 globulin, 7 per cent beta globulin and 55 per cent gamma globulin.

Therapy with melphalan, 2 mg. daily, was reinstituted and the patient noted gradual relief of pain.

Six months later she had only minor back pains. The hematocrit was 33 per cent, W.B.C. 5000 per cu.mm., and the differential count was normal. Platelets were 229,000 cu.mm. Total protein was 8.8 gm. per cent with 32 per cent gamma globulin and bone marrow aspiration revealed only 33 per cent plasma cells.

Melphalan, 2 mg. by mouth two or three times each week, depending on the degree of leukopenia, has been continued to the present.

She has remained relatively free of pain but her hematocrit has begun to fall recently. Twenty months after the onset of symptoms and 14 months after the diagnosis had been made, the bone marrow examination again revealed 65 per cent plasma cells and the total protein had risen to 10.7 gm. per cent with 50 per cent gamma globulin. Fractionation of the gamma globulin by immunoprecipitation revealed: $\gamma G = 5600$ mg. per cent, $\gamma A = 37$ mg. per cent, $\gamma M = 21$ mg. per cent. (Normal values: $\gamma G = 800-1680$ mg. per cent, $\gamma A = 140-420$ mg. per cent, $\gamma M = 53-193$ mg. per cent.) No protein was detected in the urine until it was concentrated 200 X. Electrophoresis of the concentrated urine revealed a single band in the gamma region.

In view of the evidence of increased activity of the disease, the dose of melphalan was increased to 2 mg. daily.

Comment. This patient illustrates many features that occur commonly in multiple myeloma. Back pain and anemia in a middle-aged patient should always raise the question of multiple myeloma. Admission to the hospital was occasioned by an upper respiratory infection so commonly seen in this group of patients. X-rays revealed typical "punched out" osteolytic lesions in the skull, ribs, and clavicles. The diagnosis was established by the finding of great numbers of immature plasma cells in the marrow aspirate, and of plasma cells on peripheral blood smear, and an increase in total plasma proteins due almost entirely to elevated gamma globulin. As is true in about half the patients with this disease, Bence Jones protein was not demonstrated in the urine by the usual tests; it can be demonstrated in nearly all cases by special tests.

The patient had a significant response to the administration of melphalan, manifested by a 50 per cent decrease in plasma cells in the marrow, a fall in the abnormal protein, improvement in the anemia, and relief from pain. Melphalan, used intermittently or cyclically, appears to be beneficial in many patients.

Heavy Chain Diseases

Recently, several variants of malignant monoclonal gammopathy have been described. These disorders are characterized by the appearance of a protein antigenically related to the Fc fragment of the H chain in both the serum and urine without any reaction to anti-light chain antisera. To date, γG, γA, and γM heavy chain diseases have been described.

γG TYPE

Franklin[79] described a patient with a malignant proliferative disorder of the reticuloendothelial system in whom asynchronous production of a protein which was antigenically like the Fc fragment of γG was present as a monoclonal spike in both serum and urine.[79] Other cases have since been reported.[143]

Clinical findings. The reported patients with γG heavy chain disease have been male and have ranged from 43 to 71 years of age. Lymphadenopathy, splenomegaly, fever, and anemia have been constant findings. Hepatomegaly, leukopenia, and thrombocytopenia were noted to occur. Unusual susceptibility to bacterial infection was noted in four of the five reported patients. Three patients had an unusual erythrema and edema of the palate lasting several days and subsiding spontaneously.

The bone marrow aspirate and lymph node sections revealed atypical immature plasma cells to be dominant with an admixture of other cells including atypical lymphocytes, plasma cells, reticulum cells, and eosinophils. Bence Jones negative proteinuria was present in each reported case. The urinary protein was homogeneous on electrophoresis and had fast gamma or slow beta mobility. The total serum proteins varied from 4.1 to 8.2 gm. per cent and electrophoresis revealed the presence of an abnormal homogeneous protein with fast gamma or slow beta mobility. The normal gamma globulin was decreased.

Pathologic physiology. The atypical plasma cells in the bone marrow and lymph nodes are believed responsible for the production of the abnormal protein, but techniques currently available are inadequate to correlate the basic biochemical defect with structural abnormality. The abnormal serum and urine protein of these patients had a molecular weight of about 53,000 ± 2,000. Immunologic analysis has confirmed its relationship to γG globulins and a lack of antigenic similarity to either macroglobulins, γA, or Bence Jones proteins. They are related to the F fragment of papain-digested gamma globulin and not to the S fragment.

The decrease in normal immunoglobulins demonstrated by these patients probably accounts for the increased susceptibility to bacterial infection. In one study the reduction in normal immunoglobulins was demonstrated to be the result of decreased production rather than increased destruction or loss.[79]

Treatment. The cellular infiltrates appear to be radiosensitive and the most effective form of therapy is external radiation. Short-term improvement has been noted with nitrogen mustard, cyclophosphamide, and steroids.[43]

γA TYPE

A new immunoglobulin abnormality has been recently identified and designated "α chain disease".[167] The initial patient was a young Arab woman who had chronic diarrhea and malabsorption secondary to malignant lymphoma involving the entire small intestine ("Mediterranean lymphoma"). The invasive cells were pleomorphic; plasma cells in particular, as well as medium-sized lymphocytes and reticulum cells, were frequent.

The abnormal protein, which was found in serum, urine, and saliva, was closely related to the γA₁ (LE) subclass and devoid of light chains. It is not yet certain whether this protein represents a complete alpha chain or only a portion thereof. No intracellular light chain synthesis could be demonstrated in those cells found to produce the abnormal protein.

Some normal γA globulins were demonstrated in the serum. γG and γM immunoglobulins were both abnormally low. Trace amounts of free light chains of both antigenic types were demonstrated in the urine.

γM TYPE

Recently there has been a report of a patient with a heavy chain fragment related to the μ chain of IgM. The findings in this patient differed significantly from those with a heavy chain fragment of IgG or IgA in that the urine contained Bence Jones protein. There was marked plasma cell and lymphocytic bone marrow infiltration.[9] The anomalous serum protein was demonstrated to be the H chain of IgM devoid of light chains.

The patient did not have eosinophilia, lymphadenopathy, pyrexia, recurrent infections, or edema of the uvula. Amyloid deposits were prominent during the clinical course of the patient. The major clinical features presented by the patient were those of bone pain, a lymphoproliferative disorder, amyloidosis, and bilateral carpal-tunnel syndrome.

"Benign" Monoclonal Gammopathy

Over the past several years, reports of asymptomatic patients with an increased sedimentation rate, hypergammaglobulinemia, and a tall narrow peak on serum electrophoresis have appeared. A very small percentage (2.3 per cent) have been found to have Bence Jones proteinuria.[58] The condition was termed "benign monoclonal gammopathy." [189, 191] These patients had no other evidence of myeloma, macroglobulinemia, or other serious disease, and they were well with the exception of some increase in the frequency of infection. Recently, a number of reports have described the development of clinical myeloma after many years of asymptomatic "benign" monoclonal gammopathy.[139, 175, 192] In one report, the patient developed classical multiple myeloma 18 years after the initial observation.[112]

Such reports may occur more frequently in the future, since it has been calculated that starting from a single mutant cell it would take 33 years, 21 years, and 11 years, respectively, to develop clinical γG, γA, and Bence Jones myeloma, based on the doubling times of the paraproteins.[95] Abnormalities in immunoglobulins will be exposed much earlier with the widespread use of serum electrophoresis. Perhaps "benign" monoclonal gammapathy represents a "preclinical" phase of myeloma.[139] It does not appear to be safe to assume these patients have a benign condition even after years of observation.

Macroglobulinemia

There are a number of clinical conditions in which an increase in the concentration of macroglobulins has been observed.[156, 161] The increase may be slight to moderate in cancer, syphilis, chronic infections, hepatitis, or rheumatoid arthritis. The term macroglobulinemia is usually reserved for situations in which the concentration of macroglobulin is greater than 15 per cent. Such high concentrations of macroglobulins are occasionally found in proliferative disorders involving the lymphocyte, plasma cell, or reticulum cell, such as chronic lymphocytic leukemia, lymphosarcoma, reticulum cell sarcoma, and multiple myeloma.[126, 128] More commonly these levels are found in association with the disorder known as Waldenström's macroglobulinemia.

Waldenström's Macroglobulinemia

In 1944 Waldenström[189] described two patients with marked elevation of the serum macroglobulins. Since that date, his observations have been amply confirmed and studies of this condition have contributed a great deal to our understanding of the normal plasma proteins.

CLINICAL FINDINGS

Waldenström's macroglobulinemia occurs most often in patients 50 to 70 years of age and is somewhat more common in men. It has approximately the same incidence as multiple myeloma.[190]

A history of recent weight loss, weakness, lethargy, and lowered resistance to infections and the findings of hepatosplenomegaly and slight to moderate lymphadenopathy are common. There may be retinal hemorrhages and bleeding from the mucous membranes. Less commonly, one finds Reynaud's phenomena and signs and symptoms of congestive heart failure.

X-rays of the bones often reveal generalized demineralization, but punched-out lesions similar to those of multiple myeloma are rare.

Examination of the bone marrow aspirate reveals infiltration by cells which are difficult to classify and are frequently referred to as lymphoplasmacytic cells. The cells have cytoplasm like that of a plasma cell and a nucleus like that of a lymphocyte. Similar cells are seen in the lymph nodes, spleen, and liver and, rarely, in the peripheral blood. Plasma cells and mast cells are also seen in the affected tissues. The total protein of the serum is almost always increased and associated with an elevated sedimentation rate and serum viscosity. A rather sharp peak in the beta or gamma region is found on paper electrophoresis. As the molecule is large it will not enter a starch gel and electrophoresis in this medium without special techniques is not possible.[34] Immunoelectrophoresis on agar gel is often possible and may reveal a dense γM band.[140] Cryoglobulins may be present.[122a] (F.S.: II, 98)

The Sia test, which is based on the insolubility of macroglobulins in distilled water, is often positive, but false negatives may occur. Five to 10 per cent of the patients will have Bence Jones proteins in the urine.

Although these findings are highly suggestive of macroglobulinemia, a positive diagnosis must rest on data obtained by the ultracentrifugation of the serum. High molecular weight globulins of 15S or more in concentrations greater than 5 per cent must be demonstrated.

PATHOLOGIC PHYSIOLOGY

The high concentration of macroglobulins in Waldenström's macroglobulinemia is the result of markedly increased synthesis[12] of these proteins by the lymphoplasmacytic cells found in the bone marrow, liver, lymph nodes, and spleen. A marked increase in viscosity of the plasma results from the presence of the high concentration of macroglobulins[155] and is believed to slow the flow of blood. The slowing of blood flow increases the lateral pressure in small vessels, resulting in dilatation, tortuosity, thrombosis, and hemorrhage in the retina[173] and, presumably, in small blood vessels in other parts of the body.[5] Coating of the platelets with macroglobulins has been demonstrated to interfere with the release of platelet factor III and to contribute to the hemorrhagic diathesis.[149]

The decrease in normal gamma globulins contributes to the lowered resistance to infection. Anemia is often considered secondary to the presence of large numbers of abnormal cells in the marrow but may be hemolytic, perhaps secondary to coating of the red cells by the macroglobulin, or dilutional.

TREATMENT

Macroglobulins may be removed from the blood by plasmapheresis[169] or may be reduced by depolymerization after the administration of penicillin or penicillamine.[155] The effect of both is short-lived but helpful in acute situations.

Long-term management using chlorambucil has been reported to be effective with reduction in abnormal proteins and subjective improvement.[15]

References

1. Adams, W. S., and Skoog, W. A.: The management of multiple myeloma. J. Chronic Dis., *6*:446, 1957.
2. Aisenberg, A. C.: Lymphocytopenia in Hodgkin's disease. Blood, *25*:1037, 1965.
3. Aisenberg, A. C.: Manifestations of immunological unresponsiveness in Hodgkin's disease. Cancer Res., *26*:1152, 1966.
4. Alexanian, R., Haut, A., Khan, A. U., Lane, M., McKelvey, E. M., Migliore, P. J., Stuckey, W. J., and Wilson, H. E.: Treatment for multiple myeloma. J.A.M.A., *208*:1680, 1969.
5. Argani, I., and Kipkie, G. F.: Macroglobulinemic nephropathy. Am. J. Med., *36*:151, 1964.
6. Arinkin, M. I.: Die intravitale Untersuchungsmethodik des Knochenmarks. Folia haemat., *38*:233, 1929.
7. Bain, B., Vas, M. R., and Lowenstein, L.: The development of large immature mononuclear cells in mixed leukocyte culture. Blood, *23*:108, 1964.
8. Baker, W. H.: Abnormalities in calcium metabolism in malignancy: effects of hormone therapy. Am. J. Med., *21*:714, 1956.
9. Ballard, H. S., Hamilton, L. M., Marcus, A. J., and Illes, C. H.: A new variant of heavy-chain disease (μ-chain disease). New England J. Med., *282*:1060, 1970.
10. Balner, H.: Identification of peritoneal macrophages in mouse radiation chimeras. Transplant, *1*:217, 1963.
11. Bankman, H. N., and Watchi, J. M.: Spontaneous anuria in multiple myeloma. Presse Méd., *71*:2735, 1963.
12. Barth, W. F., Wochner, D., Waldmann, T. A., and Fahey, J. L.: Metabolism of human gamma macroglobulins. J. Clin. Invest., *43*:1036, 1964.
13. Barth, W. F., Glenner, G. G., Waldmann, T. A., and Zelis, R. F.: Primary amyloidosis. Ann. Int. Med., *69*:787, 1968.
14. Bauer, D. C., Mathies, M. J., and Stavitsky, A. B.: Sequences of synthesis of γ-1 macroglobulin and γ-2 globulin antibodies during primary and secondary responses to proteins, salmonella antigens, and phage. J. Exper. Med., *117*:889, 1963.
15. Bayrd, E. D.: Continuous chlorambucil therapy in primary macroglobulinemia of Waldenström: report of four cases. Proc. Staff Meet. Mayo Clinic, *36*:135, 1961.
16. Bayrd, E. D., and Heck, J. F.: Multiple myeloma: a review of eighty-three proved cases. J.A.M.A., *133*:147, 1947.
17. Ben-Bassat, I., Frand, U. I., Isersky, C. I., and Ramot, B.: Plasma cell leukemia with IgD paraprotein. Arch. Intern. Med., *121*:361, 1968.

18. Bence Jones, H.: Papers on chemical pathology. Lancet, *2*:88, 1847.
19. Bennett, W. E., and Cohn, Z. A.: The isolation and selected properties of blood monocytes. J. Exp. Med., *123*:145, 1966.
20. Bennich, H., Ishizaka, K., Ishizaka, T., and Johansson, S. G.: A comparative antigenic study of γE-globulin and myeloma IgND. J. Immunol., *102*:826, 1969.
21. Bennich, H. H., Ishizaka, K., Johansson, S. G. O., Rowe, D. S., Stanworth, D. R., and Terry, W. D.: Immunoglobulin E, a new class of human immunoglobulin Bull. World Health Org., *38*:151, 1968.
22. Berggard, I.: On a γ-globulin of low molecular weight in normal human plasma and urine. Clin. Chim. Acta, *6*:545, 1961.
23. Berggard, I., and Edelman, G. M.: Normal counterparts to Bence-Jones proteins: free L polypeptide chains of human γ-globulin. Proc. Nat. Acad. Sci., *49*:330, 1963.
24. Bergsagel, D. E., Sprague, C. C., Austin, C., and Griffith, K. M.: Evaluation of new chemotherapeutic agents in the treatment of multiple myeloma. IV. L-Phenylalanine mustard (NSC-8806). Cancer Chemother. Rep., *21*:87, 1962.
25. Berkheiser, E. J.: Multiple myeloma of children. Arch. Surg., *8*:853, 1924.
26. Berman, L., and Stulberg, C. S.: Primary cultures of macrophages from normal human peripheral blood. Lab. Invest., *11*:1322, 1962.
27. Bernier, G. M., and Cebra, J. J.: Polypeptide chains of human gamma-globulin: cellular localization by fluorescent antibody. Science, *144*:1590, 1964.
27a. Bjorneboe, M.: Gamma globulin and colloid-osmotic pressure. In Killander, J. (Ed.): Gamma Globulins. Nobel Symposium. Interscience Publishers, Inc., New York, 1967, pp. 545–553.
27b. Blackburn, W. R., and Miller, J. F. A. P.: Electron microscopic studies of thymus graft regeneration and rejection. Lab. Invest., *16*:66, 1967.
27c. Bloom, B. R., and Bennett, B.: Mechanism of a reaction in vitro associated with delayed-type hypersensitivity. Science, *153*:80, 1966.
28. Bloom, W., and Bartelmez, G. W.: Hematopoiesis in young human embryos. Am. J. Anat., *67*:21, 1940.
29. Brook, J., Bateman, J. R., and Steinfeld, J. L.: Evaluation of melphalan (NSC-8806) in treatment of multiple myeloma. Cancer Chemother. Rep., *36*:25, 1964.
30. Brown, M., and Battle, J. D., Jr.: The effect of urography on renal function in patients with multiple myeloma. Canad. Med. Assoc. J., *91*:786, 1964.
31. Bryan, C. W., and Healy, J. K.: Acute renal failure in multiple myeloma. Am. J. Med., *44*:128, 1968.
32. Burnet, F. M.: Immunological aspects of malignant disease. Lancet, *1*:1171, 1967.
33. Burnet, M.: The clonal selection theory of antibody production. Oxford University Press, New York, 1959.
34. Butler, E. A., Flynn, F. V., Harris, H., and Robson, E. B.: Laboratory diagnosis of macroglobulinemia, with special reference to starch-gel electrophoresis. Lancet, *2*:289, 1961.
35. Butterworth, C. E., Jr., Frommeyer, W. B., and Riser, W. H., Jr.: Erythrophagocytosis in a case of plasma cell leukemia. Blood, *8*:519, 1953.
36. Carbone, P. P., Zipkin, I., Sokoloff, L., Frazier, P., Cook, P., and Mullins, F.: Fluoride effect on bone in plasma cell myeloma. Arch. Intern. Med., *121*:130, 1968.
37. Carson, C. P., Ackerman, L. V., and Maltby, J. D.: Plasma cell myeloma. A clinical, pathologic and roentgenologic review of ninety cases. Am. J. Clin. Path., *25*:849, 1955.
38. Carter, J. R.: Plasma cell hyperplasia and hyperglobulinemia in trichinosis. The duration of larviposition. Am. J. Path., *25*:309, 1949.
39. Choi, O. S., English, A., Hilton, J. H. B., Catton, G. E., and Brown, M. D.: Cyclophosphamide in the treatment of myelomatosis. Canad. Med. Assoc. J., *97*:1133, 1967.
40. Cioli, D., and Baglioni, C.: Catabolic origin of a Bence-Jones protein fragment. J. Exper. Med., *128*:517, 1968.
41. Clark, H., and Muirhead, E. E.: Plasmacytosis of bone marrow. Arch. Intern. Med., *94*:425, 1954.
42. Clawson, C. C., Cooper, M. D., and Good, R. A.: Lymphocyte fine structure in the bursa of fabricius, the thymus and the germinal centers. Lab. Invest., *16*:407, 1967.
43. Cline, M. J., and Berlin, I.: Studies of the anemia of multiple myeloma. Am. J. Med., *33*:510, 1962.
44. Cohen, A. S.: Amyloidosis. New England J. Med., *277*:522, 1967.
45. Cohen, P.: Fluoride and calcium therapy for myeloma bone lesions. J.A.M.A., *198*:583, 1966.
46. Cohen, P., Nichols, G. L., and Banks, H. H.: Fluoride treatment of bone rarefaction in multiple myeloma and osteoporosis. A review. Clin. Orthop., *64*:221, 1969.
47. Cohen, S.: Properties of the separated chains of human γ-globulin. Nature, *197*:253, 1963.
48. Cohen, S.: Annotation: the nature of myeloma proteins. Brit. J. Haemat., *15*:211, 1968.

49. Cohn, Z. A., Fedorko, M. E., and Hirsch, J. G.: The in vitro differentiation of mononuclear phagocytes. V. The formation of macrophage lysosomes. J. Exper. Med., *123*:757, 1966.
50. Cohn, Z. A., Hirsch, J. G., and Fedorko, M. E.: The in vitro differentiation of mononuclear phagocytes. IV. The ultrastructure of macrophage differentiation in the peritoneal cavity and in culture. J. Exper. Med., *123*:747, 1966.
51. Collier, F. C., and Jackson, P.: The precipitin test for Bence Jones protein. New England J. Med., *248*:409, 1953.
52. Cone, L., and Uhr, J. W.: Immunologic deficiency disorders associated with chronic lymphatic leukemia and multiple myeloma. J. Clin. Invest., *43*:2241, 1964.
53. Coons, A. H., and Kaplan, M. H.: Localization of antigen in tissue cells. J. Exper. Med., *91*:1, 1950.
54. Coons, A. H., Leduc, E. H., and Connolly, J. M.: Leukocytes involved in antibody formation. Ann. N.Y. Acad. Sci., *59*:951, 1955.
55. Cooper, M. D., Raymond, D. A., Peterson, R. D. A., South, M. A., and Good, R. A.: The function of the thymus system and bursa system in the chicken. J. Exper. Med., *123*:75, 1966.
56. Cross, R. J. (Ed.): Multiple myeloma (combined staff clinic). Am. J. Med., *23*:283, 1957.
57. Cunningham, R. S., Sabin, F. R., and Doan, C. A.: The development of leukocytes, lymphocytes, and monocytes from a specific stem-cell in adult tissues. Contrib. Embryol., Carnegie Inst., *16*:227, 1925.
58. Dammacco, F., and Waldenström, J.: Bence Jones proteinuria in benign monoclonal gammopathies. Acta. Med. Scandinav., *184*:403, 1968.
59. DePetris, S., and Karlsbad, G.: Localization of antibodies by electron microscopy in developing antibody producing cells. J. Cell. Biol., *26*:759, 1965.
60. DeVaal, O. M., and Seynhaeve, V.: Reticular dysgenesia. Lancet, *2*:1123, 1959.
61. DiGeorge, A. M.: Discussion of Cooper, M. D., Peterson, R. D. A., and Good, R. A.: A new concept of cellular basis of immunity. J. Ped., *67*:907, 1965.
62. Doan, C. A., Cunningham, R. S., and Sabin, F. R.: Experimental studies on the origin and maturation of avian and mammalian red blood-cells. Contrib. Embryol., Carnegie Inst., *16*:163, 1928.
63. Downey, H.: The occurrence and significance of the "myeloblast" under normal and pathologic conditions. Arch. Int. Med., *33*:301, 1924.
64. Downey, H.: Origin of monocytes in monocytic leukemia and leukemic reticuloendotheliosis. Anat. Rec., *48*:16, 1931.
65. Downey, H.: Handbook of Hematology. Paul B. Hoeber, New York, 1938.
66. Dumonde, D. C.: The role of the macrophage in delayed hypersensitivity. Brit. Med. Bull., *23*:9, 1967.
67. Edelman, G. M., and Gally, J. A.: The nature of Bence-Jones proteins: chemical similarities to polypeptide chains of myeloma globulins and normal γ-globulins. J. Exper. Med., *116*:207, 1962.
68. Edelman, G. M., and Poulik, M. D.: Studies on structural units of the γ-globulins. J. Exper. Med., *113*:861, 1961.
69. Edwards, G. A., and Zawadzki, Z. A.: Extraosseous lesions in plasma cell myeloma: a report of six cases. Am. J. Med., *43*:194, 1967.
70. Engle, R. L., and Wallis, L. A.: Multiple myeloma and the adult Fanconi syndrome. I. Report of a case with crystal-like deposits in the tumor cells and in the epithelial cells of the kidney. Am. J. Med., *22*:5, 1957.
71. Fagraeus, A.: Antibody production in relation to the development of plasma cells. Acta Med. Scandinav., Suppl. 204, 1948.
72. Fahey, J. L., Carbone, P. P., Rowe, D. S., and Bachmann, R.: Plasma cell myeloma with D-myeloma protein (IgD myeloma). Am. J. Med., *45*:373, 1968.
73. Fishman, M.: Antibody formation in vitro. J. Exp. Med., *114*:837, 1961.
74. Fishman, M., Hammerstram, R. A., and Bond, V. P.: In vitro transfer of macrophage RNA to lymph node cells. Nature, *198*:549, 1963.
75. Fleisher, G. A.: Peptidases in human leukocytes. Ann. N.Y. Acad. Sci., *59*:1012, 1955.
76. Forbus, W. O., Perlzweig, W. A., Parfentjev, I. A., and Burwell, J. C., Jr.: Bence Jones protein excretion and its effects upon the kidney. Bull. Johns Hopkins Hosp., *57*:47, 1935.
76a. Ford, W. L., and Gowans, J. L.: The traffic of lymphocytes. Seminars Hemat., *7*:67, 1969.
77. Franklin, E. C.: Structural units of human 7S gammaglobulin. J. Clin. Invest., *39*:1933, 1960.
78. Franklin, E. C.: Physiochemical and immunological studies of gamma globulins of normal human urine. J. Clin. Invest., *38*:2159, 1959.
79. Franklin, E. C., Lowenstein, J., Bigelow, B., and Meltzer, M.: Heavy chain disease. A new disorder of serum γ-globulins. Am. J. Med., *37*:332, 1964.

80. Friedman, H. P., Stavitsky, A. B., and Solomon, J. M.: Induction in vitro of antibodies to phage T2: antigens in the RNA extract employed. Science, *149*:1106, 1965.
81. Geschickter, C. F., and Copeland, M. M.: Multiple myeloma. Arch. Surg., *16*:807, 1928.
82. Ginsberg, D. M.: Circulating plasma cells in multiple myeloma. A method for detection and review of the problem. Ann. Int. Med., *57*:843, 1962.
83. Gitlin, D., and Craig, J. M.: The thymus and other lymphoid tissues in congenital A gamma-globulinemia. Pediatrics, *32*:517, 1963.
84. Glasgow, L. A.: Leukocytes and interferon in the host response to viral infections. J. Bact., *91*:2185, 1966.
85. Good, R. A., Peterson, R. D. A., Perey, D. Y., Frustad, J., and Cooper, M. D.: In Good, R. A., and Bergman, D. (Eds.): The immunological deficiency diseases in man. Birth Defects, *4*:17, 1968.
86. Gowans, J. L.: Life history of lymphocytes. Brit. M. Bull., *15*:50, 1959.
87. Grey, H. M., and Junkle, H. G.: Chain subclasses of human G globulin. Biochemistry, *6*:2326, 1967.
88. Hamilton, L. D.: Control and functions of the lymphocyte. Ann. N.Y. Acad. Sci., *73*:39, 1958.
88a. Hanauer, L. B., and Chrisitan, C. L.: Studies of cryoproteins in systemic lupus erythematosus. J. Clin. Invest., *46*:400, 1967.
89. Hanson, L. A.: Aspects of the absence of the IgA system. Birth Defects, *4*:292, 1968.
90. Harboe, M., Osterland, C. K., Mannik, M., and Kunkel, H. G.: Genetic characters of human γ-globulins in myeloma proteins. J. Exper. Med., *116*:719, 1962.
91. Haurani, F. I.: Effect of multiple myeloma and dysproteinemias on bone. Clin. Orthop. & Rel. Res., *52*:113, 1967.
92. Heiser, S., and Schwartzman, J.: Variations in the roentgen appearance of the skeletal system in myeloma. Radiology, *58*:178, 1952.
93. Heremans, J. F.: Immunochemical studies on protein pathology. The immunoglobulin concept. Clin. Chim. Acta, *4*:639, 1959.
93a. Herreman, G., et al.: L' hypervolemic de la macroglobulinemie de Waldenstrom. Nouv. Rev. Franc. Hemat., *8*:209, 1968.
93b. Hess, C. E., Ayers, C. R., Wetzel, R. A., and Mohler, D. N.: Mechanism of dilutional anemia in multiple myeloma. Clin. Research, *18*:41, 1970. (Abstract.)
94. Hobbs, J. R.: Immunochemical classes of myelomatosis, including data from a therapeutic trial conducted by a medical research council working party. Brit. J. Haemat., *16*:599, 1969.
95. Hobbs, J. R.: Growth rates and responses to treatment in human myelomatosis. Brit. J. Haemat., *16*:607, 1969.
96. Hobbs, J. R., Slot, G. M. J., Campbell, C. H., Clein, G. P., Scott, J. T., Crowther, D., and Swan, H. T.: Six cases of gamma D myelomatosis. Lancet, *2*:614, 1966.
97. Holland, J. F., Danielson, E., and Sahagian-Edwards, A.: Use of ethylene diamine tetra acetic acid in hypercalcemic patients. Proc. Soc. Exper. Biol. & Med., *84*:359, 1953.
98. Hoogstraten, B., Costa, J., Cuttner, J., Forcier, J., Leone, L. A., Harley, J. B., and Glidewell, O. J.: Mephalan therapy in multiple myeloma. J.A.M.A., *209*:251, 1969.
99. Hsiao, S., and Putnam, F. W.: The cleavage of human γ-globulin by papain. J. Biol. Chem., *236*:122, 1961.
100. Huber, J., Cholnoky, P., and Zoethout, H. E.: Congenital aplasia of parathyroid glands and thymus. Arch. Dis. Child., *42*:190, 1967.
101. Ishizaka, K., and Ishizaka, T.: Human reaginic antibodies and immunoglobulins E. J. Allergy, *42*:330, 1968.
102. Ishizaka, T., Ishizaka, K., Johansson, S. G. O., and Bennich, H.: Histamine release from human leukocytes by anti-γE antibodies. J. Immunol., *102*:884, 1969.
103. Ishizaka, T., Ishizaka, K., Orange, R., and Austen, K. I.: Release of histamine and slow reacting substance of anaphylaxis (SRS-A) by γE system from sensitized monkey lung. J. Allergy, *43*:168, 1969.
104. Jarrold, T., and Vilter, R. W.: Hematologic observations in patients with chronic hepatic insufficiency. Sternal bone marrow morphology and bone marrow plasmacytosis. J. Clin. Invest., *28*:286, 1949.
105. Johansson, S. G. O., Bennich, H., and Wide, L.: A new class of immunoglobulins in human serum. Immunol., *14*:265, 1968.
106. Jordan, H. E.: The significance of the lymphoid nodule. Am. J. Anat., *57*:1, 1935.
107. Jordan, H. E., and Johnson, E. P.: Erythrocyte production in the bone marrow of the pigeon. Am. J. Anat., *56*:71, 1935.
108. Kenny, J. J., and Moloney, W. C.: Multiple myeloma: Diagnosis and management in a series of fifty-seven cases. Ann. Int. Med., *46*:1079, 1957.
108a. Keller, H. U., and Sorkin, E.: Studies on chemotaxis. Int. Arch. Allergy Appl. Immunol., *31*:575, 1967.

109. Keuning, F. J., and van der Slikke, L. B.: The role of immature plasma cells, lymphoblasts, and lymphocytes in the formation of antibodies as established in tissue culture experiments. J. Lab. Clin. Med., *36*:167, 1950.

110. Killmann, S. A., Gjørup, S., and Thaysen, J. H.: Fatal acute renal failure following intravenous pyelography in patient with multiple myeloma. Acta Med. Scandinav., *158*:43, 1957.

110a. Kopp, W. L., MacKinney, A. A., and Wasson, G.: Blood volume and hematocrit value in macroglobulinemia and myeloma. Arch. Intern. Med., *23*:394, 1969.

111. Korst, D. R., Clifford, G. O., Fowler, W. M., Louis, J., Will, J., and Wilson, H. E.: Multiple myeloma II analysis of cyclophosphamide therapy in 165 patients. J.A.M.A., *189*:758, 1964.

112. Kyle, R. A., and Bayrd, E. D.: "Benign" monoclonal gammopathy: a potential malignant condition? Am. J. Med., *40*:426, 1966.

113. Lamb, D. L., Pilney, F., Kelly, W. D., and Good, R. A.: A comparative study of the incidence of anergy in patients with carcinoma, leukemia, Hodgkin's disease and other lymphomas. J. Immunol., *89*:555, 1962.

114. Levi, D. F., Williams, R. C., and Lindstrom, F. D.: Immunofluorescent studies of the myeloma kidney with special reference to light chain disease. Am. J. Med., *44*:922, 1968.

115. Lichtenstein, L., and Jaffe, H. L.: Multiple myeloma. Arch. Path., *44*:207, 1947.

116. Liebling, M. E., Grizzle, J., Hammack, W., and Rundles, R. W.: Comparison of chlorambucil and prednisone with urethan and prednisone regimens in the treatment of multiple myeloma. Cancer Chemother. Rep., *16*:253, 1962.

117. Little, J. R., and Loeb, V., Jr.: Immunoglobulin abnormalities and current status of treatment of multiple myeloma. J.A.M.A., *208*:1688, 1969.

118. LoSpalluto, J., Miller, W., Jr., Dorward, B., and Fink, C. W.: The formation of macroglobulin antibodies. 1. Studies on adult humans. J. Clin. Invest., *41*:1415, 1962.

119. Mannik, M., and Kunkel, H. G.: Localization of antibodies in group I and group II γ-globulins. J. Exper. Med., *118*:817, 1963.

120. Maximow, A.: Relation of the blood cells to connective tissue and endothelium. Physiol. Rev., *4*:533, 1924.

121. Meacham, G. C.: Plasma cell myeloma. Ann. Int.Med., *38*:1035, 1953.

122. Mellors, R. C., and Korngold, L.: The cellular origin of human immunoglobulins. J. Exper. Med., *118*:387, 1963.

122a. Meltzer, M., and Franklin, E. C.: Cryoglobulinemia—a study of twenty-nine patients. Amer. J. Med., *40*:828, 1966.

122b. Meuwissen, H. J., Stutman, O., and Good, R. A.: Functions of the lymphocytes. Seminars Hemat., *7*:28, 1969.

123. Meyer, F.: C^{14} lysine incorporation into Bence Jones protein by cultures of myeloma bone marrow. Fed. Proc., *16*:222, 1957.

124. Michels, N. A.: The plasma cell. Arch. Path., *11*:775, 1931.

125. Migita, S., and Putnam, F. W.: Antigenic relationships of Bence-Jones proteins, myeloma globulins and normal human γ-globulin. J. Exper. Med., *117*:81, 1963.

126. Miller, D. G.: Patterns of immunological deficiency in lymphomas and leukemias. Ann. Int. Med., *57*:703, 1962.

127. Miller, J. F. A. P.: Immunological function of the thymus. Lancet, *2*:748, 1961.

127a. Mitchell, J., and Abbot, A.: Ultrastructure of the antigen-retaining reticulum of lymph node follicles as shown by high resolution autoradiography. Nature, *208*:500, 1965.

128. Moore, D. F., Migliore, P. J., Shullenberger, C. C., and Alexanian, R.: Monoclonal macroglobulinemia in malignant lymphoma. Ann. Int. Med., *72*:43, 1970.

129. Mueller, A. P., Wolfe, H. R., and Meyer, R. K.: Precipitin production in chickens. J. Immunol., *85*:172, 1960.

130. Nazelof, C., Jammet, M. L., Lortholary, P., LaBrune, B., and Lammy, M.: L'hypoplasie héréditaire du thymus. Arch. Franc. Pédiat. *21*:897, 1964.

131. Neer, R. M., Zipkin, I., Carbone, P. P., and Rosenberg, L. E.: Effect of sodium fluoride therapy on calcium metabolism in multiple myeloma. J. Clin. Endo., *26*:1059, 1966.

131a. Nelson, D. S.: In Neuberger, A., and Tatum, E. L. (Eds.): Frontiers of Biology Macrophages and Immunity, Vol. 2. John Wiley and Sons, Inc., New York, 1969, pp. 63–64.

132. Nelson, D. S., and Boyden, S. V.: Macrophage cytophilic antibodies and delayed hypersensitivity. Brit. Med. Bull., *23*:15, 1967.

133. Nowell, P. C.: Differentiation of human leukemic leukocytes in tissue culture. Exper. Cell Res., *19*:267, 1960.

134. Ogawa, M., Kochwa, S., Smith, C., Ishizaka, K., and McIntyre, O. R.: Clinical aspects of IgE myeloma. New England J. Med., *281*:1217, 1969.

135. Ortega, L. G., and Der, B. K.: Studies on a gammaglobulinemia induced by ablation of the bursa of Fabricius. Fed. Proc., *23*:546, 1964.

136. Osserman, E. F.: Plasma cell myeloma. New England J. Med., *261*:1006, 1959.
137. Osserman, E. F.: Therapy of plasma cell myeloma with melphalan (1-phenylalanine mustard). Proc. Am. Assoc. Cancer Res., *4*:50, 1963.
138. Osserman, E. F., and Lawlor, D. P.: Abnormal serum and urine proteins in thirty-five cases of multiple myeloma as studied by filter paper electrophoresis. Am. J. Med., *18*:462, 1955.
139. Osserman, E. F.: Plasmocytic dyscrasias. Am. J. Med., *31*:671, 1961.
140. Osserman, E. F., and Lawlor, D.: Immunoelectrophoretic characterization of serum and urinary proteins in plasma cell myeloma and Waldenström's macroglobulinemia. Ann. N.Y. Acad. Sci., *94*:93, 1961.
141. Osserman, E. F., and Lawlor, D. P.: Serum and urinary lysozyme (muramidase) in monocytic and monomyelocytic leukemia. J. Exper. Med., *124*:921, 1966.
142. Osserman, E. F., and Takatsuki, K.: Plasma myeloma: gamma globulin synthesis and structure. Medicine, *42*:357, 1963.
143. Osserman, E. F., and Takatsuki, K.: Clinical and immunochemical studies of four cases of heavy (Hγ²) chain disease. Am. J. Med., *37*:351, 1964.
144. Osserman, E. F., Takatsuki, K., and Talal, N.: The pathogenesis of "amyloidosis." Seminars Hemat.,*1*:1, 1964.
145. Pachter, M. R., Johnson, S. A., Neblett, T. R., and Truant, J. P.: Bleeding, platelets and macroglobulinemia. Am. J. Clin. Path., *31*:467, 1959.
147. Peterson, R. D. A., and Good, R. A.: Morphology and development differences between the cells of the chicken's thymus and bursa of Fabricius. Blood, *26*:269, 1965.
148. Porter, R. R.: Hydrolysis of rabbit γ-globulin and antibodies with crystalline papain. Biochem. J., *73*:119, 1959.
149. Potter, M., Fabey, J., and Pilgrim, H. T.: Abnormal serum proteins and bone destruction in transmissible mouse plasma cell neoplasm (multiple myeloma). Proc. Soc. Exper. Biol. & Med., *94*:327, 1957.
150. Putnam, F. W.: Aberrations of protein metabolism in multiple myeloma. Interrelationships of abnormal serum globulins and Bence Jones proteins. Physiol. Rev., *37*:512, 1957.
151. Putnam, F. W.: Structural relationships among normal human γ-globulin, myeloma globulins and Bence-Jones proteins. Biochim. et Biophys. Acta, *63*:539, 1962.
152. Rebuck, J. W., and Crowley, J. H.: A method of studying leukocyte functions in vivo. Ann. N.Y. Acad. Sci., *59*:757, 1955.
153. Rebuck, J. W., Monto, R. W., Monaghan, E. A., and Riddle, J. M.: Potentialities of the lymphocyte with an additional reference to its dysfunction in Hodgkin's disease. Ann. N.Y. Acad. Sci., *73*:8, 1958.
153a. Rieke, W. O., Coffey, R. W., and Everett, N. B.: Rates of proliferation and interrelationships of cells in the mesenteric lymph node of the rat. Blood, *22*:674, 1963.
154. Remington, J. S., Merler, E., Lerner, A. M., Gitlin, D., and Finland, M.: Antibodies of low molecular weight in normal human urine. Nature, *194*:407, 1962.
154a. Reynolds, H. Y., and Johnson, J. S.: Canine immunoglobulins. J. Immunol., *104*:888, 1970.
155. Ritzmann, S. E., Coleman, S. L., and Levin, W. C.: The effect of some mercaptanes upon a macrocryogelglobulin: modifications induced by cysteamine, penicillamine and penicillin. J. Clin. Invest., *39*:1320, 1960.
156. Ritzmann, S. E., Thurm, R. H., Truax, W. E., and Levin, W. C.: The syndrome of macroglobulinemia. Arch. Int. Med., *105*:939, 1960.
157. Rivers, S. L., and Patro, M. E.: Cyclophosphamide vs. melphalan in myeloma. J.A.M.A., *207*:1328, 1969.
158. Robbins, J. H.: Tissue culture of the human lymphocyte. Science, *146*:1648, 1964.
159. Robertson, T.: Plasmacytosis and hyperglobulinemia as manifestations of hypersensitivity. Am. J. Med., *9*:315, 1950.
160. Rogentine, G. N., Jr., Rowe, D. S., Bradley, J., Waldman, T. A., and Fahey, J. L.: Human immunoglobulin D (IgD) metabolism. Clin. Res., *14*:335, 1966.
161. Rosen, F. S.: The macroglobulins. New England J. Med., *267*:491, 546, 1962.
162. Rowe, D. S., and Fahey, J. L.: A new class of human immunoglobulin. J. Exper. Med. *121*:185, 1965.
163. Rundles, R. W., Dillon, M. L., and Dillon, E. S.: Multiple myeloma. III. Effects of urethane therapy on plasma cell growth, abnormal serum protein components and Bence Jones proteinuria. J. Clin. Invest., *29*:1243, 1950.
164. Sabin, F. R.: On the origin of the cells of the blood. Physiol. Rev., *2*:38, 1922.
165. Salmon, S. E., Samal, B. A., Hayes, D. M., Hosley, H., Miller, S. P., and Shilling, A.: Role of gamma globulin for immunoprophylaxis in multiple myeloma. New England J. Med., *277*:1336, 1967.
166. Schoenberg, M. D., Mumaw, V. R., Moore, R. D., and Weisberger, A. S.: Cytoplasmic inter-

action between macrophages and lymphocytic cells in antibody synthesis. Science, *143*:964, 1964.

167. Seligmann, M., Danon, F., Hurez, D., Mihaesco, E., and Prend'homme, J. L.: Alpha chain disease: a new immunoglobulin abnormality. Science, *162*:1396, 1968.

168. Seligmann, M., Fudenberg, H. H., and Good, R. A.: A proposed classification of primary immunologic deficiencies. Am. J. Med., *45*:817, 1968.

169. Skoog, W. A., Adams, W. S., and Coburn, J. W.: Metabolic balance study of plasmapheresis in a case of Waldenström's macroglobulinemia. Blood, *19*:425, 1962.

170. Slater, R. J., Ward, S. M., and Kunkel, H. G.: Immunological relationships among the myeloma proteins. J. Exper. Med., *101*:85, 1955.

171. Snapper, I., Turner, L. B., and Moscovitz, H. L.: Multiple Myeloma. Grune & Stratton, New York, 1953.

172. Soothill, J. F.: In Good, R. A., and Bergman, D. (Eds.): The immunological deficiency diseases in man. Birth Defects, *4*:459, 1968.

173. Spulter, H. F.: Abnormal serum proteins and retinal vein thrombosis. A.M.A. Arch. Ophth., *62*:868, 1959.

174. Steinberg, A. G.: Progress in the study of genetically determined human γ-globulin types (the Gm and Inv groups). Progr. Med. Genet., *2*:1, 1962.

175. Stevens, A. R.: Evolution of multiple myeloma. Arch. Int. Med., *115*:90, 1965.

176. Stevenson, G. T.: Further studies of the gamma-related proteins of normal urine. J. Clin. Invest., *41*:1190, 1962.

177. Study Committee on Midwest Cooperative Chemotherapy Group: Multiple myeloma. J.A.M.A., *188*:741, 1964.

178. Sutton J. S., and Weiss, L.: Transformation of monocytes in tissue culture into macrophages, epithelioid cells and multinucleated giant cells. J. Cell. Biol., *28*:303, 1966.

179. Sundberg, R. D.: Lymphocytes and plasma cells. Ann. N.Y. Acad. Sci., *59*:671, 1955.

180. Takatsuki, K., and Osserman, E. F.: Demonstration of two types of low molecular weight gamma globulins in normal human urine. J. Immunol., *92*:100, 1964.

181. Tomasi, T. B., Jr., and Czerwinski, D. S.: The secretory IgA system. In Good, R. A., and Bergman, D. (Eds.): Immunological Deficiency Diseases in Man. Birth Defects, *4*:270, 1968.

182. Tomasi, T. B., Tan, E. M., Soloman, A., and Pendergast, R. A.: Characteristics of an immune system common to certain external secretions. J. Exp. Med., *121*:101, 1965.

183. Tourville, D. R., Adler, R. H., Bienenstock, J., and Tomasi, T. B., Jr. The human secretory immunoglobulin system: immunohistological localization of γA secretory "piece" and lactoferrin in normal tissues. J. Exp. Med., *129*:411, 1969.

184. Tourville, D. R., and Tomasi, T. B., Jr.: Selective transport of γA. Proc. Soc. Exp. Biol. and Med., *132*:473, 1969.

185. Trowell, O. A.: Some properties of lymphocytes in vivo and in vitro. Ann. N.Y. Acad. Sci., *73*:105, 1958.

186. Valentine, W. N., and Beck, W. S.: Biochemical studies on leucocytes. I. Phosphatase activity in health, leukocytosis, and myelocytic leucemia. J. Lab. Clin. Med., *38*:39, 1951.

187. Vaerman, J. P., and Heremans, J. F.: Subclasses of human immunoglobin A based on differences in the alpha polypeptide chains. Science, *153*:647, 1966.

188. Volkman, A., and Gowans, J. L.: The production of macrophages in the rat. Brit. J. Exp. Path., *46*:50, 1965.

189. Waldenström, J.: Incipient myelomatosis or "essential" hyperglobulinemia with fibrinogen-openia—a new syndrome? Acta Med. Scandinav., *137*:216, 1944.

190. Waldenström, J.: Diseases associated with abnormal plasma proteins. Proc. Roy. Soc. Med., *53*:789, 1960.

191. Waldenström, J.: Studies on conditions associated with disturbed gamma globulin formation (gammopathies). Harvey Lect., *56*:211, 1960–61.

192. Waldenström, J.: The occurrence of benign essential monoclonal (M type) non-macro-molecular hyperglobulinemia and its differential diagnosis. Acta Med. Scandinav., *176*:345, 1964.

193. Wallerstein, R. S.: Multiple myeloma without demonstrable bone lesions. Am. J. Med., *10*:325, 1951.

194. Ward, P. A., Remold, H. G., and David, J. R.: Leukotactic factor produced by sensitized lymphocytes. Science, *163*:1079, 1969.

194a. Webb, T., Rose, B., and Sehon, A. H.: Biocolloids in normal human urine. II. Physicochemical and immunochemical characteristics. Canad. J. Biochem., *36*:1167, 1958.

194b. Weiss, L.: Electron microscopic observations on the vascular barrier in the cortex of the thymus of the mouse. Anat. Rec., *145*:413, 1963.

195. White, A.: Effects of steroids on aspects of the metabolism and functions of the lymphocyte; a hypothesis of the cellular mechanism in antibody formation and related immune phenomena. Ann. N.Y. Acad. Sci., *73*:79, 1958.

196. Williams R. C., Jr., Brunning, R. D., and Wollheim, F. A.: Light chain disease: an abortive variant of multiple myeloma. Ann. Int. Med., *65*:471, 1966.

197. Wochner, R. D., Strober, W., and Waldmann, T. A.: The role of the kidney in the catabolism of Bence-Jones proteins and immunoglobulin fragments. J. Exper. Med., *126*:207, 1967.

198. Wolf, J., and Worken, B.: Atypical amyloidosis and bone marrow plasmacytosis in a case of hypersensitivity to sulfonamides. Am. J. Med., *16*:746, 1954.

199. Wright, J. H.: A case of multiple myeloma. Trans. Assoc. Am. Physicians, *15*:137, 1900.

200. Wulff, H. R., and Sparrevohn, S.: The origin of mononuclear cells in human skin windows. Acta Path. Micro. Scand., *68*:401, 1966.

201. Yoffey, J. M.: The present status of the lymphocyte problem. Lancet, *1*:206, 1962.

202. Yoffey, J. M., Hanks, G. A., and Kelly, L.: Some problems of lymphocyte production. Ann. N.Y. Acad. Sci., *73*:47, 1958.

203. Zawadski, J. A., and Rubini, J. R.: D myeloma. Arch. Int. Med., *119*:387, 1967.

204. Zucker-Franklin, D.: Structural features of cells associated with the paraproteinemias. Seminars Hemat., *1*:165, 1964.

XVI / *Therapeutic Agents Used in the Treatment of Hematologic Disorders*

The principal agents used to treat leukemia, myeloma, and lymphoma are ionizing radiation, alkylating agents, antimetabolites, oncolytic alkaloids, adrenocortical hormones, antibiotics, enzymes, and uricosuric agents. All of them may produce serious side effects. They are rarely curative, yet they often induce hematologic and clinical remission when employed properly. Support of patients with hematologic disorders often necessitates administration of whole blood or blood products. These patients may require restoration of the blood volume, the oxygen-carrying capacity of the blood, platelets, or some plasma fraction or fractions. There are major hazards associated with the administration of blood or its components that must be balanced against the expected results.

Radiation

Ionizing radiation may be administered from an external source by use of roentgen rays or cobalt,[1] or from an internal source by the administration of a radioactive isotope, such as radioactive phosphorus (P^{32}). The effects produced by the irradiation of tissue cells have been studied extensively but the site of the primary biochemical lesion has not been established. A variety of enzymatic

611

changes have been demonstrated in the cell after irradiation but these occur late and may be secondary to some disturbance in cellular metabolism.[5, 54, 116, 143] Inhibition of the synthesis of both deoxyribonucleic acid (DNA) and ribonucleic acid (RNA) has been demonstrated, but protein synthesis by the cell seems unaffected.[1, 200, 201] It has been demonstrated that small doses of radiation produce a delay in the onset of DNA synthesis[143] but do not inhibit DNA synthesis once it has been initiated. At the present time it is not known whether these changes represent a primary effect of ionizing radiation on the biochemical sequence leading to nucleic acid synthesis or an effect that is secondary to mitotic inhibition.[116, 200] Studies of the effect of x-radiation of regenerating rat liver during the first cycle of DNA synthesis indicate marked depression of DNA synthesis and suggest that this is related to cell death from radiation.[152] It has been shown that main polynucleotide chains of DNA are broken by the direct action of ionizing radiations. If this effect is relatively unselective, as it appears to be, any cellular function in which DNA is involved may be affected.[5] It has been postulated that the primary effect of radiation on the cell may be so small as to be undetectable at present. As the result of the initial disturbance the metabolic activities of the cell may function incompletely and produce the biochemical and anatomic changes which can be demonstrated.[5]

Because ionizing radiation interferes with deoxyribonucleic acid synthesis, it produces damage in any tissue composed of dividing cells. The damage is most apparent in the tissues with active cellular proliferation. Therapeutic radiation aims at destroying the rapidly proliferating tumor cells while sparing the normal cells of the body as far as possible. Ionizing radiation from an external source is directed in such a manner that the amount of normal tissue in its path is as small as possible. This is accomplished by careful positioning of the patient and the use of protective shielding. The use of multiple portals of entry for the ionizing radiation when a large dose is required in the body cavity reduces the effects on the normal skin and other tissues which must be traversed to reach the lesion. The cells of the hematopoietic system, the gastrointestinal tract, and the skin, which have a high rate of turnover, are particularly susceptible to radiation damage. Damage to the cutaneous cells and depression of the bone marrow frequently limit the amount of radiation the patient can receive.

Ionizing radiation has been used extensively in the treatment of diseases of the lymphoma group and the chronic forms of leukemia but is not employed in the uncomplicated acute forms of leukemia, since its use often results in a more rapid course. It was used first for the treatment of Hodgkin's disease between 1902 and 1905.[163] Since that time it has been used more than any other form of treatment for all of the diseases in the lymphoma group. It is more effective than the radioactive isotopes in the control of these disorders.[153, 163] The diseases of the lymphoma group are radiosensitive and they often undergo striking regression after exposure to a small amount of radiation. Unfortunately, the remissions are usually temporary and the disease eventually becomes resistant to additional intensive therapy. However, it has been recognized in recent years that the probability of recurrence of Hodgkin's disease (and perhaps other lymphomas) in a radiation-treated field is a function of the dose given. This observation has stimulated aggressive therapy with equipment capable of producing mega voltage energy beams, since the doses required cannot be delivered with ordinary

250-Kv conventional x-rays. The results indicate that relatively high-dose, wide field radiotherapy may cure some patients with this disorder.[128, 179]

The use of high-energy beams has made it possible to deliver large doses of radiation to a tumor without excessive damage to the skin. Unfortunately, normal tissues in the area of the tumor are being heavily irradiated and have been found to be unexpectedly radiosensitive. Heart disease has been found to be a complication of irradiation of the thoracic cavity. The clinical incidence of this complication is on the order of 4 to 5 per cent, but acute pericarditis, chronic pericardial effusion, chronic constrictive pericarditis, diffuse myocardial fibrosis, and myocardial infarction have been reported.[45, 127, 161, 171] Connective tissue proliferation appears to be the hallmark of these late radiation lesions. Organizing pericarditis with extensive fibrosis is the most frequent alteration, but diffuse interstitial myocardial fibrosis is common.[75] These complications must be recognized and treated appropriately; it should not be assumed that the manifestations are the result of the underlying neoplastic disease.[168]

A variety of other complications have been noted. A late developing radiation nephritis with associated hypertension has been reported.[211] Radiation therapy of abdominal Hodgkin's disease has been associated with perforation of the bowel;[47] radiation pneumonitis may be another complication of irradiation of the thoracic cavity.[14] A transient radiation-induced myelitis may occur after a latent period of 3 to 4 months; this is an entirely subjective sensory disorder and spontaneously subsides in 2 to 4 months. A progressive, permanent myelitis may occur after a latent period of 9 to 12 months and is believed to be mediated by vascular injury.[49, 214] Radiation hepatitis and local damage to bone have been reported.[13, 129]

The use of radioactive phosphorus (P^{32}), which was introduced in 1936 as a source of ionizing radiation, has been reviewed.[191] This method of treatment offers certain advantages over roentgen ray therapy in that generalized radiation of the hematopoietic system may be obtained with relative ease without the production of radiation sickness.[148] P^{32} emits beta radiation which produces ionization within an area limited to its maximal range of 0.7 cm. It has a 14.3 day half-life and decays to stable sulfur. Since the sensitivity of a cell to ionizing radiation seems related to its mitotic stage, the continuous radiation provided by P^{32} may have a distinct advantage over intermittent therapy from an external source in the treatment of a growing tissue that contains cells asynchronously undergoing cell division. Following administration P^{32} is concentrated in tissues composed of rapidly metabolizing cells which have a high phosphorus turnover, such as the bone marrow, lymph nodes, spleen, and liver; later the P^{32} enters the osseous tissue of the skeleton. Because of the selectivity provided by its distribution within the body the chief value of radioactive phosphorus has been in the treatment of chronic leukemias and polycythemia vera.

Because of the depressant effect that all ionizing radiation exerts on the bone marrow, frequent leukocyte counts and hematocrit determinations are performed while the patient is undergoing therapy. The level of the leukocytes that is considered a contraindication to further therapy depends on details of the individual case and no fast rules can be stated. The development of leukopenia, thrombocytopenia, and anemia demands caution and careful evaluation before proceeding with further therapy.

Alkylating Agents

Among the most effective compounds available for the treatment of chronic leukemia and lymphoma are the alkylating agents. These agents were introduced into clinical medicine as the result of extensive studies that were carried out during World War II. The chemical, pharmacologic, and clinical studies of these compounds have been summarized.[94]

One group of alkylating agents, the mustards, owe their biologic activity to the presence of the *bis*, beta-chloroethyl grouping.[98] In neutral or alkaline aqueous solution the nitrogen mustards are highly reactive. The tertiary amine undergoes intramolecular transformation to form a cyclic ionium cation with liberation of a chloride ion. This cyclic ethylenimonium cation reacts readily with inorganic anions, water, and organic radicals.[98] These compounds limit

$$\begin{matrix} CH_2CH_2Cl & & CH_2 \\ | & & | \diagdown \\ R-N & \longrightarrow R-\ ^+N-CH_2 + Cl^- \\ | & & | \\ CH_2CH_2Cl & & CH_2CH_2Cl \end{matrix}$$

tissue growth by inhibiting mitotic activity and cell division. Although the nitrogen mustards are capable of inactivating many enzyme systems, the evidence appears to indicate that these compounds do not act in vivo by inhibiting intracellular enzymatic activity.[94, 98, 193] Considerable work along different lines has led to the hypothesis that alkylating agents, which are active in aqueous solution, produce their antitumor effect by esterifying ionized acid groups rather than by reacting with sulfhydryl groups or free amino groups.[193]

A reaction with nucleic acids, especially the inactivation of deoxyribonucleic acid, would have a profound effect on cell division. In vitro experiments have demonstrated that alkylating agents cause marked alterations in the physical properties of nucleic acids. These include changes in the shape of the macromolecules and in the ability to combine with basic material.[193] It has been demonstrated that nitrogen mustard produces a marked decrease in the viscosity of dilute solutions of deoxyribonucleic acid.[95, 96] Other in vitro studies that have utilized the electron microscope have demonstrated intramolecular cross-linking and coiling up of deoxyribonucleic acid molecules after exposure to nitrogen mustard.[204] The alkylating agents appear to act by producing cross-linking of the different DNA molecules via their phosphate groups, which renders them inactive.[5]

The alkylating agents that have been used most widely in clinical practice are:

1. Methyl-*bis* (β-chloroethyl) amine hydrochloride (nitrogen mustard, HN₂).

2. Triethylene melamine (TEM).

3. *p*-(Di-2-chloroethylamine)-phenylbutyric acid (chlorambucil, CB 1348).

4. 1-4-Dimethanesulfonyloxybutane (busulfan).

5. 2-[bis(2-chloroethyl)amino]-1,3,2-oxazaphosphoridine,2-oxide (cyclophosphamide, cytoxon).

6. p-di(2-chloroethyl)-amino-L-phenylalanine (1-phenylalanine mustard) (melphalan).

These compounds differ in their effectiveness against different strains of cells, different types of lesions, and in their toxic effects.

NITROGEN MUSTARD

Nitrogen mustard has been studied more extensively than the other alkylating agents. The histologic changes in the lymphoid tissue and marrow that occur in rats after the injection of mustard were studied by Kindred.[136] He found that lymphocytes were more sensitive than the granulocytes or the red cell precursors; reticulum cells and megakaryocytes were much less sensitive.

For clinical use nitrogen mustard is made up in a fresh solution of physiologic saline and is administered intravenously by injecting it into the tubing of an intravenous saline infusion. Local thrombophlebitis sometimes develops and a severe local reaction occurs if the nitrogen mustard is extravasated into the tissue. Approximately 80 per cent of the patients who receive the drug develop nausea and vomiting.[131]

The most important toxic effect is exerted on the bone marrow. This is manifested within 7 to 10 days by a fall in the leukocyte count followed by a decrease in the platelets that generally reaches its lowest level within 2 or 3 weeks. In order to avoid serious damage to the bone marrow an interval of at least 6 weeks is allowed between courses of therapy whenever possible. When the patient has extensive involvement with lymphosarcoma, smaller doses spaced several days apart are advisable because the rapid destruction of tissue may cause hyperuricemia and renal impairment[131] or even, as the authors have seen, vascular collapse. Evidence of impaired bone marrow function is also an indication for smaller doses spaced at longer intervals.

Nitrogen mustard has found its greatest usefulness in Hodgkin's disease, in which it often produces a prompt remission in fever, sweats, anorexia, pruritus, and weakness, accompanied by a decrease in the size of the spleen, liver, and lymph nodes. In lymphosarcoma, reticulum cell sarcoma, and giant follicular lymphoma the response to treatment with nitrogen mustard varies greatly in different patients but in general the response is not as good as in Hodgkin's disease.[98, 121, 131, 140, 224] Nitrogen mustard has not been used widely in the treatment of chronic leukemia though it has been suggested that it might be effective if a satisfactory plan of administration could be worked out.[17]

TEM

Triethylene melamine (TEM) is converted in an acid medium to a reactive quaternary ethylenimonium compound and produces therapeutic effects similar to those produced by nitrogen mustard. Since it is transformed into its active form in an acid medium, it may be administered by mouth. Because TEM will be inert by the time it is absorbed if the stomach contents are too acid, it is usually administered with sodium bicarbonate. It is often difficult to determine how much active compound has been absorbed and, in addition, there seems to be considerable individual variation in response to the drug. For these reasons the drug must be administered with great caution. In some patients an initial dose of 2.5 mg. produces a marked effect on hematopoiesis that persists for months. Although the effects of TEM are similar to those produced by nitrogen mustard, better clinical results have been obtained with TEM in lymphosarcoma and giant follicle lymphoma than in Hodgkin's disease and reticulum cell sarcoma.[195] Good clinical results have been obtained in the treatment of both chronic myelocytic leukemia and chronic lymphocytic leukemia with TEM.[17]

CHLORAMBUCIL

Chlorambucil (CB 1348), a water soluble aromatic nitrogen mustard, is also administered orally and is much less toxic to hematopoietic tissue than nitrogen mustard or TEM. It can produce marrow aplasia, however, and blood counts should be performed at intervals of not less than 3 weeks while the patient is receiving the drug.[119] Improvement generally occurs in 3 or 4 weeks if the drug is effective, and the usual course of treatment lasts from 4 to 8 weeks. Gastrointestinal disturbances are mild and infrequent. This drug is more effective in diseases characterized by abnormal lymphocyte proliferation, such as lymphosarcoma and giant follicle lymphoma, than in reticulum cell sarcoma and Hodgkin's disease.[119] Nevertheless, remissions were obtained in 22 of 47 patients with Hodgkin's disease and in 12 the remission lasted 5 to 12 months.[64] Chlorambucil is effective in the treatment of chronic lymphocytic leukemia but is ineffective in chronic myelocytic leukemia.

BUSULFAN

Busulfan is a sulfonic acid ester and in low doses selectively depresses granulocytopoiesis. This alkylating agent is an effective agent in the treatment of chronic myelogenous leukemia and other "myeloproliferative" disorders[56, 90] but has not been effective in other forms of malignant disease.[90] The ease of administration and the relatively high therapeutic index of busulfan make it the agent of choice in chronic myelogenous leukemia. Busulfan was administered to a pregnant woman with chronic granulocytic leukemia after the eighth week of gestation without apparent effect on the child.[66] The most serious toxic effects of busulfan that occur in some patients are bone marrow depression, hyperpigmentation of the skin, testicular atrophy, and pulmonary fibrosis.

CYCLOPHOSPHAMIDE

The demonstration of increased amounts of phosphamidase in malignant tissue[97] prompted a search for inactive cyclic phosphamide esters of nitrogen mustard which would transport the β chloroethyl group and be activated by phosphamidases in tumor tissue.[103] Cyclophosphamide was developed as the result of these studies and after the demonstration of an antitumor effect in animals received extensive clinical trials.

Reports of various groups[18, 96, 103, 115, 199] have indicated that this alkylating agent is most effective against reticulum cell sarcoma and lymphosarcoma and moderately effective in Hodgkin's disease. The mechanism of its anti-tumor activity is believed to be similar to that of nitrogen mustard. The drug may be given orally or parenterally. Cyclophosphamide has recently been shown to be as effective as 6-mercaptopurine in the treatment of acute leukemia in childhood. No significant difference was observed in the rate or duration of remission effected by the two drugs.[84] It is also effective in the treatment of early relapse of acute leukemia in children.[181]

Some of the toxic side effects of cyclophosphamide are similar to those of nitrogen mustard.[172] Anorexia and nausea occur in nearly all patients while the drug is being administered, and are difficult to control. Leukopenia occurs in most patients, but anemia and reticulocytopenia are rare. Thrombocytopenia does not appear to be a problem. Alopecia occurs in approximately 25 to 40 per cent of patients while receiving the drug. Regrowth of hair has been reported to occur after the drug is discontinued.[103] Hemorrhagic cystitis caused by the excretion of active breakdown products of cyclophosphamide develops in a significant percentage of patients.[44, 194] While most patients respond to symptomatic therapy, some progress to a chronic fibrosing or hemorrhagic cystitis severe enough to produce urinary obstruction and exsanguinating hemorrhage.[92]

MELPHALAN

Melphalan is the L-isomer of phenylalanine mustard. The racemic (DL-) form is known as merphalan. The compound may be involved in intracellular protein synthesis and carry the alkylating fraction into the cells. Melphalan remains active in the blood for 2 hours and is believed to exert its cytotoxic effect by crosslinking DNA in the resting stage. The effect of melphalan on a variety of tumors has been investigated[43] and it has found wide use in the treatment of multiple myeloma.[29] The toxicity of this compound is similar to that of the other mustards.

Antimetabolites

FOLIC ACID ANTAGONISTS (AMINOPTERIN AND AMETHOPTERIN)

Folic acid antagonists were introduced in the treatment of acute leukemia by Farber, who in 1947 noted the acceleration of the leukemic process in patients receiving folic acid. He suggested that "antifolic" compounds might be of benefit, and the following year reported the production of a temporary remission in 10 of 16 children with leukemia who were treated with an antifolic compound, aminopterin, an observation which ushered in the present era of chemotherapy in leukemia.[81] The use of these agents, which interfere with the metabolism of neoplastic cells to a greater extent than they do with the metabolism of normal cells, has not yet resulted in the cure of leukemia but it has produced striking temporary remissions in the disease.[80, 130]

The antifolic compounds are derived by substitutions in the folic acid molecule. The hydrogen atoms in the structure may be replaced, as may the hydroxyl

Folic acid

on the pyrimidine ring, or the glutamic acid may be replaced in its entirety by another amino acid or polypeptide chain. Aminopterin is produced by substitution of an amino group for the hydroxyl group. Amethopterin (methotrexate) is formed when, in addition to the amino group substitution, a methyl group is substituted at position 10.

The mechanism by which the folic acid antagonists exert their effect is not understood completely. Folic acid is essential for the synthesis of nucleic acid as a result of its effect on formate metabolism. The antifolic acid compounds inhibit the conversion of folic acid to citrovorum factor (folinic acid) and thus limit formate metabolism; formate, along with CO_2, NH_3, and glycine, is essential for the synthesis of deoxyribonucleic acid and ribonucleic acid. The antifolic compounds may also interfere with the synthesis of thymine,[205] which is used in the synthesis of nucleic acid. It is probable that folic acid antagonists are effective because they disrupt the metabolic pathways that lead to the formation of nucleic acid.[32] These drugs exert their greatest effect on cells which are dividing rapidly and have the greatest demand for nucleic acid. Ordinarily the cells of the bone marrow, lymph follicles, and gastrointestinal tract are the first that are affected. Leukemic cells, which have an extremely high proliferative rate, are affected to a greater extent than normal cells. It is only the difference in the rate of proliferation that makes leukemic cells more sensitive to these drugs than normal cells. Since normal cells are also affected there is a definite limit to the amount of the drug that can be administered.

A number of investigators have reported their results with the antifolic compounds.[35, 78, 81, 109] Of a group of 425 children with acute leukemia, 68 per cent received some benefit and 30 to 50 per cent obtained good clinical and hematologic results. Since these preparations are beneficial in only about 14 per cent of the adults,[35] their chief use is in the treatment of leukemia in children. Amethopterin is usually preferred to aminopterin because there is a wider range of safety between the effective therapeutic dose and the dose that produces severe toxic effects.[70] Both compounds are administered by the oral route.

Amethopterin alone or in combination with other drugs is effective in inducing and maintaining a remission in acute lymphoblastic leukemia, and it is the most effective agent currently available for the treatment of meningeal leukemia.[88] It is also often used for maintenance therapy in lymphoma.

The major toxic effects of these preparations are bone marrow depression with pancytopenia and megaloblastic erythropoiesis, stomatitis, and gastroenteritis.

PURINE AND PYRIMIDINE ANALOGS

Because investigations of nucleic acid synthesis revealed a close relationship between folic acid, purine, and thymine metabolism, efforts have been made to find analogs of purine and pyrimidine compounds which would block nucleic acid synthesis, particularly in malignant cells.[32, 111] For years it was thought that dietary purines and pyrimidines could not enter into the formation of nucleic acids.[182] After the demonstration of the incorporation of adenine into nucleic acid in 1948 this concept was modified.[33] This observation stimulated the search for purine analogs which might effectively interfere with cellular metabolism. Each of the naturally occurring purine and pyrimidine bases has been investigated systematically and new compounds have been produced by altering the basic chemical composition of the naturally occurring compounds.[111] These compounds have been tested in microbiologic systems and those that showed promise have been tested against tumors or leukemia in rodents. These purine antagonists are believed to interfere with nucleic acid metabolism, perhaps by becoming incorporated into nucleic acid and rendering it biologically ineffective.[32] It has been suggested that a hypoxanthine-containing compound that is an intermediate in the conversion of adenine to guanine may be the site of action.[68]

6-Mercaptopurine (6-MP). The first clinical trials with 6-mercaptopurine were encouraging. In 1953 it was reported that 15 of 45 children with acute leukemia underwent a good clinical and hematologic remission and another 10 had a partial remission. Resistance to therapy appeared to develop more rapidly than with the antifolic compounds but it was observed that patients who had become resistant to the antifolic acid compounds were still sensitive to treatment with 6-mercaptopurine.[16, 36] A review of the results obtained with 6-MP indicates that remission will occur in approximately one-third of the children with acute leukemia and in about one-seventh of the adults.[31] Remission may occasionally be obtained in children who have become resistant to steroid and antifolic acid compounds;[16] currently initial treatment in children usually is prednisone combined with 6-MP or vincristine. After relapse occurs the subsequent remissions that are obtained with any of these drugs are less complete and of shorter duration than the initial response.

6-mercaptopurine alone or in combination has a significant incidence of induction of remission in children. It is much less effective in adults, but is used for the treatment of acute granulocytic leukemia. The major toxic effects of 6-MP are nausea, vomiting, and marrow depression.

AZATHIOPRINE

Azathioprine 6 [(1-methyl-4-nitro-5-imidazolyl)thio] purine was developed as part of a program to present the thiopurines in a masked but metabolically active form.[69] Metabolic studies have shown that the drug is well absorbed from the gastrointestinal tract and converted to free 6-MP; its oxidation product is 6-thiouric acid.[196]

The toxic effects of the drug are similar to those of 6-MP and include nausea and vomiting, and bone marrow depression. Rarely, liver damage has been reported and patients with liver disease should probably not receive the drug. Chromosomal breakage has been reported in humans and lymphomas have been observed in mice with auto-immune disorders after treatment with azathioprine.[40, 123] These reports emphasize the need to exercise caution when antimitotic therapy is given, especially in conditions not already neoplastic. The drug should not be given during pregnancy.[10]

Azathioprine alone or in combination with steroids or antilymphocyte serum is used primarily for immunosuppression following homotransplantation. More recently it has been used in a variety of disorders for which altered immunologic mechanisms are believed responsible,[10, 155, 164, 219] including several hematologic disorders.[24, 206]

8-AZAGUANINE

8-Azaguanine, a compound similar to guanine in chemical structure, has been reported to be effective in acute leukemia.[80] The compound is interesting because it has been shown to inhibit adenosine deaminase in vitro.[83] This observation suggests that compounds may interfere with nucleic acid metabolism by inhibiting essential enzymes. It appears that leukemic cells are much more sensitive to 8-azaguanine than are normal cells. Toxic manifestations, such as dermatitis, nausea, vomiting, and diarrhea, have limited the amount of the drug that can be administered.

CYTOSINE ARABINOSIDE (ARABINOSYLCYTOSINE, ARA-C)

Cytosine arabinoside is a synthetic pyrimidine nucleoside differing in the sugar moiety from the normal metabolites cytidine and deoxycytidine. The exact mechanism of its action is not known, but cytosine arabinoside triphosphate is an inhibitor of cytosine ribonucleotide reductase, the enzyme involved in the conversion of cytosine diphosphate to deoxycytidine diphosphate. Inhibition of the formation of deoxycytidine diphosphate results in inhibition of the synthesis of DNA and a decrease in cellular proliferation.[41, 73] The incorporation of cytosine arabinoside triphosphate into nucleic acids may also cause acute cell death separate from the slower destruction due to inhibition of cytosine ribonucleotide reductase.[41] It has also been reported to be a competitive inhibitor of deoxycytidine triphosphate and thus an inhibitor of DNA polymerase.[89] Recent studies have shown that cytosine arabinoside tends to synchronize the mitotic cycle of the abnormal cells of patients with acute leukemia. Such information may be of value in the choice of drugs and the timing of their administration in the future.[144]

Although this drug is also effective in the treatment of acute leukemia in children,[117] its effect on adult acute leukemia has excited greater interest.[22, 53, 71] Cytosine arabinoside has been shown to be effective against acute lymphocytic leukemia and acute myelocytic leukemia in adults of all ages. The effect of the drug has not been shown to be influenced by pre-treatment leukocyte counts, but thrombocytopenia reduces the chance of a favorable response.[71]

Toxic effects of the drug include marrow depression, particularly thrombocytopenia, and disturbances of the gastrointestinal tract. The drug induces marked megaloblastic change in the erythroid precursors of the bone marrow with mitotic abnormalities similar to those seen in megaloblastic anemia.[210] Nausea and vomiting and oral ulceration may occur. Since severe thrombocytopenia occurs in a high percentage of patients receiving cytosine arabinoside, it is imperative that platelet transfusions be immediately available when the drug is used.[22, 91, 210]

6-AZAURIDINE

6-Azauridine is an interesting investigative drug which is converted in mammalian tissues to 6-azauridylic acid and binds orotidylic acid decarboxylase. The conversion of orotidylic acid to uridylic acid is blocked and the utilization of orotic acid as a source of nucleic acid pyrimidines is inhibited.[106] A pronounced orotic acid and uric acid crystalluria sometimes accompanies the administration of 6-azauridine. Apparently both 6-azauridine and orotic acid have a uricosuric action.[76]

Though no remissions have been reported, 6-azauridine has been shown to have an effect on acute myelogenous leukemia, and it is possible that it will be useful in combination with other antimetabolites. The clinical investigation of this drug is continuing.[110, 218]

The most striking toxicity reported has been somnolence associated with a diffuse slow wave dysrhythmia on electroencephalography. The neural toxicity is similar to that noted with 6-azauracil. There is no evidence of myelosuppression or gastrointestinal toxicity.

Oncolytic Alkaloids

A large number of alkaloids have been extracted from the periwinkle plant (vinca rosea Linn.) and some demonstrated to have oncolytic activity. Only two, vinblastine and vincristine, have had intensive clinical evaluation.[208]

Biochemical investigation has not uncovered any effect on cell metabolism or protein or nucleic acid synthesis, and their mechanism of action remains unknown.[124]

Vinblastine and vincristine are useful in the treatment of Hodgkin's disease and other lymphomas.[124, 216, 221] Vincristine produces striking remissions in a high percentage of childhood acute lymphocytic leukemia but is ineffective in sustaining the remission.[132] Serious side effects from the use of these agents are prominent. Both produce alopecia, severe paralytic ileus, and moderate reticulocytopenia and anemia. Platelets are usually unaffected by either drug. The major limiting toxic effect of vinblastine is leukopenia; that of vincristine is central nervous system toxicity and peripheral neuropathy which may persist for months after the drug has been discontinued. Despite the toxic side effects these drugs are valuable when used properly.[124, 220]

ANTIBIOTICS

Certain antibiotics have a profound effect on the metabolic activities of mammalian cells, and some are proving to be of therapeutic interest.

Streptonigrin.   The antibiotic streptonigrin is a metabolite of the *Strepto-myces flocculus* which exhibits striking antitumor activity in animals and man.[108, 188] It is a potent inhibitor of DNA production, causing chromosomal breakage and, possibly, degradation of formed DNA.[190] Various studies have indicated that streptonigrin given orally or intravenously has a significant effect on lymphomas, mycosis fungoides, and chronic lymphocytic leukemia.[108, 133]

Immediate toxicity to the drug includes nausea, vomiting, diarrhea, alopecia, depigmentation, and thrombophlebitis. The most profound toxic effect is marrow depression, which reaches a maximum 3 to 4 weeks after the start of treatment.[223]

The methylester of streptonigrin also shows antitumor activity in a variety of lymphomas and chronic lymphocytic leukemias. Further studies of these drugs are needed.[108, 190]

Daunomycin.   Daunomycin (Rubidomycin, Daunorubicin) is a new antibiotic isolated from cultures of *Streptomyces peucetius.* It is a tetracycline quinone (daunomycinone) and an amino sugar, 2,3 dideoxy-3 amino-1-fucose (daunosamine).[61]

Daunomycin is the first antibiotic shown to have an effect on acute leukemia. It inhibits cell growth, decreases the mitotic index, and produces chromosomal aberrations of HeLa cells in vitro by its action on DNA polymerase or by the direct physicochemical changes which occur in DNA structures following link-age with the antibiotic. There is also marked inhibition of nucleolar RNA syn-thesis.[62] Interest in daunomycin was stimulated by its effectiveness in the treat-ment of acute myelogenous leukemia in adults. It also has low-grade activity for induction of remission in children with advanced leukemia. Combination with prednisone may enhance its effect.[114]

Daunomycin is a very toxic drug which can cause rapid and profound marrow aplasia and oral ulceration. Evidence of severe cardiotoxicity, which may occur without warning, is growing. There may be a short period of tachycardia, arterial hypotension, and dyspnea followed suddenly by cardiac decompensation and death. The extreme cardiac toxicity appears to occur more frequently and at lower drug levels in older patients.[15, 23, 157] There appears to be less toxicity if the drug is given on an intermittent schedule rather than daily.[157]

ENZYMES

L-asparaginase (l-asparagine aminohydrolase).   In 1953 it was noted that regression of transplanted lymphomas in rats and mice could be obtained in vivo by the administration of normal guinea pig serum.[134] Later it was found that the l-asparaginase activity of guinea pig serum was responsible for the anti-lymphoma effect.[30] Cultures of the coliform bacillus *Escherichia coli* are an ex-cellent source of l-asparaginase.[160]

Some malignant cells are unable to synthesize l-asparagine and require an exogenous source of this amino acid. Since l-asparagine is degraded to aspartic acid and ammonia by l-asparaginase, the dependent cell is deprived of l-asparagine in the presence of this enzyme. Tumor cells which are not sensitive to the enzyme have the ability to make l-asparagine and are independent of exogenous sources. Sensitive cells can be made resistant in vitro by treatment with subeffective doses of the enzyme. These cells develop l-asparagine syn-thetase activity and no longer require exogenous l-asparagine for growth in vitro.[2] These findings make it possible to predict in advance which patients have malignant cells that will respond favorably to l-asparaginase.[173]

L-asparaginase is the first therapeutic agent used in the treatment of neo-plastic disease in man which has an action based on a specific metabolic defect of certain malignant cells. Optimal therapeutic trials have not been possible be-cause the enzyme is in short supply, but patients with acute lymphoblastic leukemia and acute myelogenous leukemia have been found to respond. In vitro tests have had predictive value in distinguishing those who would respond.[8, 42, 174, 209]

Toxic side effects, which include chills, fever, nausea, and vomiting, may be due to residual bacterial products. Some patients have become sensitized to the enzyme, usually in the second or third course. Liver damage and pancreatitis have been recorded accompanied by marked changes in serum protein and cholesterol.[8] Serum albumin fell to 30 to 50 per cent of pretreatment levels with 14 days of treatment; globulins and cholesterol also decreased.[39, 174]

Procarbazine. Procarbazine (Natulan, Matulane), a synthetic methyl-hydrazine derivative, is a new class of antitumor agent. Its mode of action has not been elucidated completely, but many of its effects resemble those of ionizing radiation.[203a] Its main use thus far has been in treating patients with Hodgkin's disease; although it is used most often as a drug in "quadruple" therapy or the MOPP regime, it is also effective when given alone. Numerous toxic effects, including nausea and vomiting, leukopenia, thrombocytopenia, and emotional disturbances, have been reported; these, however, are often mild, and alopecia and peripheral neuritis appear to be rare.

Adrenocortical Steroids

The initial report of the use of adrenocortical steroid compounds in the treatment of a child with acute leukemia was encouraging. Administration of the drug was followed by a remission that lasted 2 months.[82] In one series of cases, hematologic improvement was noted in 44 per cent of the patients with acute leukemia treated with adrenocorticotropic hormone and 52 per cent of those treated with cortisone. From 60 to 70 per cent of the patients obtained some im-provement from both drugs, but adults did not respond as well as children. Following relapse, subsequent remissions became more difficult to achieve. Larger series have not revealed such good results. In a series of 425 patients only 30 per cent had a good remission and another 24 per cent obtained a partial remission.[85] The remission rate was higher in patients with acute lymphoblastic or undifferentiated leukemia. Remissions were not observed in myeloblastic or monocytic leukemia and in some patients the disease seemed to be made worse. Others report that occasional remissions that do not differ from those seen in other forms are seen in the myeloblastic and monocytic leukemia.[70] A recent study of 391 children with acute leukemia who were given prednisone as initial treatment revealed that complete remission occurred in 40 per cent and good partial remission in another 34 per cent. Complete bone marrow remission occurred in 63 per cent. Remission was maintained without treatment for a median duration of 58 days, and few subjects had much longer or much shorter remissions. Infants under 1 year, those with an initial diagnosis or acute granulocytic leukemia, and those with initially marked leukocytosis did not do so well.[225] Prednisone by itself or in combination with other antileukemic agents is used most commonly to induce remission. Alone it is not effective in the maintenance of remission though it is often included with other drugs when combined therapy is administered for that purpose.[34, 107, 122, 207] These preparations may be beneficial in the treatment of an associated bleeding tendency or hemolytic anemia even when they produce no striking change in the leukocyte count.

Although adrenocortical steroids may occasionally produce a remission in diseases of the lymphoma group, they are not as effective as ionizing radiation or the alkylating agents and complications may plague their use. The administration of high doses of steroids on an intermittent schedule to patients unable to tolerate or resistant to alkylating agents and radiotherapy has resulted in maximal benefit with minimal complications.[38] They are particularly useful in the treatment of the auto-immune hemolytic anemias which may accompany these disorders. They are also effective when used with other agents to induce remission.

Complications of steroid hormone therapy were more common when only cortisone and adrenocorticotropic hormone were available. Electrolyte disturbances with excessive potassium loss and sodium retention were a constant problem. Dietary sodium restriction and the administration of oral potassium chloride minimized these dangers but did not remove them. With the advent of the newer adrenal steroid analogs, the problem of electrolyte imbalance has ceased to be of clinical importance. However, other dangers, common to all of the adrenocortical hormones, remain. These compounds may so alter the usual body responses to infection or to peritoneal soiling that the occurrence is masked. An increased incidence of peptic ulceration has been observed, and in some patients severe gastrointestinal hemorrhage occurs. Because of the reports of activation of tuberculous foci in some patients and the development of mucosal ulcerations in the gastrointestinal tract of others, patients on these drugs for more than a few weeks should receive 100 mg. of isoniazid (INH) three times a day and an antacid between meals and at bedtime. The development of serious systemic or local fungal infection is not unusual in patients receiving these compounds. Hyperuricemia has been a troublesome complication of the treatment of neoplastic diseases with steroids.[225] Changes in mood are seen commonly and major psychotic reactions may occur. The administration of adrenocortical steroids will curtail endogenous steroid production and for this reason it is advisable to reduce the drugs slowly if therapy is terminated. Weeks or months after cessation of therapy with these preparations the severe stress of a surgical procedure or infection may precipitate an addisonian crisis despite the adequacy of adrenal function for ordinary day to day activities.

The possible mechanisms by which these compounds might produce an effect on the hematopoietic system have received wide attention.[99] Patients with adrenal insufficiency are known to have a lymphocytosis; those with adrenal hyperplasia have a lymphopenia. The administration of adrenocorticotropic hormone or adrenocortical steroids will depress the lymphocyte count. Stress reactions in the intact animal produce a lymphopenia whereas the adrenalecto-mized animal responds to the same stimulus with a lymphocytosis.[65] Evidence has been presented which suggests that the adrenal steroids exert a destructive effect on lymphoid tissue[65] and a cytolytic effect on the individual lymphocyte,[86] or influence the distribution of the lymphocytes in the body.[99] It is possible that all of these effects contribute to the lymphopenic state that is produced by these compounds. The effect of the adrenal gland on myeloid activity is less clear. Although there have been reports that increased myeloid activity occurs as the result of the administration of adrenocortical steroids to humans,[175] a decrease in myeloid activity during prolonged administration of these compounds to laboratory animals has also been observed.[99, 100] The mechanism through which the adrenocortical hormones favorably influence the bleeding tendency and hemolytic anemia which may occur in patients with leukemia and malignant lymphoma is likewise unknown.

During the administration of these compounds a distinct elevation in the mood of the patient often occurs. Appetite improves and a sense of well-being is noted. Fever, tachycardia, and "toxicity" diminish. These improvements often allow time for one of the cytotoxic agents to exert an effect.

URICOSURIC AGENTS

Hyperuricemia is often a problem in patients with neoplastic disease, particularly those who are under treatment with radiation or chemotherapeutic agents. Agents that prevent the precipitation of urate crystals in the renal tubules on the occurrence of acute gouty arthritis are of value in the management of these patients.

Allopurinol. Xanthine oxidase is responsible for the oxidation of normal purines and converts 6-MP to 6-thiouric acid. A search was undertaken to develop a xanthine oxidase inhibitor in hopes of developing a therapeutic adjuvant of 6-MP. The hypoxanthine isomer, 4-hydroxypyrazolo (3,4-d) pyrinidine (allopurinol), was found to be a potent xanthine oxidase inhibitor in vitro and to produce a seven-fold potentiation of the antitumor effect of dif-ferent thiopurines in mice.[197]

It was soon shown that allopurinol in man would potentiate four-fold the effect of 6-MP. This does not appear to offer a therapeutic advantage.[150, 215] Allopurinol is of great use, however, in the prevention of tubular precipitation of urate crystals, which is so often encountered in patients with neoplastic disease, particularly when they are responding to therapy. Urolithiasis and renal insufficiency associated with hyperuricemia are well-known accompaniments of neoplastic disease, especially lymphoma and leukemia.[57, 104, 139] Either radiation or chemotherapy may produce an elevation of the patient's serum level of uric acid and acute uric acid nephropathy. This is a frequent cause of renal failure in patients with leukemia.

The drug has proved to be relatively non-toxic. A 3 per cent incidence of a minor erythematous pruritic rash and occasional diarrhea and leukopenia have been reported. If allopurinol is administered with 6-MP, the dose of 6-MP should be reduced to 25 per cent of its usual level because the "dose sparing" effect of allopurinol could produce a dangerous degree of myelosuppression.[57, 138]

Blood Transfusion

Increased knowledge of the numerous blood groups, improved techniques in cross-matching the donor and recipient, and the development of more efficient methods of preserving and storing blood have all combined to make progress in blood transfusion one of the foremost accomplishments of modern medicine. The important technical details related to this important subject are thoroughly covered in several monographs.[58, 167] Publications prepared by the Committee of the Joint Blood Council and the American Association of Blood Banks and by the Committee on Transfusion and Transplantation (American Medical Association) give authoritative and concise statements concerning minimal standards for processing donors and general principles of blood transfusion.[46, 46a]

HISTORY

The early history of blood transfusions has been summarized by several authors.[67, 135, 217] Authentic references to blood transfusions date from the middle of the seventeenth century. In 1667 Lower transfused blood of a lamb into a "mildly melancholy insane" man and this was considered successful. In the same year Jean Baptist Denis transfused 9 ounces of lamb's blood into a youth and the lad made a remarkable recovery from an obscure fever. Denis repeated the procedure in other patients until he encountered a fatal hemolytic reaction in a man who was given lamb's blood for insanity; this patient had received two previous transfusions without untoward effect. Denis was charged with murder but after a prolonged legal battle he was exonerated. The use of transfusion during the next 10 years was forbidden by Parliament and by a Papal Bull. In 1818 James Blundell, a London physiologist and obstetrician, used indirect blood transfusions in 10 patients with postpartum hemorrhage and five of these were successful. Interest in this field increased and by 1875 at least 347 transfusions of human blood had been recorded.

The modern era of blood transfusions began in 1900 when Landsteiner described the presence of iso-agglutinating and iso-agglutinable substances in human blood. In 1936 the first blood bank in the United States was organized at Cook County Hospital in Chicago by Fantus.[77] In recent years the operation of blood banks has led to an increasing use of blood transfusion. The availability and safety of the blood have made possible many operations and other treatments that otherwise would have been impossible. The easy availability of blood transfusion also has led to its use in situations in which it is not necessary, a procedure that subjects the patient to an unnecessary hazard.

Blood Groups

Blood groups are important in clinical medicine primarily because of their relationship to hemolytic transfusion reactions and hemolytic disease of the newborn. Blood group antigens, which are located on the cell membrane, also provide gene markers that are utilized in the study of human population genetics and in anthropology. Further study can be expected to identify the relationship of the different blood groups to differences in susceptibility to certain diseases such as duodenal ulcer, pernicious anemia, and carcinoma of the stomach, and the role of this relationship to natural selection. Determination of the blood groups is important also in legal questions concerning parentage. Excellent summaries of this complex and rapidly expanding field are available.[7, 126, 158, 167, 170, 187, 192, 222]

The important discovery that human erythrocytes belong to several different antigenic systems was made in 1900 by Landsteiner, who identified the ABO blood groups.[145] In their recent book, Race and Sanger listed well over 100 antigens that have been identified on the red blood cells.[186, 187] The same authors list 14 different antigenic systems that have been recognized: ABO (A_1A_2BO); MNSs; P; Rh; Lutheran; Kell; Lewis; Duffy; Kidd; Diego; Yt, I, Xg, and Dombrook. The blood group systems in which naturally occurring antibodies are most often found are ABO, MNSs, P, Lewis, and Wright.[167] The antigens, other than those that belong to these systems, which have been identified are classed as "public" (found almost universally) or "private" (limited to one or several families). Further investigation may prove that some of these really belong to already recognized systems and others are examples of new systems that are not yet established as such. The ABO and Rh systems are of particular importance in clinical medicine because they are responsible for nearly all instances of hemolytic transfusion reactions and hemolytic disease of the newborn. The other antigens may be responsible for severe instances of these disorders but they occur only rarely.

The ABO system consists of four main blood groups – A, B, AB, and O. The antigens, A and B, occur on the erythrocytes and the agglutinins, anti-A and anti-B, occur in the serum in a reciprocal fashion. Thus a person who belongs to the AB blood group will have the antigens A and B on the erythrocytes and no agglutinins in the serum. A person with group O blood has neither A nor B antigen on the red cells but has both anti-A and anti-B agglutinins in the serum. A person with group A blood has A antigen on the cells and anti-B agglutinins in the serum; a patient with group B blood has B antigen on the cells and anti-A agglutinins in the serum. It is thus possible to determine the blood group of an unknown blood by noting the reactions of the red cells to anti-A and anti-B sera.

It has been demonstrated that several subgroups of A exist. The most important are A_1 and A_2. Accordingly, subgroups A_1, A_2, A_1B and A_2B are recognized. About 80 per cent of persons in group A belong to subgroup A_1 and 20

Table 16–1. *The ABO Blood Groups*

NAME OF BLOOD GROUP	ANTIGENS IN RED CELLS (AGGLUTINOGENS)	ANTIBODIES IN SERUM (AGGLUTININS)	INCIDENCE IN WHITES (%)
O	none	anti-A and anti-B	45
A	A	anti-B	41
B	B	anti-A	10
AB	A and B	none	4

per cent belong to subgroup A_2; about 60 per cent of persons in group AB belong to subgroup A_1B and 40 per cent belong to A_2B.[165] The erythrocytes of subgroup A_1 are agglutinated more strongly by anti-A sera than are cells of subtype A_2. For this reason cells containing the A_2 antigen may be missed unless anti-A serum that is known to produce a strong reaction with A_2 cells is used when the blood group is determined.

About 85 per cent of persons who possess the A or B substance in their tissues secrete the substance in the saliva, urine, tears, semen, gastric juice, and milk.[58] Such persons are termed "secretors"; those who do not possess this faculty are termed "non-secretors." The ability to secrete the group specific substance is inherited as a Mendelian dominant character.[58, 165]

The MNS blood system was discovered by Landsteiner and Levine in 1927.[146] These blood group factors, which are found in the blood of every person, occur independently of factors of the ABO blood groups. The MNS system is of little importance in clinical medicine because it is very rarely associated with hemolytic transfusion reactions or hemolytic disease of the newborn. These reactions are almost non-existent because agglutinins for the MNS agglutinogens are rarely found, either as so-called "natural antibodies" or as a response to the injection of blood of a different type.

Antibodies to erythrocytes are usually either γG (IgG) or γM (IgM) immunoglobulins. Antigens representing the phenotypes of all of the systems noted above are present in very large numbers on the red cell. The number of any one of these antigens varies from as few as 25,000 per red cell in the case of the Rh (D) system to as many as 1,000,000 per red cell for the ABO system.

Red cells repel one another, since they are negatively charged, and in order for agglutination to occur this charge must be overcome or reduced. γM (IgM) antibodies are large, and as few as 10 antibodies per red cell can easily bridge the "charge gap" between cells and cause visible agglutination. γG (IgG) antibodies are smaller and do not bridge the "charge gap" unless there are several thousand antibodies per cell. The heavy coat of γG antibodies mitigates the inherent negative charge of the cells, allowing them to move closer together. Agglutination therefore requires several thousand more γG antibodies than γM antibodies. If there are relatively few antigens on the red cell, direct agglutination does not occur no matter how high a concentration of γG antibody is introduced, since there will be an insufficient coating of antigen-antibody complexes to change the charge of the cell. The presence of small numbers of γG antigen-antibody complexes can be detected if the "charge gap" can be overcome. This may be accomplished in several ways. The charge itself may be dispersed by lowering the ionic strength of the supporting medium or may be reduced by enzymatic removal of the neuraminic acid residues responsible for the negative charge. High-speed centrifugation may be used to physically overcome the "charge gap" and force the cells into close proximity. The "charge gap" may be bridged by adding an intermediate antibody attachment, as in the Coomb's test, which uses a rabbit anti-human γG to agglutinate γG coated cells.[167]

Specific isoimmune antibodies which occur in human serum may be of the "immune antibody" or "natural antibody" type. Immune antibodies arise as the result of transfusions from a blood donor or, in the case of a pregnant female, from a fetus. Natural antibodies may be present in the serum of an individual with no history of transfusion, pregnancy, or other specific opportunities for immunization. The natural antibodies are assumed to form in response to "accidental" immunization by cross-reacting antigens from the environment. A and B antigens, for example, are ubiquitous in nature. Since they are present in dust and many foods, virtually all individuals lacking one of these antigens will have formed an antibody to it by the end of the first year of life. Antibodies of a single specificity may occur as a mixture of γM and γG immunoglobulins or as either type alone. Generally, natural antibodies are of the γM type and immune antibodies are of the γG type, but there are numerous exceptions. An extensive discussion of this subject may be found in the recent book by Mollison.[167]

The Rh factor was discovered by Landsteiner and Wiener in 1940.[147] They observed that serum from rabbits that had been injected with erythrocytes of the rhesus monkey caused agglutination of the red cells from about 85 per cent of human beings without relation to their other blood groups. The new system was termed the Rh system. The rapid discovery of several different antigens in this system and the introduction of different terminologies for the antigens have led to some confusion. The equivalent gene symbols used by Wiener[222] and by Fisher and Race[187] and the approximate incidence of each are shown in Table 16–2 prepared by Dr. O. B. Bobbitt. According to the Fisher-Race concept, there are three sets of closely linked allelic genes, C and c, D and d, E and e; every person inherits one gene from each pair, a total of three genes from each parent. Everyone has paired chromosomes of eight possible types that result from different combinations of the genes. According to the Fisher-Race nomenclature these are designated as follows: cde; Cde; cdE; CdE; cDe; CDe; cDE; CDE. The corresponding symbols according to the Wiener nomenclature are r, r', r", r^y, R^0, R^1, R^2, R^z. Wiener feels that these antigens are controlled by a single gene.[222]

The importance of the Rh system in clinical medicine, particularly in

Table 16–2. The Rh Blood Types

Symbol	Genotypes (Synonyms)		Approx. Incidence (%)	
	Wiener	*English*	*White*	*Black*
	R^{1}R^0	CDe/cDe	34	23
	R^{1}r	CDe/cde		
	R^{1}R^1	CDe/CDe	18	4
	R^{2}R^0	cDE/cDe	12	12
	R^{2}r	cDE/cde		
Rh$_0$(D)	R^{1}R^2	CDe/cDE	13	3
Positive	R^{0}R^0	cDe/cDe	2	48
	R^{0}r	cDe/cde		
	R^{2}R^2	cDE/cDE	2	2
	Others		< 2	< 2
	Total Rh$_0$(D) pos.		83	93
	rr	cde/cde	16	6
Rh$_0$(D)	r'r	Cde/cde	< 2	< 2
Negative	r"r	cdE/cde		
	Total Rh$_0$(D) neg.		17	7

erythroblastosis fetalis, was first demonstrated by Levine and Stetson.[151] The natural occurrence of iso-antibody for the Rh factor is exceedingly rare. However, the introduction of erythrocytes from an Rh-positive person into an Rh-negative person may stimulate the production of the corresponding antibodies. Although there are as many different Rh antibodies as there are Rh antigens, the D (Rh_0) antigen is by far the most potent and thus the most important in clinical medicine. Persons who have the D (Rh_0) antigen are referred to as "Rh-positive," and those who lack the D (Rh_0) antigen are referred to as "Rh-negative." About 83 per cent of American whites and 93 per cent of American blacks are Rh-positive. Immunization may result from the introduction of the D (Rh_0) antigen by the transfusion of Rh-positive blood into an Rh-negative recipient or by the passage of erythrocytes from an Rh-positive fetus into the circulation of an Rh-negative mother. When Rh-positive blood is transfused into the Rh-negative recipients, about 50 to 75 per cent of the recipients become immunized, but only about 5 per cent of Rh-negative mothers are immunized by pregnancies.[165]

The isoimmunization of an Rh-negative mother by her Rh-positive fetus can now be prevented.[59, 87] Since most fetal cells gain access to the maternal circulation at the time of delivery, there is time to determine the infant's blood type and to intervene to prevent isoimmunization if necessary. If the infant is Rh-positive, concentrated gamma globulin obtained from persons hyperimmune to the D antigen is injected into the mother; the Rh immunoglobulin must be administered intramuscularly since intravenous administration of gamma globulin is unsafe. A rapid removal of fetal Rh-positive cells is effected by the Rh-immunoglobulin. The precise mechanism by which passive antibody is able to effect specific immunosuppression on the active immunity that follows injection of an antigen is not completely understood, but is believed to relate to the "walling off" of the antigen by circulating antibody so that it either fails to reach immunologically competent cells at all or reaches them only in an inactive state.[202]

Survival of Blood Components

When fresh, normal erythrocytes are transferred into a compatible recipient, the donated cells have a half-life of 60 days. When blood is stored in ACD mixture at 4° C and then transfused, a portion of the cells leave the circulation within the first 24 hours but the remainder survive fairly well. After 14 days of storage, 90 per cent of the cells survive for more than 24 hours and the survival time of these cells is almost normal; after storage for 28 days only 70 per cent of the cells survive for 24 hours and all have disappeared by 80 days.[167] Transfused leukocytes have a short survival time in the recipient, probably no more than 30 to 90 minutes, even when fresh blood is infused. The use of leukocyte transfusions is still experimental.[169] Platelets taken in a glass container and stored with ACD mixture at 4° C rapidly lose their viability; after 24 hours their survival time in the recipient is negligible. In order to preserve platelets for transfusion, careful attention must be paid to adequate mixing of anticoagulant with the blood as it is being drawn. Venipuncture must be clean and there must be no admixture of tissue juices which would stimulate clotting in the extrinsic system. When platelets are transfused, whole blood is usually collected in plastic bags, although there is a difference of opinion regarding the effect that contact with glass has on the platelets. It appears that the most important factor in platelet survival is the freshness of the blood that is transfused. Platelets have been found to survive better at room temperature than at 4° C. They should be prepared, left uncooled, and infused within 6 hours of their drawing.[149]

Indications for Blood Transfusions

Whole blood is a mixture of erythrocytes, leukocytes, and platelets suspended in plasma. Plasma is largely water, but it contains important electrolytes and proteins. The techniques available in modern blood banks now allow the physician to administer to his patient whole blood or some component of whole blood. The physician must assess the requirements of each patient individually and use only those components indicated. If the growing needs for blood and blood products are to be met, the best possible use must be made of each donated unit of blood.

To increase oxygen-carrying capacity of blood and expand volume. Whole blood transfusion is used when the oxygen-carrying capacity of the blood and the circulating blood volume must be restored simultaneously. It is indicated in the treatment of acute severe hemorrhage and the criteria for adequate transfusion rest primarily on the evaluation of the clinical condition of the patient, though measurement of blood volume and hematocrit may be of assistance. Seldom, if ever, is complete replacement of the lost blood necessary.[52]

To increase oxygen-carrying capacity of blood with little or no volume expansion. Packed red cells should be administered to those patients who require an increase in the oxygen-carrying capacity of their blood to prevent acute hypoxia or invalidism but who are not in need of increased blood volume. Transfusion is probably advisable for patients with severe chronic anemia if the hemoglobin level is less than 6.0 gm. per cent.[167] The use of packed red cells in transfusing patients of this type, and also those with cardiac disease, allows an increase in oxygen-carrying capacity of the blood with as small an increment in blood volume as possible. In patients with heart disease, 250 ml. of packed cells should be administered slowly over a period of about 4 hours and the patient should be watched carefully for any evidence of heart failure. The transfusion can be repeated in 24 hours if indicated, as long as no untoward event has occurred. However, many patients with chronic anemia who require blood transfusions can be given 500 ml. of packed cells in one day.

Packed red cells which have been prepared by sedimentation or centrifugation have a post-transfusion survival equivalent to those in whole blood, provided that the container is not entered during preparation. The reduction in the amount of plasma transfused with the packed cells is believed to account for the reported reduction in the incidence of hepatitis transmitted by packed red cells.[137]

To expand circulatory volume without an increase in oxygen-carrying capacity. Blood plasma has been used for many years to expand the circulatory volume. The increasing evidence of hepatitis transmission and the availability of products such as dextran and albumin have served to reduce its use for this purpose. Fresh frozen plasma and stored plasma are both useful sources of certain blood clotting factors.

Plasma protein fraction U.S.P. is a by-product of the commercial preparation of fibrinogen and gamma globulin. It contains 5 gm. per cent protein, nearly all of which is albumin, and has been useful as a plasma expander. The material is held at 60° C for 10 hours to inactivate the hepatitis virus. It is not a source of clotting factors.

Human serum albumin is fractionated from blood plasma. Its administration carries a low risk of hepatitis. It contains no blood group antibody and it fares well on storage. Serum albumin is available as a 5 per cent or 25 per cent solution. The 5 per cent solution is iso-osmotic and can be used to expand the blood volume; the 25 per cent solution is often used to treat hypoproteinemia with little risk of circulatory overload but will result in expansion of the blood volume in patients who are not dehydrated.

To provide platelets or needed components of plasma.   Plasma and fractions of plasma have long been used in the treatment of blood coagulation defects.[4] The effective treatment of deficiencies of specific coagulation factors has been difficult because their low concentration in normal plasma makes circulatory overload a constant threat; their short survival time in vivo, the necessity for repeated transfusions, and the short survival of some coagulation factors during storage make fresh preparation a necessity.

Fibrinogen was one of the first materials to become available in relatively pure form. It is prepared as a dry powder in an ampule and must be carefully mixed with distilled water before infusion; too much agitation may cause denaturation of the protein and loss of biologic activity. The administration of fibrinogen is accompanied by a high risk of hepatitis and many recommend that patients receiving it be given gamma globulin prophylactically.[180]

For many years, fresh frozen plasma or fresh plasma was the only source of the labile blood clotting factors V and VIII. A number of techniques for the concentration of Factor VIII have now been developed,[21, 48, 159, 189] but the most significant improvement has been the development of cryoprecipitation by Pool.[55, 183] The technique is simple and inexpensive and can be carried out in any well-equipped blood bank. The material prepared is an excellent source of Factor VIII, concentrated 10 to 15 times, and contains Factor V, Factor I, Factor XIII, and the bleeding-time factor and Factor VIII–stimulating factor missing in von Willebrand's disease,[9, 19, 27, 162, 177, 183, 184] but the risk of hepatitis transmission remains.

While Factor IX is relatively stable on storage, treatment of patients with Factor IX deficiency has posed problems similar to those encountered in the treatment of Factor VIII deficiency. Recently, potent, highly stable concentrates have been prepared which contain Factors II, VII, IX, and X.[26, 93, 112, 203, 212] The activity of these factors in 10 ml. of the concentrate is equivalent to that found in 250 ml. of normal plasma.[203] This development represents a great advance in the treatment of patients with single or multiple deficiencies of these factors that cannot be managed with whole plasma. The risk of hepatitis is apparently reduced but not eliminated.[93, 203]

The relatively long biologic half-life and low levels required for hemostasis make it possible to treat Factor XI deficiency with whole plasma. Although Factor XI is relatively stable on storage, fresh or fresh frozen plasma is generally used.[185]

Platelets. The use of platelet transfusions has grown in recent years because of the more vigorous treatment of leukemia and generalized neoplasia. Platelet transfusions continue to be of great importance in the treatment of bone marrow failure with thrombocytopenia, particularly in patients with significant bleeding, in the treatment of thrombocytopenia. They have been of particular importance in the treatment of neonatal thrombocytopenia and thrombocytopenia secondary to drugs, radiation, or infection. The recent use of intensive cancer chemotherapy would not have been possible without the availability of platelet transfusions.[63]

Platelets may be given in fresh whole blood to those patients who need red cells and plasma as well; if red cells are not needed, platelet-rich plasma may be prepared by proper centrifugation. Platelet concentrates are the best means of delivering platelets without the attendant risk of circulatory overload. With proper acidification and centrifugation of the platelet-rich plasma, a platelet concentrate with a yield equal to that of the original plasma can be prepared which can be administered in 20 to 30 ml. of plasma.[118] Recent advances in platelet typing may make possible the proper matching and better survival of platelets in the future.[3]

Complications of Blood Transfusions

Blood transfusions have been given for reasons that appear questionable at best. Among these are its use as a "tonic," as an aid to convalescence from some infection, or as a routine preoperative or postoperative measure. Transfusion in these circumstances is of doubtful value and every transfusion is potentially dangerous.[50, 51]

Even under the best circumstances blood transfusion is associated with some risk; for this reason the procedure should be employed only when the danger of withholding the transfusion exceeds the risk of complications from the transfusion. The complications that can follow blood transfusions are hemolytic, febrile, and allergic reactions, and the transmission of disease. The incidence and severity of the various types of reactions are difficult to state with exactness and probably vary from one institution to another. The mortality rate has been quoted as being 0.16 per 1000 in 1949[58] and in 1960 was estimated to be as low as one in 250,000 or 350,000 transfusions.[125] In the University of Virginia Hospital between 1955 and 1958 there was one fatal reaction in 25,465 transfusions, an incidence of about 0.04 per thousand. In the period 1958 to 1964 there were three fatal reactions in 59,441 transfusions, an incidence of about 0.05 per thousand. Three of these four deaths followed hemolytic reactions that were caused by clerical errors made by peronnel in or out of the blood bank; the other fatality was the result of serum hepatitis.

HEMOLYTIC TRANSFUSION REACTIONS

One of the most serious complications of transfusions is the occurrence of intravascular hemolysis that results from the administration of incompatible blood. Although any antigen-antibody may be involved in these reactions, those involved in the ABO, Rh, and Kell systems are of greatest significance clinically.[226] In the most severe reactions, the antigen is on the donor's red cell and the antibody is in the recipient's plasma; usually less severe reactions occur when an antibody in the donor's plasma reacts with an antigen on the recipient's red cells or on other donor red cells transfused to the patient. Reactions of this type are usually manifested by burning along the course of the vein being used for infusion, flushing of the face, pain in the lumbar region, a sense of constriction in the chest, chills, hemoglobinemia, and hemoglobinuria, but serious hemolytic reactions can present with nothing more than urticaria or low-grade fever, especially if the patient is under an anesthetic. Any unusual reaction in a patient receiving a transfusion must be considered a hemolytic reaction, and treated accordingly, until it is proven otherwise.

Symptoms of this type do not occur if a similar amount of hemolyzed compatible blood is injected, and for this reason it is assumed that the symptoms are caused by some substance that is released by the combination of antigen and antibody.[167] Following acute intravascular hemolysis, free hemoglobin is released and bound by serum haptoglobin. The hemoglobin-haptoglobin complex is cleared by the reticuloendothelial system. If the amount of hemoglobin released exceeds the capacity of the plasma haptoglobin, free hemoglobin will appear in the plasma. As an early step in the catabolism of hemoglobin, the iron-porphyrin compound heme is cleaved from globin. Methemalbumin may be formed by the binding of albumin to hematin and can be observed from 5 to 24 hours after the hemolytic episode.[74]

Hemoglobin appears in the urine after the reabsorption capacity of the proximal renal tubules is exceeded. Some of the hemoglobin reabsorbed by the renal tubules is deposited as hemosiderin. As these renal tubular cells are sloughed for the next several days, they can be identified in a centrifuged specimen of urine. The finding of hemosiderin is proof that intravascular hemolysis has taken place. The appearance of jaundice is generally delayed for more than 12 hours. A significant increase in the serum bilirubin level within 24 hours after the transfusion is good evidence of a rapid (1 to 2 hours) release of a large amount of hemoglobin, whereas a rise of 1 mg. in the bilirubin level within 4 to 6 hours can be considered to be within the range usually seen after the administration of 500 ml. of blood.

Some patients develop renal failure following a hemolytic transfusion reaction. The precise mechanism responsible for this serious turn of events is not known, but it is believed to be related to the occurrence of shock at the time of hemolysis and perhaps the release of some toxic substance by the antigen-antibody reaction.

Intravascular hemolysis may also result in diffuse intravascular coagulation, with excessive utilization of blood clotting factors, and secondary fibrinolysis. This condition, known as the defibrination syndrome, may first be manifested by abnormal bleeding and requires immediate treatment.[141, 226]

Management of hemolytic transfusion reaction. When a hemolytic transfusion reaction is suspected, the blood transfusion should be stopped immediately. The seriousness of the reaction is often directly related to the amount of incompatible blood administered. Serious renal damage is infrequent in adults if less than 200 ml. of incompatible blood is given.[58]

Osmotic diuresis should be initiated with mannitol.[12] An intravenous infusion of 10 per cent mannitol at a rate titrated to give a urine output of 100 ml. per hour has proved effective. One thousand ml. mannitol infusions may be alternated with 1000 ml. Ringer's lactate or 5 per cent glucose and water. Diuresis should be maintained until free hemoglobin is no longer visible in the patient's plasma. Vasopressor drugs should not be given, as they have not proved effective and may produce further vasoconstriction in the kidneys.

If the patient does not respond and urine output decreases, excessive fluid administration must be avoided. Fluids are restricted to 500 ml. plus visible output in a 24-hour period. One hundred gm. of carbohydrate should be given at a constant rate to avoid hypoglycemia and to decrease catabolism.[12] The serum electrolytes must be followed closely, and if marked derangement occurs despite the use of ion exchange resins, particularly in the potassium level, dialysis should be performed. Measures such as renal decapsulation, spinal anesthesia, intravenous procaine hydrochloride, and alkalinization are probably of no value.[158]

Mollison has listed indications for hemodialysis as follows: (1) blood urea more than 400 mg. per 100 ml., (2) plasma bicarbonate less than 12 mEq. per liter, (3) plasma potassium more than 7.5 mEq. per liter, (4) electrocardiographic evidence of intraventricular block, widening of QRS complexes from hyperkalemia, (5) uremic stupor, vomiting, cough, or fits.[167] Indications for dialysis vary somewhat from hospital to hospital. At the University of Virginia Hospital in general the same guides are followed but usually dialysis is performed if the blood urea level is 300 mg. per 100 ml.; a potassium level of 6.5 mEq. per liter despite the use of ion exchange resins is considered another indication. Also an effort is made to perform dialysis before the clinical features of the uremic syndrome become prominent.

An important part of the management of a hemolytic transfusion reaction is the effort to determine the cause of hemolysis. Investigation of the reaction is facilitated if a sample of blood is drawn from each patient immediately before transfusion and a few ml. of blood from each transfusion bottle is saved for several days. The following procedures are followed at the University of Virginia Hospital:

1. The patient and bottle are checked for clerical error, and the bottle is returned to the blood bank for retyping and bacteriologic investigation (stain of uncentrifuged plasma for bacteria and culture of specimen).

2. Typing and cross-matching are repeated using the patient's pre-transfusion blood.

3. A direct antiglobulin (Coombs) test is performed on the patient's post-transfusion blood.

4. An immediate check of patient's plasma for free hemoglobin is made; 1 hour and 24 hour post-transfusion urine specimens are examined for hemoglobin and determinations of bilirubin are made on 6 hour and 24 hour sera.

5. Specimens of blood from the donor and recipient are held for 6 days

after transfusion; the patient can be tested for immune response (i.e., high titers of anti-A or anti-B or for other acquired antibody).

Febrile reactions. Febrile reactions, which are reported to have an incidence of 18 per 1000 transfusions,[58] may develop from pyrogens, or from the lysis of erythrocytes or leukocytes. Pyrogens, which are bacterial polysaccharides, are contaminants introduced in the chemical substances used in the preparation of the solutions or the apparatus. The use of disposable transfusion sets has greatly reduced the incidence of this type of reaction. A febrile reaction usually accompanies a severe hemolytic reaction and may occur after hemolysis of mild degree. Since a febrile reaction may herald the onset of a hemolytic reaction, the transfusion must be stopped and an investigation undertaken. A frequent cause of febrile reactions in patients who receive repeated transfusions over a long period is the destruction of transfused leukocytes.[28] The reactions, which may be severe, usually occur only after the patient has received seven or more transfusions. Patients who have repeated febrile reactions to transfusions should be studied for this type of reaction. Such reactions usually can be prevented if the buffy coat is removed by centrifugation. After a febrile reaction has occurred aspirin, 1.0 gm., is usually effective treatment.

Allergic reactions. Allergic reactions, such as urticaria, asthma, or facial edema, occur as the result of abnormal reactions on the part of the patient. An incidence of about 8 per 1000 transfusions has been reported.[58] The transfusion is stopped as soon as the reaction occurs, as it may become more severe or may be a sign of an impending hemolytic reaction. The patient should be given an antihistamine drug intramuscularly. In patients who have frequent allergic reactions administration of an antihistaminic drug 1 hour before the transfusion usually suppresses the reaction. It is poor practice to add antihistamine drugs to the blood to be transfused.

INFECTION

Syphilis. Syphilis is transmitted only rarely by blood which has been stored. The use of the blood bank has probably been the greatest single factor in the reduction of the transmission of this disease by transfusion. Storage of blood at 4° to 6° C for 4 to 5 days is usually sufficient to render it noninfectious. The chance of transmission of the disease by fresh blood and fresh blood products remains.[118]

Malaria. The possibility of the accidental transmission of malaria by the transfusion of fresh or stored blood has long been recognized. Storage of blood at 4 to 6° C for days or even weeks fails to destroy the malarial parasite. Most of the reported cases have been due to *P. malariae* and *P. vivax* but a few cases caused by *P. falciparum* have been recorded. In each instance, the donors of the blood had been residents for a period of time in malarious areas. Some had lived outside of these areas for as long as 20 years without symptoms of the disease, and in many no parasites could be detected in their blood.[20, 102]

The return of many servicemen from malarious areas and the increase in worldwide civilian travel will make prevention of transfusion malaria more difficult. All persons who have traveled or lived in malarious areas must be considered potential carriers.[102] Of importance is the fact that malaria has been transmitted by fresh plasma, which usually contains some red cells.[60]

The incubation period of transfusion malaria has been reported to vary between 5 and 74 days.[213] Malarial infection should be considered a possibility if fever of uncertain origin occurs following transfusion.[176]

Viral hepatitis. Probably the greatest single problem of blood transfusion at the present time is the transmission of viral hepatitis. Viral hepatitis may occur as the result of infection with the virus of infectious hepatitis, which has an incubation period of 15 to 50 days, or the virus of serum hepatitis, which has an incubation period of 50 to 160 days. The virus of infectious hepatitis may be transmitted by the fecal-oral route or by injection, whereas that of serum hepatitis is transmitted only by injection. The incidence of carriers has been placed at 1 in 200 and the incidence of serum jaundice at 0.5 per cent in patients who receive two bottles of blood.[167] The frequency of serum hepatitis may vary in different localities and from one blood bank to another. The incidence in the United States has been reported as 0.7 per 1000 units of blood,[142] and as high as 3 per cent of transfused patients who averaged 3.4 units each.[6] A recent study using sensitive enzyme determinations to detect non-icteric hepatitis revealed an incidence of 8.76 per 100 units transfused.[105] The incidence of hepatitis rises with the number of transfusions given and the death rate from hepatitis increases dramatically in the older age groups.[101] In one study, all deaths occurred in patients over 35 years of age.[6]

The prevention of viral hepatitis remains a problem. Careful screening of donors for a past history of hepatitis is essential; liver function tests are unsatisfactory because they will not detect all carriers of the virus. The discovery of an antigenic lipoprotein associated with virus-like particles in the serum of some patients with hepatitis and some carriers of the infection offers hope for the development of a laboratory screening test capable of eliminating carriers from blood bank donor lists.[198] The virus-like particles in the serum samples of patients with hepatitis appear to be identical with the Australia, SH, or hepatitis-associated antigen.[11] They have been shown to persist for long periods in the serum of patients following clinical or subclinical infection and appear to be capable of transmitting disease in concentrations too low to be detected by current methods.[11] The limited sensitivity of current methods precludes detection of the agent in all infectious material, but it is possible to detect high levels, which might serve to reduce the incidence of the disease.[11, 198]

One study indicated that the administration of 10 ml. of gamma globulin within 1 week after transfusion and again 1 month later prevents three-fourths of the expected icteric post-transfusion hepatitis but did not change the incidence of non-icteric hepatitis.[166] Minor variations in this regimen have not shown the same results,[113, 156] and more experience is needed.

Bacterial infection. Transmission of bacterial infection by transfusion is seldom seen at present. However, certain saprophytic bacteria may enter the blood to be transfused. The gram-positive organisms, such as diphtheroids, have produced only fever with no serious constitutional symptoms. The gram-negative organisms have been responsible for a type of overwhelming shock that is almost invariably fatal. The syndrome is characterized by chills, fever, hypotension, severe pain in the abdomen and extremities, dryness and flushing of the skin. Symptoms usually occur within 30 minutes of the start of the transfusion and may follow the administration of but 50 ml. of blood. Treatment with broad spectrum antibiotics, vasopressors, and massive doses of steroids must begin as soon as the syndrome is recognized. The outlook for these patients is poor.[25] Scrupulous care must be taken in collection, storage, and administration of blood and blood products in order that they may not become contaminated.[118]

OTHER PROBLEMS

Pulmonary edema may occur as the result of circulatory overload. Tourniquets should be applied at the upper portion of the four extremities without delay and should be rotated in such a manner that none remains in place longer than 15 minutes. Phlebotomy with the removal of 500 ml. of blood is advisable and the administration of morphine may be desirable. Even if the patient responds well to these measures he should be observed carefully and any other treatment necessary should be given. Pulmonary edema, which is most likely to occur in elderly patients with severe chronic anemia and in those with heart disease, can be avoided if the patient is transfused slowly with packed red cells. Whole blood is to be avoided.

When a large number of units of stored blood are given, citrate and potassium toxicity are potential hazards. Citrate toxicity results in a depression of ionization of the divalent cations, such as Ca^{++}. The excitable tissues of the body are susceptible to such depression, the effect on the cardiac muscle being most important. Hypothermia or liver disease may augment the problems by slowing the metabolism of citrate. Citrate toxicity may be treated by the administration of appropriate solutions of calcium chloride or calcium gluconate intravenously.[154, 226]

Since the plasma potassium gradually increases on storage as the result of the breakdown of red cells, the transfusion of stored blood may result in an acute rise in serum potassium in the recipient. This is particularly hazardous to patients already hyperkalemic and can be avoided by the administration of fresh blood to such patients.[226]

Massive transfusions of blood may result in the development of thrombocytopenia. The thrombocytopenia is probably a dilution effect that is the result of using large quantities of blood that contain no viable platelets.[120] The administration of 500 ml. of fresh blood, not more than 3 to 4 hours old, for each three or four units of bank blood may prevent this complication.[226]

References

1. Abrams, R.: Effect of x-rays on nucleic acid and protein synthesis. Arch. Biochem., *30*:90, 1951.
2. Adamson, R. H., and Fabro, S.: Anti-tumor activity and other biologic properties of l-asparaginase (NSC-109229)—a review. Cancer Chemother. Rep., *52*:617, 1968.
3. Adner, M. M., Fisch, G. R., Starobin, S. G., and Aster, R. N.: Use of "compatible" platelet transfusions in treatment of congenital isoimmune thrombocytopenic purpura. New England J. Med., *280*:244, 1969.
4. Aggler, P. M.: Physiological basis for transfusion therapy in hemorrhagic disorders: a critical review. Transfusion, *1*:71, 1961.

5. Alexander, P., and Stacey, K. A.: Comparison of the changes produced by ionizing radiations and by the alkylating agents: evidence for a similar mechanism at the molecular level. Ann. N.Y. Acad. Sci., *68*:1225, 1958.

6. Allen, J. G., and Sayman, W. A.: Serum hepatitis from transfusions of blood: epidemiologic study. J.A.M.A., *180*:1079, 1962.

7. Andresen, P. H.: The Human Blood Groups. Charles C Thomas, Springfield, Ill., 1952.

8. Asparaginase. Brit. Med. J., *2*:465, 1969.

9. Amris, C. J., and Hilden, M.: Treatment of factor XIII deficiency with cryoprecipitate. Thromb. et Diath. Haemorrh., *20*:528, 1968.

10. Azathioprine. Brit. Med. J., *2*:1378, 1966.

11. Barker, L. F., Shulman, N. R., Murray, R., Hirschman, R. J., Ratner, F., Diefenbach, W. C. L., and Geller, H. M.: Transmission of serum hepatitis. J.A.M.A., *211*:1509, 1970.

12. Barry, K. G., and Crosby, W. H.: The prevention and treatment of renal failure following transfusion reactions. Transfusion, *3*:34, 1963.

13. Bell, E. G., McAfee, J. G., and Constable, W. C.: Local radiation damage to bone and marrow demonstrated by radioisotopic imaging. Radiology, *92*:1083, 1969.

14. Bennett, D. E., Million, R. R., and Ackerman, L. V.: Bilateral radiation pneumonitis—a complication of the radiotherapy of bronchogenic carcinoma. Cancer, *23*:1001, 1969.

15. Bernard, J.: Acute leukemia treatment. Cancer Res., *27*:2565, 1967.

16. Bernard, J., and Seligmann, M.: A study of 61 leukemias treated with 6-mercaptopurine. Ann. N.Y. Acad. Sci., *60*:385, 1954.

17. Bethell, F. H.: The relative frequency of the several types of chronic leukemia and their management. J. Chronic Dis., *6*:403, 1957.

18. Bethell, F. H., et al.: Phase II. Evaluation of cyclophosphamide. Cancer Chemother. Rep., *8*:113, 1960.

19. Biggs, R.: Fractions rich in factor VIII. Biblio. Haematol., *29*:1122, 1968.

20. Black, R. H.: Investigation of blood donors in accidental transfusion of malaria-*Plasmodium vivax, falciparum* and *malariae* infections. Med. J. Aust., *2*:446, 1960.

21. Bloom, A. L., and Emmanuel, J. H.: Use of cryoprecipitate antihaemophilic factor for the treatment of haemophilia. Quart. J. Med., *37*:(N.S.)291, 1968.

22. Bodey, G. P., Freireich, E. J., Monto, R. W., and Hewlett, J. S.: Cytosine arabinoside (NSC-63878) therapy for acute leukemia in adults. Cancer Chemother. Rep., *53*:59, 1969.

23. Bonadonna, G., and Monfardini, S.: Cardiac toxicity of daunorubicin. Lancet, *1*:837, 1969.

24. Bouroncle, B. A., and Doan, C. A.: Refractory idiopathic thrombocytopenic purpura treated with azathioprine. New England J. Med., *275*:630, 1966.

25. Braude, A. I.: Transfusion reactions from contaminated blood. New England J. Med., *258*:1289, 1958.

26. Breen, F. A., and Tullis, J. L.: Prothrombin concentrates in treatment of Christmas disease and allied disorders. J.A.M.A., *208*:1848, 1969.

27. Brinkhous, K. M., Shanbrom, E., Roberts, H. R., Webster, W. P., Fekete, L., and Wagner, R. H.: A new high potency glycine-precipitated antihemophilic factor (AHF) concentrate. J.A.M.A., *205*:613, 1968.

28. Brittingham, T. E., and Chaplin, H., Jr.: Febrile transfusion reactions caused by sensitivity to donor leukocytes and platelets. J.A.M.A., *165*:819, 1957.

29. Brook, J., Bateman, J. R., and Steinfeld, J. L.: Evaluation of melphalan (NSC-8806) in treatment of multiple myeloma. Cancer Chemother. Rep., *36*:25, 1964.

30. Broome, J. D.: Evidence that the l-asparaginase activity of guinea pig serum is responsible for its anti-lymphoma effects. Nature, *191*:1114, 1961.

31. Bross, I. D. J.: Statistical analysis of clinical results from 6-mercaptopurine. Ann. N.Y. Acad. Sci., *60*:369, 1954.

32. Brown, G. B.: The biosynthesis of nucleic acids as a basis for an approach to chemotherapy. Ann. N.Y. Acad. Sci., *60*:185, 1954.

33. Brown, G. B., Roll, P. M., Plentl, A. A., and Cavalieri, L. F.: The utilization of adenine for nucleic acid synthesis and as a precursor of guanine. J. Biol. Chem., *172*:469, 1948.

34. Brubaker, C. A., Gilchrist, G. S., Hammond, D., Hyman, C. B., Shore, N. A., and Williams, K. O.: Induction of remission in acute leukemia with prednisone and intravenous methotrexate. J. Ped., *73*:623, 1968.

35. Burchenal, J. H.: Clinical effects of analogs of folic acid, purines, pyridines and amino acids. Fed. Proc., *13*:760, 1954.

36. Burchenal, J. H., et al.: 6-Mercaptopurine in the treatment of leukemia and allied diseases. Blood, *8*:965, 1953.

37. Burchenal, J. H., et al.: Clinical evaluation of 6-mercaptopurine in the treatment of leukemia. Am. J. Med. Sci., *228*:371, 1954.

38. Burningham, R. A., Restrepo, A., Pugh, R. P., Brown, E. B., Schlossman, S. F., Khuri, P. D., Lessner, H. E., and Harrington, W. J.: Weekly high-dosage glucocorticosteroid treatment of lymphocytic leukemias and lymphomas. New England J. Med., *270*:1160, 1964.

39. Canellos, G. P., Haskell, C. M., Arsenlau, J., and Carbone, P. P.: Hypoalbuminemic and hypocholesterolemic effect of l-asparaginase (NSC-109229) treatment in man—a preliminary report. Cancer Chemother. Rep., *53*:67, 1969.

40. Casey, T. P.: The development of lymphomas in mice with autoimmune disorders treated with azathioprine. Blood, *31*:396, 1968.

41. Chu, M. Y., and Fischer, G. A.: A proposed mechanism of action of l-β-D-arabinofuranosyl-cytosine as an inhibitor of the growth of leukemic cells. Biochem. Pharmacol., *11*:423, 1962.

42. Clarkson, B., Krakoff, I., Burchenal, J., Karnofsky, D., Golbey, R., Dowling, M., Oettgen, H., and Lipton, A.: Clinical results of treatment with *E. coli* l-asparaginase in adults with leukemia, lymphoma and solid tumors. Cancer, *25*:279, 1970.

43. Clifford, P., Clift, R. A., and Gillmore, J. H.: Oral melphalan therapy in advanced malignant disease. Brit. J. Cancer, *17*:381, 1963.

44. Coggins, P. R., Ravdin, R. G., and Eisman, S. H.: Clinical evaluation of a new alkylating agent —Cytoxan (cyclophosphamide). Cancer, *13*:1254, 1960.

45. Cohn, K. E., Stewart, J. R., Fajardo, L. F., and Hancock, E. W.: Heart disease following radiation. Medicine, *46*:281, 1967.

46. Committee of the Joint Blood Council and American Association of Blood Banks: Standards for a Blood Transfusion Service. Joint Blood Council, Washington, D.C., and American Association of Blood Banks, Chicago, Ill., 1958.

46a. Committee on Transfusion and Transplantation (American Medical Association): General Principles of Blood Transfusion. American Medical Association, Chicago, Ill., 1970.

47. Conger, J. D., Castell, D. O., and Jacoby, W. J.: Hodgkin's disease of the jejunum. Perforation during radiation therapy. Arch. Intern. Med., *121*:174, 1968.

48. Cooke, J. V., Holland, P. V., and Shulman, N. R.: Cryoprecipitate concentrates of factor VIII for surgery in hemophiliacs. Ann. Int. Med., *68*:39, 1968.

49. Coy, P., Baber, S., and Dolman, C. L.: Progressive myelopathy due to radiation. Canad. Med. Assoc. J., *100*:1129, 1969.

50. Crosby, W. H.: Misuse of blood transfusion. Blood, *13*:1198, 1958.

51. Crosby, W. H.: The single unit transfusion. Transfusion, *4*:329, 1964.

52. Crosby, W. H., and Howard, J. M.: The hematologic response to wounding and to resuscitation accomplished by large transfusions of stored blood. A study of battle casualties in Korea. Blood, *9*:439, 1954.

53. Cytosine arabinoside. Brit. Med. J., *4*:305, 1968.

54. Dale, W. M.: The effects of ionizing radiations on enzymes in vitro. Ciba Symposia on Ionizing Radiation and Cell Metabolism. J. A. Churchill, Ltd., London, 1956.

55. Dallman, P. R., and Pool, J. G.: Treatment of hemophilia with factor VIII concentrates. New England J. Med., *278*:199, 1968.

56. Dameshek, W., Granville, N. B., and Rubio, F., Jr.: Therapy of the myeloproliferative disorders with Myleran. Ann. N.Y. Acad. Sci., *68*:1001, 1958.

57. DeConti, R. C., and Calabresi, P.: Use of allopurinol for prevention and control of hyperuricemia in patients with neoplastic disease. New England J. Med., *274*:481, 1966.

58. DeGowin, E. L., Hardin, R. C., and Alsever, J. B.: Blood Transfusion. W. B. Saunders Co., Philadelphia, 1949.

59. Diamond, L. K.: Protection against Rh sensitization and prevention of erythroblastosis fetalis. Pediatrics, *41*:1, 1968.

60. Dike, A. E.: Two cases of transfusion malaria. Lancet, *2*:72, 1970.

61. DiMarco, A., Silverstrini, R., Gaetani, M., Soldati, M., Orezzi, P., Dasdia, T., Scarpinato, B. M., and Valentini, L.: "Daunomycin," a new antibiotic of the rhodomycin group. Nature, *201*:706, 1964.

62. DiMarco, A., Silverstrini, R., DiMarco, S., and Dasdia, T.: Inhibiting effect of new cytotoxic antibiotic daunomycin on nucleic acids and mitotic activity of HeLa cells. J. Cell Biol., *27*:545, 1965.

63. Djerassi, I.: The role of platelet administration in a blood transfusion service. Transfusion, *6*:55, 1966.

64. Doan, C. A., Wiseman, B. K., and Bouroncle, B. A.: Clinical evaluation of CB 1348 in leukemias and lymphomas. Ann. N.Y. Acad. Sci., *68*:979, 1958.

65. Dougherty, T. F.: Effect of hormones on lymphatic tissue. Physiol. Rev., *32*:379, 1952.

66. Dugdale, M., and Fort, A. T.: Busulfan treatment of leukemia during pregnancy. J.A.M.A., *199*:131, 1967.

67. Editorial: Blood banks. Virgina M. Monthly, *78*:275, 1951.

68. Elion, G. B., Singer, S., and Hitchings, G. H.: The purine metabolism of 6-mercaptopurine resistant Lactobacillus casei. J. Biol. Chem., *204*:35, 1953.

69. Elion, G. B., Callahan, S., Bieber, S., Hitchings, G. H., and Rundles, R. W.: A summary of investigations with 6-[(1-methyl-4-nitro-5-imidazolyl)thio] purine (BW 57-322). Cancer Chemother. Rep., *14*:93, 1961.

70. Ellison, R. R., and Burchenal, J. H.: Therapy of acute leukemia in adults. J. Chronic Dis., *6*:421, 1957.

71. Ellison, R. R., et al.: Arabinosylcytosine: a useful agent in the treatment of acute leukemia in adults. Blood, *32*:507, 1968.

72. Evans, A. E., Farber, S., Brunet, S., and Mariano, P. J.: Vincristine in the treatment of acute leukemia in children. Cancer, *16*:1302, 1963.

73. Evans, J. S., Musser, E. A., Mengel, G. D., Forsblad, K. R., and Hunter, J. H.: Antitumor activity of l-β-D-arabinofuranosylcytosine hydrochloride. Proc. Soc. Exp. Biol. & Med., *106*:350, 1961.

74. Fairley, N. H.: Methaemalbumin. Quart. J. Med., *10*:95, 1941.

75. Fajardo, L. F., Stewart, J. R., and Cohn, K. E.: Morphology of radiation-induced heart disease. Arch. Path., *86*:512, 1968.

76. Fallon, H. J., Frei, E., III, Block, J., and Seegmiller, J. E.: The uricosuria and orotic aciduria induced by 6-azauridine. J. Clin. Invest., *40*:1906, 1961.

77. Fantus, B.: The therapy of the Cook County Hospital: blood preservation. J.A.M.A., *109*:128, 1937.

78. Farber, S. (Ed.): Proceedings of the Second Conference on Folic Acid Antagonists in the Treatment of Leukemia. Blood (suppl.), 7:97, 1952.

79. Farber, S.: Summary of experience with 6-mercaptopurine. Ann. N.Y. Acad. Sci., *60*:412, 1954.

80. Farber, S.: The treatment of acute leukemia. J. Chronic Dis., *3*:455, 1956.

81. Farber, S., Diamond, L. K., Mercer, R. D., Sylvester, R. F., and Wolff, J. A.: Temporary remissions in acute leukemia in children produced by folic acid antagonist 4-aminopteroyl-glutamic acid (Aminopterin). New England J. Med., *238*:787, 1948.

82. Farber, S., et al.: In Mote, J. R. (Ed.): Proceedings of the First Clinical ACTH Conference. The Blakiston Co., Philadelphia, 1950, p. 328.

83. Feigelson, P., and Davidson, J. D.: The inhibition of adenosine deaminase by 8-azaguanine in vitro. J. Biol. Chem., *223*:65, 1956.

84. Fernbach, D. J.: Chemotherapy for acute leukemia in children: comparison of cyclophosphamide (NSC-2671) and 6-mercaptopurine (NSC-755). Cancer Chemother. Rep., *51*:381, 1967.

85. Fessas, P., Wintrobe, M. M., Thompson, R. B., and Cartwright, G. E.: Treatment of acute leukemia with cortisone and corticotropin. Arch. Int. Med., *94*:384, 1954.

86. Frank, J. A., and Dougherty, T. F.: Cytoplasmic budding of human lymphocytes produced by cortisone and hydrocortisone in in vitro preparations. Proc. Soc. Exper. Biol. & Med., *82*:17, 1953.

87. Freda, V. J., Gorman, J. G., Pollack, W., Robertson, J. G., Jennings, E. R., and Sullivan, J. F.: Prevention of Rh isoimmunization: progress report of the clinical trial in mothers. J.A.M.A., *199*:390, 1967.

88. Freireich, E. J., and Frei, E., III: Recent advances in acute leukemia. Progr. Hemat., *4*:187, 1964.

89. Furth, J. J., and Cohen, S. S.: Inhibition of mammalian DNA polymerase by the 5-triphosphate of 1-β-D-arabinofuranosylcytosine and the 5-triphosphate of 9-β-D-arabinofuranosyladenine. Cancer Res., *28*:2061, 1968.

90. Galton, D. A. G., Till, M., and Wiltshaw, E.: Busulfan (1,4-dimethanesulfonyloxybutane, Myleran): summary of clinical results. Ann. N.Y. Acad. Sci., *68*:967, 1958.

91. Gee, T. S., Yu, K.-P., and Clarkson, B. D.: Treatment of adult acute leukemia with arabinosylcytosine and thioguanine. Cancer, *23*:1019, 1969.

92. George, P.: Haemorrhagic cystitis and cyclophosphamide. Lancet, *2*:942, 1963.

93. Gilchrist, G. S., Ekert, H., Shanbrom, E., and Hammond, D.: New concentrate for treatment of factor IX deficiency. New England J. Med., *280*:291, 1969.

94. Gilman, A., and Philips, F. S.: The biological actions and therapeutic applications of B-chlorethyl amines and sulfides. Science, *103*:409, 1946.

95. Gjessing, E. C., and Chanutin, A.: The effect of nitrogen mustards on the viscosity of thymonucleate. Cancer Res., *6*:593, 1946.

96. Gold, G. L., Salvin, L. G., and Shnider, B. E.: A comparative study with three alkylating agents: mechlorathamine, cyclophosphamide and uracil mustard. Cancer Chemother. Rep., *16*:417, 1962.

97. Gomori, G.: Histochemical demonstration of sites of phosphamidase activity. Proc. Soc. Exper. Biol. & Med., 69:407, 1948.

98. Goodman, L. S., and Gilman, A.: The Pharmacological Basis of Therapeutics. 2nd Ed. The Macmillan Co., New York, 1955, p. 1416.

99. Gordon, A. S.: Some aspects of hormonal influences upon the leukocytes. Ann. N.Y. Acad. Sci., 59:907, 1955.

100. Gordon, A. S., Piliero, S. J., and Landau, D.: The relation of the adrenal to blood formation in the rat. Endocrinology, 49:497, 1951.

101. Grady, G. F., Chalmers, T. C., and the Boston Inter-Hospital Liver Group: Viral hepatitis in a group of Boston hospitals. New England J. Med., 272:657, 1965.

102. Grant, D. B.: Perinpanayagam, M. S., Shute, P. G., and Zeitlin, R. A.: A case of malignant tertian (Plasmodium falciparum) malaria after blood transfusion. Lancet, 2:469, 1960.

103. Haar, H. G., Marshall, J., Bierman, H. R., and Steinfeld, J. L.: The influence of cyclo phosphamide upon neoplastic diseases in man. Cancer Chemother. Rep., 6:41, 1960.

104. Hall, T. C.: Treatment of hyperuricemia of neoplastic diseases. J. Clin. Pharm., 7:156, 1967.

105. Hampers, C. L., Prager, D., and Senior, J. R.: Post-transfusion anicteric hepatitis. New England J. Med., 271:747, 1964.

106. Handschumacher, R. E., Calebresi, P., Welch, A. D., Bono, V., Fallon, H., and Frei, E.: Summary of current information on 6-azauridine. Cancer Chemother. Rep., 21:1, 1962.

107. Hardisty, R. M., McElwain, T. J., and Darby, C. W.: Vincristine and prednisone for the induction of remissions in acute childhood leukemia. Brit. Med. J., 2:662, 1969.

108. Harris, M. N., Medrek, T. J., Golomb, F. M., Gumport, S. L., Postel, A. H., and Wright, J. C.: Chemotherapy with streptonigrin in advanced cancer. Cancer, 18:49, 1965.

109. Haut, A., Altman, S. J., Cartwright, G. E., and Wintrobe, M. M.: The influence of chemotherapy on survival in acute leukemia. Blood, 10:875, 1955.

110. Hernandez, K., Pinkel, D., Lee, S., and Leone, L.: Chemotherapy with 6-azauridine (NSC-32074) for patients with leukemia. Cancer Chemother. Rep., 53:203, 1969.

111. Hitchings, G. H., and Elion, G. B.: The chemistry and biochemistry of purine analogs. Ann. N.Y. Acad. Sci., 60:195, 1954.

112. Hoag, M. S., Johnson, F. F., Robinson, J. A., and Aggeler, P. M.: Treatment of hemophilia B with a new clotting-factor concentrate. New England J. Med., 280:581, 1969.

113. Holland, P. V., Rubinson, R. M., Morrow, A. G., and Schmidt, P. J.: γ-globulin in the prophylaxis of post-transfusion hepatitis. J.A.M.A., 196:471, 1966.

114. Holton, C. P., Lonsdale, D., Nora, A. H., Thurman, W. G., and Vietti, T. J.: Clinical study of daunomycin (NSC-82151) in children with acute leukemia. Cancer, 22:1014, 1968.

115. Hoogstraten, B., et al.: Cyclophosphamide (Cytoxan) in acute leukemia; preliminary report. Cancer Chemother. Rep., 8:116, 1960.

116. Howard, A.: Influence of radiation on DNA metabolism. Ciba Symposia on Ionizing Radiations and Cell Metabolism. J. A. Churchill, Ltd., London, 1956.

117. Howard, J. P., Albo, V., and Newton, W. A., Jr.: Results of a cooperative study in acute childhood leukemia. Cancer, 21:341, 1968.

118. Huestis, D. W., Bove, J. R., and Busch, S.: Practical Blood Transfusion. Little, Brown and Company, Boston, 1969.

119. Israels, L. G., Galton, D. A. G., Till, M., and Wiltshaw, E.: Clinical evaluation of CB 1348 in malignant lymphoma and related diseases. Ann. N.Y. Acad. Sci., 68:915, 1958.

120. Jackson, D. P., Krevans, J. R., and Conley, C. L.: Mechanism of the thrombocytopenia that follows multiple whole blood transfusions. Trans. Assoc. Am. Physicians, 69:155, 1956.

121. Jacobson, L. O., et al.: Nitrogen mustard therapy. J.A.M.A., 132:263, 1946.

122. James, K. W., and Kay, H. E. M.: Some aspects of current therapy in acute leukemia. Lancet, 1:206, 1967.

123. Jensen, M. K.: Chromosome studies in patients treated with azathioprine and amethopterin. Acta Med. Scand., 182:445, 1967.

124. Johnson, T. S., Armstrong, J. G., Gorman, M., and Burnett, J. P., Jr.: The vinca alkaloid: a new class of oncolytic agents. Cancer Res., 23:1390, 1963.

125. Joseph, J. H.: Mortality due to blood transfusion. Lancet, 2:709, 1960.

126. Kabat, E. A.: Blood Group Substances. Their Chemistry and Immunochemistry. Academic Press, Inc., New York, 1955.

127. Kagan, A. R., Morton, D. L., Hafermann, M. D., and Johnson, R. E.: Evaluation and management of radiation-induced pericardial effusion. Radiology, 92:632, 1969.

128. Kaplan, H. S.: Clinical evaluation and radiotherapeutic management of Hodgkin's disease and the malignant lymphomas. New England J. Med., 278:892, 1968.

129. Kaplan, H. S., and Bagshaw, M. A.: Radiation hepatitis: possible prevention by combined isotopic and external radiation therapy. Radiology, 91:1214, 1968.

130. Karnofsky, D. A.: Chemotherapy of neoplastic disease. New England J. Med., *239*:226, 260, 299, 1948.

131. Karnofsky, D. A.: Summary of results obtained with nitrogen mustard in treatment of neoplastic disease. Ann. N.Y. Acad. Sci., *68*:899, 1958.

132. Karon, M.: Preliminary report on vincristine (Oncovin) from acute leukemia group B. Am. Assoc. Cancer Res., *4*:33, 1963.

133. Kaung, D. T., Whittington, B. M., Spencer, H. H., and Patno, M. E.: Comparison of chlorambucil and streptonigrin (NSC-45383) in the treatment of chronic lymphocytic leukemia. Cancer, *23*:597, 1969.

134. Kidd, J. G.: Regression of transplanted lymphomas induced in vivo by means of normal guinea pig serum. J. Exp. Med., *98*:565, 1953.

135. Kilduffe, R. A., and DeBakey, M.: The Blood Bank and the Technique and Therapeutics of Transfusion. C. V. Mosby Co., St.Louis, 1942, pp. 1–45.

136. Kindred, J. E.: Histologic changes occurring in the hemopoietic organs of albino rats after single injections of 2-chloroethyl vesicants. Arch. Path., *43*:253, 1947.

137. Kliman, A.: Low risk of hepatitis after packed red cells. New England J. Med., *277*:1320, 1967.

138. Krakoff, I. H.: Clinical pharmacology of drugs which influence uric acid production and excretion. Clin. Pharm. Ther., *8*:124, 1966.

139. Krakoff, I. H., and Meyer, R. L.: Hyperuricemia in leukemia and lymphoma. J.A.M.A., *193*, 1, 1965.

140. Krebs, H. A.: The effects of extraneous agents on cell metabolism. Ciba Symposia on Ionizing Radiation and Cell Metabolism. J. A. Churchill, Ltd., London, 1956.

141. Krevans, J. R., Jackson, D. P., Conley, C. L., and Hartman, R. C.: The nature of the hemorrhagic disorder accompanying hemolytic transfusion reactions in man. Blood, *12*:834, 1957.

142. Kunin, C. M.: Serum hepatitis from whole blood: incidence and relation to source of blood. Am. J. Med. Sci., *237*:293, 1959.

143. Lajtha, L. G., Oliver, R., Kumatori, T., and Ellis, F.: On the mechanism of radiation effect on DNA synthesis. Radiation Res., *8*:1, 1958.

144. Lampkin, B. C., Nagao, T., and Mauer, A. M.: Drug effect in acute leukemia. J. Clin. Invest., *48*:1124, 1969.

145. Landsteiner, K.: Zur Kenntnis der antifermentativen, lytischen und agglutinierenden Wirkungen des Bluxserums und der Lymphe. Zentralbl. Bakt., *27*:357, 1900.

146. Landsteiner, K., and Levine, P.: A new agglutinable factor differentiating individual human bloods. Proc. Soc. Exper. Biol. & Med., *24*:600, 1927.

147. Landsteiner, K., and Wiener, A. S.: An agglutinable factor in human blood recognized by immune sera for rhesus blood. Proc. Soc. Exper. Biol. & Med., *43*:223, 1940.

148. Lawrence, J. H., Dobson, R. L., Low-Beer, B. V. A., and Brown, B. R.: Chronic myelogenous leukemia: a study of 129 cases in which treatment was with radioactive phosphorus. J.A.M.A., *136*:672, 1948.

149. Levin, R. H., Freireich, E. J., and Chappell, W.: Effect of storage up to 48 hours on response to transfusions of platelet rich plasma. Transfusion, *4*:251, 1964.

150. Levine, A. S., Sharp, H. L., Mitchell, J., Krivit, W., and Nesbit, M. E.: Combination therapy with 6-mercaptopurine (NSC-755) and allopurinal (NSC-1390) during induction and maintenance of remission of acute leukemia in children. Cancer Chemother. Rep., *53*:53, 1969.

151. Levine, P., and Stetson, R. E.: An unusual case of intragroup agglutination. J.A.M.A., *113*:126, 1939.

152. Looney, W. B., Chang, L. O., Williams, S. S., Foster, J., Haydock, I. C., and Banghart, F. W.: An autoradiographic and biochemical study of the effects of irradiation on deoxyribonucleic acid synthesis in the intact animal. Radiation Res., *24*:312, 1965.

153. Low-Beer, B. V. A., Lawrence, J. H., and Stone, R. S.: The therapeutic use of artificially produced radioactive substances. Radiology, *39*:573, 1942.

154. Ludbrook, J., and Wynn, V.: Citrate intoxication. A clinical and experimental study. Brit. Med. J., *2*:523, 1558.

155. MacKay, I. R.: Chronic hepatitis: effect of prolonged suppressive treatment and comparison of azathioprine with prednisolone. Quart. J. Med., *37*:379, 1968.

156. Mainwaring, R. L., and Brueckner, G. G.: Fibrinogen-transmitted hepatitis. J.A.M.A., *195*:437, 1966.

157. Malpas, J. S., and Scott, R. B.: Daunorubicin in acute myelocytic leukemia. Lancet, *1*:469, 1969.

158. Manuila, A.: Blood groups and disease. Hard facts and delusions. J.A.M.A., *167*:2047, 1958.

159. Marder, V. J., and Shulman, N. R.: Major surgery in classic hemophilia using fraction I. Am. J. Med., *41*:56, 1966.

160. Mashburn, L. T., and Wriston, J. C.: Tumor inhibitory effect of l-asparaginase from *Escherichia coli.* Arch. Biochem. Biophys., *105*:450, 1964.

161. Masland, D. S., Rotz, C. T., and Harris, J. H., Jr.: Postradiation pericarditis with chronic pericardial effusion. Ann. Int. Med., *69*:97, 1968.

162. Masure, R.: Human factor VIII prepared by cryoprecipitation. Vox Sanguinis, *16*:1, 1969.

163. Meyer, O. O.: Treatment of Hodgkin's disease and the lymphosarcomas. J.A.M.A., *154*:114, 1954.

164. Michael, A. F., Vernier, R. L., Drummond, K. N., Levitt, J. I., Herdman, R. C., Fish, A. J., and Good, R. A.: Immunosuppressive therapy of chronic renal disease. New England J. Med., *276*:817, 1967.

165. Miller, S. E.: Textbook of Clinical Pathology. 5th Ed. Williams and Wilkins Co., Baltimore, 1955, p. 296.

166. Mirick, G. S., Ward, R., and McCollum, R. W.: Modification of post-transfusional hepatitis by gamma globulin. New England J. Med., *273*:59, 1965.

167. Mollison, P. L.: Blood transfusion in clinical practice. F. A. Davis Co., Philadelphia, 1967.

168. Morphology of radiation-induced heart disease. J.A.M.A., *206*:2309, 1968.

169. Morse, E. E., Freireich, E. J., Carbone, P. P., Bronson, W., and Frei, E., III: The transfusion of leukocytes from donors with chronic myelocytic leukemia to patients with leukopenia. Transfusion, *6*:183, 1966.

170. Mourant, A. E.: The Distribution of the Human Blood Groups. Charles C Thomas, Springfield, Ill., 1954.

171. Muggia, F. M., and Cassileth, P. A.: Constructive pericarditis following radiation therapy. Am. J. Med., *44*:116, 1969.

172. Nissen-Meyer, R., and Höst, H.: A comparison between the hematological side effects of cyclophosphamide and nitrogen mustard. Cancer Chemother. Rep., *9*:51, 1960.

173. Oettgen, H. F., et al.: Inhibition of leukemias in man by l-asparaginase. Cancer Res., *27*:2619, 1967.

174. Oettgen, H. F., et al.: Toxicity of *E. coli* l-asparaginase in man. Cancer, *25*:253, 1970.

175. Palmer, J. G., Cartwright, G. E., and Wintrobe, M. M.: The effects of ACTH and cortisone on the blood of experimental animals. In Mote, J. R., Ed.: Proceedings of the Second Clinical ACTH Conference. I, 1951. The Blakiston Co., New York, 1951, p. 438.

176. Pantelakis, S. N., Karaklis, A., and Doxiadis, S. A.: Transfusion malaria. Clin. Ped., *5*:543, 1966.

177. Perkins, H. A.: Brief report: correction of the hemostatic defects in Von Willebrand's disease. Blood, *30*:375, 1967.

178. Personal Observations.

179. Peters, M. V.: Radiation therapy. J.A.M.A., *191*:28, 1965.

180. Phillips, L. L.: Homologous serum jaundice following fibrinogen administration. Surg. Gynec. & Obstet., *121*:551, 1965.

181. Pierce, M., Shore, N., Sitarz, A., Murphy, M. L., Louis, J., and Severo, N.: Cyclophosphamide therapy in acute leukemia of childhood. Cancer, *19*:1551, 1966.

182. Plentl, A. A., and Schoenheimer, R.: Studies in the metabolism of purines and pyrimidines by means of isotopic nitrogen. J. Biol. Chem., *153*:203, 1944.

183. Pool, J. G., Hershgold, E. J., and Pappenhagen, A. R.: High potency antihemophilic factor concentrate prepared from cryoglobulin precipitate. Nature, *203*:312, 1964.

184. Prentice, C. R. M., Breckenridge, R. T., Foreman, W. B., and Ratnoff, O. D.: Treatment of hemophilia (Factor VIII deficiency) with human antihemophilic factor prepared by the cryoprecipitate process. Lancet, *1*:457, 1967.

185. Purcell, G., Jr., and Nossel, H. L.: Factor XI (PTA) deficiency—surgical and obstetric aspects. Obstet. & Gynec., *35*:69, 1970.

186. Race, R. R., and Sanger, R.: The inheritance of blood groups. Brit. Med. Bull., *15*:99, 1959.

187. Race, R. R., and Sanger, R.: Blood Groups in Man. 5th Ed., Blackwell Scientific Publications, Oxford, 1968.

188. Rao, K. V., Bieman, K., and Woodward, R. B.: The structure of streptonigrin. J. Am. Chem. Soc., *85*:2532, 1963.

189. Ratnoff, O. D., Kass, L., and Lang, P. D.: Studies on the purification of antihemophilic factor, Factor VIII. J. Clin. Invest., *48*:957, 1969.

190. Rivers, S. L., Whittington, R. M., and Medrek, T. J.: Treatment of malignant lymphomas with methyl ester of streptonigrin (NSC-45384). Cancer, *19*:1377, 1966.

191. Reinhard, E. H., Moore, C. V., Bierbaum, O. S., and Moore, S.: Radioactive phosphorus as a therapeutic agent. A review of the literature and analysis of the results of treatment of 155 patients with various blood dyscrasias, lymphomas, and other malignant neoplastic diseases. J. Lab. & Clin. Med., *31*:107, 1946.

192. Roberts, J. A. F.: Some associations between blood groups and disease. Brit. Med. Bull., *15*:129, 1959.

193. Rose, W. C. J.: In vitro reactions of biological alkylating agents. Ann. N.Y. Acad. Sci., *68*:669, 1958.

194. Rubin, J. S., and Rubin, R. T.: Cyclophosphamide hemorrhagic cystitis. J. Urology, *96*:313, 1966.

195. Rundles, R. W., Coonrad, E. V., and Willard, N. L.: Summary of results obtained with TEM. Ann. N.Y. Acad. Sci., *68*:926, 1958.

196. Rundles, R. W., Laszlo, J., Itoga, T., Hobson, J. B., and Garrison, F. E., Jr.: Clinical and hematologic study of 6-(l-methyl-4-nitro-5-imidazolyl)thio-purine (BW-57-322) and related compounds. Cancer Chemother. Rep., *14*:99, 1961.

197. Rundles, R. W., Wyngaarden, J. B., Hitchings, G. H., Elion, G. B., and Silberman, H.: Effects of a xanthine oxidase inhibitor on thiopurine metabolism, hyperuricemia and gout. Trans. Assoc. Am. Phys., *76*:126, 1963.

198. Saravis, C. A., Trey, C., and Grady, G. F.: Rapid screening test for detecting hepatitis-associated antigen. Science, *169*:298, 1970.

199. Shnider, B. I.: Preliminary studies with cyclophosphamide. Cancer Chemother. Rep., *8*:106, 1960.

200. Skipper, H. E.: A review: On the mechanism of action of certain temporary anticancer agents. Cancer Res., *13*:545, 1953.

201. Skipper, H. E., and Mitchell, J. H.: Effect of roentgen-ray radiation on the biosynthesis of nucleic acids and nucleic acid purines. Cancer, *4*:363, 1951.

202. Snell, G. D.: The homograft reaction. Ann. Rev. Microbiology, *11*:439, 1957.

203. Soulier, J. P., Josso, F., Steinbuch, M., and Cosson, A.: The therapeutical use of fraction P.P.S.B. Biblio. Haemat., *29*:1127, 1968.

203a. Spies, S. K., and Synman, H. W.: Procarbazine (Natulan) in the treatment of Hodgkin's disease and other lymphomas. S. Afr. Med. J., *40*:1061, 1966.

204. Stacey, K. A., Cobb, M., Cousens, S. F., and Alexander, P.: The reactions of the "radio-mimetic" alkylating agents with macromolecules in vitro. Ann. N.Y. Acad. Sci., *68*:682, 1958.

205. Stokes, J. L.: Substitution of thymine for "folic acid" in the nutrition of lactic acid bacteria. J. Bact., *48*:201, 1944.

206. Sussman, J. N.: Azathioprine in refractory idiopathic thrombocytopenic purpura. J.A.M.A., *202*:259, 1967.

207. Sutow, W. W., Vietti, T. J., Fernbach, D. J., Lane, D. M., Donaldson, M. H., and Berry, D. H.: Combination of vincristine and prednisone in therapy of acute leukemia in children. J. Ped., *73*:426, 1968.

208. Svoboda, G. H., Neuss, N., and Gorman, M.: Alkaloids of Vinca rosea (Catharanthus roseus G. Don.). V. Preparation and characterization of alkaloids. J. Am. Pharm. Assoc., *48*:659, 1959.

209. Tallal, L., Tan, C., Otteger, H., Wollner, N., McCarthy, M., Nelson, L., Burchenal, J., Karnofsky, D., and Murphy, M. L.: *E. coli* l-asparaginase in the treatment of leukemia and solid tumors in 131 children. Cancer, *25*:306, 1970.

210. Talley, R. W., and Vaitevicius, V. K.: Megaloblastosis produced by a cytosine antagonist, l-β-D-arabinofuranosyl-cytosine. Blood, *21*:352, 1963.

211. Thompson, P. L., and MacKay, I. R.: Radiation nephritis after gastric irradiation for peptic ulcer. Gastroenterology, *56*:816, 1969.

212. Tullis, J. L., and Melin, M.: Management of Christmas disease and Stuart-Prower deficiency with a prothrombin-complex concentrate. (Factor II, VII, IX & X.) Biblio. Haemat., *29*:1134, 1968.

213. Vartan, A. E.: Transfusion malaria in a man with Christmas disease. Brit. Med. J., *4*:466, 1967.

214. Verity, G. L.: Tissue tolerance: central nervous system. Radiology, *91*:1221, 1968.

215. Vogler, W. R., Bain, J. A., Huguley, C. M., Palmer, H. G., and Lowrey, M. E.: Metabolic and therapeutic effects of allopurinol in patients with leukemia and gout. Am. J. Med., *40*:548, 1966.

216. Warwick, O. H., Darte, J. M. M., and Brown, T. C.: Some biological effects of Vincaleukoblastine an alkaloid in Vinca rosea Linn. in patients with malignant disease. Cancer Res., *20*:1032, 1960.

217. Wedgwood, R. J., and Riese, G. R.: Touching a cure of an inverterate phrensy by the transfusion of blood. New England J. Med., *248*:902, 1953.

218. Welch, A. D., Handschumacher, R. F., Finch, S. C., Jaffe, J. J., Cardoso, S. S., and Calabresi, P.: A synopsis of recent investigations of 6-azauridine (NSC-32074). Cancer Chemother. Rep., *9*:39, 1960.

219. White, R. H. R.: Cytotoxic drug therapy in steroid-resistant glomerulonephritis. Proc. Roy. Coll. Med., *60*:1164, 1967.
220. Whitelaw, D. M., Cowan, D. H., Cassidy, F. R., and Patterson, T. A.: Clinical experience with vincristine. Cancer Chemother. Rep., *30*:13, 1963.
221. Whitelaw, D. M., and Teasdale, J. M.: Vinca leukoblastine in the treatment of malignant disease. Canad. Med. Assoc. J., *85*:584, 1961.
222. Wiener, A. S., and Wexler, I. B.: Heredity of the Blood Groups. Grune and Stratton, New York, 1958.
223. Wilson, W. L., Labra, C., and Barrist, E.: Preliminary observation on the use of streptonigrin as an antitumor agent in human beings. Antibiot. Chemother., *9*:147, 1961.
224. Wintrobe, M. M., and Huguley, C. M.: Nitrogen-mustard therapy for Hodgkin's disease, lymphosarcoma, the leukemias and other disorders. Cancer, *1*:357, 1948.
225. Wolff, J. A., Brubaker, C. A., Murphy, M. L., Pierce, M. I., and Servero, N.: Prednisone therapy of acute childhood leukemia: prognosis and duration of response in 330 treated patients. J. Ped., *70*:626, 1967.
226. Young, L. E.: Complications of blood transfusions. Ann. Int. Med., *61*:136, 1964.

Index

ABO blood groups, 627–629
ABO incompatibility, erythroblastosis fetalis due to, 222
AC globulin. See *Factor(s), coagulation, Factor V.*
Acanthocytes, 23
Accelerator, globulin. See *Factor(s), coagulation, Factor V.*
  prothrombin. See *Factor(s), coagulation, Factor II.*
  serum prothrombin conversion. See *Factor(s), coagulation, Factor VII.*
Acquired fibrinogen deficiency, 402
Acquired (toxic) porphyria, 44
Acute iron intoxication, 150
Adenosine diphosphate (ADP), 40, 181, 306–309
Adenosine triphosphate (ATP), 3, 34, 40, 179–182, 188, 309
Adrenocortical steroids, 623–625
  complications, 624
  in acute leukemia, 483–485, 623–624
  in aplastic anemia, 168
  in autoimmune hemolytic anemia, 237–238, 495
  in chronic erythrocytic hypoplasia, 168
  in chronic lymphocytic leukemia, 495
  in idiopathic thrombocytopenic purpura, 362–363
  in leukemia, 483–485, 495, 504, 509, 623–624
  in malignant lymphomas, 555–558, 624
  in multiple myeloma, 597
  in myeloid metaplasia, 516
Agnogenic myeloid metaplasia, 513
Agranulocytosis, 442–448
  bone marrow in, 444
  causes, 445
  clinical manifestations, 445

Agranulocytosis (*Continued*)
  diagnosis, 446
  history, 442
  illustrative case, 447
  laboratory examination, 445
  mechanism of disease, 443
  prognosis, 446
  treatment, 446
AHF (antihemophilic factor). See *Factor(s), coagulation, Factor VIII.*
Alder's anomaly, 10
Alkaline phosphatase, activity in granulocytes, 288, 500
Alkylating agents, 614–617
Allergic purpura, 370–371
Allergic reactions following transfusion, 636
Allergies, eosinophilia in, 440
Allopurinol, 625
Amethopterin, 617–618. See also *Methotrexate.*
Amidopyrine, agranulocytosis and, 443
Amniocentesis, in erythroblastosis fetalis, 228
Amyloidosis, in multiple myeloma, 588
Androgens, 28, 166, 520
  in aplastic anemia, 166, 173
  in myeloid metaplasia, 520
Anemia
  alcoholism, and, 273, 274
  aplastic, 74, 157–170
    androgens in, 166
    causes, 158–161
    chloramphenicol in, 159
    clinical manifestations, 162
    course, 167
    diagnosis, 164
    idiopathic, 161
    in children, 172
    mechanism, 157
    oxymetholone in, 166

647

Anemia (*Continued*)
  aplastic, paroxysmal nocturnal hemoglobin-
    uria, 169
    pure red cell, 170
    secondary to infectious hepatitis, 158
    treatment, 165
  blood loss, and, 62, 266
  classification of, 56–58
  diagnosis of, 68–73
    history in, 68
    laboratory tests in, 72
    physical examination in, 70
  hemolytic, 178–245
    acquired, 222–245
    autoimmune, 64, 232–239
      adrenocorticosteroid drugs in, 237
      antibodies in, 233
      classification, 185
      clinical manifestations, 235
      combination hemoglobinopathies, 219
      Coombs antiglobulin test, 236
      history, 232
      in leukemia, 493
      in lymphoma, 543
      pathogenesis, 233
      prognosis, 238
      splenectomy in, 237
      treatment, 237
    due to burns, 67
    due to chemical agents, 66
    due to drugs, 195, 230–232
    due to enzyme deficiencies, 194–198
      factors in anemia, 195
      G-6-PD deficiency, 194
      others, 198
      pyruvic kinase deficiency, 197
    due to hemoglobinopathies, 198
    due to hypersplenism, 67
    due to infectious agents, 66
    due to methyldopa, 231
    due to quinidine, 230
    due to penicillin, 231
    due to physical agents, 67
    due to primaquine, 194
    due to vegetable poisons, 67
    erythroblastosis fetalis, 222–229
      amniocentesis in, 228
      blood groups and, 223
      clinical manifestations of, 224
      diagnosis of, 225
      history in, 222
      mechanism of, 223
      prevention of, 226
      Rh factor in, 223
      treatment of, 227
    hemoglobin C disease, 212
    hemopathic, 68
    hereditary, 186–222
    hereditary elliptocytosis, 193
    hereditary spherocytosis, 186–193
      clinical manifestations, 188
      diagnosis, 191
      erythrocyte membrane in, 188

Anemia (*Continued*)
  hemolytic, hereditary spherocytosis, history,
    186
      osmotic fragility test in, 190
      pathogenesis, 186
      spleen in, 187
      treatment in, 191
    mechanical, 242
      cardiac hemolytic anemia, 243
      causes of, 242
      march hemoglobinuria, 242
      microangiopathic, 244
    sickle cell, 199–212
      clinical manifestations, 201
      course, 208
      crisis, 201
      diagnosis, 208
      history, 199
      in infants, 205
      pathogenesis, 200
      prognosis, 208
      treatment, 209
    thalassemia, 213–219
      alpha type, 214
      beta type, 214
      clinical manifestations, 215
      diagnosis, 217
      history, 213
      mechanism, 214, 215
      treatment, 218
  iron deficiency and, 129–138
  leukoerythroblastic, 277
  macrocytic, 73
    in aplastic anemia, 74
    in cirrhosis of liver, 272
    in folate deficiency, 73
    in hemolytic anemia, 75
    in myxedema, 75
    in pregnancy, 267
    in vitamin B_{12} deficiency, 73
  megaloblastic, 92
    ascorbic acid deficiency and, 111
    chronic liver disease and, 273
    dietary, 107
    excessive demands for folate, 112
    fish tapeworm and, 107
    folate antagonists and, 111
    malabsorption and, 107, 108, 110
    pernicious anemia and, 93
    postgastrectomy, 106
    pregnancy and, 112, 268
    sprue and, 110
  microcytic, 78
  normocytic, 75
    in acute blood loss, 77
    in deficient blood production, 78
    in hyperhemolysis, 75
    in iron deficiency, 78
  pernicious, 93–104
    autoimmunity in, 95
    carcinoma of stomach in, 103
    clinical manifestations, 95
    differential diagnosis, 98

Anemia (*Continued*)
pernicious, history, 93
juvenile, 103
laboratory examination, 96
megaloblastic erythropoiesis in, 97
prognosis, 103
Schilling test in, 100
treatment, 101
vitamin B_{12} deficiency in, 94
pyridoxine responsive, 140, 145
sideroblastic (iron loading), 138–150
acquired, 143
classification, 141
enzymatic defects in, 139–140
hereditary, 141
pyridoxine responsive, 145
secondary to chemicals, 143
secondary to other diseases, 144
splenomegaly and, 274–276
with chronic blood loss, 62, 266
with chronic disease, 262
with chronic liver disease, 68, 272–274
with chronic renal disease, 270
with iron deficiency, 129–138
with iron loading, 138–150
with lead poisoning, 44, 144
with myxedema, 75, 263
with pregnancy, 267
with splenomegaly, 274
Angina, agranulocytic. See *Agranulocytosis.*
Anisocytosis, 22
Antibody(ies)
leukocytes, agranulocytosis and, 444
low molecular weight, 579
opsonic function of, 432
Anticoagulants, 327–332
antithrombin, 327
circulating, 390–392
heparin, 328
action, 329
administration, 329
antidotes, 329
pharmacologic, 328–332
contraindications to, 328
coumarin-indanedione drugs, 330–332
antidote, 332
complications of, 331–332
dosage schedules of, 332
physiologic, 327
Anticonvulsants, as cause of hematologic
abnormalities, 111, 159, 445
Antiglobulin (Coombs) test in autoimmune
hemolytic anemia, 233–234
Antihemophilic factor. See *Factor(s), coagulation, Factor VIII.*
Antihemophilic globulin. See *Factor(s), coagulation, Factor VIII.*
Antimetabolites
antifolic acid compounds, 617
8-azaguanine, 620
azathioprine, 619
6-azauridine, 621

Antimetabolites (*Continued*)
cytosine arabinoside, 620
purine analogs, 619
pyrimidine analogs, 619
Antiplasmin, 322
in platelets, 322
Anti-Rh gamma globulin, 226
Aplastic anemia, 157–175. See also *Anemia, aplastic.*
Apoferritin, 126
Arvin, 319
Ascorbic acid, 47
deficiency, folic acid deficiency and, 111
Aspirin, and purpura, 374, 413
ATP, 3, 34, 40, 179, 182, 188, 309
Auer bodies, 8, 480, 481, 512
Australia antigen, 637
Autoimmune hemolytic anemia, 64, 232–239

Bacterial infections, in chronic lymphocytic
leukemia, 493
leukocyte response to, 439
Band cells (stab cells), 9
Bantu, iron overload in, 149
Barometric pressure, low, and secondary polycythemia, 292
Bartonella bacillus, 66
Basophil, 11
count, 437
Basophilia, diffuse, 22
Basophilic normoblast, morphology, 21
Bean, fava, hemolytic anemia due to, 67
Bence Jones protein, 585, 586–587
Benign monoclonal gammopathy, 601
Big spleen disease (tropical splenomegaly),
274, 276
Bilirubin, 39, 40, 178
Biopsy, lymph node, in diagnosis of patient
with enlarged lymph nodes, 532
Blackwater fever, 66
Blast cells, with Auer bodies, 8, 480, 481
Bleeding
acute, hematologic response, 266, 267
anemias due to, 62, 266–267
gastrointestinal, in iron deficiency anemia,
130
in polycythemia vera, 284
neutrophilic leukocytosis in, 266, 439
Bleeding time, determination of, in hemorrhagic diathesis, 336
Blood, cells, chemistry, 1–5
origin and relationship, 17
Blood groups, 626–630
ABO, antibodies in serum, 627
antigens in erythrocytes, 627
incidence, 627
antigenic systems, 627
MNS, 628
Rh (and others), 627
incompatible, hemolytic reactions following transfusions, 634–636

Blood loss, acute, anemia due to, 266–267
  chronic, anemia due to, 62–63
Blood transfusion(s)
  hepatitis and, 637
  history of, 626
  indications for, 631
  of blood components, 631
  reactions in, 633–638
Bone marrow, examination of, 80–83
  differential cell counts, 82
Bone marrow failure, 61, 156–177
  classification of, 157
Brill-Symmers disease (giant follicular lymphoma), 543
Burkitt's lymphoma, 545–546
Burr cells, 23, 244
Bursa of Fabricius, 434, 581
Busulfan (Myleran), 616
  in chronic granulocytic leukemia, 503
  in hemorrhagic thrombocythemia, 522
  in myeloid metaplasia, 520

Cabot rings, 23
Calcium, 307, 309, 312, 317
Cardiovascular symptoms, in polycythemia vera, 284
Celiac disease, anemia associated with, 108
Cell(s)
  anatomy of, 1–5
  blood, 6
  classification, morphology and origin, 7–24
  erythrocytic series, 17
  granulocytic series, 7
  lymphocytic series, 11
  monocytic series, 13
  plasmacytic series, 16
  stem, 6
  target, 23, 212
  thrombocytic series, 14, 303–305
Chediak-Higashi syndrome, 10, 451
Chemotaxis, 432, 436
Chemotherapy
  in acute leukemia, 482–485
  in chronic lymphocytic leukemia, 494–495
  in chronic myelocytic leukemia, 503–504
  in malignant lymphomas, 553–558
  in multiple myeloma, 596–597
  in polycythemia vera, 290
Chlorambucil (Leukeran), 616
  in chronic lymphocytic leukemia, 495
  in lymphoma, 555, 558
Chloramphenicol, in aplastic anemia, 159
Chloroma, 480
Chlorosis. See *Anemia, iron deficiency*.
Cholelithiasis, in hereditary spherocytosis, 189
  in sickle cell anemia, 203
Christmas disease, 387
Christmas Factor. See *Factor(s), coagulation, Factor IX*.
Chromosome, Philadelphia, 288, 476, 500

Chronic granulomatous disease, 450
Circulating anticoagulants, 390
Cirrhosis of liver, anemia in, 272
Citrovorum factor (Leucovorin), 618
Clot retraction, estimation, in hemorrhagic diathesis, 336
Coagulation, 309–320
  conversion of fibrinogen to fibrin, 318
  conversion of prothrombin to thrombin, 317
  development of thromboplastin activity, 312
  extrinsic system, 312
  factors of. See *Factor(s), coagulation*.
  history, 310
  intrinsic system, 313
  pathologic, 323
  venom coagulant system, 319
Coagulation time test, 336
Cobalt, in erythropoiesis, 46
Cold hemoglobinuria, paroxysmal 239–240
Congenital erythropoietic protoporphyria, 42
Congenital fibrinogen deficiency, 401
Consumption coagulopathy, 326, 402
Convulsions, leukocytosis due to, 438
Cooley's anemia, 63, 213
Coombs test, 66, 232, 236
Copper, in erythropoiesis, 45
Coproporphyria, hereditary, 43
Coproporphyrin, 35–36
Coproporphyrin I, 35, 45
Coproporphyrin III, 35, 45
Corticosteroids. See *Adrenocortical steroids*.
Coumarin-indanedione compounds, 330
Crisis, in hereditary spherocytosis, 189
  in sickle cell anemia, 201–203
CRST syndrome, 374
Cryoglobulinemia, in multiple myeloma, 587, 588
Cryoprecipitate, 384
  by Pool, 632
Cyanide-ascorbate test, 196
Cyclic neutropenia, 448
Cyclophosphamide (Cytoxan), 616
  in acute leukemia, 483
  in chronic lymphocytic leukemia, 495
  in lymphoma, 557, 558
  in multiple myeloma, 596
Cytoplasm, cell, 3
Cytosine arabinoside, 620
  in acute leukemia, 483

Daunomycin, in acute leukemia, 484
Deferoxamine, in acute iron intoxication, 150
Defibrination syndrome, 326, 402
Delta aminolevulinic acid, 36
Deoxyribonucleic acid (DNA), 3, 33
  action of chemotherapeutic agents on, 614, 618, 619, 622
  effect of radiation on, 612
  folate and vitamin B_{12} metabolism in, 90–92
  in aplastic anemia, 160

Diagnosis, of anemia, 68–83
    errors in, 84
Diet
  and anemia, 60
  and folate deficiency, 60, 89, 92, 107
  and iron deficiency, 130
  sources of folate, 89
  sources of iron, 117
  sources of vitamin B_{12}, 87
DiGeorge's syndrome, 582
Di Guglielmo syndrome, 143, 511, 512
Diphyllobothrium latum infestation, megaloblastic anemia in, 107
Disseminated intravascular coagulation, 326,
  402
  associated conditions, 326
  diagnosis of, 326, 403
  treatment of, 327, 403
DNA. See *Deoxyribonucleic acid.*
Döhle bodies, 10
Donath-Landsteiner test, 240
Downey cells, 460
DPG (2,3-DPG), 182

Edema, in erythroblastosis fetalis, 228
  pulmonary, following transfusion, 638
Elliptocytes, 23, 193
Elliptocytosis, hereditary, 193
Embden-Myerhof pathway, 181
Eosinophil, 11
Eosinophilia, causes, 440
Epsilon-aminocaproic acid, 321, 327
Epstein-Barr virus (EB virus), in infectious
  mononucleosis, 454
Erythremia. See *Polycythemia vera.*
  myelosis. 511–512
Erythroblastosis fetalis, 222–229
Erythrocyte(s)
  anerobic glycolysis in, 182
  antigenic systems, 627
  ATP, in, 179
  chemistry, 33–38
  deformability, 179
  destruction of, 38, 178
  diameter, 22
  Embden-Myerhof pathway in, 181–182
  enzymes, 180, 194
  function, 183
  glucose metabolism by, 181–182
  gluthathione, 180
  hemoglobin content, anemia classification
    by, 57
  in peripherial blood, 22
  in pernicious anemia, 98
  in sickle cell anemia, 199
  life span, 178
  maturation factor, 94
  membrane, 179
  metabolism, 179
  methemoglobin reductase systems, 183
    deficiency of, 183
  morphology, 22

Erythrocyte(s) (*Continued*)
  normal, in peripheral blood, 22
  origin, 17
  osmotic fragility test, in hereditary sphero-
    cytosis, 190
  pencil forms, 22
  pentose shunt, 180
  size of, 57
Erythrocytic hypoplasia, 170
  chronic, 157
    prednisone in, 168
  drugs as causes, 171
  mechanism, 171
  thymoma in, 170
Erythrocytic series, 19–24
Erythroleukemia, 511, 512
Erythropoiesis
  control of, 26
  factors needed for, 45
  site of in fetus, 18
Erythropoietin, 27–31
Excessive proteolysis, 325
Exchange transfusions in erythroblastosis
  fetalis, indications for, 227
Exercise, leukocytosis following, 438
Extrinsic factor. See *Factor(s), extrinsic.*
Extrinsic system in thromboplastin activity
  development, 312

Fabricius, bursa of, 434, 581
Factor(s)
  coagulation, 309, 318
Factor(s), antihemophilic, 310, 314
  Factor I, 309, 318
  Factor II, 309, 317
    deficiency, 397
  Factor III, 309, 313
  Factor IV, 317
  Factor V, 310, 316
    deficiency, 392
  Factor VII, 310, 313
    deficiency, 395
  Factor VII, IX and XI deficiency, 377
  Factor VIII, 310, 314
    deficiency, 378
  Factor IX, 310, 314
    deficiency, 387
  Factor X, 310, 316
    deficiency, 394
  Factor XI, 310, 314
    deficiency, 389
  Factor XII, 310, 313
    deficiency, 376
  Factor XIII, 310, 318
    deficiency, 407
  erythrocytic maturation, 94
  extrinsic, 94
  intrinsic, 87, 94
  leukocyte inducing, 430
  platelet clotting, 305, 315
  Rh, 629
Fanconi's syndrome, 172
Favism, 67

Fecal urobilinogen, 39, 76
Felty's syndrome, 277
Ferritin, 120, 125, 126
Ferrokinetics, 127–129
Ferrous salts, in iron deficiency anemia, 136
Fever, glandular. See *Infectious mononucleosis.*
Fibrin, chemistry of, 318
Fibrin stabilizing factor. See *Factor(s), coagulation, Factor XIII.*
Fibrinogen, 309, 318
    acquired deficiency of, 402
    congenital deficiency of, 401
Fibrinolysis, 320–323
Fish, tapeworm infestations in, and megaloblastic anemia, 107
Folic acid (folate), 46, 89–92
    absorption, 89
    antagonists, 111
    deficiency, 107–112
    metabolism, 89–92
    methyl trap hypothesis, 91
Formula, Wintrobe's, for determination of size and hemoglobin content of erythrocytes, 57
Franklin's disease, 599

G-6-PD (glucose-6-phosphate dehydrogenase), deficiency of, 194–197
Gaisböck's syndrome, 294
Gammopathy, 580
Gastrectomy, partial, iron deficiency following, 130–131
    total, megaloblastic anemia following, 106–107
Gastric analysis, in differentiation of vitamin B$_{12}$ and folic acid deficiency, 98–99
Gastric secretion in pernicious anemia, 97
Genetic factors in leukemia, 475–477
Giant follicular lymphoma, 543
Gingival hyperplasia, in acute monocytic leukemia, 509
Glandular fever. See *Infectious mononucleosis.*
Glanzmann's disease (thrombasthenia), 412
Globulins, 574
Glucose metabolism, and heme degradation, 40
    by erythrocytes, 180–183
Glucose-6-phosphate dehydrogenase (G-6-PD), deficiency of, 194–197
Glutathione, erythrocyte, 180–182
Glycolytic and pentose phosphate shunt pathways, 181
Golgi apparatus, cell, 2, 5
Graft vs host reaction, 569
Granulocytes, 9–11, 428–433
Granulomatous disease, chronic, 450

Hageman deficiency, 376
Hageman factor. See *Factor(s), coagulation, Factor XII.*

Ham's test, 241
Haptoglobin, 39–40
Heavy (H) chain disease, 599–601
Heinz bodies, 23, 182, 199, 221
Helmet cells, 23, 67
Hematopoiesis, 26–31
Hematuria, in sickle-cell trait, 202, 205
Heme, 35
    degradation of, 38
    synthesis of, 140
Hemochromatosis, idiopathic, 147
Hemodilution, during pregnancy, 267
    with multiple myeloma, 588
    with splenomegaly, 68, 274, 276
Hemoglobin(s)
    alpha chain, 33, 64
    abnormal, 198–222
    Bart's, 214
    catabolism of, 38
    chemical characteristics of, 33–35
    degradation of, 38–40
    determination of, in anemia diagnosis, 71
    function of, 31, 183
    in erythrocytes, anemia classification by, 57
    metabolism of, 31–48
    molecular weight of, 33
    protein synthesis and, 33–34, 213–215
    quantity of, determination of, 31–32
    reductase systems in, 183
    role of, 31–35
    sickle cell, 199–201
    synthesis of, 33–38
Hemoglobin A$_2$, 64, 214
Hemoglobin C disease, homozygous, 212–213
    sickle cell disease, 219–220
Hemoglobin D disease, homozygous, 221
    sickle cell disease, 220–221
Hemoglobin electrophoresis, 65, 208
Hemoglobin F, in thalassemia, 214
Hemoglobin H disease, 215
Hemoglobin Lepore, 214
Hemoglobin M, 184, 293
Hemoglobin S disease, homozygous, 199. See also *Anemia, sickle cell.*
Hemoglobinopathies, 64, 198–222
Hemoglobinuria, cold paroxysmal, 66, 239–240
    march, 242
    nocturnal, paroxysmal, 64, 169, 240–242
Hemolytic anemia. See *Anemia, hemolytic.*
Hemolytic index, 76
Hemophilia, 378–386
    clinical manifestations of, 382
    inheritance of, 378
    surgery on, 385
    treatment of, 383
Hemorrhagic diathesis, 333–341
    diagnosis of, 333
    history, 333
    laboratory examination for, 335
        bleeding time, 336
        coagulation time, 336
        platelet count, 336
        partial thromboplastin time, 337

Hemorrhagic diathesis (*Continued*)
  laboratory examination for, prothrombin
      time, 336
    thromboplastin generation test, 337
    tourniquet test, 336
  physical examination, 334
Hemorrhagic telangiectasia, hereditary, 374
Hemorrhagic thrombocythemia, 522
Hemosiderinuria, 179
Hemosiderosis, 149
Hemostasis, 302–340
  abnormal, 324
  biochemical phase of, 309
  disorders of, 353–414
  normal, 302
  vascular platelet phase of, 303
Henoch-Schönlein syndrome, 370–371
Heparin, 328–330
Hereditary coproporphyria, 43
Hereditary hemorrhagic telangiectasia, 374–
  376
Hereditary spherocytosis, 63, 186–193
Herpes zoster, in chronic lymphocytic leu-
    kemia, 488
  in lymphoma, 537
Heterophil agglutination test, 453, 461
Histiocytic medullary reticulosis, 546
Hodgkin's disease, 535–540
  clinical manifestations, 535–539
    eosinophilia, 539
    fever, 536
    herpes zoster in, 537
    jaundice, 538
    marrow, 540
    of central nervous system, 536–537
    treatment, 553–556
  diagnosis of, 529–533
  histologic types, prognosis and, 552–553
  laboratory examinations in, 539–540
  lymph nodes in, 535–536
  prognosis in, 553–556, 560–561
  staging, 548–552
Hypercalcemia, in multiple myeloma, 588
Hypercoagulable state, 324
  conditions associated with, 324
Hyperhemolysis, 75–77
Hyperplasia, megaloblastic, in pernicious
    anemia, 20, 97
Hypersplenism, 67–68, 274–277
Hypochromia, 22
Hypofibrinogenemia, acquired, 339, 402
Hypoplasia, erythrocytic, chronic, 157
Hypoprothrombinemia, 397
Hyposthenuria, in sickle cell disease, 202

Idiopathic thrombocytopenic purpura, 360–
  364
Immerslund's syndrome, 104
Immunoglobins, 573–584
  deficiencies of, 582–584
  H chains in, 575
  L chains in, 575

Immunoglobins (*Continued*)
  low molecular weight, 579
  model of, 577
  nomenclature, 579
Indanedione compounds, 330
Infectious mononucleosis, 452–464
  cause of, 454
  clinical manifestations of, 455–459
    cardiac, 458
    hematologic, 459
    hematuria, 459
    hepatic, 457
    neurologic, 458
    skin, 456
    spleen, 459
  course of, 463
  diagnosis of, 462
  E-B virus in, 454
  history of, 452
  incidence of, 454
  laboratory examination in, 459
  prognosis in, 463
  treatment of, 463
Inferior vena cavogram, 533, 549, 550
  complications of, 552
Intra-uterine transfusion, in erythroblastosis
    fetalis, 228
Intrinsic factor, 87, 94
Intrinsic system, in thromboplastin activity
    development, 313
Iron
  absorption of, 118–122
  deficiency of, 129–138
    causes of, 130, 131
    clinical manifestations of, 131–133
    diagnosis of, 132
    treatment of, 135
  dietary, sources and requirements for, 117
  excretion of, 127
  ferrokinetics, 127–129
  in erythropoiesis, 45, 124
  in mitochondria, 139
  metabolism of, 116–129
  mucosal block theory, 120
  overload of, 147–150
  plasma, normal and in disease, 125
  storage of, 125
  transport of, 122
Isoimmune hemolytic disease, 66, 223
Isoniazid (INH), in sideroblastic anemia, 141,
  144

Jaundice
  in hereditary spherocytosis, 190
  in Hodgkin's disease, 538
  in sickle cell anemia, 204
Juvenile cell (metamyelocyte), 9
Juvenile pernicious anemia, 103

Kernicterus (in erythroblastosis fetalis), 223
Kidney
  chronic disease and anemia, 270

Kidney (*Continued*)
  erythropoietin and, 28
  function of, in sickle cell anemia, 203
  hemodialysis, 635
  insufficiency of, in multiple myeloma, 589
  nephrotic syndrome and lymphoma, 542
Koilonychia, in iron deficiency, 132

L-asparaginase, 622
L chains (light chains), 575, 586
Laboratory procedures helpful in diagnosis
    of anemia, 72
Laki-Lorand factor. See *Factor(s), coagulation,
    Factor XIII.*
Lead poisoning, anemia of, 144
  heme synthesis, and, 44
Leptocytes, 63
Leukanemia. See *Myeloid metaplasia.*
Leukemia, 471–511
  acute, 478–487
    anemia in, 480
    Auer rods in, 480
    central nervous system involvement, 484,
        497
    chromosomal abnormalities in, 476
    clinical course, 482
    clinical manifestations, 478
    diagnosis, 481
    hypertrophied gums in, 509
    illustrative case, 485–487
    incidence, 472
    laboratory manifestations, 490
    monocytic, 507
    peroxidase stain in, 480
    prognosis, 484
    transformation from chronic, 479
    treatment, 482–485
    types, 478
  chromosomal abnormalities, 476
  chromosome, Philadelphia, 476
  chronic reticulolymphocytic, 491
  classification, 472
  cutis, 489
  eosinophilic, 506
  etiology, 473
    drugs, 474
    genetics, 475
    infections, 474
    radiation, 473
  familial, 477
  genetic, 475
  granulocytic (myelocytic), chronic, 496–
      504
    anemia in, 498
    blast crisis in, 504
    clinical course, 500
    clinical manifestations, 496
    incidence, 496
    laboratory manifestations, 498
    leukocyte alkaline phosphatase, 500
    Philadelphia chromosome, 500

Leukemia (*Continued*)
  granulocytic (myelocytic), prognosis in,
      500–501
    treatment, 501–504
      busulfan, 503
      dibromomannitol, 503
      hydroxyurea, in, 504
      6-mercaptopurine, 503
      radiotherapy, 502
      supportive measures, 501
    vitamin B_{12} level in plasma, 500
  historical aspects of, 471
  incidence of, 472
  lymphocytic, chronic, 487–496
    anemia in, 490
    autoimmune hemolytic anemia, 490, 493
    bacterial infections in, 493, 505
    cutis, 489
    clinical course of, 492
    clinical manifestations of, 488
    diagnosis of, 490
    herpes zoster, 488
    laboratory manifestations of, 490
    prognosis in, 492
    surgical operations in, 504
    treatment for, 494–495
      adrenocortical steroids in, 495
      chlorambucil, 495
      cyclophosphamide, 495
      radiotherapy, 494
  lymphosarcoma cell, 491
  monocytic, 507–512
    acute, 507
    age incidence, 508
    clinical course of, 509
    clinical manifestations of, 508
    histiocytic leukemia, 508
    hyperplasia of gums, 509
    laboratory manifestations of, 508
    Naegeli type, 507
    Schilling type, 507
    treatment of, 509
  myeloblastic, acute, 478, 483
  treatment of, special problems and, 504–505
Leukemic hiatus, 441
Leukemic reticuloendotheliosis, 492
Leukocytes, 428–464
  granulocytes, antibodies to, 440
    defects, 449
    disorders associated with qualitative de-
        fects, 449
    function, 431
    killing of organisms, 432
    leukopoiesis, 428–431
    life span, 430
  leukemoid reactions, 441, 481
  lymphocytes, 433–435
  monocytes, classification of, 13
    function of, 435
    relation to macrophages, 435, 572
  normal values, 437
  physiologic variations, 438
  variations and disease, 438–442

Leukocytes (*Continued*)
  variations and disease, causes of eosino-
    philia, 440
    causes of lymphocytosis, 439
    causes of monocytosis, 440
    causes of neutropenia, 441
    causes of neutrophilic leukocytosis, 439
Leukoerythroblastic anemia, 277
Leukopheresis, leukocyte response to, 429
Leukopoiesis, 428–431
Leukosarcoma, 547
Liver disease, chronic, anemia associated with,
  272–274
Lymph nodes, biopsy, in diagnosis of patient
  with enlarged lymph nodes, 532
  enlargement of, diagnosis of patient with,
    529
    monocytosis and, 531
    in chronic lymphocytic leukemia, 489
    in disseminated lupus, 530, 547
    in Hodgkin's disease, 530
    in lymphoma, 531
    in metastatic carcinoma, 530, 547
Lymphangiograms, 533, 549–552
  complications of, 552
Lymphoblast, morphology, 12
Lymphocytes, 12–13
Lymphocytosis, causes, 439
Lymphoma, malignant, 529–565
  classification, 534
Lymphosarcoma
  anemia associated with, 543
  blood abnormalities in, 542–543
  chest roentgenograms in, 542
  clinical features of, 540–542
  fever in, 540
  illustrative case, 563
  leukemia and, 534
  marrow abnormalities in, 542, 543
  prognosis in, 556–558
  treatment of, 556–560
Lysosomal enzymes, 5
Lysosomes, 4

"M" spike, in electrophoresis, 593
Macrocytes (macrocytic erythrocytes), in peri-
  pheral blood, 23
Macroglobulinemia, 601–603
Macrophages, 435, 572
Macropolycytes, 97, 98
Malabsorption syndrome, 108
Malayan pit viper venom (Arvin), 319
Malignant lymphoma, 529–565
Marchiafava-Micheli syndrome, 240
Marrow. See *Bone marrow.*
Marschalko's plasma cell, 16
May-Heggelin anomaly, 11
Mean corpuscular volume, determination, 57
Measles, thrombocytopenic purpura second-
  ary to, 359, 367
Mediterranean anemia. See *Thalassemia.*
Megakaryoblast, 14
Megakaryocyte, 15

Megaloblast, 19, 21
Melphalan (phenylalanine mustard), 617
  in hemorrhagic thrombocythemia, 522
  in multiple myeloma, 596
Membrane, cell, 1
Menadione, in Factor II deficiency, 397
Meningeal leukemia, 479
6-Mercaptopurine, 619
  in acute leukemia, 483
  in chronic meylocytic leukemia, 503
Messenger RNA, 3, 33
Metamyelocyte, 9
Methemoglobin reduction test, 196
Methemoglobinemia, 183
  due to hemoglobin M, 184
  toxic, 184
Methotrexate, 617–618
  in acute leukemia, 484
  in lymphoma, 557
Microangiopathic hemolytic anemia, 244–245
Microcyte (microcytic erythrocyte), 22
Migration inhibitory factor (MIF), 572
Mikulicz's syndrome, 488
Mitochondria, cell, 4–5
Monoblast, 13
  in acute monocytic leukemia, 509
Monocyte, 13, 14, 435, 572
Monocytosis, causes of, 440
MOPP, in Hodgkin's disease, 556
Mott cells, in multiple myeloma, 591–592
Mucosa, gastrointestinal, regulation of iron
  absorption by, 118–122
"Mucosal block" theory, 120
Mycosis fungoides, clinical features of, 544
Myeloblast, 7
Myeloid metaplasia (myelofibrosis), 512–522
  primary, 513
    anemia in, 520
    bone marrow in, 517
    clinical course, 519
    clinical manifestations, 515
    diagnosis, 518
    etiology, 513
    laboratory findings, 516
    leukocyte alkaline phosphatase, 516
    myeloproliferative disorder, 514
    Philadelphia chromosome, 518
    prognosis, 520
    relation to leukemia, 514
    treatment, 519–520
      androgens, 520
      busulfan, 520
      prednisone, 520
      radiotherapy, 519
      splenectomy, 519
  secondary, 513
  synonyms, 513
Myeloma, multiple, 584–599
  adrenocortico-steroids in, 597
    amyloidosis in, 588
    anemia in, 588
    blood abnormalities in, 591
    clinical manifestations, 588
    course, 593

Myeloma (*Continued*)
  multiple, cryoglobulinemia in, 587, 588
    diagnosis, 594
    EDTA in, 597
    hemorrhages in, 597
    historical aspects, 585
    hypercalcemia in, 588, 594
    in mice, 585
    marrow, 591
    melphalan in, 596
    Mott bodies in, 591–592
    myeloma cells in, 591
    pathogenesis, 585
    pathologic physiology, 585
    plasmablast in, 591
    plasmacytes in, 591
    pneumonia in, 589
    prognosis in, 595
    proteins of serum and urine in, 592
    renal insufficiency in, 589
    skeletal lesions in, 590, 591
    skull in, 590
    treatment of, 596–597
Myelosis, aleukemic. See *Myeloid metaplasia.*
Myxedema, and anemia, 263–265
    clinical manifestations, 264
    diagnosis and prognosis in, 265

NADH, 180, 183
NADPH, 180, 183
Naegeli type of monocytic leukemia, 507
Neonatal thrombocytopenic purpura, 364
Neurologic findings in pernicious anemia, 96
Neutropenia, 448
  causes, 441
  chronic idiopathic, 449
  cyclic, 448
  familial, 449
Neutrophil(s), 9–11
  classification, morphology, and origin of, 9
  function of, 431
  life span of, 430–431
Nitrogen mustard, 615
  in Hodgkin's disease, 555
  in leukemia, 615
  in malignant lymphoma, 558, 615
  mechanism of action, 614
Nocturnal hemoglobinuria, paroxysmal, 64, 169, 240–242
Normoblast, classification, morphology, and origin of, 19–21, 31, 82
Nucleic acid synthesis, folic acid in, 90, 91
  vitamin B_{12} in, 91
Nucleus, cell, 3
Nurse cells, 124
Nutrition. See *Diet.*

Oncolytic alkaloids, 621
Opsonins, 432, 436
Oroya fever, 66

Osler-Weber Rendu syndrome, 374–376
Osmotic fragility test, in hereditary spherocytosis, 187, 190–191
Osteosclerosis. See *Myeloid metaplasia.*
Ovalocytes, 23, 193
Oxymetholone, in aplastic anemia, 166

Parahemophilia, 392
Parasites, infestations, eosinophilia in, 440
Paroxysmal cold hemoglobinuria, 66, 239
Paroxysmal nocturnal hemoglobinuria, 64, 169, 240–242
  acetylcholinesterase in, 241
  in aplastic anemia, 169, 241
Partial thromboplastin time, 337
Paul-Bunnel test, in infectious mononucleosis, 453, 461
Pel-Ebstein fever, in Hodgkin's disease, and malignant lymphomas, 536
Pelger-Huet anomaly, 10
Pentose phosphate shunt, 180–182
Peptide chains, alpha and beta, 33
Pernicious anemia. See *Anemia, pernicious.*
Peroxidase stain for leukocytes, in acute leukemia, 480
  in normal cells of the granulocytic series, 9, 10
Petechiae, in idiopathic thrombocytopenic purpura, 356, 362
Phagocytosis, 431–433, 436, 572
Philadelphia chromosome, 476, 500
Phosphatidyl ethanolamine, 313, 315
Phosphatidyl serine, 315
Phosphorus, radioactive (P^{32}), 613
  in treatment of granulocytic leukemia, 502
  in treatment of lymphocytic leukemia, 494
  in treatment of polycythemia vera, 289
Phototherapy, in hyperbilirubinemia of the newborn, 228
Phytohemagglutinin, 571
Pica, in iron deficiency, 131
Pinocytosis, 436
Plasma
  iron levels, 124
  iron turnover rate, 128
  volume, normal, 285
Plasma cell, 16, 571
  in peripheral blood, 16, 17
  production of antibodies, 571, 580
Plasmablast, in multiple myeloma, morphology, 16, 591
Plasmin, 322
Plasminogen, 320
  activators, 321
  inhibitors, 321
Platelet(s), 15, 303–309
  adhesion of, 309
  aggregation, 306
    ADP in, 307
    ATP in, 304
  count, 336
  disorders of, 411–413

Platelet(s) (*Continued*)
  function of, 306
  metabolism of, 303
  morphology of, 304
  origin of, 303
  proteins in, 303
  transfusion of, 166, 633
Pneumonia, in multiple myeloma, 589
Poikilocytosis, 22
Polycythemia, 281–297
  absolute, 281
  benign familial, 294
  classification of, 282
  relative, 281
  secondary, 291–293
    cardiac malformation and, 292
    hemoglobin M, 293
    low barometric pressure, 292
    pulmonary disorder, 292
    with excess steroids, 293
    with inappropriate erythropoietin production, 293
  vera, 282–291
    blood volume in, 283
    clinical manifestations of, 283
    complications of, 285
    course and prognosis in, 285
    diagnosis, 286
    history of, 282
    laboratory findings in, 285
    leukemia and, 287, 288, 290
    pathogenesis of, 282
    Philadelphia chromosome and, 288
    thrombosis in, 286
    treatment of, 288
      chemotherapy, 290
      radioactive phosphorus, 289
      venesection, 288
Porphobilinogen, 36, 37
Porphyria, 41–45
  acquired toxic, 44
  acute intermittent, 43
  cutanea tarda, 43
  erythropoietica, 41–42
  hepatica, 43
Porphyrins, chemistry of, 35–38
  metabolism, abnormal, 41
    diseases of, 41
    light sensitivity and, 42–43
Porphyrinurias, 44
Postperfusion syndrome, 463
Prednisone. See *Adrenocortical steroids.*
Pregnancy, anemia in, 112, 267
Preleukemia, 476, 511
Priapism
  in leukemia, 497
  in sickle cell anemia, 203, 210
Primaquine sensitivity, 64, 194
Proaccelerin. See *Factor(s), coagulation, Factor V.*
Procarbazine (Natulan, Matulane), 556, 623
  in Hodgkin's disease, 556
Proconvertin. See *Factor(s), coagulation, Factor VII.*
Proconvertin and prothrombin (P and P) test, 331

Progranulocyte (promyelocyte), 9
Prolymphocyte, 12
Promegakaryocyte, 15
Promyelocyte, 9·
Pronormoblast, 19
Proplasmacyte, 16
Prorubricyte, 21
Protamine sulfate, 329
Protein(s)
  abnormalities of, in Hodgkin's disease, 540
    in lymphosarcoma, 543
    in reticulum cell sarcoma, 543
  Bence Jones, 585, 586–587
    in serum in multiple myeloma, 586
    in urine in multiple myeloma, 586–587
  plasma, 573–579
    synthesis of, 580
  synthesis of, 33, 34
Prothrombin. See also *Factor(s), coagulation, Factor II.*
Prothrombin and proconvertin (P and P) test, 331
Prothrombin time, 337
  one stage determination, in hemorrhagic diathesis, 336
Protoporphyria, 42
Protoporphyrin, 36
PTA. See *Factor(s), coagulation, Factor XI.*
PTC. See *Factor(s), coagulation, Factor IX.*
Pteroylglutamic acid. See *Folic acid.*
Purpura, 353–374
  fulminans, 372
  non-thrombocytopenic, 370
    allergic, 370
    caused by aspirin, 374
    senile, 373
  thrombocytopenic, 353
    clinical examination for, 355
    illustrative case, 367
    laboratory examination for, 356
    management of, 360, 365
    mechanism of, 355, 357, 365
    rubella syndrome and, 364
    syndromes of, idiopathic, 360
      neonatal, 364
      secondary, 357
      thrombotic, 365
    treatment of, 362, 365
Pyridoxine, 46
  in anemia, 140, 145
Pyruvate kinase deficiency, 197–198

Qualitative platelet defects, 411–413
  thrombasthenia, 412
  thrombocytopathy, 412
  thrombopathia, 413

Radiation, ionizing, 611–613
Radioactive phosphorus. See *Phosphorus, radioactive.*
Radiotherapy
  complications of, 613

Radiotherapy (*Continued*)
    in acute leukemia, 484
    in chronic leukemia, 494, 502
    in myeloid metaplasia, 519
Red cell mass, normal, 285
Red cell membrane, 179
Reed-Sternberg cells, in Hodgkin's disease, 540, 552
Refractory anemia. See *Anemia, aplastic.*
Renal erythropoietic factor (REF), 28
Reticulocyte(s)
    after acute blood loss, 266
    hemolytic anemia, 190
    morphology, 22
    response, in iron deficiency, 135
        in pernicious anemia, 99
Reticulosis, histocytic medullary, 546
Reticular cell, 573
Reticulum cell sarcoma, 540
    clinical manifestations of, 540–543
    diagnosis of, 529, 547
    prognosis in, 560
    treatment of, 556
Rh blood types, 629–630
Rh factor, 223, 629
Ribonucleic acid (RNA), 33, 90, 612, 614, 618, 620, 622
    synthesis of, vitamin B_{12} in, 90, 91
Ribosomes, cell, 3
Rider cell, 8
"Ringed sideroblast," 139
Roentgen therapy, 611–613
Ropheocytosis, 124
Rubidomycin, 622
Rubriblast, 19
Rubricyte, 21
Russell bodies, in multiple myeloma, 591
Russell viper venom, 319

Salicylates, hazards of, 328, 334, 385, 413
Sarcoma, Hodgkin's, 552, 553
Schilling test, in pernicious anemia diagnosis, 100
Schilling type of monocytic leukemia, 507
Schistocytes, 23, 67
Schönlein-Henoch syndrome, 370–371
Secondary thrombocytopenic purpura, 357
Segmented cell, 9
Senile purpura, 373
Serotonin in hemostasis, 303, 306
Serum bilirubin level, in erythroblastosis fetalis, 225
Sia water test, in macroglobulinemia, 602
Sickle cell disease, 199–212
Sickle cell–hemoglobin C disease, 219–220
Sickle cell–hemoglobin D disease, 220–221
Sickle cell test, technique, 207
Sickle cell–thalassemia disease, 220
Sideroblasts, 139, 142
    normal values in bone marrow, 133, 142
Siderocytes, 23
Skeleton, involvement of, in Burkitt's tumor, 545
    in hemophilia, 382

Skeleton (*Continued*)
    involvement of, in leukemia, 478, 489, 497
        in lymphoma, 538, 543
        in multiple myeloma, 590
        in myeloid metaplasia, 518
        in sickle cell anemia, 205
Skin disease, eosinophilia in, 440
SPCA. See *Factor(s), coagulation, Factor VII.*
Spherocytosis, hereditary, 63, 186–193
Spleen, rupture of, in infectious mononucleosis, 459
Splenectomy, in myeloid metaplasia, 519
Splenomegaly, as mechanism in neutropenia, 441
    in big spleen disease, 274
    in Felty's syndrome, 277
Sprue, non-tropical, 108–110
    tropical, 110
Stem cells, 6–7, 26
Stercobilin, 39
Stippling, 22
Stomach, carcinoma of, pernicious anemia and, 103
Stomatocytosis, 194
Storage
    of folate, 89
    of iron, 125
    of vitamin B_{12}, 88
Streptokinase, 321
Stress polycythemia, 281
Stuart-Prower factor. See *Factor(s), coagulation, Factor X.*
Succinyl-CoA, 36, 139
Sugar water (Hartman-Jenkins) test, 241
Sulfhemoglobin, 184
Surgery
    in patients with hemophilia, 385
    in patients with leukemia, 504–505
    in patients with polycythemia vera, 286
Swiss type agammaglobulinemia, 583
Syndrome. See names of specific syndromes.

Tapeworm, fish, megaloblastic anemia and, 107
Target cells, 23, 212, 216
Telangiectasia, hemorrhagic, hereditary, 374–376
Test(s)
    antiglobulin (Coombs), in autoimmune hemolytic anemia, 233, 234
    Davidson differential absorption, in infectious mononucleosis, 461
    Donath-Landsteiner, 240
    Ham's, 241
    Kahn, in infectious mononucleosis, 462
    liver function, in infectious mononucleosis, 461
    osmotic fragility, in hereditary spherocytosis, 190–191
    Paul-Bunnell, in infectious mononucleosis, 461
    prothrombin and proconvertin (P and P), 331
    Schilling, in pernicious anemia diagnosis, 100

Test(s) (*Continued*)
  Sia, in macroglobulinemia, 602
  thromboplastin generation, 337
  tourniquet, of capillary fragility, technique, 336
    in hemorrhagic diathesis, 336
    positive, in thrombocytopenic purpura, 356
Thalassemia (Cooley's anemia), 63, 213
Thalassemia–hemoglobin C disease, 221
Thalassemia–hemoglobin E disease, 221
Thalassemia–sickle cell disease, 220
Thrombasthenia, 412
Thrombin
  chemistry, 317
  conversion from Factor II, 317
  time, 339
Thrombocyte. See *Platelet.*
Thrombocytic series, 14–15
Thrombocytopathy, 412
Thrombocytopenia, 354
Thrombokinase, 311
Thrombopathia, 413
Thromboplastin, 312
Thromboplastin generation test, 337
Thrombosis, 320–323
Thrombotic thrombocytopenic purpura, 365
Thymoma, in erythrocytic hypoplasia, 170
Tissue thromboplastin, 309, 313
Tourniquet test, in hemorrhagic diathesis, 336
Toxic granulation, 10
Transfer RNA, 33
Transferrin, 122–125
  function, 123
  variations in disease, 125
Transfusion(s)
  exchange, in erythroblastosis fetalis, 227
    indications, 227
  history, 626
  in sickle cell anemia, 209
  incompatible, thrombocytopenia following, 634
  indications for, 631
  reactions, 633–638
    citrate toxicity, 638
    hemolytic, 634
      cause of, determination of, 634
    incidence, 633
    management, 635
    pulmonary edema, 638
    pyrogenic, 636

Transfusion(s) (*Continued*)
  survival of blood components, 630, 638
  transmission of infection by, 636, 638

Ulcer(s), of legs, in sickle cell disease, 202, 203
Uremia, anemia of, 270–272
Urethan, in multiple myeloma, 596
Urobilinogen, fecal, 39
  excretion, 39
  hemoglobin, daily amount, formula, 76
Urokinase, 321
Uroporphyrin, 35

Vascular lesions, as factors in secondary polycythemia, 292
  in hereditary hemorrhagic telangiectasia, 374
  in purpura, 356
Vena cavogram, inferior, in Hodgkin's disease, 549
Venesection, in polycythemia vera, 288
Vinblastine, 621
Vincristine, 621
Virocytes, 460
Viruses, role in leukemia, 474–475
  role in thrombocytopenia, 359
Vitamin B_6. See *Pyridoxine.*
Vitamin B_{12}, 46, 86
  absorption, 87
  deficiency, 93–107
  formula, 86
  in nucleic acid synthesis, 90–92
  metabolism of, 86–107
  serum levels in chronic granulocytic leukemia, 500
  transport, 88
Vitamin E, 47
Vitamin K, 330
  as antidote to coumarin-indanedione drugs, 332
von Willebrand's disease, 407–411

Waldenstrom's macroglobulinemia, 602
Wassermann test, in infectious mononucleosis, 462

Zieve's syndrome, 273